MOSBY'S
NEUROLOGY
PSYCHIATRY
ACCESS SERIES

Child and Adolescent Psychiatry

OTHER BOOKS IN MOSBY'S NEUROLOGY PSYCHIATRY ACCESS SERIES

Guze, Washington University Adult Psychiatry

David, Child and Adolescent Neurology

Corey-Bloom, Adult Neurology

MOSBY'S
NEUROLOGY
PSYCHIATRY
ACCESS SERIES

Child and Adolescent Psychiatry

Dean X. Parmelee, MD
Editor

Chairman
Child and Adolescent Psychiatry
Associate Professor of Psychiatry and Pediatrics
Medical College of Virginia
Virginia Commonwealth University
Richmond, Virginia

Ronald B. David, MD
Series Editor

Children's Neurological Services
Associate Clinical Professor of Pediatrics
Medical College of Virginia
Virginia Commonwealth University
Richmond, Virginia

Mosby

St. Louis Baltimore Boston Carlsbad Chicago Naples New York Philadelphia Portland
London Madrid Mexico City Singapore Sydney Tokyo Toronto Wiesbaden

Mosby
Dedicated to Publishing Excellence

A Times Mirror Company

Vice-President and Publisher: Anne S. Patterson
Editors: Laura DeYoung and Michael Brown
Editorial Assistant: Alicia Moten
Project Manager: Deborah L. Vogel
Production Editor: Karen L. Allman
Designer: Pati Pye
Manufacturing Manager: Theresa Fuchs
Cover art: Bob Cass

Printed in the United States of America
Composition by Clarinda Company
Printing/binding by Maple-Vail Book Mfg Group

Mosby-Year Book, Inc.
11830 Westline Industrial Drive
St. Louis, Missouri 63146

Library of Congress Cataloging in Publication Data

Child and adolescent psychiatry / Dean X. Parmelee, editor.
p. cm. — (Mosby's access series)
Includes bibliographical references and index.
ISBN 0-8151-6809-8
1. Child psychiatry. 2. Adolescent psychiatry. I. Parmelee, Dean X., 1947- . II. Series.
RJ499.C48228 1996
618.92'89—dc20 95-52516
CIP

96 97 98 99 00 / 9 8 7 6 5 4 3 2 1

Contributors

Cheryl Al-Mateen, MD, is Assistant Professor of Psychiatry and Pediatrics at the Medical College of Virginia/Virginia Commonwealth University and Medical Director of the Adolescent Program at the Central State Hospital in Petersburg, Virginia. She graduated from Howard University College of Medicine and completed her residencies in general and child and adolescent psychiatry at Hahnemann University. Her special interest is the effects of violence on children and adolescents.

Kelly N. Botteron, MD, is Assistant Professor of Psychiatry (Child) at the Washington University School of Medicine and Assistant Professor of Radiology at the Mallinckrodt Institute of Radiology. She is also Director of the Psychiatry Center at St. Louis Children's Hospital. She completed her internship in pediatrics at Children's Mercy Hospital in Kansas City, Missouri, her residency in general psychiatry at Washington University, and her fellowship in child psychiatry at Washington University.

Richard R. Brookman, MD, is Professor of Pediatrics, Director of Residency Training in Pediatrics, and Chairman of the Division of Adolescent Medicine at Virginia Commonwealth University/Medical College of Virginia. He is a graduate of Tufts University School of Medicine, completed his residency in pediatrics at Montefiore Hospital Medical Center, Bronx, New York, and completed his fellowship in adolescent medicine at the University of Cincinnati. His areas of special interest are adolescent sexuality, teen pregnancy, sexually transmitted diseases, health education, and health professional education.

Debbie R. Carter, MD, is Assistant Professor of Psychiatry and Director of the Collaborative and Consultation Mental Health Services Office of Youth Services, Programs for Public Psychiatry, University of Colorado Health Sciences Center. She graduated from the Jefferson Medical College in Philadelphia and completed her residencies in general, child, and adolescent psychiatry at the Thomas Jefferson University in Philadephia. Her areas of special interest are adolescent identity synthesis, normal sexual development, and comorbidity issues in juveniles with mental health problems.

Ronald B. David, MD, is a child neurologist who has practiced in Richmond, Virginia since 1970. He is a graduate of the Medical College of Virginia/Virginia Commonwealth University and completed his fellowship in pediatrics and neurology at the Mayo Clinic in Rochester, Minnesota. Dr. David's interests relate to the study and broad practice of child neurology but also focus on the area of developmental cognitive neuroscience. He has a keen interest in classification issues. His interest in developmental cognitive neuroscience and classification became intertwined in 1985 when he initiated and became principle investigator for a multicenter National Institute of Neurologic Disease and Stroke Program Project, *Nosology: Higher Cerebral Function Disorders in Children.* Believing classification and structure as key to communication and understanding, Dr. David then developed a child neurology textbook that has a unique format and incorporates classification skills developed in association with the many colleagues with whom he worked during the period of the National Institutes of Health grant. Beyond this series, Dr. David is now working with the Child Neurology Society to develop a curriculum for training child neurologists in the area of developmental cognitive neuroscience.

Daniel N. Davidow, MD, is Medical Director of Cumberland Hospital for Children and Adolescents, New Kent, Virginia, and Clinical Associate Professor of Pediatrics at the Medical College of Virginia/Virginia Commonwealth University. He completed his medical degree at the Medical College of Georgia and his Pediatrics training and 2 years of adolescent medicine fellowship at Children's Hospital National Medical Center, Washington, D.C. His special interests are chronic illnesses and neurobehavioral disturbances in children and adolescents.

John Diamond, MD, is Director of Training in Child and Adolescent Psychiatry and Associate Professor at the East Carolina University School of Medicine in Greenville. He is a graduate of Howard University School of Medicine, and he completed 1 year of pediatrics training at the Medical College of South Carolina in Charleston and his general and child and adolescent psychiatry residencies at the University of Pittsburgh.

Craig L. Donnelly, MD, is Assistant Professor of Psychiatry at Dartmouth Medical School. He is a graduate of the University of Vermont School of Medicine and completed his postgraduate training in general psychiatry and child and adolescent psychiatry at Duke University Medical Center. His special interests are developmental psychopathology, child and adolescent anxiety disorders, and psychopharmacology.

Cynthia R. Ellis, MD, is Director of the Child Development Clinic and Assistant Professor of Pediatrics and Psychiatry at the Medical College of Virginia/Virginia Commonwealth University. She graduated from the University of Nebraska Medical School and completed her pediatrics residency and a child and adolescent psychiatry fellowship at the Medical College of Virginia/Virginia Commonwealth University. Her areas of special interest are developmental disabilities, psychopharmacology, and behavioral pediatrics.

Graham J. Emslie, MD, is Associate Professor of Psychiatry at the University of Texas Southwestern Medical Center at Dallas, where he also holds the Charles E. and Sarah M. Seay Chair in Child Psychiatry. He is a graduate of the Aberdeen University College of Medicine in Scotland, completed his general psychiatry training at the University of Rochester School of Medicine and Dentistry, and completed his training in child and adolescent psychiatry at Stanford. His special interests are depression in children and adolescents and sleep polysomnography.

Katherine Grimes, MD, is Child Psychiatry Training Director at the Harvard Community Health Plan and is on the Clinical Faculty of the Department of Psychiatry at Harvard Medical School. She graduated from the College of Human Medicine of the Michigan State University, completed her general psychiatry training at the Menninger School of Psychiatry, Topeka, Kansas, and completed training in child and adolescent psychiatry at the Children's Hospital/Judge Baker Guidance Center of Harvard Medical School, Boston. Her special interests are clinical guidelines, outcomes research, child abuse, and eating disorders.

James C. Harris, MD, is Director of Developmental Neuropsychiatry and Associate Professor of Psychiatry, Pediatrics, and Mental Hygiene at the Johns Hopkins University School of Medicine. He is a graduate of the George Washington University School of Medicine, completed pediatrics training at the University of Southern California, the University of Rochester, and Johns Hopkins University School of Medicine, and completed training in general and child and adolescent psychiatry at Johns Hopkins University School of Medicine. His special interest is developmental neuropsychiatry, for which he has recently published a two-volume text with Oxford Press. He is a former physician to the Peace Corps in Thailand and the U.S. Representative for the International Society for the Study of Behavioral Phenotypes, and he continues his interest in international health issues.

Myla Harrison, MD, is an Instructor of Psychiatry and Pediatrics with the Division of Child and Adolescent Psychiatry at the Mt. Sinai Medical Center in New York. She completed her medical education and a year of training in general pediatrics at the State University of New York Health Sciences Center at Brooklyn and the Triple Board Program at Mt. Sinai Medical Center. Her special interest is chronic illness in children and adolescents.

Stanley E. Hemsley, Jr., MD, MBA, is Craig-Delsimer Fellow in Adolescent Medicine at the Children's Hospital of Philadelphia and Clinical Instructor in Pediatrics and Internal Medicine at the University of Pennsylvania School of Medicine. He is a graduate of Harvard Medical School and completed pediatrics training and a fellowship in adolescent medicine at St. Christopher's Hospital for Children in Philadelphia. His areas of interest are health-care delivery in the juvenile justice system, obesity and other eating disorders, and high-risk youth. His MBA is with Specialty in Health Administration from Temple University.

Robert L. Hendren, DO, is Director of the Division of Child and Adolescent Psychiatry and Professor of Psychiatry and Associate Professor Pediatrics at the University of New Mexico Health Sciences Center. He is a graduate of the Kirksville College of Osteopathic Medicine, and he completed his general psychiatry residency at the Mayo Graduate School of Medicine and his child and adolescent psychiatry training at the Yale Child Study Center. His special interests are adolescent impulse control disorders, neurodevelopment, and neuroimaging.

E. Vennecia Jackson, MD, recieved her medical degree from the East Carolina University School of Medicine and completed her pediatric residency and a fellowship in developmental pediatrics at the Medical College of Virginia/Virginia Commonwealth University. She is currently practicing at the Texas Scottish Rite Hospital for Children in the Child Development Division in Dallas, Texas. Her special interests are communication disorders, dsylexia, and other learning disorders.

Steven Jaffe, MD, is Associate Professor of Psychiatry at Emory University, Clinical Professor of Psychiatry at Moorehouse Medical School, and Director of the Child and Adolescent Program at Brawner Hospital in Atlanta. He is a graduate of the Albert Einstein College of Medicine, served as an intern in Pediatrics at UCLA, completed training in general psychiatry at the Massachusetts Mental Health Center, and was a Teaching Fellow at Harvard Medical School. He also completed child and adolescent psychiatry training at Emory University. For

6 years, he was Editor of the American Academy of Child and Adolescent Psychiatry Newsletter, Chair of the Work Group for Practice Guidelines (first one in the field), and the 1993 Psychiatrist of the Year, awarded by the Georgia Psychiatric Physicians Association.

Betsy D. Kennard, PsyD, is Director of Psychological Services at the Children's Medical Center of Dallas and Assistant Professor of Psychiatry at the University of Texas Southwestern Medical Center at Dallas. She completed her doctoral program in clinical psychology at Baylor University and her internship in clinical psychology at Southwestern and Terrell State Hospital. Her special interests are cognitive therapy with depressed adolescents and pediatric psychology.

Robert A. Kowatch, MD, is Assistant Professor of Psychiatry at the University of Texas Southwestern Medical Center at Dallas. He is currently a recipient of the National Institutes of Mental Health Child and Adolescent Clinical Mental Health Academic Award. He graduated from the Chicago Medical School, completed training in general psychiatry at the Hospital of the University of Pennsylvania and training in child and adolescent psychiatry at Hahnemann University. His special interests are child and adolescent bipolar disorders and brain imaging.

Vladimir Maletic, MD, is a child and adolescent psychiatrist who was trained at the Duke University Medical Center. He is currently in private practice in Greenville, South Carolina.

John S. March, MD, is Director of the Program in Child and Adolescent Anxiety Disorders at Duke University Medical Center. He received his bachelor's degree at the University of California Riverside, a Master of Science degree in Molecular Biology at the University of California Berkeley, and his medical degree and master's degree in Public Health at the UCLA School of Medicine. He completed a family medicine residency at UCLA and then went to Montana for several years of general practice. Then he went to the University of Wisconsin for residency training in general and child and adolescent psychiatry. He is board certified in all three areas of medicine. He was a member of the DSM-IV Advisory Subcommittee of PTSD, a current member of the OCD Foundation Scientific Advisory Board, and a recent recipient of the Norbert and Charlotte Reiger Award of the American Academy of Child and Adolescent Psychiatry for his work on the behavioral treatment of OCD. His special interests are the developmental neuropsychology of childhood onset anxiety disorders, patterns of comorbidity in anxious children, and behavior and pharmacologic therapies for these conditions.

Åke Matteson, MD, is Director of Child and Adolescent Psychiatry and Professor of Psychiatry and Pediatrics at the East Carolina University School of Medicine. He received his medical education at the Karolinska Institute in Sweden, his pediatrics training at Vanderbilt University, and general and child and adolescent psychiatry training at Case Western Reserve in Cleveland. He is a native of Sweden.

David J. Mullen, MD, is Assistant Professor of Child and Adolescent Psychiatry and Director of the Adolescent Inpatient Unit at the University of New Mexico Health Sciences Center. He received his medical degree at the University of Oklahoma College of Medicine and completed his residencies in general and child and adolescent psychiatry at the University of New Mexico. His special interests are conduct disorders, mood disorders, and schizophrenia. He is also the Psychiatric Consultant to the Bernalillo County Juvenile Detention Center.

Jeffrey Newcorn, MD, is Director of Child and Adolescent Psychiatry and Associate Professor of Psychiatry at the Mt. Sinai Medical Center in New York. He is a graduate of the University of Rochester School of Medicine and Dentistry, and he completed his general and child and adolescent psychiatry residencies at the Tufts New England Medical Center in Boston. He has served as Consultant to the American Academy of Pediatrics for their DSM-Primary Care Project, Member of the Advisory Committee for the DSM-Primary Care Project, and Member of the Child Disorders Workgroup for DSM-IV. His special interests are ADHD and disruptive behavior disorders, the nature and diagnosis of psychopathology in children, and the neurobiologic disorders.

Donald P. Oswald, PhD, is Assistant Professor of Psychiatry at the Medical College of Virginia/Virginia Commonwealth University. He received his doctorate in psychology at Virginia Polytechnic Institute and completed his clinical internship at the Yale Child Study Center. His areas of special interest are behavior therapy with children and families and developmental disabilities.

Dean X. Parmelee, MD, is Chairman of Child and Adolescent Psychiatry and Associate Professor of Psychiatry and Pediatrics at the Medical College of Virginia/Virginia Commonwealth University. He is also the Director of the Second Year Medical School Curriculum and the M-1 Behavioral Sciences Course at the Medical College of Virginia. He is a graduate of the University of Rochester School of Medicine and Dentistry and completed his general psychiatry training at the Massachusetts General Hospital/Harvard Medical School and child and his adolescent psychiatry training at McLean Hospital/Harvard Medical School. He is especially interested in the education of medical students and neuropsychiatric disorders of children.

Joan Plotkin, MD, is in private practice in Richmond, Virginia with Horizons, Inc. She completed medical school at the Medical College of Virginia/Virginia Commonwealth University and an obstetric-gynecology internship at the State University of New York-Buffalo. She continued in an obstetrics-gynecology residency at the Eastern Virginia Medical School in Norfolk until she entered general and child and adolescent psychiatry training at the Medical College of Virginia/Virginia Commonwealth University. Her special interests include issues pertaining to reproduction and birth and parenting of infants and toddlers.

Debora L. Scheffel, PhD, is an Assistant Professor at Fort Hays State University at Hays, Kansas and a consultant in Colorado and western Kansas on the diagnosis and education of learning disabled children and adolescents. She received her doctoral degree from Northwestern University in Evanston, Illinois, in Communicative Disorders and completed an NIMH post-doctoral fellowship in Cognitive Psychology at the University of California, San Diego. Her areas of special interest are psycholinguistics and neuropsychology.

Nirbhay N. Singh, PhD, is Professor of Psychiatry and Pediatrics and Director of Research at the Commonwealth Institute for Child and Family Studies at the Medical College of Virginia/Virginia Commonwealth University. He recieved his training in psychology and psychopharmaclogy at the University of Auckland in New Zealand. His special interests are the civil rights of individuals with developmental disabilities and pediatric psychopharmacology. He is the Editor of *The Journal of Child and Family Studies* and *The Journal of Behavioral Education.*

Mae S. Sokol, MD, is Assistant Professor of Psychiatry and Medical Director of the Center for Overcoming Problem Eating at the University of Pittsburgh School of Medicine-Western Psychiatric Institute and Clinic. She completed her medical education at the University of Louvain in Belgium, a residency year in internal medicine at Long Island College Hospital in New York, and general and child and adolescent psychiatry residencies at the NYU Medical Center-Bellevue. Her areas or special interest are eating disorders and the inpatient care of severely disturbed children.

Aradhana A. Sood, MD, is Director of Training in Child and Adolescent Psychiatry and Associate Professor at the Medical College of Virginia/Virginia Commonwealth University in Richmond. She completed her medical Education at the Gajra Raja Medical College in India, her general psychiatry training at the University of Missouri at Kansas City, and her child and adolescent psychiatry training at Ohio State University. Her areas of special interest are depression in children and adolescents, attention deficit disorder in children and adults, and the psychopharmacology of aggression.

David Waller, MD, is Director of Child and Adolescent Psychiatry and holds the Sarah M. And Charles E. Seay Chair in Child Psychiatry at the University of Texas Southwestern Medical Center and Children's Medical Center, Dallas, Texas. He is a graduate of Harvard College and the Johns Hopkins University School of Medicine, and he completed residencies in pediatrics at Johns Hopkins University School of Medicine, in general psychiatry at the Massachusetts General Hospital, and in child and adolescent psychiatry at Children's Hospital in Boston. Eating disorders is an area of special interest.

Isaac K. Wood, MD, is the Director of the Neuropsychiatry Program at Cumberland Hospital for Children and Adolescents in New Kent, Virginia and Assistant Professor of Psychiatry and Pediatrics at the Medical College of Virginia/Virginia Commonwealth University. He completed medical school and all of his residencies at the Medical College of Virginia. His special interests are conduct disorders and behavioral neurology.

Foreword

Each book in this series is built on a structural framework that was well received by critics and readers alike in David, *Pediatric Neurology for the Clinician.* Each volume is divided into three sections:

- Tools for diagnosis
- Diseases and disorders
- Common problems

Also included to facilitate a physician's use of this book are:

- Diagnostic tables
- "Pearls and Perils" boxes
- "Consider Consultation When . . ." boxes
- Selected annotated bibliographies
- A complete bibliography

Diagnostic tables are based on a discriminator model to promote clearer understanding and are superior to a criterion-based model and others that lack similar specificity. Classification systems induce an orderliness in thinking and enhance our ability to communicate effectively. A review of the most enduring hierarchial classification systems, particularly that of Linnaeus (that is, phyla, genera, species), makes clear the value of grouping according to discriminating features, as well as the value of simplicity, expandability, and dynamism.

The goal, whatever the classification system, is to seek the most powerful discriminating features that produce the greatest diagnostic clarity. Much of the confusion that arises in diagnosis may be the result of the clinician who unwittingly crosses the anatomic, pathologic, pathophysiologic, phenomenologic, and etiologic classification domains used in medicine (for example, the inclusion of anatomically-oriented "temporal lobe seizures" in a phenomenologically based classification system that includes complex partial seizures). Some conditions, such as brain tumors, are classified according to their histopathology and lend themselves well to this classification system. Others, such as headaches and movement disorders, are classified phenomenologically and are therefore much less easily classified. In other cases, discriminators must encompass inclusionary as well as exclusionary features. At times, we can only use a criterion-based system or construct tables to compare features. Discriminating features should avoid crossing domains. Arbitrarily, we label as consistent features those that occur more than 75% of the time; features are considered variable when they occur less than 75% of the time. The diagnostic tables should be viewed, therefore, only as a beginning in the extremely difficult effort to make diagnosis more precise and biologically based. How well this book accomplishes the goals of identifying the most powerful discriminating features for maximum diagnostic clarity is limited by the current state-of-the-art in child and adolescent psychiatry. In some areas, several features, when clustered together, serve to discriminate.

> Whoever having undertaken to speak or write hath first laid for themselves some [basis] to their argument such as hot or cold or moist or dry or whatever else they choose, thus reducing their subject within a narrow compass.
>
> Hippocrates

As Hippocrates has suggested, structure is the key to learning. Unless there is a structure onto which knowledge can be built, confusion and disorganization are the inevitable consequences. Although each text in this series reflects appropriate stylistic differences among content editors, each is built on the same structural framework; hence the value of these texts to the users. It is therefore my fondest wish that these texts be on your desk rather than on your bookshelf.

As a part of this foreword, I would like to acknowledge some of the people who have made key contributions to this effort. They include Craig Percy, who initially saw the potential of this effort; the National Institute of Neurological Disease and Stroke (NINDS)* for their support in nosologic research and to the investigators who were involved with this NINDS project; Dr. Grover Robinson, a long-time friend (who suggested the "Consider Consultation When . . ." boxes for the present series); Ms. Laura DeYoung, Mr. Michael Brown, and all of the Mosby team who made this vision a reality; and Dr. Dean Parmelee, who accepted the challenge of "reconstructing" *Child and Adolescent Psychiatry* to fit this format.

Ronald B. David, MD

*NINDS 1PO1NS20489-01A1

Preface

When Dr. Ron David and Mosby asked me to edit this text, I was very interested in providing a teaching text in child and adolescent psychiatry for physicians who are most involved on a daily basis with the comprehensive health needs of children and youth. It is these physicians who are in a position to identify mental health problems and to intervene at an early stage. The book reflects my commitment to those who want to help children with emotional and behavioral problems. It also reflects Dr. David's commitment to creating a series of texts that foster greater diagnostic clarity and practice efficiency in our related fields of psychiatry and neurology.

The contributors were selected because of their abilities to apply clinically the findings from research in the field and experience from their busy clinical practices. Section One consists of three chapters that provide a foundation for understanding the diagnostic process in child and adolescent psychiatry. Section Two consists of chapters for each of the major diagnostic categories with current (DSM-IV) nosology and treatment aproaches. Section Three presents common clinical problems and ways of managing them.

There are tools throughout the text that should help in understanding and remembering key points. Diagnostic tables highlight the discriminating, consistent, and variable features of a diagnosis. "Pearls and Perils" boxes succintly reiterate salient facts and admonitions. The "Consider Consultation When . . ." feature assists the primary care physician in determining which clinical conditions and situations warrant referral to the child and adolescent psychiatrist. These tools will all help to access the information both more easily and more quickly.

Dean X. Parmelee, MD

Acknowledgments

I co-edited another textbook just after my residency training and concluded that it would have been easier to have written the entire book with the co-editor because we spent so much energy encouraging contributors to finish and then did much of the final writing. This project has not been the same experience: the contributors have met deadlines and have written well. Drs. Al-Mateen, Brookman, and Wood have edited for consistency within sections, and the entire texts reads well from their enthusiastic and attentive endeavors. We all appreciate the developmental and organizational work of Alicia Moten and the copyediting by Karen Allman of Mosby.

Contents

Section One — Assessment and Evaluation, 1

Editor — Dean X. Parmelee, MD

1 Psychiatric Examination and Diagnosis in Children and Adolescents, 3
Myla Harrison, MD and Jeffrey Newcorn, MD

2 Diagnostic Instruments, 19
Aradhana A. Sood, MD and Nirbhay N. Singh, PhD

3 Brain Imaging in Child and Adolescent Psychiatry, 33
Robert A. Kowatch, MD and Kelly N. Botteron, MD

Section Two — Diagnostic Categories, 47

Editor — Isaac K. Wood, MD

4 Pervasive Developmental Disorders, 49
James C. Harris, MD

5 Attention-Deficit/Hyperactivity Disorder, 69
John Diamond, MD and Åke Mattsson, MD

6 Conduct Disorder and Oppositional Defiant Disorder, 83
Isaac K. Wood, MD

7 Anxiety Disorders in Children and Adolescents, 97
Craig L. Donnelly, MD, Vladimir Maletic, MD, and John S. March, MD

8 Mood Disorders, 121
Robert A. Kowatch, MD, Graham J. Emslie, MD, and Betsy D. Kennard, PsyD

9 Eating Disorders, 141
David Waller, MD

10 Schizophrenia in Children and Adolescents, 153
Mae S. Sokol, MD

11 Learning Disorders, 169
Debora L. Scheffel, PhD

Section Three — Clinical Conditions and Situations, 187

Editors — Cheryl Al-Mateen, MD and Richard R. Brookman, MD

12 The At-Risk Infant, 189
Joan Plotkin, MD

13 Aggressive Behavior, 211
Donald P. Oswald, PhD

14 The Suicidal Child or Adolescent, 225
David J. Mullen, MD and Robert L. Hendren, DO

15 The Substance-Abusing Youth, 237
Steven Jaffe, MD

16 Children and Abuse, 245
Cheryl Al-Mateen, MD and Stanley E. Hemsley, Jr., MD

17 Problem Behaviors in Children with Developmental Disabilities, 263
Cynthia R. Ellis, MD, Nirbhay N. Singh, PhD, and E. Vennecia Jackson, MD

18 Chronic Illness in Children and Adolescents, 277
Daniel N. Davidow, MD

19 Sexuality, 287
Debbie R. Carter, MD, Cheryl Al-Mateen, MD, and Richard R. Brookman, MD

20 Common Behavioral Problems and Reactions to Stress, 305
Katherine Grimes, MD

Bibliography, 321

Index, 345

section one

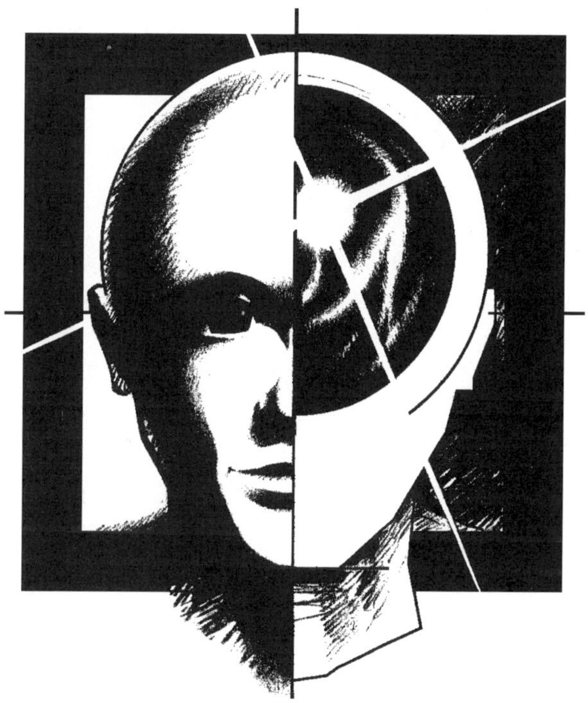

Assessment and Evaluation

Dean X. Parmelee, MD

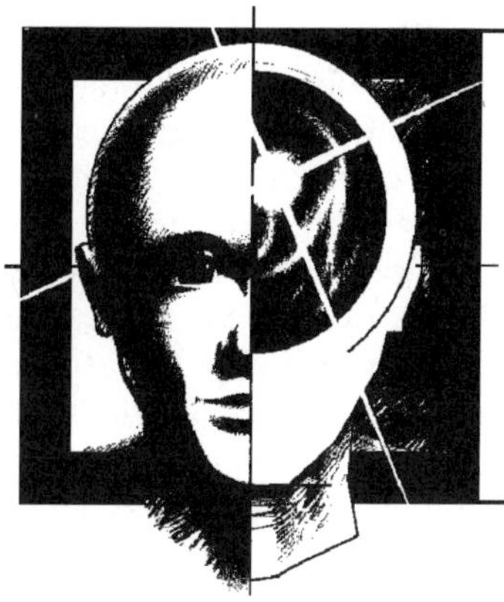

chapter 1

Psychiatric Examination and Diagnosis in Children and Adolescents

Myla Harrison, MD and Jeffrey Newcorn, MD

Complexities of Assessment in Child and Adolescent Psychiatry
The Psychiatric Examination
Diagnostic Formulation and Treatment Planning
Diagnosis in Children and Adolescents
Child Psychiatry and the Primary Care Physician
Summary

Psychiatric assessment of children and adolescents is a multifaceted process that includes interviewing parents, children, and families, obtaining current and past histories from other sources, assessing the severity of symptoms and overall levels of functioning, and synthesizing this information into comprehensive psychiatric formulations and treatment plans. The goals of this chapter are to describe the content and process of a psychiatric assessment, as well as to provide an overview of the diagnostic formulation and treatment planning process with children and adolescents. The psychiatric examination and diagnostic process are closely interwoven. Although an accurate diagnosis depends on information collected in the psychiatric interviews and in the mental status examination, it is also the case that knowledge regarding diagnostic categories affects the content and flow of clinical data collection. Nevertheless, for purposes of exposition, the clinical and diagnostic processes are described separately. This chapter considers assessment from the perspective of the child and adolescent psychiatrist, and it is intended for physicians who want to improve their skills in the evaluation of mental health functioning in children and youth. It also includes a section on the role of the primary care physician in psychiatric screening and assessment.

Complexities of Assessment in Child and Adolescent Psychiatry

There are several complex features of the psychiatric assessment of children that differ from the assessment of adults and that warrant special consideration. In children and adolescents, assessment of developmental functioning is of utmost importance. The physician must understand normal development in children of different ages, genders, and sociocultural backgrounds. Children and adolescents of different ages and developmental stages differ in their physical, cognitive, and emotional capacities. Therefore the clinician must carefully assess the ways a patient's problems reflect or deviate from normal development. The breadth of normality and the large amount of individual variation must be emphasized. For example, temper tantrums in a 2-year-old child are considered a normal part of development; however, continued temper tantrums at age 13 likely indicate a significant problem. Fears of the dark and of monsters are relatively common in 4- to 6-year-old children, and one generally does not diagnose a phobic disorder in a child of this age. In adolescents, questions regarding identity development and separation from the family are important developmental processes and should not necessarily be viewed as symptoms of psychiatric disturbance.

The fact that childhood and adolescence entail constant change also contributes to the complexities of the assessment. The presence of developmental delays or areas of precocious functioning must be determined, and the physician must decide whether intervention is useful or warranted. There are times when intervention may not be needed even though a developmental delay is present, because it is expected that a child's continued growth and development will alleviate the problem.

The child is a valuable source of information for the physician, and he is interviewed as part of the assessment. However, children are vastly different in their abilities to tell the examiner about their peer and family relationships, moods, and how they conceptualize the reason for the evaluation. Many children, especially younger ones, may only provide an indirect glimpse into this material. They may be limited in their abilities to verbalize their feelings and describe their social interactions. As a result, the use of interactive play and projective techniques are often required to obtain this information. Play with dolls that represent family figures, puppets, or drawing may take on greater importance in the assessment for a younger child than for an older child. However, the verbal expression of feelings may also be difficult for an older child or adolescent, and other, less directive procedures are often helpful.

It is important to remember that the psychiatric examination assesses a child's or adolescent's functioning at a single point in time. Therefore one cannot necessarily assume that the results of such an assessment are representative of the child's general functioning. It is possible that the physician may not see the symptoms described by the referring source in one or more evaluation sessions. Additionally, symptoms may change during the assessment process. However, even seemingly minor behaviors that may be observed during the evaluation can be highly indicative of problems in day-to-day life. For instance, some children are reluctant to participate in the individual session with the psychiatrist if it requires that their parents are left in the waiting room. Whereas this degree of difficulty separating might reflect a normal degree of anxiety in an initial appointment with a young child, it could also indicate the presence of separation anxiety disorder. On the other hand, a child with oppositional defiant disorder (ODD) may be on his best behavior with the interviewer; only by carefully listening to the child's responses to direct questions about his relationships with authority figures is it possible to develop an understanding of the problem. Because of such special considerations, a full range of information from multiple informants must be elicited and considered when formulating a diagnosis and treatment plan in children.

The psychiatric evaluation of children further differs from that of adults in that the child can only provide a limited amount of historic information. A child cannot relate the circumstances of his birth or his developmental history. A younger child is also not cognitively capable of relating symptoms in a temporal sequence. Therefore the physician must turn to other sources for a comprehensive picture of the child. This includes the parents, other relatives, teachers, pediatricians, guidance counselors, and camp counselors, as well as sources of objective information, such as the results of psychologic testing and rating scales. A review of the pediatrician's records can often provide information about the child's early developmental history, and school report cards can show the early cognitive and behavioral development of the child.

A complete picture of the child's strengths and the nature of the problem arises from the various sources of information. There are times when different informants provide conflicting data, and it can be difficult to know whom to believe. The physician must then use his judgment to assess this information variance. It is important to remain mindful of how well the various informants know the patient and to know which observers are best able to evaluate which symptoms. For instance, it is not unusual for a child to admit to mood or anxiety symptoms of which the parent is unaware; therefore such reports should be taken seriously even if they are not confirmed by the parent. Conversely, teachers' reports of inattention and overactivity should be given the highest priority when evaluating a child for attention-deficit/hyperactivity disorder (ADHD), because teachers see the child in a structured setting and are therefore considered the best informants regarding this behavior. A general rule is that children are essential sources for reporting internalizing symptoms such as anxiety and mood symptoms, whereas adults are often better informants about the presence of externalizing behaviors such as conduct problems. When parents and teachers differ in their accounts of a child, clinical judgment must be applied to discern the reasons for this disparity. Differences may not only result from the different perspectives of the informants but also from the child actually exhibiting different behavior in various settings.

It is important to supplement the information derived from the history and the mental status examination with additional data from rating scales, psychologic and neuropsychologic tests, and any requisite medical evaluation or laboratory tests. Clinically useful and easy-to-administer rating scales are Achenbach's Child Behavior Checklist (CBCL) for parents and Teacher Report Form (TRF) for teachers and the Conners rating scales for teachers and parents (see Chapter 2). These rating scales have been standardized and normed for age and gender, and therefore they provide comprehensive tests for the presence or absence of symptoms. Psychologic testing is necessary to diagnose mental retardation and learning disorders. The battery may include tests of verbal and nonverbal cognitive abilities, achievement tests (to assess academic functioning), and projective tests (to assess reality testing and interpersonal functioning). A significant discrepancy between a child's measured intelligence quotient (IQ) and his performance on a standardized academic achievement test is indicative of a learning disability, whereas an IQ below 70 may lead to a diagnosis of mental retardation. Specific neuropsychologic tests may suggest organic pathologic conditions or localizing lesions.

PEARLS & PERILS

CONDUCTING A PSYCHIATRIC EXAMINATION

- It is important that parents prepare the child for the visit and not "trick" him into coming.
- Behaviors appropriate at one age are not necessarily so at another age.
- The school, the pediatrician, and other family members have important information for the diagnostic process.
- All presenting problems are best viewed within the context of the child's family and their ethnicity, culture, and values.
- When the evaluation is complete, communicate helpful information to the referral source (with permission).

The Psychiatric Examination

Overview

The psychiatric assessment is the comprehensive clinical evaluation used to determine whether a psychopathologic condition is present, whether treatment is indicated, and what treatment should entail. The emotional and behavioral functioning of the child are evaluated and placed in the context of the child's current developmental level and expected developmental gains.

Before the evaluation begins, the parents should be informed about the assessment process and given help to prepare the child for the evaluation. This process is normally fraught with anxiety, and if the child is not properly prepared, he may not be as cooperative during the interview as he might otherwise have been. Therefore it is also important to find out what the parent has told the child about the upcoming evaluation. Parents often ask for the physician's opinion regarding how to prepare a child for an evaluation. The response to this question should be at least partially related to the nature of the impairment. For example, a parent might tell the child that he is going to see a talking (or playing) doctor who will find out how to help him improve his school performance or his behavior. Parents should also be given specific information about the length of the evaluation, the cost, and what they can expect when the evaluation is complete (such as a formal report or an informing session).

During the assessment, the physician gathers information about a child's problem, his past psychiatric history, his present and past medical history, his family history, his current developmental status, his early developmental history, his school history, and his mental status (Box 1-1). When performing the assessment, the physician should not just consider the child's pathologic condition and which symptoms are present or absent, but she must also find areas of strength in both the child and the family. When developing this profile, it is important to consider the child's age as well as his physical, cognitive, and social capabilities. The physician uses his knowledge of normal development and psychopathologic conditions to formulate a working diagnosis based on the information gathered and on the observations made. Ultimately a treatment plan is developed, and it is shared with the child and the family.

There are many approaches to the parent interview. To avoid making younger children wait excessively, it is helpful to gather a child's history from the parents in a separate appointment before the child is seen. However, regardless of the method, it is helpful to have time with the parents apart from the child and, if possible, to interview each parent separately. In the event of divorced or separated parents, it is particularly important to have both parents participate in the assessment of the child. It is often helpful to meet with the entire family together at least once during the assessment to understand what each member of the family sees as the problem and what each person sees as a realistic solution.

The parent interview provides the physician with information regarding the existing problem; the child's psychiatric, medical, and developmental histories; the family and social history; and the school history. It should include a review of past physical and psychologic stresses, adjustments to school and social situations (past and current), and the patient's relationships with siblings and with each parent or caregiver. Requests for release of information from pediatricians, school personnel, and previous treatment providers should also be obtained at the time of the initial parent interview.

BOX 1-1

COMPONENTS OF A PSYCHIATRIC EXAMINATION

Reason for referral
History of present illness
Past psychiatric history
Medical history
Developmental history
- Milestones for pregnancy, birth, and the neonatal period; infancy; toddlerhood; preschool age; school age; and adolescence

School history
Family history
Mental status
- Appearance, behavior, relatedness, speech and language, mood and affect, thought process and content, and cognitive and developmental assessment

Formulation
Diagnosis
Treatment plan

The Reason for Referral and the History of Present and Past Problems

When beginning the psychiatric assessment, the physician needs to consider the referral source and the reason for the referral. Often, it is the parents, primary caregivers or school officials who initiate the evaluation process, but referrals may also come from the legal or social service systems. If the referral has not come from the parents, the physician must find out whether they see a problem and if so, how they can be engaged in the treatment process. If they do not feel that there is a problem, then the physician must base the assessment on data from other sources and suggest that further discussion is necessary.

As with the traditional medical history, the physician first determines the chief complaint and the history of the present illness, as stated in the words of the child or a parent. There must be descriptions of the development of the symptoms and of the historical context of the problem. The patient or a parent should also explain what has happened recently to prompt the appointment. The presenting problem may be a behavioral problem, an emotional or mood problem, a specific or a pervasive developmental disability, a psychotic disorder, a reaction to an adverse life event, or some combination of these. Many dimensions used to elucidate symptoms in the medical model are also useful for gathering information about the history of the present illness in the field of child and adolescent psychiatry. The physician should gather information about the chronology (onset, duration, periodicity, and course), quality, quantity (intensity, degree of functional impairment, frequency), setting, aggravating or alleviating factors, and associated manifestations of the problem. The course of the symptoms should be recorded, but not necessarily gathered, in chronologic order from the onset of the symptoms to the time of the evaluation. A child's level of adjustment; developmental status; and social, academic, and family functioning relative to the presenting problem are also recorded in this section. It should also be noted whether a child is taking any psychotropic medications or any other medication that may affect his mental status.

The past history includes information about previous psychiatric evaluations and treatment, either for the same problem or any other psychiatric condition. Past use of psychotropic medication is highlighted, and dosages, responses, adverse effects, and duration of use are noted. If permission from the parent (and for older children and adolescents, from the patient as well) can be obtained, it is often helpful to contact physicians who have previously treated the patient.

When gathering the history of the presenting problem, it is important to include a "psychiatric review of systems." This allows the physician to obtain additional data that may not have been revealed spontaneously but may be relevant to the history and clinical presentation of a particular child. This information can be extremely useful in differential diagnosis and in determining whether co-morbidity is present. The psychiatric review of systems includes questions regarding all major areas of function, such as the child's general level of function, developmental delays or deviations, anxiety symptoms, mood symptoms, attention or behavior problems, learning problems, somatic complaints, psychotic symptoms, and drug or alcohol use. Specific questions should be geared to assess the presence of suicidal or homicidal thoughts, as well as disturbances in social, academic, or family functioning.

Medical History of the Child

The medical history of the child is obtained from the primary caregivers or the pediatrician. Pediatric records are also commonly available to complement the history obtained from the family. The psychiatrist should note any current or past medical conditions and previous hospitalizations (including any surgery). If there have been any major illnesses, the child's emotional and behavioral reactions should be recorded. Children who have had multiple hospitalizations for a chronic illness may show a range of developmental problems as a result of altered environmental stimulation, direct effects of the illness, or an interplay between variables involving the parent and the child. For example, bed wetting in a 5-year-old child hospitalized for asthma who had previously obtained bladder continence might be viewed as an expected developmental regression in a child who was otherwise developing normally.

The use of medications to treat general medical conditions and the development of allergies to medications should also be noted in this section, since the behavioral symptoms presented by the family and the child in the history of the present illness may be related to prescribed medications. For example, steroids are an integral part of medical management after an organ transplantation and can have important emotional and behavioral manifestations, such as severe agitation and psychosis.

It is important to remember that the psychiatric problem may be a direct effect of a congenital or an acquired medical illness or an indirect manifestation of the stress caused by a medical illness. Fetal alcohol syndrome is an example of a disorder that may be accompanied by psychiatric symptoms. Children with fetal alcohol syndrome have mental retardation and facial dysmorphism, and they may also have learning disorders and ADHD. Additionally, general medical conditions not directly associated with psychiatric disturbances may also cause psychiatric symptoms. For example, a child with acute lymphocytic leukemia may show the symptoms of decreased energy, anhedonia, and a poor appetite disproportionate to what is normally expected from the medical illness or the chemotherapeutic agents used in its treatment. This child may possibly be suffering from a superimposed major depressive episode or an adjustment disorder with a depressed mood. As with the psychiatric history, a general medical review of systems should be included, so the possibility that a medical condition that may be contributing to the psychiatric symptoms will not be overlooked. For example, vision or hearing deficits may be related to psychiatric or cognitive problems. Thus if a preschool child is brought to the physician with problems in language acquisition and a history of recurrent otitis media, it is important to ask about the child's hearing and to consider obtaining additional assessments to determine whether a hearing disorder may be contributing to the language delay.

Developmental History

The child's developmental history should be gathered during the parent interview, and supplemental information should be obtained from the pediatrician. When taking the developmental history, the psychiatrist must be aware of the range of individual variations in normal development. Any delays in achieving milestones, interruptions, or set-backs in the child's expected developmental progression should be noted. This information can be especially helpful when it is compared with similar data from siblings or other peers of the same age as the patient. Of course, parents may be unaware of developmental delays or deviations, so additional historians or old family videotapes may be required to supplement the information provided by the parents. In addition to developmental delays, areas of precocious development or unusual strengths and capacities should be noted. When writing up the developmental history, it is helpful to organize the material by developmental stage. Each of the relevant developmental stages is described in detail in the following sections.

Pregnancy, Birth, and the Neonatal Period

Inquiring about the events preceding and surrounding the pregnancy of the mother is often a comfortable way to begin the developmental history. It is useful to learn whether the pregnancy was planned, and if so, how long it took for the parents to conceive. If the pregnancy was unplanned, what was the parents' reaction to learning about it? Ask about the nature of any medical complications during the pregnancy or after delivery, how the pregnancy was tolerated, and whether there were any complicating events in the mother's life during the pregnancy. Pertinent information about labor and delivery should be noted, and the presence of any medical complications should also be recorded. The birth weight, the APGAR scores, and the parents' feelings at the time of birth may all be revealing. The mother's use of cigarettes, alcohol, and any over-the-counter, prescription, or illicit drugs taken during pregnancy should be determined, as should the presence of problems in the prenatal and perinatal periods (such as eclampsia or postpartum depression).

Infancy

The period from birth through about 18 months is referred to as infancy. By the end of infancy, children can walk and begin to demonstrate behaviors that indicate independence from the caregiver. It is important to know whether there were any parent-child attachment problems during this period. Such problems might occur in an infant who was in a neonatal intensive care unit for an extended period or in an infant whose mother suffered a medical or psychiatric illness after the birth of the child and was unable to provide the requisite care and attention. The presence of stranger anxiety or early separation difficulties are often important indicators of bonding. Stranger anxiety begins at approximately 8 months and often lasts several months; separation anxiety is often present when the child is between 10 and 18 months old. Both of these behaviors are normal and expected developmental markers, but they may not be present in all children. It is also important to ask about the presence of medical problems during infancy, as well as developmental competency in regulatory functions, such as eating or sleeping, and the presence of temperamental qualities such as irritability or avoidance. Specific areas of development to assess include the development of gross motor function, fine motor function, language development (not just speech), adaptive behaviors, and social skills. A variety of screening examinations can be used to assess normal development. The Denver II, a recent revision and restandardization of the Denver Developmental Screening Test, is one screening test that is commonly used by pediatricians to estimate a child's developmental status until age 6. A child's developmental level on this test can often be obtained from pediatricians and can be used to retrospectively evaluate the presence of developmental problems.

Toddlerhood

Toddlerhood begins with the child's first steps—usually around the first birthday—and lasts until approximately 36 months of age. The landmarks of this stage are the development of autonomy and self-control. The toddler becomes proficient in the gross motor skills of walking, running, and climbing, and he also masters fine motor skills such as beginning to dress and holding utensils, toys, and crayons, as well as the sometimes unwanted behaviors of opening drawers, cabinets, and medicine bottles. Speech and language development during this period should carefully be noted. The child should master single words before the age of 2 and should be able to combine them into short sentences by the end of the toddler period. Gender identity is clearly established during this period, usually beginning in the second year. Other characteristic features of this stage are temper tantrums, the development of toilet training skills, and the development of fears such as specific phobias and separation problems. Normal disturbances in sleep may be related to fear of the dark. If this has been the case, it is important to discuss how the parents have handled this, as well as whether and when the child sleeps in the parents' bed. Common problems during the toddler period may involve family struggles with the toddler's new-found autonomy.

Preschool Age

Preschool children are approximately 3 to 5 years old. Important features of development during this stage are related to socialization, in school or other out-of-home situations, and evolving cognitive capacities. Preschool development includes successful separation from parents for short periods, development of peer relationships, and the acquisition of a variety of skills such as dressing, feeding, bladder and bowel control, and being able to regulate emotional outbursts. The child's fears and capacity for impulse control should be assessed, and the presence of nightmares or other developmental problems should be noted. It is also useful to inquire about nighttime bladder control, since many children continue to wet the bed during preschool years. (Enuresis is not diagnosed before a child is 5 years old.) The extent to which the preschool child is permitted or encouraged to sleep in the parents' bed varies considerably, but it may provide insight into the parent-child relationship. Therefore it is often useful to inquire about sleeping arrangements in the family.

School Age

The school-age period is comprised of the ages between 6 and 11. This stage of development has also been referred to as the latency stage, a term derived from the psychoanalytic formulation that the sexual drive is quiescent after resolution of the Oedipus complex. However, this term is less often used at present, reflecting our current understanding that sexuality is not latent in the school-age years.

For the school-age child, the process of the history gathering often involves the child as well as the parent, although younger children in this age range are still not able to give a history. Play is an important means of communication, but there is often a mixture of talk and play. Inquiring about the school-age child's hobbies and interests is a good way to engage him in the evaluation process. Peer relationships are an important focus for school-age children. This is the time children develop "best" friends, so it is especially important to ask them about activities such as sleep-overs with friends. School-age children develop the ability to play cooperatively, and can be questioned about their involvement in after-school or team sports activities. School performance and school difficulties should be evaluated, and their effects on the child's developing sense of competence and self-esteem should be noted. Other important areas of development are related to impulse control, coordination, clumsiness, separations, and reactions to them.

Adolescence

It is often said that adolescence begins with a biologic event (puberty) and ends with a psychologic event (transition to adulthood). Thus the duration of this stage is variable and dependent on biologic, psychologic, and life-circumstance variables. The developmental challenges in this period are negotiating puberty, developing a cohesive sense of self, and psychologically and physically forming a separation from the parents and family. More than any other stage, adolescence is affected by cultural norms and expectations. It is important to consider the impact of ethnic and cultural factors in evaluating these developmental tasks. It is also essential to learn about the adolescent's reactions to the onset of puberty and to take a good psychosexual history. Sexual preference is generally well established by the adolescent period. Therefore it is important to be mindful of the needs of homosexual as well as heterosexual adolescents in the assessment process. When taking a sexual history, the physician should remain unbiased and extremely careful not to assume the adolescent has a heterosexual orientation. Inquiry regarding sexual identity and orientation should begin in an open-ended format and proceed to direct, matter-of-fact questions. This way the adolescent will sense that the interviewer is accepting and nonjudgmental, and the adolescent may be more comfortable sharing information about fears, worries, or alienation related to sexual identity.

Alcohol, tobacco, and drug usage are also key areas to include in the history of a patient in this age group. Academic or learning problems, quantity and quality of peer relationships, and symptoms of depression or identity disturbance should also be noted.

The evaluation of adolescents requires less input from parents and more direct history from the adolescent. To successfully engage the adolescent and obtain an accurate history often requires considerable skill and experience, particularly when there is resistance to participation in the assessment. An attitude that fosters openness and honesty in the dialogue is most helpful. Adolescents are much more aware of their feelings than younger children and are usually good reporters, provided they are positively engaged in the process. Depending on the specific content of the history and the goals of the evaluation, providing the adolescent with the opportunity to meet apart from the parents and the rest of the family can be very helpful in forming an alliance. Often, adolescents are seen alone as a first step in the process, with parent and family interviews coming later on. With the younger adolescent, play, in the form of drawing or table games such as cards, can help develop the relationship.

School History

The school history should be taken chronologically, beginning with organized daycare or preschool experiences and continuing through the time of the interview. Emphasis should be placed on learning, behavioral and social competencies, and problems that arise in school. Reactions of the child to separations, such as the beginning of school, and transitions to different schools should be noted. This is the section of the history in which general cognitive capacities are described. It is important to consider the child's strengths as well as his weaknesses. Note whether the child is in a special education program, has repeated a grade, or has received extra help or tutoring for any reason. Assessment of academic achievement often requires contact with the child's current teacher. Standardized reading and arithmetic tests are usually administered in school and may be available in the records. Old report cards may also be used to supplement retrospective accounts. For children of all ages, it is important to inquire about the peer group at school and the child's participation in extracurricular activities. This may include religious instruction, clubs, scouts, or school teams.

If there are school-related problems, it is important to learn how the problems began and what factors have maintained them. For example, an 8-year-old child who has attentional problems and hyperactive behavior in the third grade may be experiencing increased demands to sit, focus, and learn in school as the curriculum becomes more difficult. Therefore the assessment should attempt to elucidate whether this child's problems are related to a learning disorder, ADHD, or both.

Family History

The family history section of the assessment involves obtaining each parent's personal history, including the level of education, vocation, and presence of medical and psychiatric problems. Relevant medical and psychiatric histories of the child's siblings, grandparents, the parent's siblings, and their children should also be obtained. It is helpful to ask if there is anyone else in the family who has had similar problems to the patient.

Obtaining a sociocultural history is also important. Any migrations or relocations should be noted, and attention should be given to the impact this has had on the family and the child. Additional information of interest might include the languages spoken at home, the religion of the family, and the impact of these on the child. Cultural differences regarding child-rearing and discipline should be considered, since individuals of different ethnic groups often have different expectations regarding their children's behavior and how to manage it. The meaning of having a child evaluated by a mental health provider may also need to be explored in the context of cultural differences. It is especially important to understand the family's ideas and value judgments regarding psychiatric treatment before presenting the results of the evaluation and the treatment plan. This will prevent an otherwise good plan from being doomed to failure because it is at variance with culturally determined values.

Interview with the Child or Adolescent

Overview

The purpose of the interview with the child (in this section, the term *child* refers to both children and adolescents) is to clarify the differential diagnosis through direct observation, questioning, or play. This session is often used to confirm hypotheses generated from the parent interview or to generate additional diagnostic hypotheses, although it occasionally provides more definitive information. History-taking from the child should include questions about the present and past aspects of the child's life and overall functioning. During the child interview, the physician also attempts to learn about the child's feelings and internal states. However, this may require patience on the part of the interviewer and may not happen at the beginning of the interview.

The first task is to engage the child in the process. It is this aspect of the examination that often makes beginning child psychiatrists the most uncomfortable. Nevertheless, it is important that the beginning psychiatrist interact with the child without conveying his own sense of anxiety about the interview. In general, skills used to develop a relationship with a child in the pediatric setting are applicable. Telling the child why he is being seen and requesting his assistance is paramount, just as if the physician were seeing the child for abdominal pain. However, it is also important to indicate how this visit differs from a visit to the pediatrician. It is often useful to indicate at the outset that there will be no injections or other procedures during the evaluation. The format of the interview invariably differs with respect to the individual child and the style and temperament of the interviewer. Approaches used with the same child may also vary from session to session. The structure and flow of the child interview varies by necessity as a function of the child's age and developmental level. For example, adolescents are often seen before their parents to solidify the relationship with the interviewer and to demonstrate their centrality in the evaluation process. The preschool child is often seen with the parent present, especially if there are separation problems or questions about the parent-child interaction.

Children are often quite anxious when beginning the evaluation process. They are usually aware that they are going to the doctor because of unpleasant or unwanted feelings (such as sadness, anxiety, fear, or anger) or problem behaviors (for instance, biting other children, having tantrums, or skipping school). The physician should communicate early that he does not consider the child to be bad but that some of the child's behaviors are problematic. In this way, the interviewer distinguishes between self-worth and behavior problems. It may also be helpful to indicate that there may be different ways to behave that are more socially acceptable.

The observation of the child commonly begins in the waiting room. The physician should take note of the child's behavior, including how the child relates to his parents, his general level of anxiety, and how he separates from the caregiver. Usually the child will have been told about the appointment by the parent before the interview. Ideally, the parent will have given the child information regarding the purpose of the assessment and how the child may be helped. However, it is important to review this information at the beginning of the interview. Also at the beginning of the interview, the physician should introduce himself to the child and tell the child what type of psychiatric clinician he is (a psychiatrist or other health care provider), the amount of time the child will be in the office to play or talk, and that the parents or caregivers will be in the waiting room at the conclusion of the session.

In the same way that a physician engages conversation with a new pediatric patient, the psychiatrist begins by gathering neutral data, such as who the child lives with, how old he is, his grade in school, where he attends school, and his interests or hobbies. Taking an active interest in who the child is and what he likes to do helps reduce anxiety. It may also be reassuring to the patient if the physician shares what has been learned from the parent about the reason for the visit at that time. However, it is essential to inquire about what the child sees as the problem, and how he is coping. Young children should not be expected to give a factual and chronologic account of their behavior; it is better to obtain this information from other sources.

When interviewing the child, it is important to interact in a manner that is appropriate to the child's level of development. Depending on the age of the child, the interview may be more or less verbally oriented. Most adolescents have no trouble speaking directly with the interviewer. However, a young child is more likely to use play as an important means of communication. It is helpful to have paper, pencil, crayons, and some age-appropriate toys available for the assessment. Family figures and a doll house can be especially useful in allowing a child to express issues about his family. The use of projective techniques with puppets and dolls can be a less threatening way for the child to convey his feelings, perceptions, and means of regulating impulses. This play can be used to build rapport, as well as for diagnostic purposes. Additionally, the child may be asked to draw a picture of his choosing or to draw something specific, such as a person or his family. In either case, care must be taken not to distort the child's play with unjustified assumptions or overly intense interpretations regarding its "true meaning." Other commonly used projective techniques are to have the child say what his three wishes would be if he could have anything in the world, or what animal he would like to be. Finally, it is useful to ask what the child's future plans are. For example, the physician could ask what the child would like to do or be when he is older. This will give information about the child's sense of self, future goals, values, and concerns.

Another important aspect of the child interview is the evaluation of the child's capability to engage in a particular type of treatment. It is important to assess the child's insight into the presenting problems and his desire for change, as well as his verbal skills and capacity for abstract reasoning. This is especially important in older children, who generally assume a greater responsibility for coming to treatment and in determining the process of treatment.

Mental Status Examination

The mental status examination is comprised of the physician's observations regarding the child's psychologic process and level of functioning, which are based on the child's overall level of relatedness and responses to specific objective and subjective questions. It is the psychiatric equivalent of the physical examination. It is important to remember that the mental status examination is a cross-sectional profile, and may vary from day to day. Examples and descriptions should be used in the write-up as much as possible.

The mental status examination contains the following domains of assessment: appearance, behavior, relatedness, speech and language, mood and affect, thought process and content, and cognitive and developmental assessment.

Appearance

The general appearance of the child is noted, and attention is given to the way he is dressed and groomed. The presence of any unusual physical marks or dysmorphic features should be noted. Scars or bruises may indicate accident-prone behavior or physical abuse. Dysmorphic features may indicate the presence of genetic or prenatal syndromes that may be related to the child's symptoms. Dysmorphic features should be described specifically. Examples include "low-set ears" or "a flat philtrum."

Behavior

The level of motor activity should be noted, and attention should be given to the presence of any purposeless movements such as tics, stereotypies, or other involuntary movements. Tics are involuntary, sudden, nonrhythmic motor activities or vocalizations. Stereotypies are repetitive, nonfunctional motions such as hand waving, head banging, body rocking, or hitting one's own body. Observations should be made about the child's ability to sit still, his level of attentiveness or distractibility, and any mannerisms or habits that may be present, such as hand wringing, nail biting, or thumb sucking. Note whether the child can regulate his own behavior or whether he requires considerable structure.

Relatedness

When assessing the child's relatedness to the interviewer, it is important to keep in mind the level of anxiety that is often present in the initial evaluation session. However, most children make meaningful contact with the interviewer if they are given enough time. If this does not occur, it might signal the presence of a pervasive developmental disorder (PDD) or an anxiety disorder. Consider the length of time required for the child to warm up and his responsiveness to reassurance, both of which may constitute important temperamental features. Relatedness is described according to the child's ability to maintain eye contact, establish rapport, and engage in meaningful play or dialogue with the interviewer.

Speech and Language

Speech is the actual production of words. Language is the entire process of understanding communication and expressing one's own thoughts and ideas. Speech should be evaluated for stuttering or other phonologic problems. Note the volume and quality of speech and whether it is loud, soft, whining, or monotonal. Also note the child's fluency and competence in English, as well as whether he speaks other languages. Language has both verbal and nonverbal components. Both expressive and receptive language should be assessed. Pointing to pictures and drawing can be useful techniques in the assessment of receptive language in a child with expressive language problems.

Mood and Affect

Mood is defined as the internal emotional state of a person (that is, how the patient feels). It is often helpful to ask the child to describe his general mood. If that does not elicit a response, providing examples of moods such as mad, sad, or happy can be helpful. With young children it may be helpful to draw or point to pictures that describe these feelings. Affect is the overall expression of the present emotional content (how the patient presents himself to another individual). The description of the child's affect should include an assessment of the range of affect, its appropriateness to the situation, its quality, and its intensity. A child may look frightened or display a constricted range of affect during the early part of the interview, but as he relaxes, his affect may be more complete and appropriate.

Thought Process and Content

The process of thought is evaluated through the child's spontaneous verbalizations and through play. Some children may initially be reluctant to talk but have no difficulty drawing or playing. If a child is given items such as paper and pencil or crayons, or a dollhouse with figures, the play that follows may be indicative of the child's inner world. The thought process is described according to the coherence, goal-directedness, logic, rate, and sequence of thoughts. In adolescents, thought process can usually be assessed directly. However, it must often be inferred from the logic and coherence of a younger child's imaginative play. For example, if a child is playing with family figures in a doll house, it is important to see whether there is an identifiable beginning, middle, and end to the story-telling or play. Of course, the child's developmental level has an impact on his ability to present a coherent story.

The content of the child's thoughts includes what he chooses to talk about as well as any fantasies that may be enacted. Fantasies may be inferred from the child's drawings or play, but they are best learned from what the child actually says about his productions. A variety of open-ended, projective techniques can be useful. For example, the physicians can ask the child to describe three wishes he would make, or special powers he would want to have if the interviewer had the power to grant them. Suicidal or homicidal ideation are noted here, and all pertinent details are described (such as the nature of a plan, if there is one).

The child's reality testing should be assessed, and the presence of delusions or perceptual disturbances should be noted. There are many ways to assess reality. Children can be asked about ideas they may have that other people do not believe. They can be asked whether they feel they have special powers or whether they think that people are purposely out to get them. The presence of any perceptual disturbances, such as auditory or visual hallucinations, or any other unusual sensory phenomena should also be assessed. When asking children about hallucinations, it may be helpful to say, "Some children hear voices (or see things) that other people don't. Does that ever happen to you?" Or, "Are there ever times when your eyes or ears seem to play tricks on you?" It is important to distinguish hallucinations from illusions. Note the timing of hallucinations if they are present, and determine whether they are related to sleep, stressors, or particular events. If the child's reality testing seems impaired, question him about how firmly his beliefs are held and about the possibility that these ideas are pretend or make-believe. However, care must be taken before labeling a child psychotic, because some aspects of impaired reality-testing may be developmentally appropriate. For example, it is often developmentally appropriate for children to have imaginary friends. It is also not unusual for children to have hallucinations or altered sensory perceptions upon falling asleep or awakening, referred to as hypnagogic or hypnopompic hallucinations, respectively. Finally, many children who do report hallucinations have language problems and should not be viewed as psychotic. This latter condition is rare in prepubertal children.

Cognitive and Developmental Assessment

The evaluation of cognitive function should include an assessment of the child's general fund of knowledge, memory, reasoning ability, vocabulary, and conceptualization ability. These assessments should reflect the child's age and developmental level. A variety of techniques, such as the use of vocabulary, level of comprehension, curiosity, digit span, and drawing ability can be used. The cognitive exam should include the evaluation of age-appropriate developmental skills. Can the child copy shapes (such as a circle, square, or triangle) at ages 3, 4, and 5, respectively? What is the child's fund of knowledge? Does the child know colors or body parts? How is language development proceeding? How well developed are fine and gross motor function? Psychometric tests may also provide useful information about cognition, but testing is expensive and not readily available in some settings. Additionally, whereas psychometric testing is required to accurately diagnose a learning disability (by calculating a discrepancy score), the clinical evaluation can often indicate that a learning problem is present.

Diagnostic Formulation and Treatment Planning

Organization of Data

After all the relevant informants have been contacted and interviewed, and after the history has been supplemented with appropriate reports, rating scales, and laboratory tests, the physician must synthesize the information into a working diagnosis. The physician should begin by considering whether a general medical condition that could account for the presenting problem is present before making a psychiatric diagnosis. The range of normal developmental deviation should also be considered. In children who do have a psychiatric diagnosis, symptoms of multiple conditions may be present. In such cases, all relevant diagnoses need to be recorded. For example, a child may have ADHD and a developmental reading disorder.

It is often useful to develop an initial working assessment and differential diagnosis while the history is being gathered. For example, if after talking with the parents, the physician suspects that the child may have a disruptive behavior disorder, a subsequent conversation with the child's teacher can be used to ask specific questions about the child's school behavior and attentional performance. In this way, the physician can better determine whether the child meets criteria for ADHD or for conduct disorder (CD) or ODD. Establishing a working diagnosis is important because it allows the physician to use deductive reasoning while taking the history or writing it up.

Formulation

The diagnostic formulation provides an opportunity to develop a comprehensive framework for understanding a child's symptomatic presentation in the context of his strengths, risk factors, and life events. Additionally, it allows the physician to describe the severity of the disorder and the level of function. As a general rule, the physician's formulation should follow the biopsychosocial model, which stresses that biologic, psychologic, and social factors all be taken into account when studying the emergence of the psychopathologic condition. The formulation section of the case summary need only be a paragraph long, but it is the only place for the physician to integrate all the information that has been gathered. The formulation should always provide a statement regarding the current developmental status, but it may also include a summary of the hypothesized source of the psychiatric problems that are observed, the coping and adaptive mechanisms of the child, and the adequacy of family and social supports.

Treatment Plan

In current psychiatric practice, the cause of a disorder cannot necessarily be inferred from the diagnosis, and treatment practices are often not specific to particular diagnoses. However, the combination of the diagnosis, the overall level of functioning, and the modifying effects of risk and protective factors can be used to develop a specific treatment plan appropriate to the child's problem.

The treatment plan is an individualized recommendation for care. The goal of the treatment plan is to facilitate the child's development and alleviate symptoms. For the treatment plan to succeed, both the primary caregiver and child need to understand the plan and be willing to participate in its implementation. A child's ability to participate depends on a variety of factors such as the age of the child and the nature of the plan. When constructing a treatment plan, all the relevant data from the assessment should first be incorporated into a comprehensive multidimensional problem list. Each entry on this list should point to a target intervention; multiple treatment modalities are often required. The specifics of the plan depend on the nature and severity of the impairment, as well as a variety of mediating factors. Unfortunately, it is not always feasible for the optimal treatment plan to be enacted. There may be constraints on any one of numerous levels; these should be anticipated as much as possible when preparing the treatment plan and discussed in realistic terms with the family. Financial resources need to be considered, since treatment recommendations that do not correspond to a family's economic circumstances are not likely to be employed.

Psychiatric Diagnosis in Children and Adolescents

The development of a comprehensive nosology for psychiatric disorders in children is a relatively recent phenomenon, although tremendous gains have been made since the publication of the *Diagnostic and Statistical Manual of Mental Disorders, Third Edition* (DSM-III) in 1980. DSM employs a multiaxial system consisting of five parts. It encourages the use of more than one diagnosis when appropriate and provides a format for recording information about the context of disorders and general level of impairment, as well as for the description of symptoms. Axis I is used to describe clinical syndromes such as disruptive behavior disorders, mood and anxiety disorders, specific and pervasive developmental disorders, and other conditions that may be a focus of clinical attention but do not represent a psychiatric disorder (for example, conditions such as parent-child relational problem and bereavement). Axis II is used to record mental retardation or personality disorders. (Personality disorders are often not diagnosed in children and adolescents, but there may be traits present, particularly in adolescents.) Axis III is used to code general medical conditions, and axis IV helps the physician describe the psychosocial and environmental context with respect to the illness. Examples include parental divorce or chronic medical illness in the child. Axis V is used to code the global assessment of functioning. The patient is rated on a scale of 1 to 100 on social, occupational (school), and psychologic functioning, where 100 describes superior functioning and 1 signifies seriously impaired functioning. A score of 60 to 70 is most often consistent with the presence of a psychiatric diagnosis.

As in previous editions, the fourth edition of DSM (DSM-IV) begins with a chapter devoted to disorders that begin in infancy, childhood, and adolescence. The following disorders are included in that section: mental retardation, learning disorders, motor skills disorders, communication disorders, pervasive developmental disorders (such as autistic disorder and Asperger's disorder), attention-deficit and other disruptive behavior disorders (such as CD and ODD), feeding and eating disorders of infancy or early childhood, tic disorders, elimination disorders, and other disorders such as separation anxiety disorder (SAD), selective mutism, and reactive attachment disorder of infancy or early childhood. However, many disorders described in other sections of the manual may also be present in children and adolescents. These include mood and anxiety disorders, schizophrenia, somatoform disorders, and eating disorders. Therefore it is important that physicians who work with children and adolescents not restrict themselves to the so-called "child disorders" section. Additionally, physicians who work with adults would be well served to familiarize themselves with the disorders that first appear in childhood, since many of these disorders persist into adulthood. The following paragraphs briefly describe the diagnostic categories most often used with children and adolescents. Section 2 of this book reviews most of these conditions in greater detail.

Disorders of development and attachment are most often present at an early age. Examples include mental retardation, pervasive developmental disorders, and reactive attachment disorder. Mental retardation is defined as general intellectual functioning that is significantly below average. It is coded on axis II, and it is separated into mild, moderate, severe, and profound subgroups based on the degree of intellectual impairment defined by the IQ and the level of adaptive functioning. An IQ score below 65 to 70 (that is, 2 standard deviations below the mean) is the upper limit of mental retardation. Parallel impairments in adaptive functioning are also required to fulfill the criteria.

The PDDs are defined by impairments in reciprocal social interaction and communication and by a restricted range of behavior, interests, and activities. Autistic disorder, Asperger's disorder, Rett's disorder, childhood disintegrative disorder, and pervasive developmental disorder not otherwise specified (PDD-NOS) are all identified. Children with these disorders exhibit varying abnormalities of language function that may profoundly affect their abilities to communicate with others and to make their wishes and needs known. There is also a qualitative impairment in reciprocal social interaction and relatedness, even with primary caregivers. Additionally, these children often have an inability to play symbolically, so pretend play is limited or nonexistent. Stereotyped movements such as hand flapping or head banging may be present, or there may be a fascination with parts of objects, such as the wheels on toy cars. There is often, but not always, an associated degree of mental retardation in individuals with autistic disorder (approximately two-thirds have an IQ below 70). The onset of autistic disorder is usually evident in the first years of life and, by definition, occurs before age 3.

Reactive attachment disorder is another disorder that is present in preschool children. The features of this disorder begin before a child is 5 years old with disturbed and developmentally inappropriate social relatedness (for example, a child may be overly friendly with strangers or withdrawn). By definition, the unrelatedness is associated with pathogenic care of the child. Children who come to the physician with failure to thrive often qualify for this diagnosis.

There are more diagnostic categories that may apply to the school-age child. The most prominent among these are ADHD and disruptive behavior disorders. However, a variety of cognitive and learning disorders, such as specific developmental or communication disorders, may also become apparent at this age. ADHD is a disorder characterized by a pattern of inattention and hyperactivity-impulsivity that is excessive relative to the behavior of other children of the same age and gender. Children with this disorder may have difficulty remaining seated, waiting their turn, completing assignments, sustaining attention, or organizing their work. By definition, some of these symptoms must be present before a child reaches 7 years of age, and there must be some symptoms causing impairment in more than one setting (for example, at home, at school, or in clubs). ADHD often begins in preschool years and commonly extends into adolescence or adulthood, but the largest number of cases can be found in school-age children. Individuals with this disorder are commonly both inattentive and hyperactive-impulsive, although a smaller number of children may have disturbances in only one of these domains. Many children with ADHD show symptoms of aggression and defiance; co-morbid learning, behavior, mood, and anxiety disorders are often present. However, although these conditions may coexist with ADHD, they must be distinguished from it. When multiple disorders are present, they should all be diagnosed.

ODD and CD are the other disruptive behavior disorders listed in DSM-IV. ODD is defined by the presence of persistent minor violations of age-appropriate social norms. Children with ODD often argue with adults, lose their tempers, refuse to follow rules, deliberately annoy people, and blame others for their actions. They are often angry and resentful. Exclusionary criteria for this disorder include the presence of a psychotic, mood, or conduct disorder. CD is a behavior pattern in which the basic rights of others or major age-appropriate societal norms are violated. Examples include aggression directed toward people and animals, destruction of property, deceitfulness or theft, and serious violation of rules. This diagnosis takes precedence over ODD if criteria for both diagnoses are met, since approximately 90% of children with CD also meet criteria for ODD. There is good evidence that ODD represents a developmental precursor to CD in a subgroup of children.

Learning disorders are defined by academic functioning that is significantly below what is expected for an individual's chronologic age, measured intelligence, and age-appropriate education. These disorders may involve deficits in reading, mathematics, and written expression. The accurate diagnosis of learning disorders requires the use of standardized intelligence and achievement tests to establish a discrepancy score. (That is, the score on a standardized achievement test is below what would be expected from the level of intellectual functioning as measured on a standardized IQ test.)

The communication disorders, which are characterized by difficulties in speech or language, include expressive language disorder, mixed receptive-expressive language disorder, phonological disorder, and stuttering. Communication disorders often appear in preschool years, but they may not be properly identified until the child is in a school setting. Expressive language disorder is characterized by lower than expected abilities in vocabulary, use of tenses, production of complex sentences, and word recall. Mixed receptive-expressive language disorder involves an impaired understanding of language and a concomitant difficulty with expressive language. Phonological disorder consists of errors in sound production and substitutions or omissions of sounds that would be developmentally expected. Stuttering is a disturbance of the fluency and time patterning of speech.

There are several tic disorders in DSM-IV. By far, the most common is transient tic disorder, which involves the transient presentation of single or multiple motor or vocal tics. A tic is a sudden, rapid, recurrent, nonrhythmic, stereotyped movement or vocalization; tics may be simple or complex. Tourette's disorder is the least common but most dramatic of the tic disorders. The diagnosis is made when there is a history of multiple motor tics and at least one vocal tic. The average age of onset of tics is 7 years. Approximately 40% to 50% of children with Tourette's disorder in clinical samples also have symptoms of ADHD. Tourette's disorder is also often co-morbid with obsessive-compulsive disorder (OCD). However, it is not clear to what extent Tourette's disorder causes impairment in nonreferred samples, since referral bias as a function of psychiatric co-morbidity is not uncommon. (That is, cases with co-morbidity and cases of greater impairment are more likely to be referred for treatment.)

Enuresis and encopresis comprise the elimination disorders in DSM-IV. These disorders have a minimum age threshold defined by the child's chronologic age or equivalent developmental level. Encopresis is the repeated passage of feces in inappropriate places by a child who is at least 4 years old. Enuresis is the repeated voiding of urine into the bed or clothes by a child who is at least 5 years old.

SAD is a condition in which there is developmentally inappropriate and extreme anxiety about separation from home, parents, or primary caregivers. This is the most common anxiety disorder in childhood. It can have such symptoms as school avoidance or phobia, sleep disturbance, and nightmares. This disorder commonly follows an acute life event such as the medical illness of the child or parent, the loss of a close family member, parental separation, or the birth of a new sibling. Most often, separation anxiety disorder lasts for a limited time and good return to normal function results from the use of simple behavioral measures and encouragement. However, some children develop more chronic symptoms and impairment.

Disorders that are often diagnosed in children and adolescents that are not described in the childhood section of DSM-IV include schizophrenia and other psychotic disorders, mood disorders, other anxiety disorders (such as OCD and generalized anxiety disorder [GAD]), eating disorders, substance use disorders, and gender identity disorder. Schizophrenia is phenotypically similar in children and adults, although children may have a less pronounced onset of symptoms and may not meet the full criteria for months or years after they are first brought to a physician. Children with schizophrenia have blunted or inappropriate affect, isolation, withdrawal, auditory and visual hallucinations, and thought disorders. There is some indication that the "negative symptoms" (such as thought disorder and isolation) predominate over "positive symptoms" (such as hallucinations and delusions). However, the only diagnostic criterion that actually differs in children is that they may fail to reach expected levels of social and academic functioning (rather than deteriorate from a predetermined level). Schizophrenia is rare before puberty and must be aggressively distinguished from the PDDs when it occurs in this age group.

Since the 1980s, there has been considerable interest in the subject of mood disorders in children and adolescents. Although it is now recognized that children of all ages become depressed and often show the same symptoms as adults, major depressive disorder (MDD) is still not common until after puberty. There are only minor differences in the diagnostic criteria for the mood disorders in children and adolescents when compared with adults. A child or adolescent with MDD may have an irritable rather than depressed mood, and he may fail to make expected weight gain instead of having a significant weight loss. In children or adolescents with dysthymia, the mood may again be irritable rather than depressed, and the duration of the mood need only be 1 year, as compared with 2 years for adults. There are no differences in the criteria for bipolar disorder as a function of age. Again, whereas bipolar disorder can exist in prepubertal children, it is not often present in its full form until after puberty.

The "adult" anxiety disorders include panic disorder, specific phobias, social phobia, OCD, posttraumatic stress disorder (PTSD), acute stress disorder, and GAD. These disorders may be present in children and adolescents as well as adults, and they do not appear to be particularly different in children. OCD is characterized by recurrent intrusive thoughts or behaviors. OCD symptoms often have their onset in childhood or adolescence, although the specific disorder may not be identified for several years. Common signs of OCD in children are excessive handwashing and avoidance of supposedly contaminated objects.

Adolescents may have any of the disorders that begin in childhood, or they may have the initial onset of any of the disorders commonly seen in adults. Developmental differences related to a psychopathologic condition must be considered. For example, ADHD is often seen in adolescents, but there are usually fewer hyperactivity and impulsivity symptoms than in the school-aged child. Symptoms of several of the personality disorders may become clinically apparent in the adolescent period, although they are not usually diagnosed until an adolescent reaches 18 years of age. Disorders that are common in adolescents include the eating disorders, anorexia nervosa and bulimia nervosa, and the substance-related disorders.

The substance-related disorders include disorders of drug use and abuse; they may involve the use of alcohol, cannabis, and cocaine. Substance abuse is defined as substance use that interferes with a person's capacity to meet obligations in work, school, or home and that results in a physically dangerous situation, legal problems, or continued use despite recurrent problems. Substance dependence pre-empts a diagnosis of abuse. Dependence involves a long-standing pattern of abuse that shows tolerance, withdrawal, and a lack of control over the substance.

The eating disorders involve severe disturbances in eating behavior and perceptions of body shape and weight. These disorders have received considerable attention since the late 1970s, and there has been a resultant increase in case identification. Anorexia nervosa is the refusal to maintain a minimally normal body weight accompanied by an unshakable fear of gaining weight or becoming fat. Bulimia nervosa involves repeated episodes of binge eating and purging behavior in an attempt to control weight gain. Self-induced vomiting, use of laxatives or diuretics, and compulsive exercising may all be seen. The most common age of onset of anorexia nervosa is in the mid-teenage years, and the disorder is much more common in females. Bulimia nervosa has a later age of onset and often begins in the late teens or 20s. Both disorders may be characterized by serious medical complications and co-morbid psychopathologic conditions.

Child Psychiatry and the Primary Care Physician

Recently, there has been increasing interest in the role of the primary care physician in the arena of child and adolescent mental health. This is important, because there are few child and adolescent psychiatrists relative to the number of children in need and because the vast majority of children see a primary care physician. The primary care physician is well suited for screening and early intervention in children's mental health problems. Some of these problems may also be treated by primary care physicians, although referral to specialists and collaborative case management is still the norm.

Screening is the process by which the existence of a problem becomes known. To successfully screen for mental health problems, the primary care physician must be able to understand developmentally appropriate skills and functions; recognize major difficulties a child may have in school, social, or family functioning; be aware of major psychiatric syndromes; ask about the presence of symptoms; and investigate events that are known to be stressful to the child and family. Some screening can actually be done in the waiting room by using a parent rating scale such as the CBCL or Conners Parent Questionnaire. These scales provide a comprehensive profile of developmentally appropriate tasks and a range of psychiatric symptoms, and they allow the physician to note any areas of past or present difficulties. Inquiries should be made at each visit about the child's mental health functioning, level of functioning in age-appropriate activities, and general sense of well-being. Specific areas of functioning to be evaluated are the child's sleep and appetite habits, social skills (such as the presence of friends and participation in groups or clubs), academic and behavioral performance in school, and relationships within the family (how the child gets along with parents and siblings). Screening questions regarding mood and anxiety symptoms, suicidal or homicidal thoughts, and hallucinations should be included in each contact and can be helpful in identifying a problem requiring referral.

The primary care physician is also in a perfect position to make early interventions and manage risk factors when they are present. These interventions may decrease the need for an additional visit to the psychiatrist. Examples of prevention or early intervention services well suited to primary care settings include parenting classes for parents of infants and toddlers, dissemination of information regarding management of common behavior problems, and providing directive parental counselling for the management of specific problems. Teaching parents techniques they can use to manage behavior problems, such as ignoring a tantrum rather than giving in (so as not to reinforce the behavior), can be reassuring to parents, especially if techniques are discussed in a conversational and nonjudgmental manner.

There are many types of events that may place a child at increased risk for behavioral or psychiatric problems. Primary care physicians should be alerted to the possible consequences of these events. Some of the more common events are parental divorce or separation, a death in the family, a move to a new home or school, a change in the parent's employment status, or a medical illness of the child or a family member. The occurrence of such events can be determined during the beginning of a routine visit by asking open-ended questions about the family's circumstances. If significant events or changes in the family are identified, then more specific questions can be asked. Once a profile of risk is elicited, supportive management techniques can often help alleviate more significant problems.

There can be no simple rule about when to refer. Some pediatricians are comfortable managing certain conditions, but they are more likely to refer others to a specialist. The primary care physician needs to know when a problem is interfering with a child's development and functioning, as well as when early intervention has not been successful. In this case, referral for more extensive treatment is generally appropriate. Once a referral has been made, it is essential that there be collaboration between the primary care physician and the mental health specialist. This contact maximizes the likelihood that the referral will be successfully negotiated by the patient and family.

Summary

The psychiatric assessment of children and adolescents is a complex process. However, it can be made less intimidating when a basic framework is followed. The components of the examination include meeting with the parents and the child to gather a complete history, obtaining the mental status examination of the child, developing a treatment plan, and presenting the results of the evaluation to the family. Yet, within this framework, it is necessary to account for individual differences in children and parents, as well as for stylistic differences among physicians. The basic issues that should be addressed in the assessment process are: whether the child has a problem that significantly interferes with his normal development, whether there are problems in social, academic, or family functioning, and whether there is effective treatment that will allow the child to reach his potential free of interference from psychiatric morbidity. More effective recognition of mental health problems in children is needed, and closer collaboration between primary care providers and mental health specialists is imperative in this regard.

Annotated Bibliography

Canino IA: *Taking a history.* In Shaffer D, Ehrhardt AA, Greenhill LL, editors: *The clinical guide to child psychiatry,* New York, 1985, The Free Press.

This is a comprehensive and practical chapter on history-taking in child psychiatry.

Lewis M: *General psychiatric assessment of children and adolescents.* In Solnit AJ, Cohen DJ, Schowalter JE, editors: *Child psychiatry,* vol 6, Michels R, chairman, editorial board: *Psychiatry* series, Philadelphia, 1986, JB Lippincott Co.

This chapter is on assessment and gives attention to the mental status examination.

Simmons JE: *Psychiatric examination of children,* ed 4, Philadelphia, 1987, Lea & Febiger.

This is an easy-to-read book that covers many aspects of the complete psychiatric examination in children.

chapter 2

Diagnostic Instruments

Aradhana A. Sood, MD and Nirbhay N. Singh, PhD

Choosing Diagnostic Instruments
Clinical Judgment
Ecologic Context of Assessment
Types of Instruments Used with Children and Adolescents
General Instruments
Disorder-Specific Instruments
Summary

Psychiatric assessment is both a science and an art, and it is the clinician who has to integrate the two in practice. Many assessment instruments are grounded in empirical research and have robust psychometric properties, well-validated cutoff scores, and computerized scoring and interpretation methods. Others have less of an empirical basis and are more subjective, relying on the clinician's training and experience for interpretation of the findings. Assessment is an art because it involves clinical judgment, an appreciation of the individual within an ecologic context, and the use of intuition to integrate clinical knowledge and data from various assessment instruments. Furthermore, the mere fact that the clinician chooses which assessment instruments should be used to answer specific questions that will lead to a diagnosis and treatment means that a subjective element is introduced in the assessment process. Additionally, the clinician is interested in providing an evaluation of the individual in as efficient yet effective a manner as possible.

The contents and the process of psychiatric assessment were presented in Chapter 1. The goals of this chapter are to briefly present the issues that a physician must address when selecting an instrument, to briefly discuss the various types of diagnostic instruments that are available, and to provide an overview of the most commonly used instruments in child and adolescent psychiatry. The instruments are discussed within the context of specific disorders of children and adolescents taken from the *Diagnostic and Statistic Manual of Mental Disorders, Fourth Edition* (DSM-IV). They were chosen with the intention of providing clinicians and primary care physicians a guide to instruments that are of practical use within a clinical context. Some instruments, such as intelligence, achievement, and neuropsychologic tests, are not presented here because advanced training in psychologic measurement is required before they can be used. Psychiatric clinicians and primary care physicians are advised to refer the child or adolescent to a licensed clinical psychologist for such testing. In this chapter, the term *child* is used to include children and adolescents.

Choosing Diagnostic Instruments

There are several issues that a physician must consider before selecting a diagnostic instrument or a battery of instruments for use with children and adolescents. Of these, the four most important areas are practical considerations, standardization, reliability, and validity.

Practical Considerations

The choice of diagnostic instruments is first and foremost dependent on practical considerations related both to the physician and the patient. Instruments that provide the best clinical picture of the child must be chosen. The usefulness of the instrument depends on the specific questions to be asked and the specific problems of the patient to be solved. Thus there should be a good match between the selected instruments and the purpose for which they are chosen. It is also important to know whether the physician needs additional training to use the test or whether the patient should be referred to another professional who is trained to use the instrument (for example, in the case of an achievement or intelligence test). If a self-report measure is to be used, the physician must be certain that the child's reading level matches the level required by the test. Furthermore, the length of each test is a consideration, because time is at a premium and lengthy instruments do not necessarily provide more relevant information than shorter ones.

Standardization

The physician must be certain that the instruments being considered for use have adequate norms for the population that is being assessed. This means that a child's scores on an instrument are meaningful only if there is a good deal of similarity between the child and the sample on which the instrument was standardized. There are three critical issues that merit consideration. First, the sample used to standardize the instrument should be representative of the population that the physician would like to evaluate. Second, the size of the sample used to standardize the instrument should be large enough to give stable estimates of the variable being tested; small samples have the problem of random fluctuation within the group. Third, the instrument should have broad national norms as well as specialized subgroup norms. The subgroup norms may be based on a number of variables, including gender, age, race, school grade, and living environment (for example, rural vs. urban). Physicians may find that their patients match subgroups better than the overall population on which the instrument was standardized. Thus subgroup norms may be more appropriate than the national norms for specific children. Additionally, a well-standardized instrument provides a set of administration procedures that the physician must know and adhere to closely.

Reliability

Reliability refers to the extent that the scores obtained by a child on a specific instrument remain the same when the child is tested on different occasions. In technical terms, reliability refers to the degree of stability, consistency, predictability, and accuracy of the scores obtained on diagnostic instruments. Physicians must remember that there is rarely 100% reliability because of natural variation in the child's performance on an instrument. Additionally, psychiatric and psychologic testing methods are imprecise, and many factors are inferred rather than directly measured. There are several types of reliability, including test-retest reliability (repeated administration of the same test with the same child), alternate forms (parallel forms of the same test), split-half reliability (correlation between the two halves of a single test), and inter-rater reliability (administration of the same test by two or more clinicians). Current consensual agreement is that a reliability of over 70% is acceptable, although many physicians expect about 90% reliability on pivotal tests used for making treatment decisions. Data on reliability are presented in the administration manual of an instrument.

Validity

From the psychiatrist's perspective, validity is probably the most important aspect of an instrument. That is, does the instrument measure what it purports to measure, and does it provide clinically useful information? A valid instrument reliably measures the variable that it is intended to measure. Validity is established by correlating the test scores with some external, independently observed event. There are three ways of establishing validity: through content (how well the instrument covers the major aspects of the content area being measured), through criterion (how well the scores on this instrument correlate with other instruments that measure the same or a totally different variable), and construct validity (the extent to which the instrument measures the variable of interest). Clinicians may also be interested in incremental validity, or the ability of an instrument to produce new information.

Clinical Judgment

Regardless of the scientific basis of the instruments used, it is the clinician who has to synthesize the information, and thereby the very important element of clinical judgment is introduced into the evaluation process. Astute clinical judgment is required at all phases of assessment and particularly during data gathering and data synthesis. During data gathering, it is essential that the physician develop an optimum level of rapport with the child if the data to be obtained is to be reliable and valid. Additionally, the physician should be aware of possible factors that may make a child's responses unrepresentative of his typical behavior. Some such factors may be transient conditions (such as test anxiety or lack of sleep) and conscious or unconscious faking.

The physician should also be conscious of the fact that she is influenced by various cultural and personal factors and that the questions she asks during unstructured and semistructured interviews may be influenced by factors other than those related to the child. Data gathering and data analysis are interactive processes that are guided by the child's response, as well as the clinician's clinical judgment and theoretical orientation. Therefore bias is introduced at several points, including during the choice of instruments, in the questions asked, in the initial impressions of the psychiatrist, in the level of rapport, in the psychiatrist's theoretical assumptions, and in the weight given to information obtained through different sources (for example, the child's vs. the parent's response, or direct observations vs. teacher reports).

When all the data have been gathered and analyzed, the physician has to judge what the data show. The accuracy of this judgment may be compromised if the physician fails to take into account the base rate of the disorder in question (that is, the rate at which the particular disorder occurs in the general population of children) or the developmental level of the child. Furthermore, the data must be interpreted within the ecologic and cultural contexts of the child—variables that have not received enough emphasis in the past. A child's behavior does not occur in a vacuum; thus it is imperative that the context in which the behavior occurs (such as family, school, and community contexts) is considered in the clinical judgment. Physicians can increase the accuracy of their clinical judgments by combining different methods of data gathering (for example, interviews and formal assessment) and by following statistical interpretive rules. The fact that physicians feel confident about the accuracy of their clinical judgments does not necessarily lead to more accurate clinical judgments. Indeed, as physicians increase their knowledge and experience, they typically show less confidence in their clinical judgments!

Ecologic Context of Assessment

The social ecology of the child is an important consideration in psychiatric assessment because a child's behavior maintains a dynamic relationship with his environment. Inherent in this view is the emphasis that a child's behavior is shaped by and interacts with the social contexts and physical environments in which his behavior occurs. The general principle is the interrelatedness of all phenomena. Thus the physician should realize that making a change in the behavior of a child inevitably leads to a change in not only other aspects of the child's behavior but also in some aspects of his social and physical environments.

This poses a unique problem in assessment, since no battery of instruments can encompass the totality of a child's social ecology. However, an approximation can be made by using an ecobehavioral approach to assessment. This type of approach provides a methodology for describing the interactions and interrelationships that occur between individuals, behavior, physical and social settings, and a child's internal state. In traditional assessment practices, these contextual conditions are often viewed as confounding variables, or noise, but our view is that greater emphasis on these variables during assessment provides a closer approximation of the nature of a child's problems.

In practice, this involves gathering sociodemographic data on the child (such as age, race, gender, school, grade level, history of mental illness, and achievement

PEARLS & PERILS

ASSESSMENTS

- Assessment is always undertaken within an ecologic context; be wary of assessments that do not specify the parameters of this context.
- Assessment instruments must be chosen to answer specific questions.
- Assessment instruments must have good psychometric properties, such as validity and reliability, to be useful.
- Assessment instruments should have adequate norms for the target population.
- Even the best quantitative assessments can be meaningless unless they are artfully interpreted by the physician with reference to each child within his or her natural environment.
- All assessments are culturally biased; choose instruments that have been validated on the target population.
- All phenomena are interrelated and are constantly changing; an assessment is a snapshot that is anchored in time and therefore less accurate with the passage of time. Be wary of dated assessments!

scores) and family (for example, race, age, and other standard sociodemographic variables, as well as family income, maternal education, family size, source of referral, area of residence, parental psychopathologic states, and an index of socioeconomic disadvantage). Similarly, if the child is in school, a number of school variables, including the instructional environment, a record of the child's school history, and the teacher's expectations and standards for the children in the target child's class, may need to be considered. Although it is not possible to assess each contextual variable that is in a dynamic relationship with the child and her behavior, physicians should attempt to gather as much information about the ecologic context of the child as possible.

Types of Instruments Used with Children and Adolescents

The types of diagnostic instruments used with children and adolescents are the same as those used for adults: structured interviews, checklists and rating scales, direct behavioral observations, intelligence and achievement tests, physiologic tests, neuropsychologic tests, and projective tests. As the objective diagnostic criteria for psychiatric disorders have been developed and refined, diagnostic instruments are increasingly based on the International Classification of Diseases (ICD) and DSM diagnostic classification systems. Furthermore, there has been an unevenness in the development of instruments for assessing various psychiatric disorders; there are several types of instruments for some disorders and very few for others. We neither believe nor suggest that because many instruments are available for a disorder, it is necessary to use them all to accurately assess a given disorder. Certainly, it would be an overkill to use each type of diagnostic instrument listed with any one child at any one time. Indeed, the selection of different types of instruments should be guided by the types of questions being asked rather than the mere availability of well-validated instruments.

Diagnostic instruments suitable for use with children and adolescents are designed to assess several disorders or a specific disorder. Furthermore, there are several checklists, rating scales, and observational measures that provide a broad range of data on various intervening variables (for example, sociodemographic and ecobehavioral variables) that affect the child's behavior and are of interest to the physician because they provide the context in which the child functions. In this chapter we briefly discuss instruments that provide a broad range of data, and then we discuss disorder-specific instruments.

General Instruments

Diagnostic Interviews

For the physician, the diagnostic interview is the most important source of data on the child; data that are often unobtainable through formal testing can be collected at this time. This interview can be used to gather information about the nature and history of the child's problem, level of adjustment, and strengths; to collect diagnostic information; and to uncover unique aspects of the child's history in a flexible, open-ended manner. Although the interview format has many strengths, it has been criticized with regard to its reliability and validity, particularly when it has been used as the basis to diagnose a child's problems. The two most important problems contributing to the lack of diagnostic reliability include information variance (that is, differences between physicians in the amount and kind of information obtained during diagnostic interviews) and criterion variance (differences between physicians in their use of inclusionary and exclusionary criteria when they summarize a child's data into a psychiatric diagnosis). To help solve these problems, a number of investigators have developed explicit criteria and classification schemes, as well as structured interviews that include standardized questions for systematically eliciting data from both children and adults.

In a structured interview, the interview process is limited to the sequence and flow of questions that are included in the diagnostic instrument. It serves as a method to obtain unbiased information in a standardized manner and to reduce subjective and, by inference, inaccurate gathering of data. Most of the diagnosis-generating interviews fall into this category of instruments. The advantage of using structured interviews is that a person with little or no training in mental health can be trained in a short time to reliably and inexpensively gather clinical information. Additionally, some structured interviews can be administered and scored by a computer. Disadvantages of these instruments include their length and their tendency to be overinclusive.

Interviews that are semistructured by design also specify the content and items that are to be included, but they provide more flexibility in terms of wording and the sequence of the interview. They are intended to be conducted by physicians who are well versed in diagnostic issues in children and adolescents, because they allow the interviewer to probe the child to obtain more sensitive and valid data. Thus semistructured interviews require the use of clinical judgment throughout the interview process.

There has been a proliferation of structured and semistructured interviews since the first one was published in 1981. We provide an overview of five of the most commonly used interviews for children. However, physicians must remember that all such instruments are continually being revised as new data are gathered and the diagnostic criteria for psychiatric disorders are refined. Thus it is the physician's responsibility to ensure that the most recent versions of these interviews are used.

Structured Interviews

Diagnostic Interview for Children and Adolescents-Revised

The Diagnostic Interview for Children and Adolescents-Revised (DICA-R), one of the earliest structured interviews to be developed, is designed for children age 6 to 12 and adolescents age 13 to 17. A version for parents is also available. Administration of either version takes about 60 to 90 minutes. The interviewer systematically questions the child or parent on various symptoms that correlate to DSM-III-R diagnostic criteria for mental disorders. The presence or absence of these symptoms is documented and coded; the scoring can be done manually or by using computer-generated scoring algorithms. Although the interview format is highly structured, there are provisions for the interviewer to provide examples if the question is not understood and for follow-up questions. Additionally, instructions are provided for skipping irrelevant items.

Data on the psychometric properties of the DICA-R are not available, but earlier versions of the instrument have good test-retest and inter-rater reliability for diagnostic concordance. Parent-child agreement for internalized symptoms, such as anxiety and depression, is poor. Validity of diagnosis, in terms of agreement with chart diagnosis, is good for conduct disorders, depression, and attention-deficit/hyperactivity disorder (ADHD), but it is relatively poor for anxiety disorders. The DICA-R provides information on a range of symptoms, including their onset and duration, as well as limited information on severity.

Diagnostic Interview Schedule for Children-Revised

The Diagnostic Interview Schedule for Children-Revised (DISC-R) was developed for use by lay interviewers in epidemiologic studies of psychiatric disorders in children and adolescents. It can be used with children between the ages of 6 and 18. There are parallel child and parent versions of the original DISC and of subsequent revisions (such as the DISC-2.1 and the DISC-R). Both versions are highly structured, requiring the interviewer to follow the order of questions and method of recording exactly as prescribed by the developers of the interview. However, there is a skip structure that allows the interviewer to skip irrelevant items. Manual and computer scoring can be used with DISC-2.1 and DISC-R to make diagnostic determinations based on DSM-III-R criteria. Physicians and lay interviewers are required to undergo 2 to 3 days of training before using this interview. The psychometric properties of this instrument are comparable to other child diagnostic interviews, with each revision producing an instrument with better reliability and validity.

Semistructured Interviews

Child Assessment Schedule

The Child Assessment Schedule (CAS) was originally designed for use with children age 7 to 12, but it has also been found to be useful with younger children (5 to 7 years old) and adolescents (up to 16 years old). Parallel forms of the interview for parents are available, and the administration of either version takes about 60 minutes. The CAS is more structured than other semistructured diagnostic interviews, making it easier for novice clinicians. The interview is divided into three sections. The first section includes 75 content-area questions that are given scores of positive, negative, ambiguous, not applicable, or no response. The second section includes onset and duration questions, which are scored to generate DSM-III diagnoses. In the third section the interviewer is required to rate a number of observational items. Manual or computer scoring can be used to derive scale scores for the total interview, for diagnostically related symptom scales, and for 11 content areas (such as school, friends, or family).

The inter-rater reliability of the CAS for total symptoms score and content areas are excellent, but it is only fair for individual items. The total score test-retest reliability for children between ages 6 and 12 are excellent for conduct disorder (CD), depression, anxiety, and ADHD. The CAS has good validity when it is compared with specific scales in other instruments, such as the overanxious scale of the State-Trait Anxiety Inventory for Children, or to disorder-specific scales, such as the Child Depression Inventory. Furthermore inpatient, outpatient, and normal controls can be differentiated on the basis of total symptoms scores on the CAS. Generally, this instrument has more psychometric validation than any other semistructured interview and appears to be a useful instrument for physicians.

Schedule for Affective Disorders and Schizophrenia for School-Age Children

The Schedule for Affective Disorders and Schizophrenia for School-Age Children (K-SADS) is designed for use with children age 6 to 17. It has been revised a number of times, with the most recent version incorporating the DSM-III-R diagnostic criteria. Two forms of the interview are available; the K-SADS-E is an epidemiologic version that assesses the past and most recent episodes of each disorder, and the K-SADS-P is a present-episode version that assesses existing disorders. An experienced interviewer is needed to administer this interview, because the interviewer may adjust the questions to suit the child and ask additional questions as needed. Typically, the items are rated for severity on a 6-point scale. A skip structure is used, so questions irrelevant to the child can be omitted. It takes up to 90 minutes to administer the interview. Both the parent and the child are interviewed, with the parent being interviewed first. The diagnosis is based on an integration of both interviews, as well as on all other information available.

The test-retest reliability of the K-SADS is good for diagnosis and symptom scales related to depression and conduct disorders but relatively poor for anxiety disorders. The issue of validity of this interview remains to be determined in formal studies. This interview was designed primarily to provide a mechanism by which children meeting the criteria for an affective disorder could be included in a research protocol. For this purpose, the K-SADS is an excellent tool, but its usefulness in clinical practice remains to be demonstrated.

Interview Schedule for Children

The Interview Schedule for Children (ISC) was developed specifically for a longitudinal study of childhood depression and has undergone various revisions. It is designed for children age 7 to 18. The same physician is required to interview both the parent and the child, with the parent interview taking about 90 to 120 minutes and the child interview taking 45 to 60 minutes. Additionally, a follow-up version of the interview can be used to determine changes over time. The interview is flexible in its structure, requiring the interviewer to be highly trained on the interview, as well as knowledgeable about the DSM-III-R criteria.

Little formal psychometric assessment has been undertaken with this interview, but the information that is available suggests that the ISC may have adequate reliability. No validity data are currently available. Physicians wishing to use a semistructured interview that primarily focuses on anxiety or depressive symptoms of children will find the ISC to be useful if they do not mind the time it takes to administer it.

Summary

The advantage of structured and semistructured interviews is that they provide a method for gathering diagnostic information in a thorough and standardized manner. However, because they are overly inclusive and time consuming, their practical use may be limited in a busy clinic. Of course, specific modules from these interviews can be used to gather data on disorders of interest, and computer algorithm scoring programs can be used for scoring. Furthermore, physicians must remember that these interviews are based on either DSM-III or DSM-III-R diagnostic criteria and all of them will undergo major revisions to keep current with the refinements in diagnostic criteria introduced in the DSM-IV.

Rating Scales and Behavior Checklists

Rating scales have been used for a number of purposes in child and adolescent psychiatry, including the diagnosis and classification of psychiatric disorders, the measurement of severity of psychopathologic conditions, the prediction of the response to treatment, and the evaluation of treatment outcome. Furthermore, rating scales can be classified in terms of the purpose for which they were developed. For example, there are scales to measure clinical disability, social functioning, and clinical discomfort, as well as a global rating scale and a diagnostic rating scale. Regardless of the type of rating scale needed, physicians should consider the following variables when making a selection: comprehensiveness (for example, how well do the subscales cover the areas of interest?); administration of the instrument (is the scale self-reported or observer-reported?); norms (does the scale include the age, race, sex, and other characteristics of the patients in the normative sample?); and psychometric characteristics (how reliable and valid is this test?).

Rating scales are often used to complement the information obtained through diagnostic interviews. They are particularly useful for providing a global measure of the severity of a disorder, as well as for categorizing the symptoms in terms of subscales. Although a few broad-based diagnostic rating scales are available, most have been designed to provide a rapid assessment of a specific disorder or specific subsets of psychiatric symptoms. Examples of broad-based scales include the Child Behavior Checklist (CBCL), the Conners Parent Rating Scale-Revised, the Conners Teacher Rating Scale-Revised, and the Revised Behavior Problem Checklist (RBPC). Each of these rating scales contains a number of factors derived through factor analysis that provide information on specific subsets of psychiatric symptoms. Of these scales, the CBCL is probably the best-known and most-used rating scale in child and adolescent psychiatry. It has two broad-band factors (internalizing and externalizing) and eight or nine narrow-band factors or specific scales, depending on the age group used. The CBCL has excellent reliability and validity, and it can also be used with children from diverse cultures.

Self-Reports

Self-reports are used to complement other sources of information, such as the rating scales completed by parents and teachers and the physician's own observations. With children, they offer the physician a peek at the child's perception of reality and conception of her problems. Self-reporting is a particularly suitable method for probing into internalized problems, such as depression and anxiety, because it involves subjective emotional states of the child. Additionally, self-reports can be used to gather information on a range of behaviors or disorders, or they can be used to obtain detailed information on just one problem area. The Youth Self-Report is an excellent example of a broad-based self-report that provides information on two competence scales and seven problem scales.

Potential problems with the use of self-reports include the issue of competence (that is, is the child able to fully express her feelings?), accuracy and social desirability (is the child providing only socially desirable responses?), self-disclosure (what factors limit self-disclosure?), and various psychometric considerations (such as reliability, validity, and norms of the instruments). As a general rule, the younger the child, the more cautious physicians should be in drawing specific conclusions from self-reports. Additionally, the choice of instruments is important, and physicians should be wary of using instruments that do not have adequate psychometric properties or instruments with norms that are not current.

Disorder-Specific Instruments

Information obtained through diagnostic interviews and physician's observations can be supplemented with rating scales designed to determine the presence and severity of specific psychiatric disorders. There are a large number of behavior- and disorder-specific instruments that evaluate various aspects of childhood disorders; however, they vary tremendously in terms of their psychometric properties and clinical utility. We focus on commonly used scales that are relatively easy to administer in clinical settings.

Pervasive Developmental Disorders

Pervasive developmental disorders (PDDs) are characterized by delayed and deviant development of social reciprocity and relatedness, language, symbolic development, and communication; an unusual responsiveness to the environment expressed as unusual interests and repetitive, ritualistic, stereotyped behaviors; and a need for sameness. The PDDs included in DSM-IV are: autistic disorder, Rett's disorder, childhood disintegrative disorder, Asperger's disorder, and pervasive developmental disorder not otherwise specified (PDD-NOS). With the exception of autistic disorder, these disorders are relatively rare but qualitatively different enough to be classified as separate disorders. We present instruments that focus on autistic disorder.

Childhood Autism Rating Scale

The Childhood Autism Rating Scale (CARS) can be used to screen for the presence and severity of autistic disorder and is best used as part of a full diagnostic evaluation. It consists of 15 subscales or dimensions of behavior that are rated along a 7-point scale and summarized to provide one of three classifications: not autistic, mildly to moderately autistic, or severely autistic. The CARS has good inter-rater reliability and validity in terms of concordance with clinical diagnosis. The CARS can be used in several settings and is based on a number of sources of information (such as a parent interview and direct observations in the clinic, home, and school). Novice interviewers can be trained with relative ease, or the CARS can be used by experienced physicians, teachers, or psychologists in a variety of situations.

Ritvo-Freeman Real Life Rating Scale

The Ritvo-Freeman Real Life Rating Scale is a brief scale that can be used to assist in the diagnosis of autistic disorder. It provides data on five dimensions of child behavior, including sensorimotor functions, social relationships, affect, sensory responses, and language. It has good reliability and validity and can be used by both clinicians and nonclinicians.

Behavior Rating Instrument for Autistic and Atypical Children

The Behavior Rating Instrument for Autistic and Atypical Children (BRIAAC) consists of eight dimensions of behavior that are rated on a 10-point scale. The behavioral dimensions that are assessed include relationship to adults, communication, drive for mastery, vocalization, expressive speech, sound reception, speech reception, social responsiveness, body movement, and psychobiologic development. Unlike the other instruments, the BRIAAC is useful mainly for assessing the effectiveness of various treatments.

Anxiety Disorders

A variety of methods can be used to measure anxiety in children. These methods include diagnostic interviews, self-report measures, parent and teacher checklists, direct behavioral observations, and physiologic measures. For example, structured and semistructured diagnostic interviews such as the DISC-R, the CAS, the ISC, and the K-SADS can be used for this purpose. We briefly discuss two new semistructured interviews and a few commonly used rating scales developed specifically to assess anxiety disorders in children. Physicians should note that although they are not widely used, parent and teacher ratings can be used to complement self-report measures of anxiety in children. The anxiety or withdrawal subscales of such instruments as the Conners Teacher Rating Scale-Revised, the CBCL, the Teacher Report Form (TRF), and the RBPC can be used for this purpose.

Anxiety Disorders Interview Schedule for Children

The Anxiety Disorders Interview Schedule for Children (ADIS-C) is a semistructured interview designed for children age 6 to 18 and is based on DSM-III-R criteria for anxiety disorders. Preliminary data indicate that the interview is fairly reliable for the overall category of anxiety, as well as for most subcategories of anxiety (for example, simple phobia or school phobia). However, both reliability and validity data are limited, and the psychometric robustness of this instrument remains to be determined. A parallel parent version is also available.

Children's Anxiety Evaluation Form

The Children's Anxiety Evaluation Form (CAEF) is also a semistructured interview for children age 7 to 17, but it is not based on DSM classification. Instead, the questions are based on observable signs, symptoms, and history of anxiety. The inter-rater reliability for this diagnostic interview is high, and it has good concordance with the trait subscale score of the State-Trait Anxiety Inventory for Children and the Revised Children's Manifest Anxiety Scale, two self-report measures of anxiety in children. As with the ADIS-C, there is only limited psychometric information available on this interview. There is no parallel parent version.

Revised Children's Manifest Anxiety Scale

The Revised Children's Manifest Anxiety Scale (RCMAS) is a widely used self-report scale for assessing the presence of anxiety in children. It provides a total score, as well as scores on three factors: physiologic, worry and oversensitivity, and difficulty with concentration. It has excellent reliability, but its validity is not well established.

State-Trait Anxiety Inventory for Children

The State-Trait Anxiety Inventory for Children (STAIC) consists of two self-report inventories, one for measuring anxiety proneness, or trait anxiety, and the other for measuring transitory anxiety, or state anxiety. It was originally developed for measuring anxiety in children age 9 to 12, but it can also be used with younger children if they have an above-average reading ability. The reliability and validity of the STAIC are well established, and in addition to norms for children in the general population, there are norms for children with emotional disturbance. This is a clinically useful self-report instrument for measuring anxiety in children.

Depression

Structured and semistructured interviews and self-report instruments are most often used to diagnose and assess the severity of depression in children. Parent ratings, peer nomination, and projective tests are also used but not nearly as often as these other instruments. The two structured interviews (DICA-R and DISC-R) and the three semistructured interviews (CAS, K-SADS, and ISC) have modules on depression that can be used for this purpose. Physicians may find the semistructured interviews more appropriate for their needs because these incorporate clinical judgment and flexibility in the diagnostic process. We briefly present some of the commonly used self-report measures for depression in children.

Children's Depression Inventory

The Children's Depression Inventory (CDI) is designed to measure the severity of depression in children age 8 to 17. It is one of the easiest self-report measures of depression to read and understand, because it is written at the third-grade reading level. It has good psychometric properties, but there are also some problems. For example, in some studies, group differences in CDI scores could not be detected between depressed and nondepressed control children who had other psychiatric problems. Thus physicians may wish to use the CDI only as a measure of severity of depression in children who have already been diagnosed as being depressed rather than as a diagnostic instrument.

Beck Depression Inventory

The Beck Depression Inventory (BDI) was designed for use with adults in research and clinical practice, but it has been found to be equally useful with adolescents between the ages of 11 and 18. It has good reliability and validity. The only problem with the BDI as a self-report measure is that it is written at the sixth- to eighth-grade reading level, which may be a little difficult for many adolescents. Physicians can use the BDI both as a screening instrument and as a measure of severity of depression in adolescents.

Children's Depression Rating Scale-Revised

The Children's Depression Rating Scale-Revised (CDRS-R) is a clinician-completed rating scale for children age 6 to 12. The revised scale has good reliability and concordance with psychiatrists' global rating of depression in pediatric and psychiatric inpatients. Physicians can use the CDRS-R to complement self-report scales, especially as a measure of change during treatment.

Suicidal behavior is often a part of Major Depressive Disorder in children and adolescents, and it should be assessed as well. The K-SADS contains scales to assess suicidal tendencies, the patient's intent to die, the number of previous suicide attempts, and the lethality of the most recent attempt. The Suicidal Ideation Questionnaire can be used to assess suicidal ideation in adolescents, and the Hopelessness Scale for Children can be used to measure a negative view of the future by children 6 to 13 years old. However, the best information on suicidal behavior in children and adolescents can probably be obtained through a clinical interview. Physicians who want a detailed set of questions on suicidal risk to use in a clinical interview should consult Pfeffer's book, *The Suicidal Child*.

Attention-Deficit/Hyperactivity Disorder

Structured (DICA-R DISC-R) and semistructured diagnostic interviews (CAS, ISC, and K-SADS-E) can be used to assess children with ADHD. However, physicians should remember to use the epidemiologic version of the K-SADS, because only that version contains items relevant to ADHD. Given that both structured and semistructured diagnostic interviews tend to overdiagnose "caseness," additional information derived from other sources, such as direct observations, rating scales, and psychoeducational testing, should be sought before a diagnosis of ADHD is made. Furthermore, given that the behavior of children with ADHD varies according to the environment, it is important that assessments are undertaken in socially important contexts, such as at school and at home. We provide examples of instruments that can be used in different settings to provide a broad-based ecobehavioral assessment. Physicians who want detailed information on other instruments used to assess children with ADHD should consult Barkley's chapter in *Assessment and Diagnosis in Child Psychopathology,* edited by Rutter, Tuma, and Lann.

The Instructional Environment Scale

The Instructional Environment Scale (TIES) was developed to help professionals systematically analyze a student's instructional environment. It can be used to describe the extent to which a child's academic and behavior problems are a function of the instructional environment.

Walker-Rankin Rating Scale of Adaptive and Maladaptive Child Behavior in School

The Walker-Rankin Rating Scale of Adaptive and Maladaptive Child Behavior in School provides an index of the teacher's perception of a student's adaptive and maladaptive behaviors. The first of two parts deals with behavioral skills and competencies facilitative of successful classroom adjustment and positive social relationships with peers. The second part deals with maladaptive and obnoxious social behaviors that disrupt classroom adjustment and interfere with peer relationships and the development of friendships.

Family Environment Scale

The Family Environment Scale (FES) consists of 10 subscales that measure the social-environmental characteristics of families in terms of three underlying domains: relationship, personal growth, and system maintenance. The Real Form (Form R) can be used by physicians to measure families' perceptions of their nuclear family environments. This is a widely used scale that has excellent psychometric properties. It can be used to determine the extent to which a child's behavior problems are a function of the family environment.

Conners Rating Scales

The Conners Parent Rating Scale-Revised and the Conners Teacher Rating Scale-Revised are the most widely used scales for rating children with hyperactivity disorders. The 48-item parent questionnaire yields five factor scores: conduct problems, learning problems, psychosomatic, impulsive-hyperactive, and anxiety. The revised teacher's version is a 28-item questionnaire that provides Hyperactive, Inattentive-Passive, and Conduct Problem factor scores. Both scales have good psychometric properties and norms are available for both.

IOWA-Conners Rating Scale

The IOWA-Conners Rating Scale was developed to provide independent scores for inattention/overactivity and aggression. The IOWA-Conners Rating Scale consists of 10 items, five of which are correlated to external measures of inattention/overactivity but not to measures of aggression. The other five are correlated to external measures of aggression but not to measures of inattention/overactivity. The scale has good validity, and normative data by age and gender are available.

Attention Deficit Disorder Comprehensive Teacher Rating Scale

The Attention Deficit Disorder Comprehensive Teacher Rating Scale (ACTeRS) is another commonly used teacher-report rating scale to assess children with ADHD and their responses to treatment. This scale provides scores on four subscales: Oppositional Behavior, Attention, Hyperactivity, and Social Problems. Normative data are available for 5- to 12-year-old children.

Attribution Questionnaire

The Attribution Questionnaire was developed specifically to address the issue of attributions for and self-evaluations of the behavior of children with ADHD while they are on and off medication. The questionnaire is in two parts. A set of 11 questions are presented in a

10-point Likert-type format that provides scores in three domains: attribution, behavior, and mood/self-esteem. This is followed by a set of three forced-choice questions that reflect the attributional domains of effort, medication, or teachers. Children's causal attributions of treatment effects are important to include in an ecobehavioral assessment because of the effect of cognitive-motivational factors on treatment outcome.

Achievement Tests

A number of achievement tests are typically used to assess children with ADHD. The standard battery includes the Woodcock-Johnson Psychoeducational Battery, the Peabody Individual Achievement Test-Revised, the Wide Range Achievement Test-R and the Kaufman Test of Educational Achievement (K-TEA) test battery.

Neurocognitive Tests

Neurocognitive tests are clinically administered instruments that can be used for diagnosing ADHD, as well as for assessing treatment effects in children with ADHD. The three most used instruments include the Continuous Performance Test for identifying attentional problems, the Matching Familiar Figures Test for assessing cognitive tempo and impulsivity in the context of visual problem solving, and the Paired Associate Learning Task (an "effortful" task that may be related to classroom learning).

Conduct Disorder

A child with CD has a persistent pattern of antisocial behaviors that occur beyond normative levels and cannot be controlled by parents, teachers, and significant others. These behaviors affect not only the child in terms of his academic achievement and interpersonal relationships, but they also affect the child's family and community. Thus a broad-based assessment is required to fully understand a child with this disorder. Several multidimensional rating scales, including the CBCL and the RBPC can be used with children who have CD. Direct observations can also be used, but given the low frequency and typically covert nature of the antisocial acts of children with conduct disorder, it is not a common method with these children. Additionally, institutional and community records (for example, school attendance, suspensions, and expulsions or contacts with police and arrest records) can also be used as supplementary measures of antisocial behavior. We present examples of self-report and informant rating scales that have been developed to assess antisocial behavior in children.

Children's Action Tendency Scale

The Children's Action Tendency Scale (CAT) is a self-report scale designed to assess children's responses in forced-choice interpersonal situations. It is suitable for children between the ages of 6 and 15. The scale provides subscale scores for aggressiveness, assertiveness, and submissiveness. It has good psychometric properties and can be used for initial assessment as well as for assessing treatment effectiveness.

Self-Report Delinquency Scale

The Self-Report Delinquency Scale was developed as part of the National Youth Survey, which is a longitudinal study of delinquent behavior, use of alcohol and drugs, and related problems in American adolescents. This is a self-report scale that provides a measure of the frequency with which an adolescent has committed offenses that are included in the Uniform Crime Reports during the previous 12 months. It is suitable for children age 11 to 21.

Interview for Aggression

The Interview for Aggression is a semistructured interview for children age 6 to 13 that yields three scores: severity of aggression, duration of aggression, and total aggression. Additionally, it provides a measure of both overt and covert aggressive behaviors. A parallel parent form is available.

Eyberg Child Behavior Inventory

The Eyberg Child Behavior Inventory (ECBI) was developed to provide physicians with a parental assessment of a child's behavior at home. It is suitable for assessing children age 2 to 17. The ECBI provides two scores: the number of problems the child has and the intensity of the problems. It has good reliability and validity, and it has been used extensively for research and clinical purposes. Normative data are available for children and adolescents.

Sutter-Eyberg Student Behavior Inventory

The Sutter-Eyberg Student Behavior Inventory (SESBI) is structurally similar to the ECBI and was developed to provide a teacher's assessment of a child's behavior at school. It is suitable for assessing children age 2 to 17. As with the ECBI, this instrument has good reliability and validity. Physicians can use both the ECBI and SESBI to obtain a good clinical picture of the antisocial behaviors of the child in two settings.

Eating Disorders

The two main eating disorders in children and adolescents are anorexia nervosa and bulimia nervosa. Given that these disorders are multiply-determined in terms of their predisposing, precipitating, and maintaining factors, physicians should ensure a broad-based assessment of various factors, such as becoming familiar with a patient's clinical and treatment history; learning the patient's current body weight and weight history; the frequency, intensity, and duration of various weight-controlling methods used; the nature and frequency of binge eating and eating behavior; self-perceptions of weight, shape, body-size, and body-image; physical symptoms; and psychiatric co-morbidity. Some of the information can be obtained through a detailed clinical interview and supplemented by information obtained through semistructured interviews and self-report instruments.

Eating Disorder Examination

The Eating Disorder Examination (EDE) is a semistructured diagnostic interview designed to elicit information on the clinical features and specific psychopathologic nature of anorexia nervosa and bulimia nervosa over the 4 weeks prior to the interview. It is intended for use by physicians who have experience and knowledge in the assessment and treatment of eating disorders, and it takes about an hour to complete.

Clinical Eating Disorder Rating Instrument

The Clinical Eating Disorder Rating Instrument (CEDRI) is a clinical rating scale that provides information on behavioral patterns, attitudes, and other symptoms (such as depression or self-esteem) that are associated with eating disorders. This scale has adequate inter-rater reliability, but other psychometric characteristics are yet to be determined.

Eating Attitudes Test

The Eating Attitudes Test (EAT) was designed to provide self-reported information on the symptoms of anorexia nervosa. Recent research shows that it is equally useful in providing information on bulimia nervosa. It provides a total score, as well as scores for three subscales: dieting, bulimia and food preoccupation, and oral control. This has been a widely used scale in both research and clinical practice.

Eating Disorder Inventory-2

The Eating Disorder Inventory-2 (EDI-2) is another commonly used self-report measure that was designed to provide information on psychologic, attitudinal, and behavioral traits common in both anorexia nervosa and bulimia nervosa. The original scale (EDI) included three subscales that assessed attitudes and behavior concerning eating, weight, and shape, as well as five subscales that assessed general psychologic traits related to eating disorders. The EDI-2 retains these subscales, but with the addition of more items it now includes three additional subscales (asceticism, impulse regulation, and social insecurity). Physicians will find the EDI-2 useful for determining the severity of eating disorders by comparing the child to the norms that are provided. Additionally, some of the subscales provide clinically useful information that can be used for planning treatment.

Mental Retardation

Luckasson defines mental retardation as intellectual functioning that is significantly subaverage. It exists concurrently with related limitations in at least two of the following adaptive skill areas: communication, self care, home living, social skills, community functioning, self-direction, health and safety, functional academics, leisure, and work. Furthermore, it must manifest before age 18. Although mental retardation is included in the DSM-IV classification of psychiatric disorders, it is neither a medical nor a mental disorder. Therefore, psychiatrists are rarely called on to actually provide a diagnosis of mental retardation. It is not unlikely, however, that a child with mental retardation will be referred for a psychiatric or pediatric consultation for the assessment and treatment of either behavior problems or a psychopathologic condition.

The physician may be required to provide a differential diagnosis of behavior problems and a psychopathologic condition. The initial step in a diagnostic assessment is to undertake a thorough structural and functional analysis of the behavior problem (see Chapter 16). Typically, a behavioral psychologist is the professional who is trained to undertake this task. The second step is to screen for any broad-based psychopathologic disorder that the child may have and then to follow this up with disorder-specific assessments. We present a number of diagnostic instruments that can be used to determine the child's level of adaptive and maladaptive behavior, as well as instruments that screen for psychopathologic disorders.

AAMD Adaptive Behavior Scales

The AAMD Adaptive Behavior Scales (ABS) is one of the standard instruments for assessing adaptive and maladaptive behavior in individuals with mental retardation between the ages of 3 and 69. It is an informant rating scale that is divided into two parts. Part I deals with adaptive behaviors across 10 domains, and part II deals with maladaptive behaviors across 14 domains. A school version is also available, but its psychometric properties are not robust. Data on the psychometric properties of the ABS are rather limited, but the scale appears to be clinically useful in evaluating and tracking adaptive and maladaptive behavior of specific individuals.

Vineland Adaptive Behavior Scales

The Vineland Adaptive Behavior Scales (VABS) are the most commonly used adaptive behavior scales in studies of mental retardation. It was designed for use with children from birth to age 18. It is an informant rating scale that is available in three versions: the Survey Form, the Expanded Form, and the Classroom Edition. Each version includes four domains of adaptive behavior (communication, daily living skills, socialization, and motor skills), and the Survey Form and the Expanded Form also include a domain on maladaptive behavior. The VABS has very good psychometric properties that make it a useful tool for use with this population.

Aberrant Behavior Checklist

The Aberrant Behavior Checklist (ABC) was designed to assess the effects of pharmacologic, behavioral, and other interventions on the behavior of individuals (age 5 and older) with mental retardation. It is increasingly used to assess inappropriate and maladaptive behavior in the absence of treatment in the same population. The ABC is an informant rating scale and is available in two versions: residential and community. It had good psychometric properties, and it is the most widely used rating instrument for assessing clinical effects of medications in this population.

Prout-Strohmer Assessment System

The Prout-Strohmer Assessment System (PSAS) consists of two separate rating scales that measure emotional and behavioral problems in adolescents (age 14 and older) and adults with mental retardation. The Prout-Strohmer Personality Inventory (PSPI), a self-report instrument, and the Strohmer-Prout Behavior Rating Scale (SPBRS), an informant rating scale, provide assessments of two broad-band factors (internalizing and externalizing) and 12 clinical scales. The scales appear to have reasonably good psychometric properties and may prove useful to the physician.

Reiss Screen for Maladaptive Behavior

The Reiss Screen for Maladaptive Behavior is a screening instrument designed to assess the mental health status of adolescents and adults with mental retardation. It requires ratings from at least two informants, such as teachers and caregivers. It provides a total score, as well as scores for each of eight subscales and six special symptoms (such as drug or alcohol abuse, self-injury, stealing, overactivity, sexual problems, and suicidal tendencies). Although the normative sample used was rather small, this scale has good psychometric properties. Clinically, this scale should be used only as a screening instrument for the identification of any psychopathologic condition rather than for establishing a specific diagnosis. The Psychopathology Instrument for Mentally Retarded Adults can be used for deriving more specific diagnoses for adolescents and adults, but a similar scale is not available for children. The Diagnostic Assessment for the Severely Handicapped can be used for a similar purpose with adolescents and adults who have severe and profound mental retardation, and again, a parallel version for children is not available.

Pain Disorder

Pain is one of the somatoform disorders and, in children, it can result from many sources, including accidents and trauma, recurrent pain syndromes (for example, recurrent headaches), physical disorders (such as juvenile rheumatoid arthritis), and medical procedures (such as bone marrow aspirations). Given that pain is a subjective experience that is affected by contextual variables (for example, culture and social ecology), it has been difficult to define and assess it, especially in young children. However, there are a number of behavioral and self-report measures that provide physicians systematic methods of assessing pain in children and adolescents.

Procedure Behavior Rating Scale

The Procedure Behavior Rating Scale (PBRS) was designed to assess anxiety levels in children during medical procedures such as bone marrow aspirations and lumbar punctures. The scale has been found to be sensitive to developmental changes in pain. That is, it is able to account for the changing behavioral expressions of pain as children grow older. The Observational Scale of Behavioral Distress (OSBD) is a modified version of the PBRS that includes partial-interval recording and an intensity rating of the pain. Both scales have very good psychometric properties and have been used extensively in pediatric settings. The Procedure Behavior Check List (PBCL) is a shorter version of the PBRS that includes two additional categories of the expression of distress in adolescents.

Frankl Behavior Rating Scale

The Frankl Behavior Rating Scale is a physician-rated scale that was developed to assess distress in children age 18 months to 7 years. It has good inter-rater reliability and concordance with the OSBD rating scale. Physicians typically find this scale to be easy to administer and score.

Children's Hospital of Eastern Ontario Pain Scale

The Children's Hospital of Eastern Ontario Pain Scale (CHEOPS) is a rating scale for clinicians that is designed to measure postoperative pain in children. Physicians rate a child's pain behavior every 30 seconds in six general categories: vocalizations, facial expression, child's verbal behavior, torso position, touch behavior, and leg position. The scale is valid and reliable for assessing pain in children age 1 to 7.

The intensity of pain can be measured along a continuum, from "no pain" to "very severe pain." With some advance training, VAS can be used with children as young as 7 years old. These scales are easily administered and provide a reliable and valid measure of the intensity of pain. Additionally, they can be used to assess treatment effectiveness in terms of pain intensity. The Varni/Thompson Pediatric Pain Questionnaire (PPQ) is a good example of a multifaceted pain scale that uses visual analogs to assess pain in children. Three forms of the scale are available for children, adolescents, and parents.

Child Physical Abuse and Neglect

Although child abuse and neglect is not a medical or a psychiatric disorder, it is one of those conditions that is often the focus of clinical intervention. We briefly touch on this topic because of its increasing prevalence and the need for physicians to be aware of the breadth of the assessment that may be required for intervention. Furthermore, this is a problem in which the main focus of the intervention is on the perpetrators of the abuse, although the child certainly needs some form of therapy for the effects of abuse. In families, parents are most often the perpetrators of the abuse and should be the primary focus of intervention. Physicians interested in the assessment of *parents* who engage in physical abuse and neglect of their children should consult Ammerman's chapter in the *Handbook of Child and Adolescent Assessment,* edited by Ollendick and Hersen, for more details.

Unlike childhood psychiatric disorders, which have a large number of disorder-specific instruments, there are no well-validated instruments to directly assess the emotional and psychologic consequences of physical abuse and neglect. In addition to a broad-based clinical interview with the child, the physician may use multidimensional rating scales to gather information on the child's social functioning and psychopathologic state. The CBCL and TRF are suitable for this purpose. Because children may engage in behaviors that elicit or escalate physical abuse from parents, the ECBI can be used to determine which of the child's behaviors the parents find difficult to manage. This information can be used by the physician to enhance the parents' skills in managing the child's behavior in socially accepted ways. Additionally, the physician should provide appropriate therapy to the child for the emotional and psychologic effects of physical abuse and neglect.

Summary

Although the clinical assessment of children and adolescents will, to some extent, remain an art, increasing numbers of diagnostic instruments are becoming available that make this task much easier for physicians. The refinements in the diagnostic criteria of psychiatric disorders have led to the development of several structured and semistructured diagnostic interviews and an explosion in disorder-specific rating scales. However, although there is a rating scale for virtually every behavior of children and adolescents that could possibly be of interest to mental health professionals, the lack of rigor in the psychometric properties of many of them should alert the physician that a cautious choice of instruments is warranted.

Annotated Bibliography

Canino IA, Spurlock J: *Culturally diverse children and adolescents: assessment, diagnosis, and treatment,* New York, 1994, Guilford.

This book provides an excellent introduction and practical guide to the assessment and diagnosis of children and adolescents of minority cultures. The focus is on the mental health needs of children of African-American, Latino, Asian-American, and American Indian heritage.

Ollendick TH, Hersen M: *Handbook of child and adolescent assessment,* Needham Heights, Mass., 1993, Allyn and Bacon.

This book presents the principles and procedures of child and adolescent assessment. It is divided into three major sections: fundamental issues and principles, specific assessment strategies, and the assessment of specific populations.

Reynolds CR, Kamphaus RW: *Handbook of psychological and educational assessment of children,* New York, 1990, Guilford.

This is a standard work in the field that comes in two volumes. The general areas of assessment covered include intelligence, achievement, personality, behavior, and context. This is a scholarly work that would be of interest to those who wish to read about different areas in some depth.

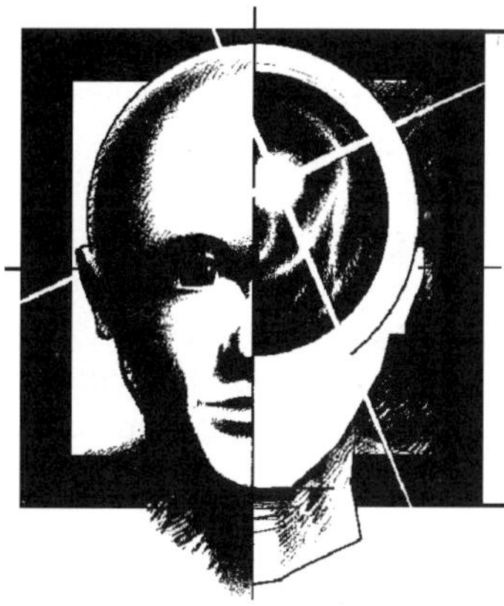

chapter 3

Brain Imaging in Child and Adolescent Psychiatry

Robert A. Kowatch, MD and Kelly N. Botteron, MD

Developmental Factors in Brain Imaging
Structural Imaging
Functional Brain Imaging Techniques
Brain Imaging Studies in Selected Child Psychiatric Populations
Summary

Brain imaging techniques such as computed tomography (CT), magnetic resonance imaging (MRI), single-photon emission computed tomography (SPECT), positron emission tomography (PET), and others have caused enormous advances in our ability to visualize both the structure and the function of the central nervous system (CNS). Structural imaging techniques such as MRI have helped physicians define regional volumetric differences in psychiatric populations, and functional imaging techniques such as SPECT and PET have provided unique methods to visualize and measure brain activity.

The purposes of this chapter are to give the reader an overview of the brain imaging techniques that are currently available to study children and adolescents with psychiatric disorders and to review selected imaging studies that have examined children and adolescents with psychiatric disorders. These technologies are evolving at a rapid rate, and although their clinical applications may not be readily apparent, these applications will hopefully be developed with further study. We do not discuss the electrophysiologic and magnetic brain imaging modalities of electroencephalography (EEG), computerized EEG, evoked potentials, or magnetoencephalography because these modalities are beyond the scope of this chapter.

Brain imaging techniques available to study psychiatric disorders may be broadly divided into two groups: those techniques that image the *structure* of the CNS—CT and MRI—and those techniques that image the *function* of the CNS—PET, SPECT, magnetic resonance spectroscopy (MRS), and functional magnetic resonance imaging (fMRI).

One of the main goals of any brain imaging technique is to provide physiologically meaningful information about the brain. Ultimately, this may be best accomplished with several imaging techniques, since they each have their separate areas of strength and weakness. For example, some MRI scanners provide a tissue resolution of less than 1 mm but do not provide any information about the function of the brain. Both PET and SPECT can provide valuable information about cerebral blood flow, but their spatial resolution is limited to 5 to 8 mm. Additionally, many of these imaging technologies are still in the early phases of development and not at the point where they can be used to diagnose childhood psychiatric disorders.

There are two concepts central to the theory and practice of brain imaging that are important to understand, since all brain imaging techniques attempt to achieve maximum levels of each of these variables. These two concepts are spatial and temporal resolution. Spatial resolution is usually measured in millimeters and refers to the degree of tissue resolution that can be acquired during an imaging procedure. Currently, the best spatial resolution for clinical studies is that of MRI, which can achieve a spatial resolution of less than 1 mm. Temporal resolution refers to the time it takes to detect a signal after it occurs in the brain. During SPECT there is a 2-minute window after a radiotracer like ^{99m}Tc HMPAO is injected. During this time, the radiotracer is taken up and trapped across the blood-brain barrier in the brain. This period is when the actual measurement of cerebral blood flow occurs. Ultimately and ideally, a combination of imaging techniques, both structural and functional, may be used in tandem to provide meaningful physiologic information about the brain.

Developmental Factors in Brain Imaging

When considering the application of structural neuroimaging techniques to child and adolescent populations, it is important to consider issues of cerebral development. Before the advent of MRI, most studies examining brain development were neuropathologic studies of neonates and young infants, and very little was known about the regional structural development of children and adolescents. Recently, a small number of studies have demonstrated that significant cerebral regional development continues through adolescence. Jernigan et al. reported changes in cerebral morphology during late childhood and adolescence, with significant but slight increases in overall cerebral volume and striking changes in cerebral gray and white matter. They reported a decline in the gray to white matter ratio from 1:8 in 8 to 10-year-old children to 1:3 in adults. This decrease in gray matter was strongly related to increased ventricular and cortical cerebrospinal fluid (CSF) over this age range. Subcortical limbic structures, such as caudate nucleus, the putamen, the globus pallidus, and the thalamus, were reported to decrease in volume with age. Other groups have also demonstrated that significant developmental changes occur in ventricular volume, in subcortical structures such as the caudate nucleus, and in the cerebellar vermi. In a quantitative MRI study of 50 normal children and adolescents between the ages of 4 and 18, Gied et al. reported gender differences in brain morphology that were most marked before puberty. They also found significant age-related changes in the head of the caudate nucleus, the posterior portion of the temporal lobe, the corpus callosum, and the pons. These examples illustrate that developmental changes in the structure of the brain can be significant and need to be considered in the evaluation of children's neuroimaging examinations.

PET and SPECT studies have also found significant developmental and gender differences that must be taken into account when the brain of a child or an adolescent is imaged and compared. Several studies of the maturational changes of regional cerebral blood flow (rCBF) and local cerebral metabolic rates for glucose (lCMRGlc) in healthy children and adolescents are available. Most of these studies have concentrated on populations of children and adolescents referred for neurologic evaluation because of "transient neurologic difficulties." Many of these subjects were being treated with anticonvulsant medications when they were imaged. In 29 subjects (age 5 days to 15 years), Chugani et al. found that by the age of 2, absolute lCMRGlc for various gray matter regions (frontal, parietal, temporal, and occipital cortices) are similar to those of adults. In most brain areas, lCMRGlc increased beyond adult values from the age of 2 until the end of the second decade and then decreased to adult levels. In a ^{133}Xe SPECT study, Chiron et al. studied 42 subjects (age 2 days to 19 years) and found global rCBF levels were lower at birth than adult rCBF levels. They reached a maximum level at 5 or 6 years that was 70% higher than adult levels. They decreased to adult levels after age 15. In their PET fluorodeoxyglucose (FDG) study comparing adolescents with no disorders with adolescents who had attention-deficit/hyperactivity disorder (ADHD), Zametkin et al. reported finding a global metabolic rate that was 18% higher in the ADHD group than in unaffected adults.

These imaging studies of brain development indicate that controls for both age and gender effects are essential before any comparisons with abnormal populations can be made using either structural or functional imaging techniques.

Structural Imaging

Structural neuroimaging techniques such as MRI and CT are useful tools for clinical diagnostic evaluation in neurology and pediatrics. They help the physician visualize gross pathologic conditions such as tumors, infarctions, or hemorrhages. However, in the evaluation of psychiatric neuropathologic states, the qualitative visual examination of MRI or CT images reveals gross structural pathologic lesions only in the minority of cases. This relative lack of information on qualitative visual review is in contrast to mounting evidence supporting quantitative differences in cerebral structures between psychiatric and normal populations. Neuromorphometry is defined as the quantification of cerebral structures and currently is only applied as a research tool. However, it is probable that in the future, neuromorphometric parameters will provide clinical information relevant to differential diagnosis, treatment response, course, and prognosis in child psychiatric patients.

Computed Tomography

The development and clinical application of CT scanners in the early 1970s revolutionized diagnostic medicine, allowing for the first time the in vivo examination of soft tissues, including the brain. CT scans are based on the same basic principle as standard radiographs: attenuation of x-ray radiation has distinct characteristics through different tissue types. A CT scanner consists of a rotating x-ray beam surrounded by a circular detection unit that contains a large number of x-ray detectors. Images are acquired in a slice-by-slice manner. For each slice, the x-ray tube and detectors rotate 360° around the head, obtaining x-ray attenuation data for that slice. A computer then digitizes the electrical impulses generated by the x-ray detectors, and the data is processed and reconstructed using mathematic tomographic reconstruction algorithms.

CT creates axial images of the entire brain parenchyma and is useful for the investigation of gross CNS lesions such as tumors, infarctions, or ventricular enlargements. It is the preferred imaging modality when bony disease or lesions involving calcified tissue are suspected. Intravenously injected contrast agents are at times used with CT to highlight areas of blood-brain barrier breakdown. CT scans have the advantage of being generally well tolerated by children and take 10 to 15 minutes to complete. However, CT has numerous disadvantages in comparison with MRI because of inferior gray to white matter contrast, radiation exposure to the child, images produced in one plane of orientation, and bony artifacts that obscure visualization of the temporal and posterior fossa regions. One substantial advantage of CT is its lower cost relative to MRI. However, MRI scans without contrast are generally only several hundred dollars more than CT, and given their other substantial advantages, they may be preferred.

Clinical Indications for Computed Tomography

CT scans have little role in the routine evaluation of child and adolescent psychiatry patients. In a mixed clinical population of 120 child and adolescent psychiatry patients, Ghaziuddin et al. reported that approximately 20 percent demonstrated clinical abnormalities on CT head examinations. These abnormalities were generally nonspecific findings that included increased ventricular size, cerebral atrophy, and focal alterations in brain density. The demonstrated findings did not lead to further clinical intervention, and they suggested that CT scanning may have very limited utility in child psychiatric practice. As reviewed on p. 42, many of the regions that demonstrate abnormalities in childhood psychiatric disorders are basal ganglia or temporal lobe structures. These regions are not well visualized on CT scans. CT scans can be useful for the detection of neoplasms, hemorrhages, large infarcts, or atrophy; however, MRI provides superior visualization in virtually all cases. Thus as with all diagnostic evaluation procedures, the risks and benefits of the study should be weighed by the physician and discussed with the family.

PEARLS & PERILS

COMPUTED TOMOGRAPHY

- CT scans are useful for gross neuropathologic lesions and can indicate the presence of abnormalities such as ventricular enlargement, ischemia, or tumors.
- CT scans are preferred for images of bony defects.
- The visualization and delineation of brain areas and gray white matter contrast is limited with CT scanning, and some areas may not be adequately visualized secondary to bony artifacts.
- CT scanning involves exposure to ionizing radiation.
- Intravenous contrast agents are associated with a risk of allergic reaction.

Magnetic Resonance Imaging

MRI is a newer imaging technique introduced into clinical practice in the late 1980s and early 1990s. MRI is especially attractive for pediatric populations because it does not involve any radiation exposure and has no significant known biologic risks. MRI provides excellent gray to white matter contrast, producing highly detailed neuroanatomic images. In addition to standard structural MRI images, a variety of different MRI techniques are currently being explored. These new methods offer the potential for providing biophysical information that cannot currently be obtained by any other manner. Two of these techniques, MRS and fMRI, are discussed on pp. 41-42 of this chapter.

Magnetic resonance (MR) images are created based on the inherent magnetic principles of atoms that are amplified and enhanced for detection and visualization by the MR scanner. A basic summary of the physical principles involved in the production of an MR signal can provide the reader with an intuitive appreciation of the principles involved. For a more detailed discussion of the physical principles, please see the writings

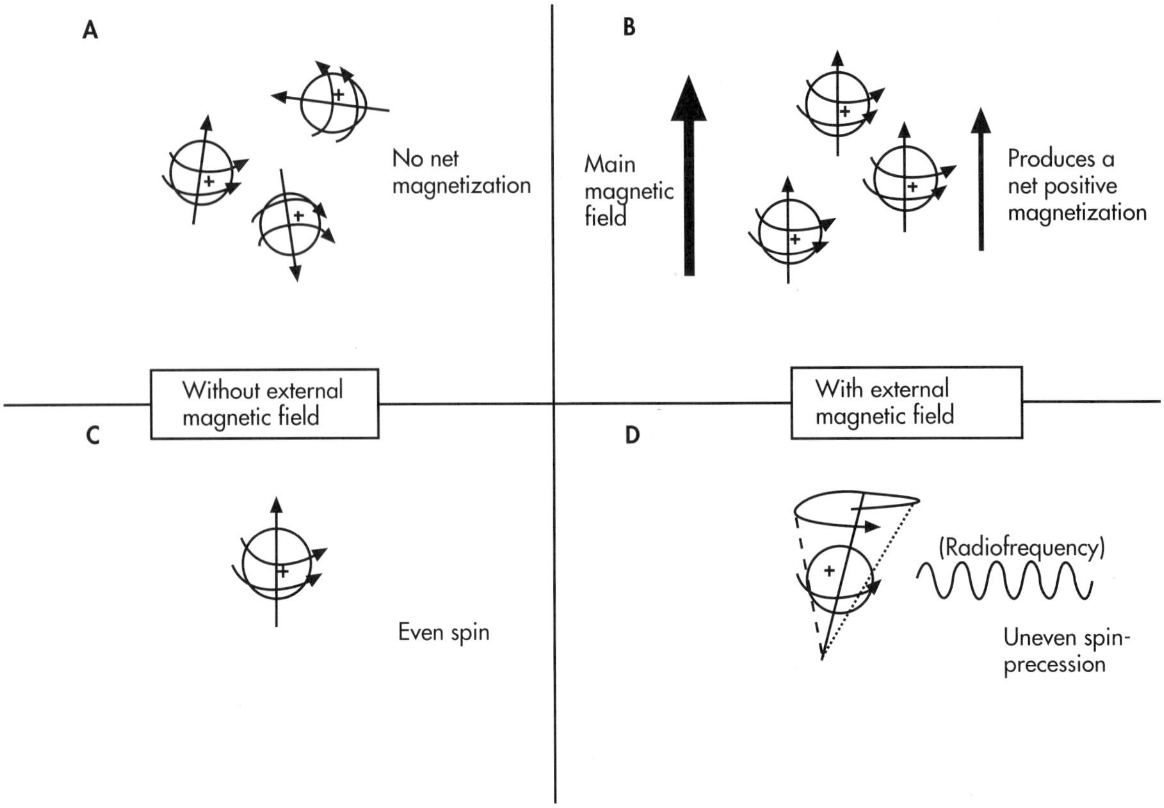

FIGURE 3-1 Physical principles of MRI. **A,** Atomic nuclei with an odd number of electrons or protons have an associated positive charge and inherent spin. In the natural state, these nuclei are randomly oriented and their positive charges cancel each other out and create no net magnetic force. **B,** When placed in an external magnetic field (such as in an MR scanner), the nuclei align parallel to the magnetic field and produce a net positive magnetization. **C,** Nuclei in their natural state spin evenly. **D,** However, nuclei within an external magnetic field precess; that is, they spin unevenly, similar to the wobble of a top, around the axis of the magnetic field. This precession releases energy in the form of a radio frequency that can be detected by the MR scanner under certain conditions.

of Newhouse and Weiner or Stytz and Frieder. When an atomic nucleus of an element has an odd number of electrons or protons, it has a charge and associated inherent spin. These spinning charged molecules create their own magnetic dipole, or minute magnetization. In their natural state, the randomly oriented dipoles cancel out each other's charges, and there is no net magnetization of tissue (Figure 3-1, *A*). However, when this tissue is placed in a magnetic field such as an MR scanner, the nuclei align parallel to the field (their lowest energy state), producing a net positive magnetization of the tissue (Figure 3-1, *B*). The nuclei in their natural state spin evenly (Figure 3-1, *C*). As the nuclei within a magnetic field spin, they wobble, or precess, like a top, and the precession of molecules releases energy in the form of a radio frequency that can be detected by the MR scanner under appropriate conditions (Figure 3-1, *D*). To detect the resonance, the nuclei are further excited through the application of an external radio frequency pulse that shifts the nuclei and net magnetization out of the plane parallel to the magnetic field (generally 90° perpendicular to the plane of magnetization) (Figure 3-2). When the radio frequency pulse is removed, the nuclei attempt to return to the original plane within the magnetic field in a process known as relaxation, and the radio frequency emitted is detected to create MR images. The rate of relaxation is detected by the receiver antenna, and the signal is transformed through a series of mathematic algorithms, or Fourier transformations, to create an MR image. MRI can generate images in any plane of orientation; the most commonly used images are in the sagittal, coronal, and axial planes (Figure 3-3).

Tissues with different compositions produce distinct resonance signals, thus creating the tissue contrast between CSF, gray matter, and white matter. Different types of relaxation parameters can be measured. T1 and T2 are commonly used terms that refer to spin-lattice relaxation and spin-spin relaxation, respectively. Gray matter, white matter, and CSF have different appearances on T1- and T2-weighted images, as outlined in Table 3-1. Because differently weighted acquisitions dif-

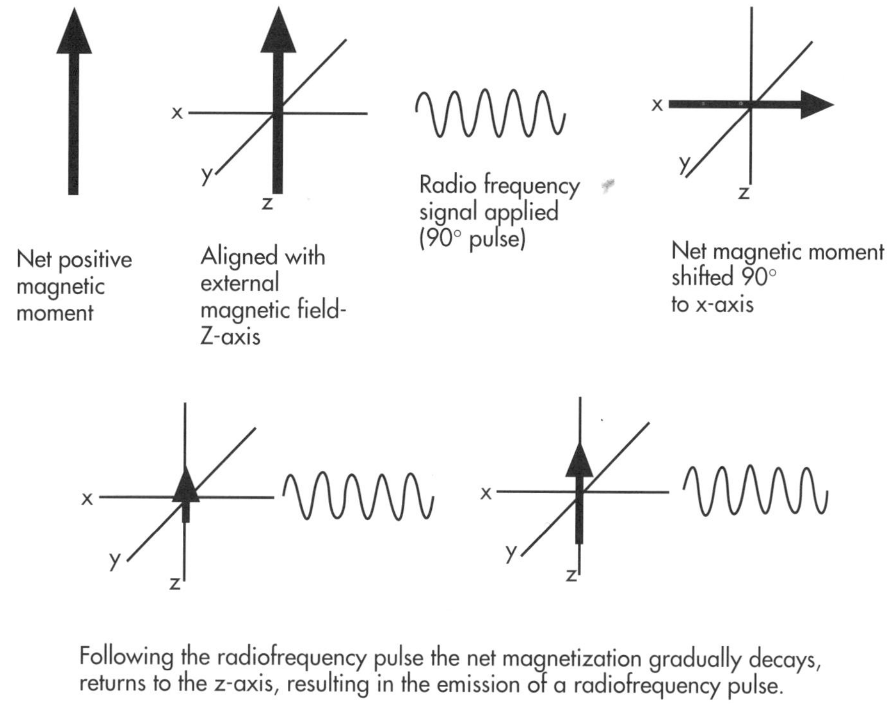

FIGURE 3-2 Physical principles of MRI. In order to detect the radio frequency generated by the nuclear resonance or precession, the nuclei are further excited by the application of an external radio frequency pulse that shifts the net plane of magnetization. When this pulse is removed, the nuclei gradually regain orientation parallel to the magnetic field through a process known as relaxation. Precessing nuclei in the process of relaxation emit a radio frequency signal that is characteristic of the nuclear species and can be detected by the MR scanner and reconstructed to create an image.

TABLE 3-1

TISSUE APPEARANCE OF MR IMAGES

	T1-weighted	T2-weighted
Gray matter	dark gray	light gray
White matter	light gray	dark gray
CSF	black	white
Inflammation or demyelination	darker	brighter
Infarction	darker	brighter
Edema	darker	brighter
Solid tremor	darker	brighter
Hemorrhage (chronic rim)	brighter	brighter

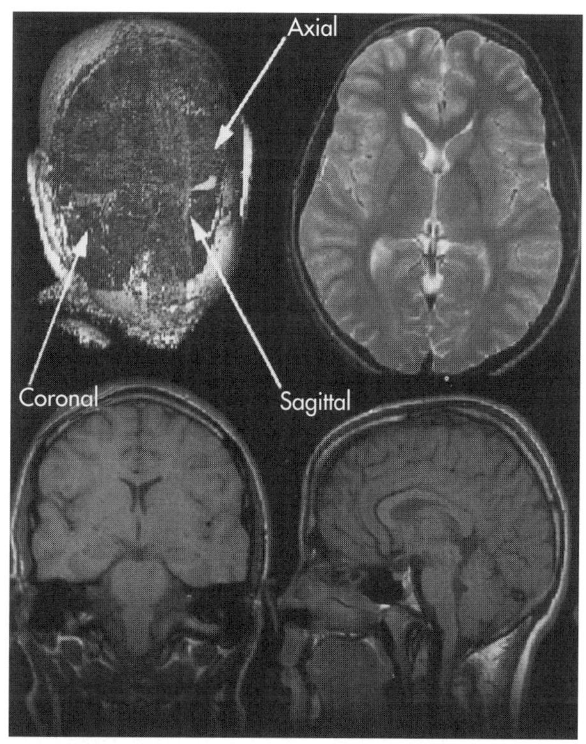

FIGURE 3-3 MRI images can be created in any plane of orientation. Clinically, images are generally obtained and viewed in the axial, coronal, and sagittal planes.

fer in their tissue contrast, they can be helpful in the examination of particular types of tissue. For example, T2-weighted images are more useful than T1-weighted images for the examination of pathologic conditions of the white matter.

Standard clinical examinations vary from center to center but generally include T1-weighted axial or coronal images and T2-weighted axial images. These clinical sequences can take from 3 to 20 minutes to complete, depending upon the MR scanner. MRI is sensitive to motion artifact, so it is important for a child to remain motionless during the entire MR acquisition. Certain patient populations may require sedation. We have found that children over age 5 generally can lay quietly and tolerate the MR scan while they are awake if the procedure has been discussed with them in detail before the examination. At many centers a child can listen to a radio or favorite tape with headphones, and in some centers a child can watch a video with reflective glasses during an examination. Both of these distractions appear to help children comply.

MRI has several advantages over CT, including the lack of radiation exposure, the ability to acquire images in any plane of orientation, superior gray to white matter contrast, superior detection of pathologic lesions in white matter, higher resolution, and more accurate volumetric measurements.

Just as there are multiple ways to acquire MR data, there are many ways to analyze MR data. Generally, clinical images are only interpreted qualitatively (except in a very few centers where quantitative measures are used in the evaluation for epilepsy surgery). However, advances in methods for quantitative analysis (such as volumetric analysis) are bringing their clinical application near. Although qualitative interpretations are intrinsically appealing and easily obtained, they are not sensitive to volumetric differences unless they are substantial and cannot reliably arrive at specific quantitative patterns or differences. Thus they are unlikely to provide ultimately useful parameters.

MRI is a generally safe, noninvasive procedure that has no known biologic risks in the clinical setting. MRI with higher field magnets than are currently used has potential hazards. With higher field magnets, the changing magnetic fields produced during the pulse sequences can induce electric currents that have been shown to interfere with nerve and cardiac conduction. Additionally, radio frequency signals can induce the heating of tissue. However, very conservative guidelines govern the clinical use of MR scanners.

Contraindications for MRI are related to the strong magnetic field that can dislodge metallic objects and interfere with the operation of mechanical devices. Surgical clips can create image artifacts that interfere with visualization; however, they are only a contraindication if they are intracranial or aneurysmal clips. Individuals who work in industrial situations or have any history of intraocular metallic objects need a thorough ophthalmologic evaluation before any further consideration of MRI, because movement of intraocular metal fragments during MRI has caused blindness. Individuals with electric or magnetically activated devices such as cochlear implants or cardiac pacemakers should not undergo MRI. These contraindications are rarely limitations in children.

Clinical Indications for Magnetic Resonance Imaging

The decision for an MR neuroimaging study should be based on the child's clinical presentation, risk factors for gross CNS pathologic conditions, and physical and neurologic examinations. There is debate regarding the current clinical utility of MRI examinations in childhood psychiatric disorders. Conservative indications for neuroimaging in clinical practice should include first onset psychosis, deteriorating cognitive abilities, focal abnormalities on the neurologic examination, EEG, or neuropsychologic testing. MRI is indicated if the physician suspects structural developmental abnormalities, degenerative disorders, or the sequelae of perinatal asphyxia or periventricular hemorrhage. In the diagnostic evaluation of children with autistic disorder, other pervasive developmental disorders, or severe mental retardation, MRI should be given consideration as a component of a comprehensive evaluation. Recent studies of children with moderate to severe developmental delays have reported gross CT abnormalities in 30% of cases and MRI abnormalities in 65% of cases. MRI was clearly superior to CT in the detection of abnormalities, including evidence on MRI of delayed myelination and white matter abnormalities that were not evident on CT. Despite the high percentage of noted abnormalities, there are conflicting views on the indications for neuroimaging in the evaluation of developmental disorders. Some authors suggest that the findings are often nonspecific and do not point to specific causes; however, others assert that some abnormalities previously identified as "nonspecific" indicate evidence of cerebral dysgenesis. The identification of cerebral dysgenesis can help the physician and family understand potential underlying causes, the prognosis, and the recurrence risk. Shaefer and Bodensteiner have noted that the presence of abnormalities suggesting cerebral dysgenesis falls in the category of sporadic cases that do not have increased genetic risk and have a nondegenerative course.

A variety of CNS lesions or insults can precipitate very similar clinical symptoms. Lesions in certain areas, such as the frontal or temporal lobes, can be notoriously difficult to detect by neurologic examination, but the patient may have symptoms of motor, cognitive, or behavioral disorders. Pathologic conditions in the frontal lobe are often associated with behavioral disinhibition, irritability, a "silly" affect, apathy, and changes in motor activity. The possibility of frontal lobe, temporal lobe, or other CNS pathologic disturbances should be considered in the evaluation of children who have symptoms atypical of classic childhood psychiatric syndromes.

PEARLS & PERILS

MAGNETIC RESONANCE IMAGING

- MRI can acquire and visualize images in any plane; for standard clinical examinations in the coronal, sagittal, and transaxial planes are visualized. Additionally, it has the ability to acquire three-dimensional data that can be manipulated and viewed in any plane or volume desired.
- MRI avoids bony artifacts associated with CT and provides detailed anatomic images of the entire cerebrum, temporal lobes, posterior fossa, and brain stem.
- There are no known clinical risks.
- MRI has improved differentiation of gray matter and white matter, and it is superior for the visualization of white matter lesions. MRI generally has superior sensitivity for the visualization of lesions, with most standard clinical MR scanners achieving resolution of 1 to 2 mm and with newer, higher power magnets achieving microscopic resolution of approximately 300 μm.
- Standard protocol scanning time is routinely less than 20 minutes, and on many clinical scanners with echoplanar capabilities it can be significantly shorter.
- The narrow cylinder shape of the scanner is difficult for some patients (generally adolescents or older) with claustrophobia to tolerate and makes the patient more inaccessible during the MR scan.
- MR images are sensitive to motion artifact, and if a patient is unable to remain motionless, she may require sedation.

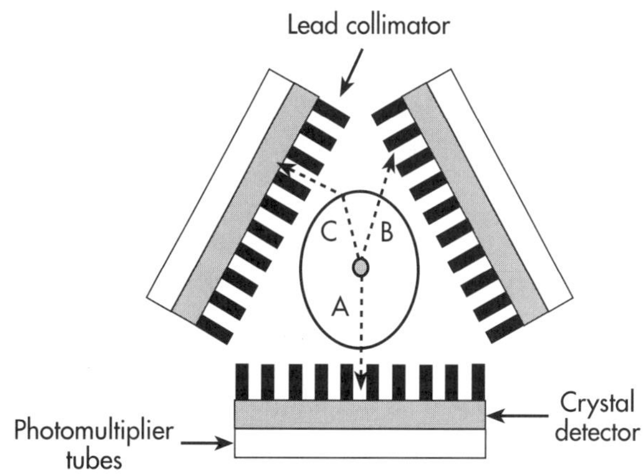

FIGURE 3-4 Camera-based SPECT scanners utilize the principle of collimation to determine the trajectory of emitted gamma rays from a patient's brain. These cameras rotate around the patient's head, acquiring multiple views of the whole brain volume. These multiple views are then reconstructed to create images in any plane. Photomultiplier tubes are used for the detection of the emitted gamma particles, and lead collimators permit only photons of parallel trajectory to pass through to the photomultiplier detectors.

Newer developments with stronger magnets and faster imaging protocols are making the field of MR microscopy increasingly possible. High-field magnet techniques (such as ≥4 tesla magnets) can currently create images with a resolution down to 300 μm, resulting in highly anatomically detailed images. These techniques will provide increasingly powerful tools for research and future clinical applications in the examination of neuropathologic conditions in childhood psychiatric disorders.

Functional Brain Imaging Techniques

Single-Photon Emission Computed Tomography

SPECT is a powerful, noninvasive method of measuring cerebral activity. Normally there is a tight coupling between rCBF, glucose metabolism, and neuronal activity in the brain. In practice, SPECT is a two-stage process. During the first stage of a SPECT brain scan, the subject is injected with or inhales a radioactively labeled compound. Radiotracers used for SPECT imaging include ^{133}Xe, ^{99m}Tc HMPAO, and ^{123}I IMP. For example, before a high-resolution SPECT brain scan, a radioactive element such as technetium (^{99m}Tc) is bound to a neutral, lipid-soluble agent, in this case hexamethylpropyleneamineoxime (HMPAO). This compound is administered intravenously to the patient. It flows rapidly into the subject's brain with arterial circulation and is trapped in the brain within 30 seconds of the initial injection. Thus a "snapshot" of brain activity at the time of injection is produced. The second stage of this procedure occurs when the subject undergoes imaging by lying within a group of gamma ray detectors arrayed around the subject's head. The bound ^{99m}Tc HMPAO emits gamma rays for several hours that are detected by one of two methods; either an array of probes that detect and register the emitted gamma rays may be positioned around the subject's head, or the subject's head may be positioned within rotating gamma cameras that detect the emitted gamma rays. Figure 3-4 illustrates a SPECT scanner with three gamma cameras that rotate around a subject's head to detect the emitted gamma rays.

Figure 3-5 shows a series of transverse oblique, sagittal, and coronal images generated by a three-head sys-

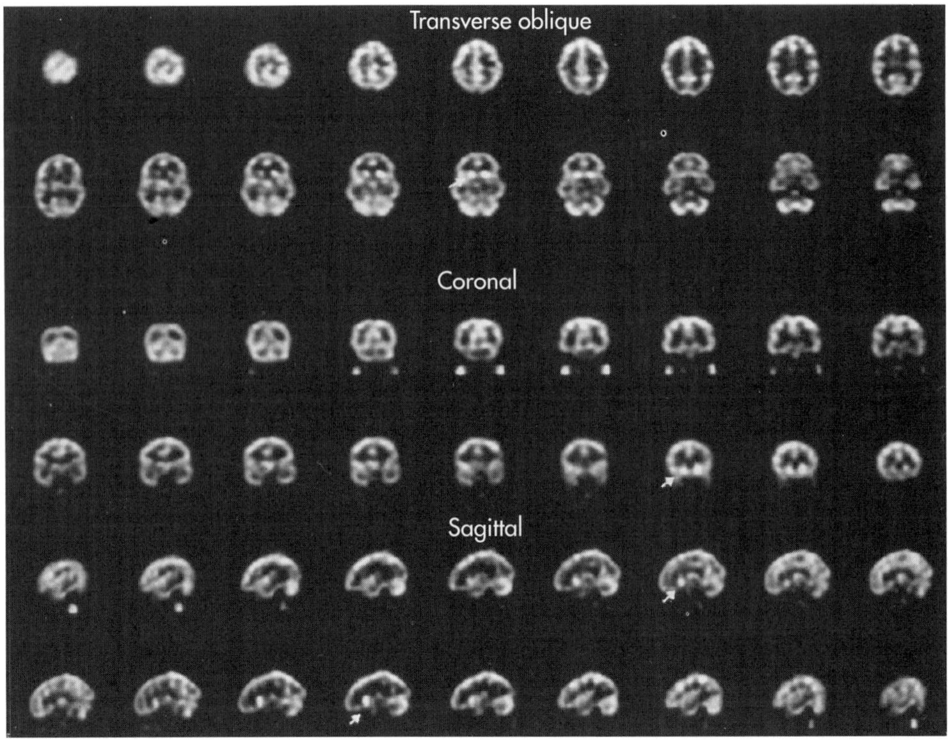

FIGURE 3-5 Transverse, coronal, and sagittal images from a three-head SPECT system (PRISM) of a 16-year-old girl with schizophrenia. In this particular patient, there was increased blood flow in both caudates; these areas of increased flow are indicated with arrows in each of the three projections shown.

tem (PRISM) from a 16-year-old girl with schizophrenia. This system is capable of resolutions in the range of 6 to 8 mm. Figure 3-6 is a three-dimensional rendering of this subject's cortical surface and selected subcortical structures.

A major advantage of SPECT is that it is widely available within most hospitals' nuclear medicine departments. This is because the radioisotopes used for SPECT do not require a cyclotron for their production and thus are easily available. It is now possible for SPECT to achieve spatial resolutions of 6 to 8 mm, and resolutions of 2 to 3 mm are expected to be achieved in the near future with fiberoptic collimation. Quantitative methods are available for measuring blood flow, and it is becoming possible to study specific neurotransmitter receptors (such as muscarinic, dopaminergic, adrenergic, and opiate receptors). Disadvantages of SPECT include extracranial contamination from background radiation, its inability to measure glucose metabolic rates, and the lack of both clinical and research experience using SPECT in children and adolescents with psychiatric disorders.

Clinical Indications for Single-Photon Emission Computed Tomography

In child psychiatry there are no known clinical indications at this time for SPECT imaging. Although the studies using ^{133}Xe SPECT by Lou et al. in ADHD have shown promising results (see p. 44), there are not enough studies of children and adolescents with or without psychiatric disorders to be able to use SPECT diagnostically. SPECT's greatest promise for child psychiatry lies in the area of challenge studies, both cognitive and pharmacologic, and in the area of measuring specific brain receptor sites.

Positron Emission Tomography

PET is one of the most versatile and powerful brain imaging techniques available to psychiatric researchers today. Unfortunately however, the high cost of creating and maintaining a PET facility makes it one of the least available and least affordable brain imaging modalities. PET imaging uses a cyclotron to produce short-lived isotopes of carbon, nitrogen, oxygen, or fluorine. These isotopes are then combined with a compound of interest and injected intravenously into the subject. The injected tracer yields a positron that collides with an electron and produces two photons that travel in exactly opposite directions. A detector coincidence circuit recognizes this simultaneous ionization and creates an image from these events by filtered back-projection methods. Figure 3-7 illustrates this process.

The advantages of PET are that many specific receptors, as well as CBF and glucose metabolism, may be imaged. Disadvantages of PET scanning are that it is expensive and requires a cyclotron, which makes its availability to physicians and researchers very limited.

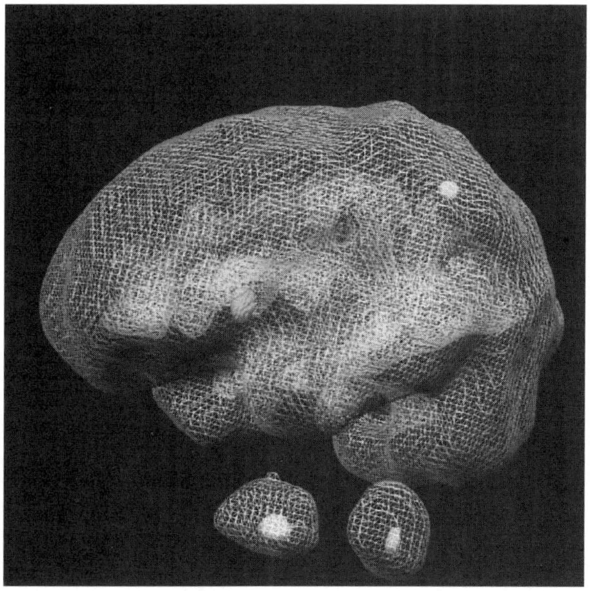

FIGURE 3-6 A computer generated three-dimensional surface-rendered image of the same patient's brain from Figure 3-5. The cortical surface is illustrated with the outer wire frame, and the head of the left caudate nucleus with relatively high blood flow is indicated subcortically. Twin spheres below the brain are from radiotracer uptake in the patients salivary glands.

Similar to SPECT, there are no known clinical indications for PET imaging in child psychiatry. We are not at the stage where either of these imaging techniques, SPECT or PET, can be used diagnostically. Both of these imaging technologies remain primarily research tools in child psychiatry. However, this should change as researchers use these technologies to learn more about the developing brain.

Functional Magnetic Resonance Imaging

Recent developments in fMRI have exciting potential for future use in research and for clinical applications in child psychiatry. Using relatively noninvasive protocols that do not have significant risk, fMRI techniques have been successfully demonstrated in adults. One imaging paradigm demonstrates vascular flow changes using a contrast agent bolus (gadopentetate dimeglumine) in conjunction with rapid acquisition MRI. Another more recent, completely noninvasive technique has demonstrated changes in CBF based on the detection and quantification of MR parameters sensitive to changes in blood oxygenation. The signal in these images is based on the differences in magnetic resonant properties of deoxyhemoglobin vs. oxyhemoglobin. With this technique, changes in brain activation during visual and motor stimulation paradigms have been demonstrated.

PEARLS & PERILS

SINGLE-PHOTON EMISSION COMPUTED TOMOGRAPHY

- It is possible to acquire excellent SPECT images in pediatric subjects using 50% of the standard adult dose of ^{99m}Tc HMPAO.
- A typical SPECT brain scan lasts 22 to 25 minutes, does not require the patient to lie in a tunnel, and is very quiet.
- It is possible to sedate patients after they have been injected with ^{99m}Tc HMPAO and not effect the measurement of rCBF.
- SPECT is readily available at most medical centers and provides functional information that CT and MRI scans do not.
- In pediatric patients who are needle phobic or very anxious, it is best to start a heparin-lock and then wait 30 minutes before injecting the radiotracer. Injecting a radiotracer into a patient who has become very anxious and upset right after the insertion of the intravenous catheter may confound the measurement of rCBF.

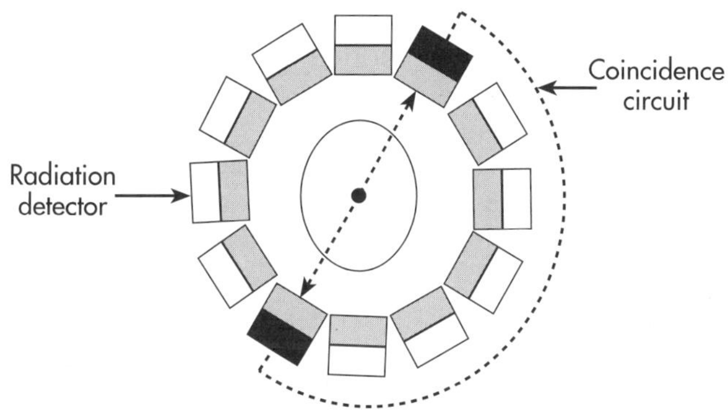

FIGURE 3-7 A PET scanner consists of a ring of radiation detectors designed to detect the simultaneously emitted dual photons that are emitted when a positron collides with an electron. A detector coincidence circuit recognizes this simultaneous ionization and creates an image from these events by filtered back-projection methods.

Functional MRI is currently being applied in preliminary functional neuroimaging studies with adult psychiatric populations. Functional neuroimaging techniques have not been used significantly in child psychiatric or neurologic populations. However, Tzika et al. studied a group of children with sickle cell anemia and demonstrated that fMRI with the gadopentetate dimeglumine bolus technique was well tolerated by children and provided quantitative blood flow information. The continued development, standardization, validation, and refinement of fMRI will provide potentially significant advances in child psychiatry, because functional imaging based on nuclear tracer techniques (such as PET and SPECT) has associated risks that limits its use for large scale studies and normal control populations or for repeated studies in longitudinal investigations.

Magnetic Resonance Spectroscopy

MRS is one of the newer imaging techniques available to psychiatric researchers. MRS is an evolving technology that could provide a tool for the investigation of underlying molecular metabolic pathologic conditions in neuropsychiatric disorders. MRS techniques can assay hydrogen or phosphorus-containing compounds; for example, phosphorus-31 (^{31}P) MRS can explore brain energy metabolism by assays of adenosine triphosphate (ATP) and related metabolites. MRS is capable of determining small variations in the resonant frequencies of different tissue compounds. A display of the MR spectrum as a function of frequency results in the different chemical forms of an element forming peaks at characteristic positions. MRS can be used to study fats, membrane lipid metabolism, high-energy phosphate metabolism, glycogen, some neurotransmitters, amino acids, the citric acid cycle, lithium, and fluorinated compounds.

The advantages of MRS are that it does not expose subjects to ionizing radiation and has no known side effects. Disadvantages of MRS are its limited spatial resolution, long acquisition times, and a limited knowledge base in its use. MRS is technically demanding, not widely available, and requires rigorous standardization for meaningful results. Thus it has received little application in the field of child psychiatry.

MRS has been used to study a small group of pediatric subjects with autistic disorder and schizophrenia. A ^{31}P MRS investigation reported significantly reduced levels of phosphocreatine and related products in patients with autistic disorder compared with control subjects. Neuropsychologic test performance in the group with autistic disorder was correlated with metabolite levels. In children with schizophrenia, differences in choline-containing compounds were suggested in a small pilot study.

Brain Imaging Studies In Selected Child Psychiatric Populations

Autistic Disorder

The current diagnosis of autistic disorder is defined by a behavioral phenotype that can be associated with multiple known causes but is most often idiopathic. Autistic disorder is a heterogeneous disorder that may be the result of multiple components acting through common neural pathways to produce autistic characteristics. Autopsy studies have suggested cerebellar abnormalities with a loss of Purkinje's and granule cells, along with a limbic system pathologic abnormality characterized by increased cell-packing density and reduced neuronal size. Three recent autopsy studies have reported a loss of Purkinje's cells in the cerebellum in a total of 12 subjects. Early MR neuroimaging investigations focused on posterior fossa structures such as the cerebellum and brain stem, and many reported decreased cerebellar vermi. Better controlled studies have reported conflicting results, with some investigators reporting hypoplasia of specific cerebellar vermi and others reporting no differences. In a study with the best matched controls for age, sex, socioeconomic status, and IQ, no differences were reported in cerebellar structure in high-functioning children with autistic disorder. However, Holttum et al. suggested that children with autistic disorder who are higher-functioning may have less irregularity in their cerebellar region. A recent reanalysis of the available data from several studies by Courchesne et al. maintains that there are differences in the cerebellar vermi of individuals who have autistic disorder, with at least 85% of subjects demonstrating hypoplasia and a small minority (10% to 15%) demonstrating significant hyperplasia. Courchesne et al. hypothesize that these extreme groups may have obscured previous mean group differences. Further research is needed to clearly define the nature and specificity of the pathologic state of the cerebellum as visualized by MRI in patients with autistic disorder.

Other MRI investigations of autistic disorder have examined brainstem structures with conflicting results. Increased fourth ventricular size and no difference in fourth ventricular size have been reported. Studies of the pons have reported both decreased size and no difference. Decreased size of the midbrain and medulla oblongata have been reported by one group. Several authors have reported an increased incidence of developmental cortical malformations, such as polymicrogyria, macrogyria, schizencephaly, and cortical atrophy of the parietal lobe, visualized on MRI.

In general, neuroimaging findings in autistic disorder have not been examined for their potential relationship to specific neuropsychologic tasks. However, atrophy of the parietal lobe was correlated with poorer performance on the Posner Test of Visuospatial Attention (a test that elicits a poor performance from adults with acquired parietal lobe damage). Further characterization of the regional abnormalities may be expected to provide additional prognostic and functional correlates for physicians and families.

Many of the structural neuroimaging studies reported in this discussion excluded subjects with autistic disorder who have clearly identified neuropathologic abnormalities such as tuberous sclerosis, neurofibromatosis, fragile X syndrome (see the following discussion), metabolic abnormalities, or congenital rubella syndrome. More specific abnormalities characteristic of each disorder can be expected to be seen on an MRI scan. Patients with tuberous sclerosis exhibit classic radiologic abnormalities of cortical tubers, white matter abnormalities, subependymal nodules, and subependymal giant cell astrocytomas. Neurofibromatosis is characterized on MRI by nonneoplastic hamartomatous lesions and an increased incidence of some neoplasms, including gliomas, neurofibromas, and neurofibrosarcomas. Congenital rubella is often characterized by delayed myelination, decreased brain size, and cortical and basal ganglia calcifications.

Zilbovicius et al. reported finding no differences in rCBF between 21 children with autistic disorder and 14 children with mixed receptive-expressive language disorder. The average nonverbal IQ in their subjects with autistic disorder was 36, whereas the average IQ in their control subjects was 96. This discrepancy may have confounded their results.

Fragile X Syndrome

Children and adults with fragile X syndrome are reported to have differences in their temporal lobe neuroanatomy compared with control subjects who have a variety of other neurobehavioral and developmental disorders. Patients with fragile X syndrome have larger right and left hippocampal volumes, an age-related increase in hippocampal volume, and an age-related decrease in superior temporal gyrus volume. Additionally, individuals with fragile X syndrome have been noted to have hypoplasia of posterior fossa structures.

Rett's Disorder

Girls with Rett's disorder have been reported to have reduced cerebral volume and subcortical atrophy. Investigations of regional neuroanatomic changes have reported significantly greater decrease in gray matter compared with white matter, with the largest decrease being in the frontal regions. There is also decreased volume of the caudate and the midbrain in comparison with normal controls. The clinical course of Rett's disorder, with developmental regression and an arrest in early brain development, suggests a possible neurodegenerative process; however, all of the existing studies have been cross-sectional in nature and have not supported any evidence for later neurodegeneration. Future longitudinal studies that begin with younger subjects should help to clarify this issue.

Dyslexia

There has long been a suggestion that people with dyslexia manifest anatomic abnormalities in the region of the planum temporale (PT). This was first demonstrated by Galaburda et al. in four young adults who had histories of reading disorders. Their postmortem neuropathologic examinations demonstrated changes in the PT with a loss of the usual pattern of asymmetry (a larger PT on the left than right) and focal cortical abnormalities. The PT is a region at the posterior pole of the temporal lobe that is important in language processing and reading, or phonologic processing. The neuropathologic reports sparked interest in neuroimaging investigations of the region of the PT. Early CT studies confirmed a lack of the normal asymmetry in aspects of the posterior occipital lobe. Several MRI studies have been completed with differing results in their examinations of the PT region. Several investigators have reported decreased left PT regions in comparison with the right. Additionally, some groups have reported a change in the asymmetry with larger right PT regions or a lack of asymmetry. Some of the discrepancy in reports appears to be related to differences in the definition of the region of the PT, as well as to difficulty with the reliability of these measurements. More recent studies examining PT regions based on area rather than linear morphometric measures have continued to note PT abnormalities. Leonard et al. examined 9 people with dyslexia, 10 of their first- and second-degree relatives, and 12 control subjects with a three-dimensional MRI acquisition to carefully quantify the temporal and parietal banks of the PT. The subjects with dyslexia had larger measures of asymmetry and an apparent shift of the right planar tissue from the temporal to the parietal region. Additionally, they reported a higher incidence of cerebral anomalies, and their phonologic decoding scores correlated with these anomalies. In contrast, Schultz et al. studied 17 children with dyslexia in comparison with 14 control children using area measurements of the PT and reported strong effects of age and sex that overshadowed any effect of diagnosis. This report again highlights the importance of developmental and sex effects, even in posterior temporal lobe and PT structures. Structural abnormalities with differences in perisylvian asymmetries have also been noted in relatives of people with dyslexia. Although conflicting results have been reported, the number of subjects studied, relative to the number of important factors that need controls, has not been adequate to clearly define potential relationships. Additionally, differences in the definitions of dyslexia or reading disability between investigations may relate to the apparent discrepancies and results. MRI quantification in dyslexia may eventually help to predict prognosis and potential genetic risks.

Attention-Deficit/Hyperactivity Disorder

Early neuroimaging investigations related to ADHD were completed on individuals with minimal brain dysfunction (MBD), an earlier diagnostic categorization that included individuals now diagnosed with ADHD. Some of these CT studies suggested that children with MBD or adults with a history of MBD may have cerebral atrophy and mild ventricular enlargement, whereas other investigators did not find significant differences.

However, more recent MRI investigations of children with ADHD have demonstrated several structural differences in comparison with normal controls. Studies examining the corpus callosum in midline sagittal images have reported regional decreases in the anterior or posterior segments of the corpus callosum. The corpus callosum is a structure that consists of fibers crossing between the right and left hemispheres. Changes in its structure are hypothesized to be indicative of an imbalance in right and left hemisphere regulation. Corpus callosal measures have been reported to significantly correlate with classroom ratings of hyperactivity. MRI studies comparing overall cerebral volume of children with ADHD to control children have reported both no significant difference and decreased overall cerebral size.

In addition to the corpus callosum findings, differences in caudate asymmetry have been demonstrated. Hynd et al. reported abnormal caudate asymmetry in 11 children with ADHD compared with control children, and Castellanos et al. demonstrated with a group of 50 boys with ADHD and matched controls that boys who had ADHD lacked expected asymmetry in caudate volumes compared with the control subjects. Additionally, boys with ADHD did not demonstrate a decrease in their caudate volumes with increasing age, as was expected and as was replicated in the control group. The researchers could not demonstrate any significant relationship in structural changes to clinical features or continuous performance task measures. Finally, Hynd et al. reported that 10 children with ADHD lacked expected frontal lobe regional asymmetry. Taken together, these findings are intriguing and consistent with hypotheses that the pathophysiology of ADHD is related to dysfunction in frontal-striatal circuits. The relationship between structural changes and impairment on specific neuropsychologic tasks remains to be defined.

In addition to the structural studies of ADHD, there have been several functional imaging studies in this disorder. Lou et al. have used ^{133}Xe SPECT to study mixed groups of children with either ADHD or ADHD with dysphasia. They found decreased blood flow to the striatal and posterior periventricular regions in the ADHD group. There was also increased flow in the primary sensory and sensorimotor cortex compared with the results from the children in the control group who were siblings of the probands. This flow pattern was reversed by treatment with methylphenidate.

Zametkin et al. reported on a PET study that compared the cerebral glucose metabolism of a group of hyperactive adolescents with that of a control group and found significant reductions of glucose metabolism in 6 of 60 specific brain regions studied. After the absolute glucose metabolic rates were normalized between subjects and controls, they found reduced glucose metabolism in the left anterior frontal area, the right posterior temporal area, the left posterior frontal area, the right temporal area, the left thalamus, and the right hippocampus.

Childhood Schizophrenia

Numerous MRI investigations have demonstrated structural abnormalities in adults with schizophrenia compared with controls. These abnormalities include enlarged cerebral ventricles and a reduced medial temporal lobe volume, as well as superior temporal gyrus, hippocampus, and amygdala volumes. A small study of 12 children with early symptoms of schizophrenia or schizotypal personality disorder reported decreased volume of the amygdala and temporal cortex, decreased corpus callosal area, and differences in symmetry measures. Preliminary investigations by McKenna et al. have reported similar findings. A small pilot study using MRS suggested that children with schizophrenia show differences in choline-containing compounds.

Tourette's Disorder

The pathophysiology of Tourette's disorder has been hypothesized to be related to basal ganglia dysfunction. Several recent MRI investigations of the basal ganglia have reported significant structural changes in patients with Tourette's disorder compared with individuals in a control group. These investigations have included adult and child populations and have demonstrated either decreased volumes on the left side or a change in the asymmetry between the right and left basal ganglia structures. Additionally, Singer et al. demonstrated that children with Tourette's disorder and ADHD had more extreme differences in globus pallidus lateralization compared to subjects with only Tourette's disorder and to controls. Yazgan et al. reported that patients with Tourette's disorder were impaired on neuropsychologic tasks believed to be related to lateralized basal ganglia function (for example, line bisection and turning preference). Although the overall group of patients with Tourette's disorder demonstrated basal ganglia differences from the control group on MRI, the neuropsychologic performance did not correlate with structural characteristics within the group of subjects with Tourette's disorder.

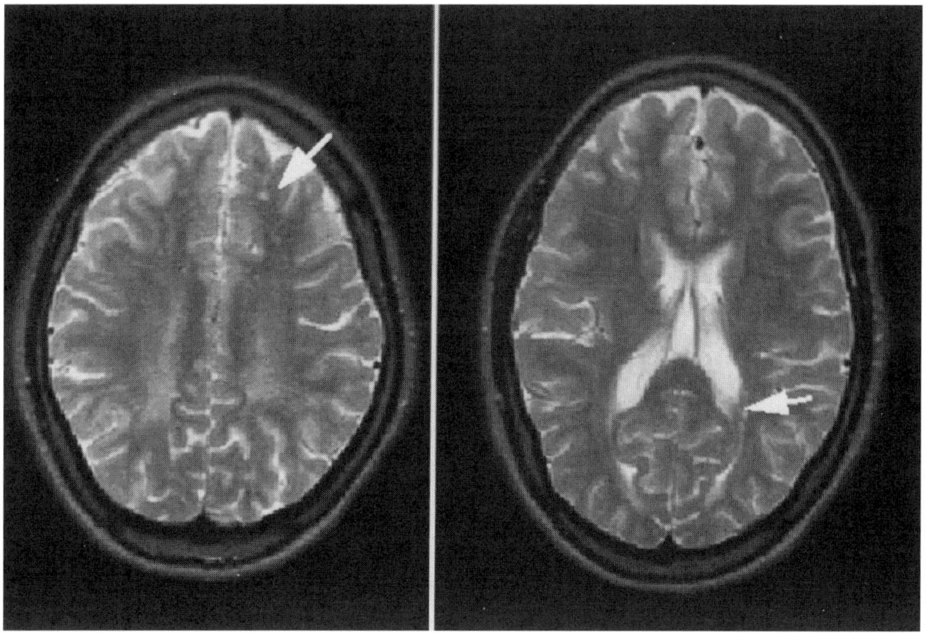

FIGURE 3-8 Deep white-matter hyperintensities as visualized on T2-weighted axial MR images in an adolescent with bipolar I disorder.

Mood Disorders

Adults with major depressive disorder (MDD) and bipolar I disorder have been reported to have a variety of neuroanatomic changes, including increased incidence of subcortical white matter hyperintensities, increased ventricular size, decreased temporal lobe volume, decreased frontal lobe volume, and changes in basal ganglia structures (for review see Coffey et al.). A pilot study of children and adolescents with bipolar disorders suggested similar changes with a 25% incidence of subcortical white matter hyperintensities (see Figure 3-8), changes in frontal asymmetry, and a trend toward increased ventricular size.

Summary

Brain imaging studies are just beginning to give us valuable information about the neurobiologic basis of a variety of childhood psychiatric disorders. With improvements in imaging hardware and software, better selection of subjects, the development of normative data bases, and the use of multimodal imaging methods, we should see significant progress in the understanding of childhood psychiatric disorders. The future holds great promise for the use of these imaging techniques to better understand the neurobiology of childhood and adolescent psychiatric disorders.

Annotated Bibliography

Andreason NC, editor: *Brain imaging: applications in psychiatry,* Washington DC, 1988, American Psychiatric Press.

This volume offers one of the best summaries of various brain imaging technologies and summarizes related literature through 1988.

Andreason NC, section editor: *Brain imaging: review of psychiatry,* vol 12, Washington DC, 1993, American Psychiatric Press.

This volume updates and expands the literature in this area.

Crease, RP: Biomedicine in the age of imaging, *Science* 261:554-561, 1993.

This article discusses some of the important issues relevant to brain imaging.

Guze BH: Magnetic resonance spectroscopy, *Arch Gen Psychiatry* 48:572-574, 1991.

This article is a nice introduction to MRS.

section two

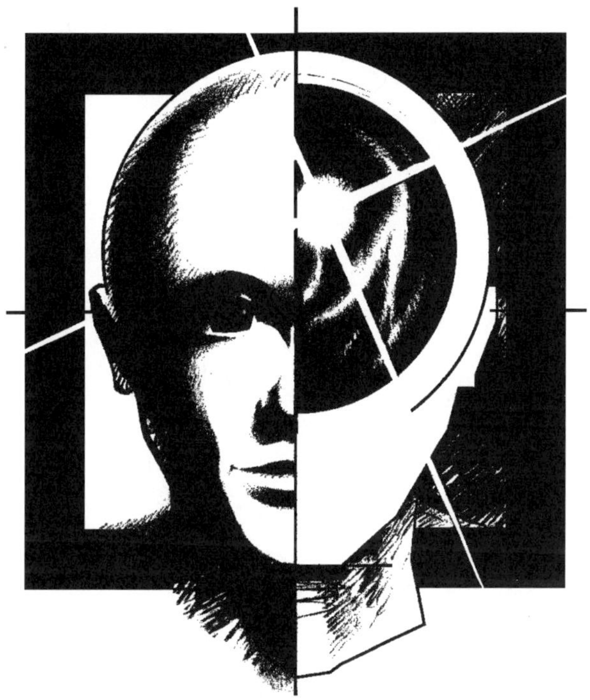

Diagnostic Categories

Isaac K. Wood, MD

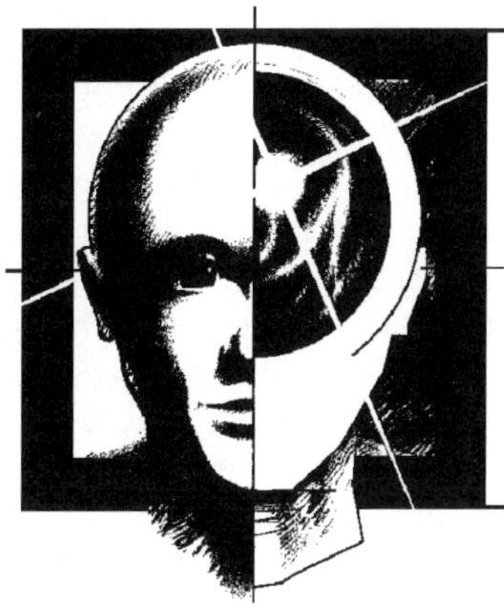

chapter 4

Pervasive Developmental Disorders

James C. Harris, MD

Pervasive Developmental Disorder
Autistic Disorder
Asperger's Disorder
Rett's Disorder
Childhood Disintegrative Disorder
Summary

"Since 1938, there have come to our attention a number of children whose condition differs so markedly and uniquely from anything reported so far, that each case merits—and I hope will eventually receive—a detailed consideration of its fascinating peculiarities." With this first paragraph of his classic 1943 paper, *Autistic Disturbances of Affective Contact,* Leo Kanner initiated clinical and research interest into conditions that would later be described as pervasive developmental disorders (PDDs).

The designation *pervasive developmental disorder* was introduced in 1980 in DSM-III to reclassify previous categories of psychoses of infancy and early childhood and childhood onset schizophrenia as developmental disorders involving deviant language, social, and behavioral development. In DSM-III, the PDD category initially included infantile autism, childhood-onset pervasive developmental disorder, residual autism, and an atypical category. As the classification system has become more refined, the initial categories that were included have been revised so that the term *PDD* is now used to designate not only infantile autism but other conditions with social communicative deficits as well. Thus the DSM-IV classification includes autistic disorder, Asperger's disorder, Rett's disorder, childhood disintegrative disorder, and a residual category, pervasive developmental disorder not otherwise specified (PDD-NOS).

In this chapter, the definition, prevalence, possible causes, natural history, diagnosis and treatment of each of these disorders is described. The primary emphasis is on autistic disorder and atypical instances of autistic disorder, since the other disorders occur less often.

Pervasive Developmental Disorders

The PDD category was initially designed to include autistic disorder, as well as a heterogeneous group of conditions that have similar features to autistic disorder. It does not suggest a particular theoretic orientation or cause for these conditions, nor does it suggest a particular kind of treatment. Generally, PDD indicates that a disturbance in development is pervasive in that it concurrently involves more than one developmental line; for example, a disorder may interfere with both language and social development. In this sense, the term *pervasive* is contrasted to *specific,* which describes developmental disorders that primarily involve one developmental line, such as cognition (mental retardation) or language and reading.

However, the term *PDD,* although officially in use for 15 years, remains controversial. Should the term be used only for children with social communicative deficits or should it be more broadly applied to emphasize profound and extensive disruption of multiple developmental lines in children whose disorders do not necessarily resemble autistic disorder? Much of the debate about the continuing use of this category results from how the diagnosis PDD-NOS, a DSM-III-R category, was used. In DSM-III-R, PDD-NOS was sometimes treated as a diagnosis in itself; that is, it was treated as a broad category of social communication disorder or atypical autism rather than as a residual category for children who have severe social communicative deficits with origins that are yet to be determined. Another objection to the term *pervasive* is related to the fact that some individuals with autistic disorder score within the normal range of intelligence on cognitive tests. This leads to questions as to whether their disorder is sufficiently pervasive to use this term. Moreover, since the term *pervasive* is nonspecific, it may be confusing to parents whose children have strengths in some areas despite their deficits in others. Hence pervasive does not imply that there are no areas of normal functioning. The decision to retain the PDD category distinguishes these disorders from specific developmental disorders and emphasizes that social, language, communicative, and cognitive skills may be deficient in varying degrees, requiring multiple services and various intervention strategies. The issue regarding social deficits is handled differently in the DSM-IV and ICD-10 classifications. In DSM-IV, social communication deficits are emphasized, whereas ICD-10 uses the term *pervasive* to include disorders with or without primary social deficits.

BOX 4-1 AUTISTIC DISORDER

DSM-IV DIAGNOSTIC CRITERIA

A. A total of six (or more) items from (1), (2), and (3), with at least two from (1), and one each from (2) and (3):

(1) qualitative impairment in social interaction, as manifested by at least two of the following:
  (a) marked impairment in the use of multiple nonverbal behaviors such as eye-to-eye gaze, facial expression, body postures, and gestures to regulate social interaction
  (b) failure to develop peer relationships appropriate to developmental level
  (c) a lack of spontaneous seeking to share enjoyment, interests, or achievements with other people (e.g., by a lack of showing, bringing, or pointing out objects of interest)
  (d) lack of social or emotional reciprocity
(2) qualitative impairments in communication as manifested by at least one of the following:
  (a) delay in, or total lack of, the development of spoken language (not accompanied by an attempt to compensate through alternative modes of communication such as gesture or mime)
  (b) in individuals with adequate speech, marked impairment in the ability to initiate or sustain a conversation with others
  (c) stereotyped and repetitive use of language or idiosyncratic language
  (d) lack of varied, spontaneous make-believe play or social imitative play appropriate to developmental level
(3) restricted repetitive and stereotyped patterns of behavior, interests, and activities, as manifested by at least one of the following:
  (a) encompassing preoccupation with one or more stereotyped and restricted patterns of interest that is abnormal either in intensity or focus
  (b) apparently inflexible adherence to specific, nonfunctional routines and rituals
  (c) stereotyped and repetitive motor mannerisms (e.g., hand or finger flapping or twisting, or complex whole body movements)
  (d) persistent preoccupation with parts of objects

B. Delays or abnormal functioning in at least one of the following areas, with onset prior to age 3 years: (1) social interaction, (2) language as used in social communication, or (3) symbolic or imaginative play.

C. The disturbance is not better accounted for by Rett's Disorder or Childhood Disintegrative Disorder

(From American Psychiatric Association: *Diagnostic and statistical manual of mental disorders,* ed 4 [DSM-IV], Washington DC, 1994, American Psychiatric Press.)

Autistic Disorder

Diagnostic Criteria

Among the DSM-IV PPDs, autistic disorder has been the most thoroughly investigated. Autistic disorder is characterized by a primary impairment in the development of social understanding and social skills. Current developmental research regarding autistic disorder addresses affective development, social cognition, and interpersonal reciprocity with the intent to better understand how an abnormality in social understanding emerges.

The diagnostic criteria for autistic disorder are based on the recognition of developmental distortions in multiple basic psychologic functions, such as attention and perception, that are involved in the development of social skills and language.

In DSM-IV, the criteria for autistic disorder are operationalized and incorporate a developmental orientation. The diagnosis requires qualitative impairments in social interaction and communication. Three broad categories are included: abnormal reciprocal social relations, disturbances in communication and imaginative play, and restricted range of activities and interests (stereotypies). To receive a diagnosis of autistic disorder according to DSM-IV, a child or adult needs to demonstrate at least 6 out of 12 criteria, with a specified distribution over the three categories. An individual with autistic disorder may receive other axis I diagnoses if the diagnostic criteria are met. For example, schizophrenia may be diagnosed if hallucinations and delusions are present; schizophreniform disorder may cooccur in a person with autistic disorder. DSM-IV uses developmentally-focused criteria and does not rely only on the current examination of the child. The diagnosis requires delays or abnormal functioning before age 3 in at least one of the following areas: social interaction, social communicative language, and symbolic or imaginative play. Moreover, with the inclusion of additional disorders in the PDD category, exclusionary criteria now include Asperger's disorder, Rett's disorder, and childhood disintegrative disorder. The DSM-IV diagnostic criteria for autistic disorder are shown in Box 4-1, and Table 4-1 shows the features of autistic disorder.

The diagnosis requires at least two items related to qualitative impairment in social interaction, one from the category of qualitative impairment in communication, and one from the category of restricted repetitive and stereotyped patterns of behavior. Since specific examples are not given in the DSM-IV criteria, it is important to consult the descriptive text for specific examples that fit under each of the categories outlined.

Atypical autism is a specific category in ICD-10 but is not a specific category in DSM-IV, where atypical autism is included under PDD-NOS. Atypical autism differs from autistic disorder in either the age of the patient when symptoms are recognized or the failure to meet all three sets of diagnostic criteria. For example, abnormal or impaired social development becomes apparent to others after age 3 when abnormalities are present in one or two, but not in all three, of the following areas: reciprocal social interaction, communication, or stereotyped repetitive behavior. The DSM-IV definition suggests that atypical autism is most often seen in profoundly retarded individuals who, possibly because of their low level of functioning, may not exhibit the specific behaviors needed for the diagnosis of autistic disorder. It may be applied to children with severe forms of specific developmental disorder of receptive language, atypical childhood psychosis, and other levels of mental retardation with autistic features. In summary, atypical autism refers to cases that do not meet the full criteria for autistic disorder because of the late age of onset, atypical symptoms, subthreshold symptoms, or all three. Moreover, criteria are not met for other specific PDDs, schizophrenia, schizotypal personality, or avoidant personality disorder. Although specific operational criteria are not given, it is suggested

DIAGNOSIS

TABLE 4-1 AUTISTIC DISORDER

Discriminating feature

1. Qualitative impairments in social interaction and communication and restricted and stereotyped behaviors

Consistent features

1. Absence of psychotic symptoms
2. Onset of symptoms prior to age 3
3. Absence of Rett's disorder and childhood disintegrative disorder
4. Higher incidence in boys than girls
5. Deficient pragmatic use of language

Variable features

1. Severe to profound mental retardation
2. Initially recognized in the second year of life
3. Family history of autistic-like behaviors
4. Difficulty in mother's pregnancy or in perinatal period
5. Impaired functioning in frontal and parietal association areas on PET scans
6. Echolalia, palilalia, and pronoun reversal
7. Congenital abnormalities including tuberous sclerosis and fragile X syndrome

that the diagnosis of atypical autism be placed in parentheses: for example, PDD-NOS (atypical autism).

However, the designation of atypical autism for children with severe and profound mental retardation remains problematic. Social deficits are commonly found in severely and profoundly retarded individuals. Wing and Gould assessed social deficits in a large sample of handicapped children and identified both children with autistic disorder and other groups of children with handicaps based on their social skills. Their categories include: (1) the aloof child who pays little attention to social exchange; (2) the passive child who is more responsive but tends to avoid social interactions unless passively engaged; and (3) the active but odd child, who may initiate interactions but does so in an inappropriate and stilted manner. The classic idiopathic autistic disorder described by Kanner may be a genetic disorder; however, the use of the term *atypical autism,* which may include multiple causes, for people who are profoundly mentally retarded may suggest a link to a genetic form of mental retardation when there is none. It is more parsimonious to describe the specific deficits that are observed. Perhaps in the next classification this group will have a new designation, such as "social communicative disorder associated with mental retardation." Considerable care is needed when diagnosing severely and profoundly mentally retarded children.

Prevalence

The incidence of autistic disorder is 4 to 5 cases per 10,000 people. When rates include children with autistic symptoms and atypical autism, the incidence increases to 12 to 15 per 10,000 individuals. The other types of PDD are less common than autistic disorder. The prevalence of autistic disorder is higher for boys than girls, with rates of 4 or 5 : 1, although girls tend to be more severely affected. The majority of individuals with autistic disorder (75% to 80%) have some degree of mental retardation. Typically, the age of initial recognition is in the second year of life. However, the diagnosis has been made in the first few months of life and after several years of normal development. Although family factors and high cognitive functioning in the child may delay case recognition, the early symptoms ordinarily are recognized when careful histories are taken. Finally, although autistic disorder was initially associated with a higher social class, it is now evident that it occurs in families at all socioeconomic levels. The recurrence risk in a family for the birth of another child with autistic disorder after the birth of one child with the disorder is approximately 3%, or 60 to 100 times the base rate in the general population.

Etiology

There is now evidence that autistic disorder can be a genetic disease. Three epidemiologic studies of identical twins found high concordance rates, ranging from 36% to 91% in contrast to a zero concordance rate among nonidentical twin pairs. LeCouteur, Bailey, and Rutter reported that 92% of identical twins were concordant for a broad cognitive or social-deficit phenotype, in contrast to 10% of nonidentical twins. Siblings and parents of a person with autistic disorder may have an increased risk for social and cognitive deficits that are mild to minimal in degree but similar in kind to those found in autistic disorder. These include disinhibited social communication, awkward or inadequate expression, and odd verbal interaction. However, the rate of mental retardation is not elevated among the siblings of children with autistic disorder.

There is little evidence that autistic disorder is linked to other genetic disorders even though autistic behaviors may occur. For example, similar behavior has been reported in patients with fragile X syndrome; yet Steffenburg et al. found fragile X syndrome in only 9% of 22 twin pairs with autistic behavior, and Piven et al. found the fragile X marker in only 2 out of 75 cases (2.7%). In fragile X syndrome, the social deficits reported do not follow the same clinical course as those found in classic autistic disorder.

Yet, the autistic spectrum of behavioral and developmental abnormalities have been reported in a variety of brain disorders. The known syndromes that are associated with autistic behavior are shown in Box 4-2.

The natural history of symptom development and outcome in these conditions does not necessarily follow the same clinical course as the classic autistic disorder described by Kanner. Therefore children with the conditions shown in Box 4-2 should be followed-up carefully to establish the course of autistic symptoms in each of them.

Difficulty in the mother's pregnancy or in the perinatal period may occur in some children who have a later diagnosis of autistic disorder; however, the occurrence of such problems is variable and is not consistently present. Early problems have not been shown to

BOX 4-2

DISORDERS ASSOCIATED WITH AUTISTIC DISORDER AND AUTISTIC BEHAVIOR

Fragile X (q27) syndrome
Tuberous sclerosis
Neurofibromatosis
Infantile spasms
Phenylketonuria (PKU)
Intrauterine rubella infection
Postnatal herpes infection
Hydrocephalus
Möbius' syndrome
Duchenne's muscular dystrophy

be causally related to autistic disorder, and there is no evidence that they provide useful indicators for the prevention of autistic disorder.

Neurochemical investigations in autistic disorder have focused primarily on neurotransmitters such as serotonin, dopamine, norepinephrine, and endogenous opiates. Thyroid hormone and cortisol production have also been evaluated. Specific endocrine abnormalities have not been found; however, dysregulation of both cortisol and melatonin rhythms have been suggested. The most consistent neurochemical finding is that of hyperserotoninemia, which has been documented in 30% to 50% of subjects with autistic disorder; whole blood serotonin levels are in the upper 5% of the normal range. However, drug treatment specifically focused on the correction of hyperserotoninemia has not led to reliable improvement in the core symptoms of autistic disorder.

Neuroanatomic studies suggest abnormalities in the emotional or limbic brain and cerebellum. The brain regions examined are important in processing environmental information, particularly social information. Initial MRI findings of hypoplasia of cerebellar lobules VI and VII, the pons, and the fourth ventricle have not been replicated in high-functioning subjects with autistic disorder when contrasted with IQ-matched control subjects. However, Piven et al. did find that 5 out of 13 subjects with autistic disorder had polymicrogyria and 1 had macrogyria, which may reflect abnormal migration of neurons to the cortex. Patients with and without these migrational abnormalities have been diagnosed with the full syndrome of autistic disorder. Although neuronal migration problems might be present more often, current techniques may not be refined enough to demonstrate them. Bauman reported autopsy findings on six individuals who were clinically diagnosed and met diagnostic criteria for an autistic disorder. These individuals had previously shown deficits in social interaction, disordered language development, and compulsive and ritualistic behavior. Neuroanatomic abnormalities were found in the amygdala, hippocampus, septum, anterior cingulum, and mamillary body—all parts of the limbic system. Many small and closely packed cells were found in limbic brain regions. When Golgi cell stains were used to study morphology, the dendrites were found to have reduced branching, especially less tertiary branching. Bauman concluded that these findings suggest a developmental curtailment in the growth of the limbic brain circuits in autistic disorder.

The developmental consequences of persistent prenatal anatomic circuits (that is, possible dysfunctional information processing) may not become apparent until the particular circuits are integrated into new systems later in development, perhaps during the second year of life. This may account for autistic symptoms generally not being recognized in the first year of life.

Functional brain imaging studies, such as PET and MRS, are also consistent with immaturity in the development of the neuronal dendritic tree. Imaging studies are consistent with incomplete development of distributed neural networks in frontal and parietal association cortex areas, which are involved in complex information processing. Such deficits may be associated with abnormalities in those executive systems and social cognitive systems that are needed for information transfer between brain regions.

Clinical Features

The essential feature of autistic disorder is qualitative abnormalities in social interaction. The severity and type of social deficit varies with the child's age and developmental level. An infant with autistic disorder may resist cuddling and may not mold to the parent. He may not initiate anticipatory gestures (such as reaching out to be picked up) when approached by or when approaching others. Moreover, in interacting with others, the infant or child with autistic disorder may lack joint attention; for example, the child may not point to objects or use eye contact to engage others' interest. The high-functioning child with autistic disorder may fail to show pride in accomplishment. During the preschool years, the child may ignore others or bump into them as if he were unaware of their existence. He may not turn when called and may not make eye contact when someone tries to engage him in conversation. The gaze avoidance may continue during the school years and even into adulthood, although these behaviors may appear in a less striking form. He may not be distressed by social isolation and seek solitude.

As he grows older, the high-functioning child may emerge from severe autistic patterns of behavior, show less social distancing, become more socially aware, and even become intrusive and perplexed about why people who do not have autistic disorder behave as they do. Yet despite this emergence, a person with autistic disorder may be unaware of others' feelings and lack understanding of the effects of his behavior on others. The ability to interpret another's emotional tone of voice or facial expression of feeling generally remains limited; consequently, the usual exchanges between child and parent that ordinarily convey wishes or show pleasure and displeasure are affected. Because of these social deficits, the high-functioning child with autistic disorder generally has difficulty making friends and engaging other children in play. When friends are sought, ostracism may be the result of awkward attempts to socialize. Because of this rigidity in social responses, a child with autistic disorder must be taught simple social norms, such as greeting another person or saying goodbye. Even when the verbal child with autistic disorder learns social norms, the newly-learned behavior may not be carried out in appropriate context and therefore may seem odd to others.

The failure to acquire language at the expected age is one of the most common presenting concerns for parents of preschool children with autistic disorder. Language impairment involves all aspects of language and not only speech. For most, language development is deviant; therefore problems occur in both the comprehension of speech and the expression of ideas in speech. Some children may be mute, whereas others may understand very little conversation that is directed toward them. Others may develop language late, have unintelligible jargon, and lack communicative intent in their speech. Such jargon may include bits and pieces of memorized information from cartoons, television commercials, or phrases that they have heard. Problems in speech fluency may sometimes mask problems in comprehension. Some may articulate more clearly but are preoccupied with a narrow range of favorite topics and show little regard for the conversational interests of the person with whom they are speaking. They may perseverate by asking the same question over and over, despite already knowing the answer. In other instances, people with autistic disorder may recite phrases that they have heard, imitating exactly the tone of voice and speech rhythm of the speaker from whom the phrase was learned. Early in life, children who have autistic disorder and are verbal may be echolalic; that is, they parrot (stereotypically repeat) a phrase rather than responding grammatically. Such echolalia may be accompanied by a reversal of pronouns (pronominal reversal); hence the child refers to himself as *you* rather than appropriately referring to himself as *I*.

Pragmatic language use, a form of nonverbal communication, is also deficient. This is most clearly seen when a person with autistic disorder does not use gestures spontaneously in conversation. Nonverbal gestures, such as shaking the head to signify no, or nodding to signify yes, may be inconsistent or absent. Instead of pointing to an object, a child may get it for himself or take a parent's hand and move it toward the preferred object to indicate his needs. If unable to use gestures to communicate effectively, he may become distressed and cry or have tantrums until an adult has guessed by trial and error what is needed. A verbal child may speak in a poorly modulated monotone or in a singsong manner. He may have an impairment in utilizing rhythm and intonation (prosody) to understand the meaning of another's speech. Verbal children must be taught how to conduct a conversation—how to maintain the conversational topic, how to take turns, and how to look at the conversational partner.

A lack of the use of imagination in play becomes apparent during the preschool years. Children with autistic disorder show repetitive patterns of movement (stereotypies and mannerisms), especially when they are excited; these include hand flapping, twirling, rocking, head banging, finger posturing, and sensory preoccupations. Commonly, they resist changes in their daily routines. The most commonly reported stereotypies with objects include flicking a string, turning light switches on and off, tearing paper into shreds, or turning a toy car over and spinning the wheels rather than rolling it appropriately. Children who are high functioning may become preoccupied with letters or numbers, for example, memorizing license plates on cars. Other children may repeat the same questions over and over again. When efforts are made to change their routines, resistance and tantrums often follow. Objects may be lined up or the same play figures may be used in repetitive ways rather than imaginatively. When high-functioning people do show some ability to pretend, such as feeding a stuffed animal or figurine and putting it to sleep, their play is repetitious and lacks flex-

PEARLS & PERILS

AUTISTIC DISORDER

- PDD indicates disturbed development involving more than one developmental line—there may be some areas of normal functioning. Problems in social awareness and social communication are the common presenting concerns.
- An individual with autistic disorder may have other major psychopathologic conditions in addition to autistic disorder.
- Children with autistic disorder usually have moderate mental retardation; only 15% to 20% test in the normal range.
- Associated seizure disorders primarily occur in people who have both autistic disorder and mental retardation.
- For autistic disorder, a child must demonstrate delays or abnormal functioning before age 3 in social interactions, social communicative language, or symbolic or imaginative play. If symptom onset is after age 3, a diagnosis of atypical autism should be used.
- Atypical autism is most often diagnosed in people who are profoundly retarded.
- The development of useful language before age 5 is a good prognostic sign in autistic disorder.
- In assessing the intelligence of an individual with autistic disorder, particular attention should be paid to the nonverbal IQ. The verbal IQ may be deflated as a result of a language impairment.
- In addressing the social skills of language in children with autistic disorder, the process of interpersonal communication should be emphasized rather than focusing on speech alone.

ibility. The high-functioning, verbal child with autistic disorder may become an expert on a limited number of topics, such as map making or time tables. Once a topic area is mastered, he may perseverate about it and want to speak about it continually.

Natural History

The child with classic autistic disorder may have a period of apparently normal early development; however, in some individuals all elements of the behavioral syndrome can be recognized in the early months of life. These include problems with feeding, lack of responsiveness to others, absent anticipatory gestures, and excessive quietness and cooperativeness.

Prognosis in autistic disorder has been linked to scores on intelligence tests and the acquisition of functional language. Language development at age 5 is a useful marker for later outcome. Although verbal and full-scale IQ scores are considered in evaluating the severity of the disorder, nonverbal IQ scores must also be taken into account. There may be differences of as much as 60 or more IQ points between nonverbal and verbal scores when testing is conducted during the preschool years, nonverbal scores being much higher than verbal scores. During the elementary school years, academic achievement for the high-functioning group may be benefitted by good memory skills. In some instances, there may be excellent word decoding ability (hyperlexia), although reading comprehension is poor. When hyperlexia is not appreciated, reading skills may be overestimated by teachers. In the later school years, academic achievement may decline when abstract reasoning is required and rote memory skills prove inadequate. Consequently, high-functioning individuals with autistic disorder may require special education classes for their learning problems, as well as for social and emotional difficulties. In some cases, high-functioning adolescents with autistic disorder who have been mainstreamed in elementary school must return to special education classes during their high school years. Mild and moderately mentally retarded people with autistic disorder do best in special education classes with teachers who have special training to work with autistic disorder.

Approximately 15% to 20% of children who show autistic behavior in their early years gradually emerge, develop social awareness, and make a limited social adjustment. Yet, they often continue to have unusual and eccentric behaviors as adults. Academic achievement by a high-functioning individual may be limited by his social deficits, difficulty in language comprehension, and poor social judgment. Moderately impaired individuals may work successfully by channeling their special preoccupations and finding jobs that require completion of repetitive tasks. Work settings that require the least interaction with others often prove most successful. Often employers do not appreciate the extent of their limitations in problem-solving and social adjustment, so ongoing contact with professionals as mediators is necessary.

Assessment

The diagnosis of autistic disorder is based on the clinical history, the neuropsychiatric interview, and observational assessment. The history of present illness focuses on characteristics that are typical of children with autistic disorder, namely the extent of sociability, the language level, play, the presence of stereotypies, and abnormal responses to sensory stimuli. The past history focuses on the mother's pregnancy and the child's early developmental milestones. Although symptoms of autistic disorder ordinarily are not linked to perinatal difficulties, the birth history and a history of infections and accidents that may involve the brain must be included in the history. Perinatal problems may affect the onset and the extent of symptoms in a vulnerable person. The family history includes information about other family members with a diagnosis of autistic disorder, other developmental disorders, and specific psychiatric disorders such as mood disorders. Mood disorders have been linked to autistic disorder in some family studies.

The physical examination looks for evidence of specific disorders listed in Box 4-2 that have been associated with autistic behavior, such as tuberous sclerosis and the fragile X syndrome. Neurologic examination emphasizes subtle (soft) signs of impairment.

The mental status examination is primarily observational for younger children. An attempt is made to engage the child in imaginative play and, for verbal children, in conversation. Although the diagnosis may be evident in those who are severely affected, for those who are less severely affected, attention must focus on more subtle difficulties in the child's relatedness and play. Gaze avoidance, difficulty in initiating social communication and sustaining conversations, and problems with joint attention and stereotypies must be assessed.

Among the psychometric instruments available for the assessment of children is the Childhood Autism Rating Scale (CARS), which is made up of 15 scales that distinguish different features of autism. The CARS requires direct observation of the child and identifies mild, moderate, and severe degrees of autistic disorder. The CARS is particularly useful for deriving a descriptive summary of the extent of autistic behavior. It is used in conjunction with diagnostic information from the child's history, and descriptions of behavior at home, in school, and in community settings. For research purposes, the most extensive interview and observation scales are the Autistic Diagnostic Interview

(ADI) and the Autism Diagnostic Observation Schedule (ADOS).

In treatment planning, various members of an interdisciplinary team test the child to plan for appropriate interventions. Psychologic tests and speech and language tests are administered to establish a base line and to clarify the extent of current deficits. Because of speech delays and language deficits, auditory testing may also be required. If the child cannot cooperate in standard behavioral audiometry, then brainstem auditory evoked response measures are conducted. Parents often ask about electrophysiologic studies, neuroimaging investigations, and blood and urine tests to establish a diagnosis. Such tests may be indicated to rule out progressive neurologic disorders or a metabolic disorder; however, only a minority of children with autistic disorder require such extensive testing.

Neuropsychologic Testing

Cognitive impairments result from the neurodevelopmental disorder. The underlying neurobiologic abnormality may involve both higher level cognitive processes and responses to affective stimuli. Specific patterns of cognitive and affective development are recognizable in people with autistic disorder. Uneven profiles on subtests of versions of the Wechsler Intelligence Scale for Children (WISC) and Wechsler Adult Intelligence Scale (WAIS), when contrasted to IQ-matched controls, are commonly found in verbal abstraction, sequencing, visual-spatial skills, and rote memory. Such deficits may be related to impaired language acquisition and social functioning.

Social cognitive functioning has been investigated in people with autistic disorder. The "theory-of-mind" paradigm is used to evaluate the extent of a person's impairments in comprehending others' mental states—in particular understanding others' beliefs—and judging others' knowledge and intentions. Theory of mind refers to the ability of unaffected children to attribute mental states (such as beliefs, desires, and intentions) to themselves and to other people as a way of making sense of and predicting behavior. It is suggested that children construct a theory of the relationship between mental states, the world, and action. Theory-of-mind describes the developmental process whereby the child comes to understand others' minds, or to anticipate what others may be thinking, feeling, or intending. Children who have autistic disorder are sometimes said to be "mind-blind," in that they may lack the ability to put themselves in the place of another person. People with autistic disorder generally also perform poorly on executive function tasks such as the Wisconsin Card-Sorting Test (WCST) and the Tower of Hanoi Test, tests designed to assess the ability to systematically plan actions or respond to novel events.

The lack of social relatedness in autistic disorder may also be linked to an inborn incapacity to recognize and respond to expressions of emotional state in others. Most children with autistic disorder are impaired in attending to and recognizing the expression of basic emotions in others and demonstrate abnormal emotional expression themselves. This may lead to a disturbance of affective contact; that is, there may be a severe disruption in the experience of "interpersonal relations as interpersonal." Affective contact refers to the affective domain where bodily inner coordination and mental inner coordination are linked, and intraindividual forms of expressed bodily feeling are recognized between persons as social experience. Stern has used the term *attunement* to describe these experiences of emotional contact, and Trevarthen refers to them as *intersubjectivity*. Since standard emotion recognition tasks are sensitive to cognitive influences, neuropsychologic tests may not identify emotion recognition deficits. The assessment of emotional responsiveness entails the evaluation of the extent of affective responsivity in a standard interpersonal situation.

Differential Diagnosis

Autistic disorder must be distinguished from other types of PDD. In Asperger's disorder, detection may occur somewhat later; children with this disorder generally have a higher intellectual level, fewer language problems, and less difficulty with communication skills. Age of onset is helpful in distinguishing childhood disintegrative disorder from autistic disorder, since behavior changes become apparent after 2 or more years of clearly normal development in childhood disintegrative disorder. Rett's disorder occurs only in girls. Children with Rett's disorder appear normal in the first months of life, but toward the end of the first year begin to show difficulty, although the diagnosis may not be made until somewhat later. In addition to other forms of PDD, the following diagnoses should be considered in the differential diagnosis: mixed receptive-expressive language disorder; reactive attachment disorder or disinhibited attachment disorder; mental retardation with an associated emotional or behavior disorder; and schizophrenia of unusually early onset.

Treatment

Successful treatment requires knowledge of the clinical features and natural history of autistic disorder, as well as an understanding of the functioning of the autistic nervous system. Treatment programs should be developmentally-based, affectively-oriented, and specifically tailored to remediate known deficits in individual children. Such programs can result in broad and positive changes in development, compensation for areas of deficit, and reduced severity of autistic symptoms.

Rutter suggests four general aims in the treatment of the person with autistic disorder. These include the promotion of cognitive development, language development, social development, and overall learning. In addition to these, behavioral reduction and behavioral enhancement strategies are often necessary, as is the use of pharmacologic interventions. The treatment aims are linked to remediation of particular impairments. Treatment programs must be sensitive to the needs of the child and provide careful guidance to parents. The overall goal of treatment is to foster normal development. In doing so, one must take into account what is known about abnormal development in autistic disorder. Despite the known neurobiologic basis of autistic disorder, intervention may be effective in helping the individual child to compensate for developmental deficits.

The promotion of cognitive development requires the facilitation of active, meaningful experiences. Common problems that require cognitive intervention include: self-isolation, which may be approached through planned periods of interaction; impaired understanding, which necessitates simplified communication; lack of initiative to interact socially, which requires structured direct learning experiences; and specific cognitive deficits, which are specifically addressed with appropriate learning tasks. Reduced cognitive capacity (that is, mental retardation) necessitates direct teaching at the appropriate developmental level.

The deficit in social communication or pragmatic language skills leads to the failure to use language socially. Language development is promoted through planned periods of interaction with the child. Limitations in social reciprocity require interpersonal exercises to enhance joint attention by structuring reciprocal language experiences. Direct teaching is needed to teach the social use of language, as is differential reinforcement of appropriate language use. Interaction should focus on the process of communication (pragmatic language) rather than on speech alone. Direct teaching takes into account the child's level of language comprehension. Pragmatic language teaching emphasizes the child's learning turn-taking and other aspects of social communication. Alternative modes of communication, such as sign language, may be needed in dealing with children with autistic disorder who also have mental retardation.

The promotion of social development involves comforting and pleasurable interpersonal experiences. The therapist must structure social contacts to help the child remain focused on the social exchange. Joint attentional exercises involve the adult's first getting the child's attention and then encouraging the child to gesture or point to what is wanted and then to look back to the adult to communicate interest. A systematic program in social skills as they relate to personal hygiene and personal care is included. Direct teaching of social skills leads to enhanced social competence.

A central problem in promoting overall learning in the child with autistic disorder is the child's difficulty understanding the meaningfulness of events. Comprehension deficits require that the teaching staff carefully monitor learning experiences. In fostering overall learning, helping the child attend to environmental cues is is essential. Children with autistic disorder lack self-direction, so structured learning is essential and learning tasks must be broken down into small steps. Children who have autistic disorder often are over-selective in their choice of activities, and considerable effort may be needed to help them remain on task. Generalization of learning to new situations is particularly important; therefore, the context in which learning takes place must be carefully considered and tasks structured so as to facilitate generalization from one situation to another. Finally, lack of persistence when challenged and negative responses to failure require that, as much as possible, the environment provide error-free learning.

Behavior modification techniques are commonly needed in the treatment of autistic disorder. The application of behavioral techniques must be based on a clear understanding of the nature of the social deficit and consider the types of abnormal behavior that are commonly associated with autistic disorder. Inappropriate use of behavior management techniques without considering the specific characteristics of the autistic nervous system can result in treatment failure or worsening of the person's behavior. Moreover, an effective behavioral program may require that the environment be adapted to the person's deficit rather than expecting the individual with autistic disorder to adapt to an unmodified environment. Since the nature of the autistic deficit makes generalization of targeted behaviors across settings difficult, a stable environmental setting and context is necessary for treatment. When this stable environment is established, it should not be changed unless careful consideration is given to the contingencies that led to improvement of the person's behavior.

Common environmental factors that are problematic for a person with autistic disorder include excessive pressure for social contact, excessive demand for change, or difficulties that result from demands made by staff members who are unfamiliar with the characteristic features of autistic disorder.

Behavior management strategies are most often used to eliminate nonspecific maladaptive behaviors. The first step is a functional analysis of behavior that involves a careful evaluation of circumstances preceding an increase or decrease in the occurrence of a maladaptive behavior. There must also be an analysis of circumstances after the behavior that might be associated with either diminution or prolongation of the behavior. For people with autistic disorder who are severely impaired, operant conditioning procedures are used, whereas for individuals who are less impaired and appreciate behavioral consequences, token reward economies may be used. Operant conditioning is a type of learning in which behaviors are altered by varying and regulating consequences that immediately follow that behavior in time. Operant behaviors may be increased or decreased in frequency depending on the consequences they produce. Token reinforcement is a process in which a desired behavior is immediately followed by the presentation of a generalized conditioned reinforcer (token). These tokens are subsequently exchanged for a variety of backup reinforcers. In any behavioral program, generalization to other settings may be limited. Behavioral programs must be individualized for each child. Identification of reinforcers can be difficult. In using tangible reinforcers, food preferences must be considered. For some children with particular preoccupations (such as spinning objects), their interests can be used as a reinforcer. In other instances, a stereotypy (for example, flicking string) may serve this purpose.

Aggressive behavior and self-injurious behavior are most commonly targeted in behavior management programs. For such disruptive behaviors, avoidance of precipitants, provision of help to establish coping skills, and differential reinforcement may be effective interventions. Differential reinforcement requires feedback to the child, offers rewards for positive behaviors, and withholds rewards when negative behaviors occur. Behavioral approaches to emotional symptoms such as fears include controlled exposure, desensitization, modeling, and the teaching of coping skills.

To be effective, the behavioral treatment must be developmentally oriented, it must recognize and target the specific deficits of an individual child with autistic disorder, and it must place those targeted skills in a meaningful developmental framework. When development is not adequately considered in the formulation of treatment goals, isolated skills may be trained that do not generalize well to other situations or to other skills. A comprehensive approach to treatment emphasizes the individual child's specific deficits and considers symbolic processes, social relationships, and communication. Functional communication training is critical in this regard.

For the older, verbal child who is no longer socially withdrawn but is socially perplexed, a social cognitive approach may be helpful. When mental state concepts can be taught, specific instructions on how to cope in a variety of social situations is given to the person with autistic disorder; in other words, he is taught social survival skills. Difficulties in reading others' intentions (theory of mind) can make the child with autistic disorder the brunt of jokes by peers; the child may not appreciate when he is being teased or deceived by others. Difficulty reading the listener's level of interest in a conversation may lead to boring monologues focused on the limited special interests of a person with autistic disorder. Individuals who have autistic disorder are generally unaware that others do not share their enthusiasm for topics that interest them. Moreover, an inability to anticipate others' responses to one's actions is commonly a problem for people with autistic disorder. Treatment based on the theory-of-mind approach might focus on compensating for and remediating possible insensitivity to others' feelings, the inability to take into account what other people know during a conversation, the inability to read others' intentions, the inability to appreciate the listener's level of interest in one's own conversation directed toward the listener, and the inability to anticipate what others might think of one's actions.

The role of the parent is crucial for any intervention with the child who has autistic disorder; the parent generally acts as a co-therapist and plays an integral role in treatment. Parent counseling begins with clarification of the diagnosis and an explanation of the characteristics of autistic disorder. To effectively participate in a behavior management program, the parents must have acknowledged the extent of the child's handicap and be able to work with their child at the appropriate developmental level. Schopler et al. have provided recommendations for working with parents derived from their experience in their Treatment and Education of Autistic and related Communication handicapped CHildren (TEACCH) program in North Carolina.

Although no specific pharmacologic treatment is available for the core deficits of autistic disorder, particular disorders and behavioral symptoms can be targeted for medication use. Such symptoms include hyperactivity, impulsiveness, inattention, aggression, affective lability, compulsive behavior, self-injurious behavior, psychotic symptoms, and depressive disorder.

Attention-deficit/hyperactivity disorder (ADHD) may be diagnosed in some children and adolescents with autistic disorder. Although the benefits of using stimulants in people who have autistic disorder have been questioned, some children do respond well to stimulants. Moreover, heterocyclic antidepressants may also be useful for attention deficit symptoms in some individuals. Clonidine has also been successfully utilized for ADHD in children who have autistic disorder.

Low-dose neuroleptic treatment may be used to target severe over-activity and aggression, as well as for brief reactive and schizophreniform psychosis. However, caution is needed when using neuroleptics; for example, Malone et al. evaluated 14 children with autistic disorder who developed repeated haloperidol-related dyskinesias while they were participating in a long-term maintenance clinical trial. The dyskinesias were seen most commonly when haloperidol was withdrawn. Autistic disorder is a lifelong condition, and the risk of tardive dyskinesia must be carefully considered, particularly when higher doses of neuroleptics are used. However, neuroleptic medications may be necessary to support a child with severe aggressive symptoms in a school program but should be used on a short-term basis.

Other medications that have been used to treat anxiety and aggression include buspirone and propranolol. Additional trials are needed to clarify their efficacy. Clomipramine has been shown to be superior to placebo and desipramine in reducing anger, compulsive, and ritualistic behavior in patients with autistic disorder. Clomipramine was equal to desipramine, and both drugs were superior to placebo in reducing hyperactivity. These results suggest controlled trials of other serotonin reuptake inhibitors (such as fluoxetine and sertraline) in the treatment of compulsive and ritualistic behavior, since the latter medications have fewer side effects. Mood stabilizers, such as lithium and carbamazepine, have been used to treat mood disorders and aggressive behavior that is related to mood lability. Finally, naltrexone, an opiate antagonist, has been successfully used as an adjunctive treatment for children with autistic disorder; its major effect was on hyperactivity. However, it is less effective than low doses of neuroleptics for target symptoms of aggression and impulsivity. In choosing the use of an opiate antagonist, it is important to consider sensory abnormalities in the child with autistic disorder. Since the opiate receptors are sensory neurotransmitters, caution is needed in their use. Some children have an enhancement of their sensitivity to sound or light as a side effect of the use of naltrexone. Although naltrexone has been used for treatment of self-injurious behavior in people with autistic disorder, results regarding its effectiveness are inconclusive.

Asperger's Disorder

Diagnostic Criteria

Asperger's disorder refers to the presence of social deficits in children and adolescents who have high cognitive functioning and apparently normal early language development. The DSM-IV recommended criteria for Asperger's disorder are listed in Box 4-3, and distinguishing features of Asperger's disorder are shown in Table 4-2.

When considering the inclusion of Asperger's disorder in the DSM-IV classification, some authors suggested that Asperger's disorder is part of an "autistic continuum" and should not be diagnosed as a separate entity. Others suggested that although there may be an autistic continuum, Asperger's disorder is sufficiently discrete to be included as a separate diagnosis. Asperger's disorder is now included as a separate entity in both DSM-IV and ICD-10. Its separate designation allows genetic studies to be carried out and provides a diagnostic category for high-functioning individuals with social deficits (the term *high-functioning autism* may be confusing). Its inclusion allows the diagnosis of school-age children, adolescents, and adults who may not have been recognized earlier. It would be best not to use an eponym to designate a diagnostic category. Kanner's syndrome was used for many years, but now autistic disorder is used. Perhaps in a future classification of social deficit disorders, another designation will be found to avoid the eponym Asperger's disorder.

Prevalence

The general population prevalence of Asperger's disorder is unknown because of the lack of availability of large-scale epidemiologic studies. The disorder appears to be considerably more common in boys than in girls and does not seem to be associated with social class or level of education of the parents. With the inclusion of this category in the diagnostic classification, epidemiologic studies can now be planned to identify its prevalence in the general population.

Etiology

Asperger felt that the syndrome he identified was genetically transmitted and suggested that the characteristic features tended to cluster in families, especially in the fathers of those with the syndrome. In regard to family studies, Ghaziuddin et al. used the ICD-10 criteria and reported the diagnosis of Asperger's disorder in three siblings. In this family study, it was proposed that Asperger's disorder may occur as a distinct clinical entity without overlapping with autistic disorder. This family report and neuropsychologic test findings provide further support for Asperger's disorder being a separate entity. Future genetic studies require more detailed evaluation of other family members, and studies of identical twins are also needed. Cases of Asperger's disorder that are associated with Tourette's disorder, aminoaciduria, and ligamentous laxity have been reported. Moreover, Gillberg found a variety of neurologic abnormalities in 60% of 23 patients with Asperger's disorder. However, Asperger's original emphasis was on an idiopathic form that was not associated with other diagnoses.

DSM-IV DIAGNOSTIC CRITERIA

BOX 4-3 ASPERGER'S DISORDER

A. Qualitative impairment in social interaction, as manifested by at least two of the following:

(1) marked impairment in the use of multiple nonverbal behaviors such as eye-to-eye gaze, facial expression, body postures, and gestures to regulate social interaction
(2) failure to develop peer relationships appropriate to developmental level
(3) a lack of spontaneous seeking to share enjoyment, interests, or achievements with other people (e.g., by a lack of showing, bringing, or pointing out objects of interest to other people)
(4) lack of social or emotional reciprocity

B. Restricted, repetitive and stereotyped patterns of behavior, interests, and activities, as manifested by at least one of the following:

(1) encompassing preoccupation with one or more stereotyped and restricted patterns of interest that is abnormal either in intensity or focus
(2) apparently inflexible adherence to specific, nonfunctional routines or rituals
(3) stereotyped and repetitive motor mannerisms (e.g., hand or finger flapping or twisting, or complex whole-body movements)
(4) persistent preoccupation with parts of objects

C. The disturbance causes clinically significant impairment in social, occupational, or other important areas of functioning.

D. There is no clinically significant general delay in language (e.g., single words used by 2 years, communicative phrases used by age 3 years).

E. There is no clinically significant delay in cognitive development or in the development of age-appropriate self-help skills, adaptive behavior (other than in social interaction), and curiosity about the environment in childhood.

F. Criteria are not met for another specific Pervasive Developmental Disorder or Schizophrenia.

(From American Psychiatric Association: *Diagnostic and statistical manual of mental disorders,* ed 4 [DSM-IV], Washington DC, 1994, American Psychiatric Press.)

Comparison of Autistic Disorder and Asperger's Disorder

Since Asperger's original description of "autistic psychopathy," similarities to autistic disorder have been reported. Although Asperger's disorder shares features with other disorders, including social-emotional learning disability and schizoid personality disorder, it is ordinarily categorized in the PDDs. However, there has been disagreement as to whether some clinical features are sufficiently distinct from high-functioning autistic disorder to justify a different disorder. Yet there are some characteristic differences between the two disorders. Patients with Asperger's disorder score within the normal range on intelligence tests, often have special abilities, first show symptoms in the third year of life, and develop grammatic speech. Asperger believed that the children he described were not as disturbed as those with autistic disorder described by Kanner. The outcome of Asperger's disorder is generally good in contrast to autistic disorder, where a good prognosis is less common and occurs in perhaps 5% to 20% of cases. Gillberg, in reviewing studies of Asperger's disorder, found a reduced capacity for an empathetic understanding of other people and odd, all-absorbing interests. In Asperger's disorder, the early development of attachment may not be quite normal, and there may be some abnormalities in language development. People with Asperger's disorder tend to be clumsy, lack coordination of movement, and may have an awkward gait. Although individuals with autistic disorder may have motor skill difficulties, those with Asperger's disorder tend to show more striking motoric involvement. These abnormalities may be different in degree and distinct from the strikingly deviant social and language development that is observed in autistic disorder.

When the early histories and outcomes of children with Asperger's disorder were contrasted with those of high-functioning children with autistic disorder, the histories of the children with autistic disorder showed

DIAGNOSIS

TABLE 4-2
ASPERGER'S DISORDER

Discriminating feature

1. Qualitative impairment in social interaction and stereotyped behaviors in the absence of delay in cognitive development

Consistent features

1. Absence of a general delay in language
2. Absence of schizophrenia
3. Age-appropriate self-help skills, adaptive behavior, and curiosity about the environment
4. More common in boys than girls

Variable features

1. Impaired use of nonverbal behaviors
2. Failure to develop peer relationships
3. Lack of social or emotional reciprocity
4. Inflexible adherence to rituals or routines
5. Normal intelligence
6. Absence of verbal memory deficits

more impairment in social responsiveness, communication, and greater restriction in the range of activities than those of the individuals with Asperger's disorder.

Assessment

A neuropsychologic distinction between autistic disorder and Asperger's disorder has been suggested based on theory-of-mind deficits found in a group of patients with autistic disorder that were not found in a comparison group with Asperger's disorder. However, the Asperger's disorder group did show abnormality on an emotional perception task. These findings, along with reports of multiple cases of Asperger's disorder in one family and a different natural history, suggest a distinction between Asperger's disorder and autistic disorder.

Individuals with Asperger's disorder, unlike those with autistic disorder, can perform adequately on theory-of-mind tests and do not demonstrate the verbal memory deficits that are found in high-functioning subjects with autistic disorder. The distinction of Asperger's disorder from high-functioning autistic disorder is important in identifying homogeneous subgroups of patients for research studies. In the future, additional research that focuses on whether subjects with autistic disorder and those with Asperger's disorder respond differently to treatment and have different prognoses is needed. Autistic disorder is recognized as a heterogeneous condition with a variety of subtypes.

PEARLS & PERILS

ASPERGER'S DISORDER

- Children with Asperger's disorder score within the normal range on intelligence tests and have a better prognosis than individuals with autistic disorder.
- Individuals with Asperger's disorder usually have more striking motoric involvement than those with autistic disorder.
- Children with Asperger's disorder do not demonstrate the verbal memory deficits found in those with autistic disorder.
- In Asperger's disorder, early language development is normal; stereotyped interests and peer-related problems ordinarily become apparent during the elementary school years, but a child may not be referred to a clinician until he reaches adolescence.

The designation of Asperger's disorder as distinct is important for future epidemiologic and outcome studies.

Treatment

Individuals with social deficits have an increased vulnerability to psychiatric disorders; the lack of recognition of their developmental disorder may complicate their treatment because neurobiologically-based symptoms may be attributed to a psychodynamic cause. The treatment of the social deficit in Asperger's disorder adheres to the same principles outlined for the social cognitive treatment of high-functioning individuals with autistic disorder. Teaching mental state concepts is of particular importance.

Rett's Disorder

Diagnostic Criteria

The inclusion of Rett's disorder among the PDDs has been controversial because of questions regarding the diagnostic validity of Rett's disorder and the suitability of classifying Rett's disorder as a mental disorder rather than a neurologic disorder.

The DSM-IV diagnostic criteria for Rett's disorder are described in Box 4-4, and Table 4-3 shows characteristic features of Rett's disorder.

The neurologic diagnostic criteria are broken down into necessary, supportive, and exclusion criteria. Moreover, the diagnosis is considered to be tentative until a child is 2 to 5 years old. The necessary criteria include apparently normal prenatal and perinatal development and apparently normal psychomotor development during the first 5 to 12 months of life, as well as normal head circumference at birth, but deceleration of head

DSM-IV DIAGNOSTIC CRITERIA

BOX 4-4 RETT'S DISORDER

A. All of the following:

(1) apparently normal prenatal and perinatal development
(2) apparently normal psychomotor development through the first 5 months after birth
(3) normal head circumference at birth

B. Onset of all of the following after the period of normal development:

(1) deceleration of head growth between ages 5 and 48 months
(2) loss of previously acquired purposeful hand skills between ages 5 and 30 months with the subsequent development of stereotyped hand movements (e.g., hand-wringing or hand washing)
(3) loss of social engagement early in the course (although often social interaction develops later)
(4) appearance of poorly coordinated gait or trunk movements
(5) severely impaired expressive and receptive language development with severe psychomotor retardation

(From American Psychiatric Association: *Diagnostic and statistical manual of mental disorders,* ed 4 [DSM-IV], Washington DC, 1994, American Psychiatric Press.)

DIAGNOSIS

TABLE 4-3
RETT'S DISORDER

Discriminating features

1. Normal prenatal and perinatal development and normal psychomotor development in the first 5 to 12 months of life
2. Deterioration in head growth and general functioning after normal development

Consistent features

1. Deceleration in head growth
2. Loss of acquired hand skills
3. Loss of social engagement
4. Poorly coordinated gait or trunk movement
5. Severely impaired expressive and receptive language
6. Absence of any known physiologic cause for symptoms

Variable features

1. Dysfunctional breathing including apnea while awake and intermittent hyperventilation
2. Abnormal EEG
3. Spasticity, dystonia, and peripheral basal motor disturbances
4. Scoliosis
5. Growth retardation
6. Poorly developed, small feet
7. Lack of recovery of lost language
8. Sleep disorders

growth between the ages of 5 months and 4 years. There is a subsequent loss of acquired, purposeful hand skills and speech by 1 to 2 years (range 6 to 30 months). This is followed by the development of stereotypical hand movements, such as hand wringing or squeezing, clapping or tapping, mouthing, and washing or rubbing automatic movements. Between 1 and 4 years, severe mixed receptive-expressive language disorder, severe psychomotor retardation with gait apraxia, and truncal apraxia or ataxia become evident. During this phase, a child with Rett's disorder may lose social interest and become socially withdrawn.

Supportive criteria for Rett's disorder are dysfunctional breathing, (including periodic apnea during wakefulness), intermittent hyperventilation, breath-holding spells, and forced expulsion of air or saliva. EEG abnormalities include a slow waking background and intermittent rhythmic slowing associated with epileptiform discharges, with or without clinical seizures. Clinical seizures occur at some point in the course, as do spasticity (with some muscle wasting), dystonia, and peripheral basal motor disturbances. Scoliosis, growth retardation, and poorly developed, small feet are reported. The diagnosis is possible, particularly in young children, without these supportive criteria.

The exclusion criteria for Rett's disorder include other conditions, such as intrauterine growth retardation, evidence of a metabolic storage disease, retinopathy at birth, evidence of perinatally acquired brain damage, identification of a known metabolic and progressive neurologic disease, and acquired neurologic disorders resulting from severe infections and head trauma. The presence of one or more of these conditions excludes the diagnosis of Rett's disorder.

Prevalence

The incidence of Rett's disorder is between 1:10,000 and 1:12,000 girls, with no confirmed male cases. Rett's disorder occurs in all ethnic groups. The diagnosis is clinical, since no consistent biochemical or physiologic markers have been identified. Although Rett's disorder occurs in girls, female sex is not indicated as a necessary criterion because of the possibility of undiagnosed cases in boys. Deviant development is apparent by 15 months in 50% of reported cases, by 18 months in 80%, and by age 2 in 100% of reported cases.

Etiology

Several genetic hypotheses have been suggested as causes for Rett's disorder. Among them, the most common is that Rett's disorder is an autosomal dominant mutation that is lethal in males. However, Zoghbi et al. suggest the possibility of nonrandom X-chromosome inactivation in putative carriers leading to an X-linked mutation, which is lethal in males. A matrilineal pattern of inheritance has been considered based on a family with affected half-sisters with the same mother and an aunt-niece pair. Although genetic research has focused on the identification and study of translocations in rare familial cases, the majority of Rett's disorder cases are thought to be sporadic.

Comparison of Autistic Disorder and Rett's Disorder

Before international diagnostic criteria for Rett's disorder were firmly established, some cases were initially diagnosed as autistic disorder. However, several reports, using both behavioral observations and family history data, have found both qualitative and quantitative differences between Rett's disorder and autistic disorder. This has led to the conclusion that Rett's disorder is distinguishable from autistic disorder in early life and is a distinct diagnostic entity.

Confusion with autistic disorder has been based on the child's loss of interest in (and lost awareness of) the environment. This symptom develops in the preschool period, primarily during the phase of rapid developmental regression in Rett's disorder. Social withdrawal is one aspect of this regressive phase. Purposeful hand movements are lost, and midline hand stereotypies that have been interpreted as autistic symptoms develop. However, these simple, central hand wringing and hand-to-mouth stereotypies differ from the typical peripheral, complex hand stereotypies seen in autistic disorder. Difficulty initiating voluntary hand movements, involuntary movements, and the extent of developmental retardation further distinguish a girl with Rett's disorder from a child with autistic disorder.

Language may develop in Rett's disorder, and the majority of girls pass through phases of babbling and jargoning, show early social reciprocity in language use, and produce single words. However, any verbal skills acquired are generally lost by 18 months and, unlike autistic disorder, there is no recovery from language loss. In autistic disorder, up to one third of the children with the disorder may use words in the first year, subsequently stop using them, and may later recover language usage.

Accompanying the regressive phase there is a deceleration in head circumference with eventual microcephaly that does not occur in autistic disorder. As the regressive phase concludes, children with Rett's disorder show a prominent gait disturbance. Those who were previously hypotonic show an increase in muscle tone and may develop hypertonia with hyperreflexia; if they walk, it is with a wide-based gait; they may become nonambulatory as early as age 4 and show fluctuations in muscle tone, scoliosis, and a movement disorder. By the third decade of life, 80% of people with Rett's disorder may be nonambulatory. In autistic disorder, ambulation is generally normal, although toe walking may be present in some individuals. Sleep disturbances are common in both autistic disorder and Rett's disorder. Eighty-five percent of girls with Rett's disorder meet diagnostic criteria for a sleep disorder with delayed sleep onset, night waking, and early morning waking.

Assessment

When girls are referred to pervasive developmental clinics because of concerns about behavior problems, behavioral regression or stereotypies, the developmental history generally suggests a diagnosis of Rett's disorder. Referral most often occurs in the second phase

PEARLS & PERILS

RETT'S DISORDER

- The diagnosis of Rett's disorder is considered tentative until a child is 2 to 5 years old.
- There are no confirmed male cases of Rett's disorder; however, female sex is not listed as a necessary criterion for the disorder.
- In Rett's disorder, there is no recovery from the language loss that occurs.
- Rett's disorder may be distinguished from autistic disorder by the presence of microcephaly, significantly impaired ambulation, and diffuse cortical atrophy on MRI.
- Lack of social interest in others, hand-wringing stereotypies, and poor functional hand use in girls suggest Rett's disorder rather than autistic disorder.

of the disease because of social withdrawal, disruptive behavior, screaming, and hand-to-mouth stereotypies. On clinical examination, hyperventilation and a clumsy, ataxic gait may be noted. The child may demonstrate midline hand-wringing stereotypies and bring her hands to her mouth often, but she will generally not bite her fingers. When the girls are placed on the floor, they may demonstrate their lack of purposeful hand movements by rocking into a sitting or standing position without using their hands to push themselves up. Older girls who have passed through the regressive phase may make eye contact and may demonstrate a social smile.

MRI abnormalities involving the cerebellum and other brain regions have been reported in some subjects with autistic disorder, whereas in Rett's disorder, imaging studies show diffuse cortical atrophy.

Childhood Disintegrative Disorder

Diagnostic Criteria

Childhood disintegrative disorder is the DSM-IV category for a syndrome previously known as Heller Syndrome, or disintegrative psychosis. It is a rare condition with distinctive clinical features and a worse prognosis than autistic disorder. The DSM-IV criteria specify the presence of age-appropriate verbal and nonverbal communication, social relationships, play, and adaptive behavior for at least the first 2 years of life. This normal developmental period is followed by a clinically-significant loss of previously acquired skills as shown in Box 4-5 and Table 4-4.

These criteria include the same qualitative impairments noted in autistic disorder: qualitative impairment in social interaction and communication, and restricted, repetitive, and stereotyped patterns of behavior, interest, and activities (including motor stereotypies and mannerisms). However, on examination the clinical presentations of these criteria are different from the way they are in autistic disorder. Other PDDs and childhood onset schizophrenia are exclusionary criteria. The inclusion in DSM-IV of the criteria for autistic disorder in this definition requires further study, since these criteria may be met only during the regressive phase of the disorder.

The DSM-IV description does not emphasize the affective symptoms and anxiety symptoms mentioned by Heller, nor does it highlight the deterioration in self-help skills that has been summarized by Volkmar. As is the case in Rett's disorder, a loss of interest in the environment during the acute, early phases of the disorder should not be confused with the classic lack of social awareness that is characteristic of autistic disorder.

Childhood disintegrative disorder resembles the diagnosis of dementia in adult life, but differs in that there is no evidence of any known neurologic disease or acquired brain damage (although brain dysfunction is usually inferred). There is a loss of skills that may be followed by some degree of recovery, and the early im-

BOX 4-5 CHILDHOOD DISINTEGRATIVE DISORDER

DSM-IV DIAGNOSTIC CRITERIA

A. Apparently normal development for at least the first 2 years after birth as manifested by the presence of age-appropriate verbal and nonverbal communication, social relationships, play, and adaptive behavior.

B. Clinically significant loss of previously acquired skills (before age 10 years) in at least two of the following areas:

(1) expressive or receptive language
(2) social skills or adaptive behavior
(3) bowel or bladder control
(4) play
(5) motor skills

C. Abnormalities of functioning in at least two of the following areas:

(1) qualitative impairment in social interaction (e.g., impairment in nonverbal behaviors, failure to develop peer relationships, lack of social or emotional reciprocity)
(2) qualitative impairments in communication (e.g., delay or lack of spoken language, inability to initiate or sustain a conversation, stereotyped and repetitive use of language, lack of varied make-believe play)

D. The disturbance is not better accounted for by another specific Pervasive Developmental Disorder or by Schizophrenia.

(From American Psychiatric Association: *Diagnostic and statistical manual of mental disorders,* ed 4 [DSM-IV], Washington DC, 1994, American Psychiatric Press.)

pairments in socialization and communication may be similar to autistic disorder and not simply a consequence of a clear-cut intellectual decline.

Clinical Features

Cognitive skills are substantially reduced, and after the onset of the disorder, children most commonly function in the severe-to-profound range of mental retardation. Stereotypical behaviors and unusual responses to the environment may occur.

Prevalence

Population studies on prevalence are not available; however, the condition is rare. Estimates are that it is one tenth as common as autistic disorder. The overall male to female ratio is approximately 4:1, which is similar to the ratio observed in autistic disorder. Although the onset is most commonly reported in the third year of life, the age range for case reports is from 1 to 9 years. The mean age of onset in a series of 76 cases summarized by Volkmar was 3.4 years. The average age of onset is later than the typical age of onset of autistic disorder, although there may be some overlap.

Etiology

An apparent association with neurologic disorders has been noted; however, the etiologic significance of association with another medical condition is not clear. Despite the fact that in a number of instances, life-change events have been reported, psychosocial stressors would not account for the severity and type of deterioration noted. The original description by Heller excluded any known neurologic disorder. Whether there is a genetic cause requires further investigation before making this diagnosis.

DIAGNOSIS

TABLE 4-4

CHILDHOOD DISINTEGRATIVE DISORDER

Discriminating features

1. Normal verbal and nonverbal communication, social relationships, play, and adaptive behavior in the first 2 years
2. Loss of acquired skills in language, adaptive behavior, bowel or bladder control, play, or motor skills before age 10

Consistent features

1. Absence of schizophrenia or another PDD
2. Qualitatively impaired social interactions
3. Qualitative impairment in communication

Variable features

1. Occurs more frequently in boys
2. Limited improvement with maturation
3. Seizure disorder

Natural History

Autistic features may be present at the onset of childhood disintegrative disorder; however, unlike autistic disorder, development is normal for at least the first 2 years of life. Although there may be an associated encephalopathy, the diagnosis is made based on the behavioral presentation. Loss of language and social skills generally occurs over several months, which are followed by a plateau and possible limited improvement with maturation. In some instances, loss of skills is progressive, but this ordinarily is associated with a diagnosable neurologic disorder.

The onset may then vary; some cases are described with an insidious onset over a period of weeks to months, and in other instances there is an abrupt onset of days to weeks. Heller described an early phase during which the child is more active, anxious, negativistic, and restless. The overall course is uniformly one of deterioration, resulting in a lower plateau of development (Table 4-4). The extent of recovery that is possible is unclear, but self-care skills have been restored in some cases. The child must be observed carefully and continually for evidence of a diagnosable, though not yet recognized, progressive neurologic disease. Childhood disintegrative disorder requires continuing care, since impairment persists throughout a person's life. The major neurologic complication is the onset of a seizure disorder.

Assessment

The assessment includes an extensive and detailed family history, with documented evidence of previous developmental milestones. Photographs and videotapes can be used to clarify early developmental milestones. Although examination of the child may be difficult because of behavioral deterioration, a complete physical examination should be carried out. During an evaluation of the child, the phase of the illness is important to consider. In the early phases of the disorder, some communication may be possible, but with continuing regression, language skills may be entirely lost. The extent of the social interactive disturbance may be less severe and pervasive than that seen in classic autistic disorder. With time, it may become apparent that autistic behavior may be linked more to the child's general lack of awareness of the environment than to the specific deficits in social reciprocity ordinarily observed in autistic disorder.

PEARLS & PERILS

CHILDHOOD DISINTEGRATIVE DISORDER

- Childhood disintegrative disorder resembles dementia but is without confirmatory evidence of neurologic disease or acquired brain damage.
- In childhood disintegrative disorder, development is normal in at least the first 2 years of life.
- When treating the child with suspected childhood disintegrative disorder, the physician should be alert to the development of any type of progressive neurologic disease that may explain the symptoms.
- The major neurologic complication in childhood disintegrative disorder is a seizure disorder.
- For the majority of individuals with childhood disintegrative disorder, the course is static.
- In autistic disorder, the age of recognition is commonly between 15 and 18 months; in Rett's disorder at the end of the first year; and in childhood disintegrative disorder after the third year.

Even though the diagnosis of childhood disintegrative disorder has been used for children with known neurologic disorders, this practice is best avoided if the child had previous social and language deficits that fit into the PDD diagnostic category. The older the child is at the time of diagnosis, the more suspicious the physician should be of a diagnosable neurologic disorder; the diagnosis of neurodegenerative diseases in childhood can be difficult. Similar concerns regarding the diagnosis have been raised for autistic disorder, since autistic disorder may be associated with a variety of medical conditions.

Differential Diagnosis

This is a diagnosis of exclusion. Autistic disorder and atypical autism are commonly the first considerations, even though the age of onset is later and the extent of deterioration in function after onset is substantially greater than that observed in children with autistic disorder. Selective mutism may be considered, but with that diagnosis, the child does not show deterioration in speech and language behavior; rather he shows communication skills selectively and only in certain interpersonal contexts.

Treatment

In his review of 76 published cases with follow-up ranging from 1.2 to 22 years, Volkmar found that the course was static for about three quarters of the patients, with minimal improvement noted in a minority. For example, when four of the published studies were combined for the purpose of follow-up statistics, 42% of the children were mute, 38% used single words or phrases, and 19% showed some capacity to speak in sentences. All children required special education services, and placement in residential settings was common. Overall function was in the moderate-to-severe range of mental retardation at follow-up. Treatment programs focus on teaching self-care skills and individualizing the educational program to the child's specific needs.

Summary

Substantial progress has been made since autistic disorder was first recognized 50 years ago; however, much remains to be done. Future research will emphasize classification, genetic aspects, and identification of better diagnostic techniques. The classification system may be modified as we learn more about the neurobiology of social cognition and developmental disorders that result in dementia-like illnesses in childhood. A future classification might include disorders of social communication and distinguish them from disorders that are pervasive but do not include autistic features throughout their course. Future classifications will benefit from outcome data on the natural history of each of the currently classified PDDs.

Better characterization of cases is essential to conduct genetic studies. For example, in autistic disorder, there seems to be a broad phenotype of social communication deficits that may include social-emotional learning disorders in siblings. This broad behavioral phenotype requires further exploration. There is considerable interest in the genetics of Asperger's disorder, but better delineation of the phenotype is required. For Rett's disorder, genetic research is under way. Continuing research is needed to establish the validity of childhood disintegrative disorder before proceeding with genetic studies.

Genetic studies will be benefitted by a better understanding of the biologic bases and identification of the underlying pathophysiologic mechanisms involved in each of these disorders. Advances in neuroimaging, particularly in MRI and functional PET scanning, and new developments in basic neuroscience may eventually provide better understanding of these perplexing conditions.

CONSIDER CONSULTATION WHEN . . .

- The diagnosis of the type of PDD is not clear
- There is a deterioration in functioning that follows a prolonged period of normal development
- Specific conditions that may be associated with the disorder, such as aggression or seizures, are not controllable with standard medical and behavioral interventions
- The child does not respond as expected to typical medical interventions
- Restrictive interventions such as hospitalization become necessary
- Psychotic symptoms are suspected or become apparent in older affected children

Annotated Bibliography

Frith U: *Autism and Asperger syndrome,* New York, 1991, Cambridge University Press.

This is an edited volume by Uta Frith that addresses the question of whether Asperger's disorder is a disorder in its own right or a form of autism. Although similar to autistic disorder, children with Asperger's disorder are more verbally articulate and socially adapted. This volume contains the first English translation of Asperger's orginal paper. Both clinical aspects and neurobiologic aspects of Asperger's disorder are considered. There is a discussion of the autobiographical writings of three adults with Asperger's disorder and their implications for theory. One chapter is devoted to living with Asperger's disorder.

Happe F et al: Is autism a pervasive developmental disorder? Debate and argument: how useful is the PDD label? *J Child Psychol Psychiatry* 7:1167-1172. 1991.

This debate discusses the origins of the term *pervasive developmental disorder* and its utility as a diagnostic term. What should be included under this designation? Should the designation PDD be abandoned? Discussants are from the United Kingdom, Sweden, and the United States.

Kanner L: Autistic disturbances of affective contact, *The Nervous Child* 2:217-250, 1943.

This is the original papar that described the syndrome that subsequently became known as infantile autism. It is a paper rich in description, and 60 years after its publication it is still current and is still stimulating new research.

Moser H: Rett Syndrome *Am J Med Gene* (Suppl 1) 1986.

In 1986 an international workshop on Rett's disorder was held at the Kennedy Institute, Johns Hopkins University. This special issue of the *Journal* includes 39 papers on Rett's disorder and provides a comprehensive overview. Dr. Andreas Rett provides a history and general overview of Rett's disorder.

Rogers SJ Pennington, BF: A theoretical approach to the deficits in infantile autism, *Dev Psychopathol* 3:137-162, 1991.

This article reviews several theoretical approaches to understanding autistic disorder, including (1) the metarepresentational theory of Frith, Leslie, and Baron-Cohen (Baron-Cohen, 1988); (2) the emotion theory of Hobson (Baron-Cohen, 1988); and (3) the intersubjectivity theory (Rogers & Pennington, 1991). References are provided to each of these theoretical approaches.

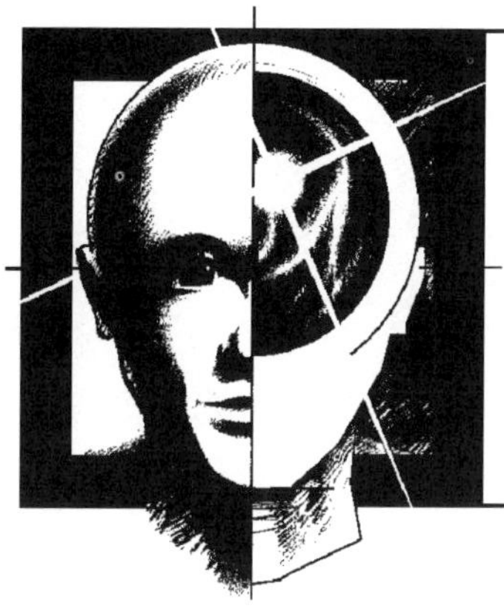

chapter 5

Attention-Deficit/ Hyperactivity Disorder

John Diamond, MD and Åke Mattsson, MD

Diagnostic Criteria
Clinical Features
Differential Diagnosis
Assessment
Treatment
Summary

Attention-deficit/hyperactivity disorder (ADHD) has been recognized as such a prevalent condition that it has generated considerable public interest. From demonstrations at psychiatric meetings by religious groups concerned about over-medication to the formation of parents' support networks such as Children with Attention Deficit Disorder (CHADD), the syndrome has received coverage in network news and in major news magazines. The clinical recognition that adolescents may have residual features and that even adults experience symptoms of ADHD makes it imperative that all physicians understand the nuances of treating this widespread disorder.

Descriptions of ADHD date back more than 100 years. By the First World War, it was observed that whereas adults suffering sequelae of von Economo's encephalitis manifested symptoms of Parkinson's disease, children with the same disorder developed a hyperkinetic behavioral syndrome. From this, it seemed clear there was an association between brain disease and behavioral pathologic abnormalities. An association between complications of pregnancy and a range of neurologic sequelae led to new postulates. Whereas severe brain damage led to overt neurologic disease, mild damage seemed to create a predisposition towards behavioral difficulties. The recognition that many children with mental retardation also showed hyperactive behavior led further to the supposition that if a child has excessive motor activity, there must be some component of brain damage. This was encapsulated in the concept of minimal brain damage (MBD). The term began to lose meaning in the 1960s when it was understood that hyperactive behavior could occur in the absence of organicity. However, the notion that subclinical brain damage can lead to behavioral disturbances is not entirely fallacious.

It was in 1980 that the DSM-III conceptualized a syndrome with deficits in attention: attention deficit disorder with hyperactivity. This new thinking arose from an appreciation that key factors in this disorder included

DSM-IV DIAGNOSTIC CRITERIA

BOX 5-1 ATTENTION-DEFICIT/HYPERACTIVITY DISORDER

A. Either (1) or (2):

(1) six (or more) of the following symptoms of **inattention** have persisted for least 6 months to a degree that is maladaptive and inconsistent with developmental level:

Inattention

(a) often fails to give close attention to details or makes careless mistakes in schoolwork, work, or other activities
(b) often has difficulty sustaining attention in tasks or play activities
(c) often does not seem to listen when spoken to directly
(d) often does not follow through on instructions and fails to finish schoolwork, chores, or duties in the workplace (not due to oppositional behavior or failure to understand instructions)
(e) often has difficulty organizing tasks and activities
(f) often avoids, dislikes, or is reluctant to engage in tasks that require sustained mental effort (such as schoolwork or homework)
(g) often loses things necessary for tasks or activities (e.g., toys, school assignments, pencils, books, or tools)
(h) is often easily distracted by extraneous stimuli
(i) is often forgetful in daily activities

(2) six (or more) of the following symptoms of **hyperactivity-impulsivity** have persisted for at least 6 months to a degree that is maladaptive and inconsistent with developmental level:

Hyperactivity

(a) often fidgets with hands or feet or squirms in seat
(b) often leaves seat in classroom or in other situations in which remaining seated is expected
(c) often runs about or climbs excessively in situations in which it is inappropriate (in adolescents or adults, may be limited to subjective feelings of restlessness)
(d) often has difficulty playing or engaging in leisure activities quietly
(e) is often "on the go" or often acts as if "driven by a motor"
(f) often talks excessively

Impulsivity

(g) often blurts out answers before questions have been completed
(h) often has difficulty awaiting turn
(i) often interrupts or intrudes on others (e.g., butts into conversations or games)

B. Some hyperactive-impulsive or inattentive symptoms that caused impairment were present before age 7 years.

C. Some impairment from the symptoms is present in two or more settings (e.g., at school [or work] and at home).

D. There must be clear evidence of clinically significant impairment in social, academic, or occupational functioning.

E. The symptoms do not occur exclusively during the course of a Pervasive Developmental Disorder, Schizophrenia, or other Psychotic Disorder and are not better accounted for by another mental disorder (e.g., Mood Disorder, Anxiety Disorder, Dissociative Disorder, or a Personality Disorder).

Attention-Deficit/Hyperactivity Disorder, Combined Type: if both Criteria A1 and A2 are met for the past 6 months.
Attention-Deficit/Hyperactivity Disorder, Predominantly Inattentive Type: if Criterion A1 is met but Criterion A2 is not met for the past 6 months.
Attention-Deficit/Hyperactivity Disorder, Predominantly Hyperactive-Impulsive Type: if Criterion A2 is met but Criterion A1 is not met for the past 6 months.

Coding note: For individuals (especially adolescents and adults) who currently have symptoms that no longer meet full criteria, "In Partial Remission" should be specified.

(From American Psychiatric Association: *Diagnostic and statistical manual of mental disorders,* ed 4 [DSM-IV] Washington DC, 1994, American Psychiatric Press.)

DIAGNOSIS

TABLE 5-1

ATTENTION-DEFICIT/ HYPERACTIVITY DISORDER

Discriminating feature

1. Significant inattention and hyperactivity-impulsivity before age 7

Consistent features

1. Occurs in two or more settings
2. Impaired social and academic functioning
3. Absence of psychotic illness
4. Absence of PDD
5. Absence of mood or anxiety disorder
6. Absence of dissociative or personality disorder
7. Absence of physiologic condition to explain symptoms

Variable features

1. Occurs more frequently in boys
2. Aggression
3. Family history of ADHD
4. Hypoperfusion of frontal lobes and striatum on PET scan
5. Abnormal quantitative EEG
6. Concomitant ODD or CD
7. Concomitant depressive disorder

PEARLS & PERILS

DIAGNOSIS OF ATTENTION-DEFICIT/ HYPERACTIVITY DISORDER

- The symptoms of ADHD must be present in at least two settings to make the diagnosis (for example, home and school).
- Symptom onset must be before age 7. If symptoms start later, consider an alternative diagnosis.
- Although the diagnosis may be made if symptoms occur any time before age 7, the diagnosis is most reliable when symptoms can be dated back to toddlerhood.
- The presence of anxiety or depression may suggest impaired attention or concentration related to a mood disorder or may be indicative of ADHDIT.

inattention and impulsivity, as well as hyperactivity. Furthermore, there was also a description of a syndrome without the presence of excessive motor activity: attention deficit disorder without hyperactivity.

ADHD, as it is known today, is a common childhood psychiatric condition. Improvements in the diagnostic criteria have led to a greater number of referrals to family physicians, pediatricians, and general and child psychiatrists.

Diagnostic Criteria

The essential features of the disorder continue to include the triad of inattention, impulsivity, and hyperactivity (Box 5-1, Table 5-1). However, this triad of behaviors has been modified from the original DSM-III criteria, with the DSM-IV criteria grouping hyperactivity and impulsivity together. Thus there are three subtypes: the predominantly hyperactive-impulsive type, the predominantly inattentive type, and the combined type. For purposes of clarity in this chapter, ADHD refers to the combined type, and ADHDIT refers to the predominantly inattentive type. There are too little data on the unique predominantly hyperactive-impulsive type for further discussion.

DSM-IV criteria indicate that symptoms are required to be present in two or more settings. This is important because the disorder is pervasive, and in the past it was probably over-diagnosed on the basis of symptoms appearing in only one setting. DSM-IV requires that the symptoms are manifested in both home and school situations.

The DSM-IV criteria pose a problem in the approach to dating the onset of symptoms. Symptoms are required to be present for at least 6 months, with onset before age 7. Therefore a child could have the first symptoms as late as age 6, and the diagnosis could be made by age 6½. This is counter-intuitive to clinical observations that show a developmental factor for the disorder, and it makes the cut-off at age 7 appear arbitrary. The diagnosis is much stronger when it is possible to document symptoms as early as toddlerhood.

There is a growing literature on the ADHDIT subgroup. Children in this group show more anxiety and more evidence of co-morbid internalizing disorders such as anxiety or depression. These children also show a more lethargic tempo, even drowsiness at times, as well as more learning problems and an older age at the time of referral. This has led to the notion that this syndrome is a unique disorder rather than a subtype of ADHD.

Clinical Features

The DSM-IV is a common source for prevalence data and cites an incidence of 3% to 5% for ADHD in school-age children. ADHD is generally reported to be more common in boys than in girls, with ratios ranging from 4:1 to 9:1. It is possible that this male bias is artifactual. On standardized behavior ratings, fewer symptoms are observed in girls. Boys with ADHD are typically more aggressive than girls. Thus boys tend to be referred more often for evaluation.

Biochemical findings have shown that girls also differ from boys because they have fewer central dopamine metabolites and greater amounts of serotonin metabolites. This suggests that girls have relatively more mature or modulated CNS functioning.

It has only been recently that prevalences have been reported to be similar in Europe and North America. For years the British held a stricter, organic definition for the disorder and placed much more emphasis on the need for pervasive symptoms. Now, similar prevalence data is even available from China.

Multiple theories have been advanced to explain the cause of ADHD. ADHD is more common among the first-degree biologic relatives and siblings of affected children than in normal boys and girls or youth with other types of psychiatric disorders. Although no single genetic marker has been found, early studies investigating parents of children with ADHD suggest a tendency for genetic transmission, and also note a greater prevalence of hysteria, sociopathy, and alcoholism in the families of identified children. The prevalence rate for ADHD in nonbiologic relatives of adopted children with ADHD is no different from a control group; this fact adds greater credence to the concept of a strong genetic contribution to the disorder. Furthermore, the increased risk of ADHD in relatives cannot be accounted for solely on the basis of gender, social class, or intactness of the family. Finally, studies of identical and fraternal twins suggest that genetic factors influence both behavioral and attentional aspects of ADHD.

There is conflicting evidence suggesting the brain-based nature of ADHD. Zametkin reviewed the numerous studies examining monoamines and their metabolites in urine, plasma, platelets, and cerebrospinal fluid. Most of these studies have not demonstrated differences between children with ADHD and children in control groups. It may be that peripheral measures of neurotransmitter metabolites are not reflecting central values. These studies may also be confounded by diagnostic heterogeneity, since children with ADHD and subtypes of CD may have alterations in dopamine-β-hydroxylase activity. Dopamine-β-hydoxylase is the enzyme responsible for converting dopamine to norepinephrine in the catecholamine synthetic pathway.

Animal studies have provided strong evidence suggesting perturbations of dopaminergic mechanisms. Rat pups depleted of brain dopamine are more active than control rats until puberty, when the activity diminishes. However, residual cognitive difficulties in maze tasks persists. This phenomena is attenuated with administration of stimulants.

In children, drugs that treat ADHD such as tricyclic antidepressants or monoamine oxidase inhibitors (MAOIs) often induce changes in noradrenergic metabolism. This suggests a noradrenergic role in the cause of ADHD.

A serotoninergic role seems plausible based on the inhibitory and sedating features of the serotoninergic system. Although this has been encouraged by anecdotal reports suggesting therapeutic efficacy for buspirone, the theory is not well substantiated. Trials with L-tryptophan, which increases serotonin levels, and fenfluramine, which decreases serotonin levels, have been unimpressive. However, there is evidence that aggressive and nonaggressive children with ADHD differ in central serotonin functioning, with aggressive children who have ADHD having significantly lower levels of this neurotransmitter than nonaggressive youth with ADHD or unaffected boys and girls. This suggests that the serotoninergic agents may well be treating comorbid conduct disorder (CD).

Most neuroanatomic and neurophysiologic studies of individuals with ADHD implicate hypoperfusion, and by inference, low metabolic activity in the white matter of the frontal lobes and in the striatum. This has been demonstrated both with PET scans on adults with hyperactivity that began in childhood and with ^{133}Xe inhalation studies in children with ADHD. However in another PET study, methylphenidate did not effect regional metabolism despite a robust clinical effect. Furthermore, the finding of reduced cerebral glucose metabolism on PET scans was not replicated in a group of adolescents with ADHD.

MRI has also been used in the attempt to localize anatomic deficits. There is evidence of abnormal frontal lobe development and a reversal in asymmetry of the head of the caudate nucleus in children with ADHD.

There are few electrophysiologic studies that focus on ADHD; most research includes a mixed group of children with MBD and learning disorders. Studies on children with MBD have found generally that the most

PEARLS & PERILS

POSSIBLE CAUSES OF ATTENTION-DEFICIT/HYPERACTIVITY DISORDER

- Structural and functional studies of the brains of children with ADHD have implicated dysfunction in the frontal lobes.
- It is likely that multiple CNS neurotransmitters are involved in the development of ADHD symptoms.
- High lead levels are associated with hyperactivity.
- Overall, there is little evidence that artificial food additives cause hyperactivity. However, diet control may occasionally be efficacious.

common abnormality was an excessive amount of slow wave activity. Other abnormalities reported include decreased alpha attenuation, absence of well-organized alpha waves, or smaller amounts of beta waves. The advent of computerized analysis of EEG, called quantitative EEG (QEEG), has begun to substantiate the early literature associating EEG abnormalities with psychiatric disorders. A QEEG study of children with ADHDIT found increases in slow-wave theta activity along with a lack of fast-wave beta activity during tasks that require focusing and concentration. This slow-wave activity was more prevalent in the frontal leads, lending support to the imaging studies. Another study on children with ADHD also found slow-wave activity, but it was associated with corresponding lesser amounts of alpha waves; the slowing was prominent occipitally. The finding of excessive theta activity has been suggested as a diagnostic marker, but this was not replicated in a subsequent study.

It has also been noted that subjects who are hyperactive have EEG abnormalities associated with their cortical evoked potentials. The abnormalities range from longer latencies and lower amplitudes for auditory evoked potentials to amplitudes and latencies that increase as visual stimuli increase in intensity. In contrast, other studies have failed to replicate evoked potential abnormalities. This is still an area of active investigation, but it has already provided further evidence for involvement of the frontal lobes.

Several toxins have been reported to impair brain function, leading to symptoms of ADHD. Lead toxicity is the most widely discussed environmental toxin. Although lead toxicity may cause inattention and hyperactivity, aggressive and antisocial behaviors have also been found to be related to high levels of lead in the blood. Serum zinc levels have been cited as low in hyperactive children, whereas high levels of hair zinc may be predictive of stimulant response.

Perhaps one of the most well-publicized and controversial issues is that of dietary intolerance or allergy leading to hyperactivity. This was popularized by the Feingold Diet, which eliminated artificial food additives. Several studies followed to refute the hypothesis about artificial additives. Yet a number of subjects within these studies showed rather robust responses to the diets, suggesting possible efficacy for some children. A study of children without ADHD showed that attention and motor behavior are quite sensitive to nutritional effects. Further studies continue to suggest some efficacy for dietary manipulation in children with ADHD, and especially among children with allergies.

Traditional conceptions of ADHD include the belief that symptoms remit by adolescence. This was supported by the concept that stimulant medication has a paradoxical effect in children that reverses by puberty. However, numerous prospective controlled reports have shown that symptoms persist into adolescence and adulthood. These follow-up studies indicate that between one third and one half of all children with ADHD continue to be impaired in adolescence. Two important caveats emerge from these studies. First, co-morbid CD indicates a worse outcome and seems largely responsible for the higher rate of antisocial behavior in patients with continued ADHD. Additionally, the greater prevalence of substance abuse in adolescents with ADHD is of concern. This is consistent with the expected co-morbidity between CD and substance-related disorders. In one study, subjects with pure ADHD showed no higher rates of substance use compared with control subjects, whereas the subjects with ADHD and CD had rates two to three times higher.

There are some optimistic outcomes. Although the work status and work record of adults who are hyperactive may be inferior to unaffected adults, the rate of full-time employment and self-sufficiency is similar. There is little evidence that children who are hyperactive are at an increased risk for adult mood or anxiety disorders.

A difficulty with the interpretation of longitudinal studies on children with ADHD is the confound of treatment intervention. Most of the attention given to treatment as a predictive outcome variable has focused on stimulant drug treatment. In fact, duration of other mental health interventions has been negatively correlated with outcome. One likely explanation is that treatment duration serves as a marker for severity of illness. Nonetheless, it appears that psychotherapeutic interventions have not been predictive of long-term outcome for hyperactive children.

Long-term outcome studies of stimulant treatment note greater differences between stimulant-treated subjects with ADHD and control subjects than between treated and untreated subjects with ADHD. Stimulant-treated subjects who were hyperactive fared better than their untreated counterparts by experiencing

PEARLS & PERILS

PROGNOSIS

- About ⅓ to ½ of children with ADHD continue to be impaired as adolescents.
- The presence of co-morbid CD with ADHD indicates the worst prognosis, including the likelihood of substance abuse.
- There is little evidence that children with ADHD are any more prone to mood or anxiety disorders in adulthood than are other boys and girls.

fewer car accidents, viewing their childhood more positively, stealing less in elementary school, and achieving better social skills and self-esteem. Stimulant treatment was not found to have deleterious physical effects, and probably decreases early social ostracism, thereby promoting a more positive outlook and self-image.

Outcome studies that show little benefit from treatment may lead to the conclusion that efforts placed on medicating these children is of little long-term consequence. This defies clinical observation and may well be a methodologic artifact. Longitudinal studies have not examined the adequacy of stimulant dosing in each subject; nor have they studied such variables as age at stimulant initiation and whether the medication was administered 2 or 3 times per day, 5 or 7 days per week, or 10 or 12 months of the year. For positive drug effects to generalize, it may be necessary to administer medication continuously. This procedure has not yet gained universal acceptance.

Differential Diagnosis

The diagnosis of ADHD is easier to make when parents recognize the disturbed behaviors early and bring their child for evaluation, and when teachers or daycare workers corroborate the signs. However, as noted in DSM-IV, one must be cautious when the children are from inadequate, disorganized, or chaotic home environments. Presumably these children have difficulty with goal-directed behavior because of these environmental factors. No research has demonstrated that ADHD can be a sequela of poorly organized family environments. Nonetheless we have experienced numerous clinical situations in which children from these environments were placed in structured group homes with one of two outcomes. In the first, medication that was judged ineffective in an outpatient clinic demonstrated efficacy in the structured environment. This scenario presumes that the chaotic environment exacerbated symptoms. In the second outcome, the symptoms of ADHD disappeared. It seems that the severity of oppositional defiant disorder (ODD) and CD symptoms render it difficult to differentiate them from ADHD symptoms. In the structured environment of a group home, these diagnostic entities are better delineated.

The disruptive behavior disorders include ADHD, CD, and ODD. These disorders coexist so often that they are viewed as related or overlapping syndromes. Parent and teacher ratings of the symptoms of these disorders show high intercorrelations. The essential feature of ODD is a recurring pattern of negativistic, hostile, and defiant behavior. The essential feature of CD is a persistent behavior pattern in which a child violates the basic rights of others, as well as major age-appropriate societal norms or rules. There seems to be consensus that ADHD is an early-onset disorder of cognitive or neuromaturational development, whereas ODD and CD reflect problems associated with temperamental factors, and family and social adversities. Thus if ADHD occurs in the presence of severe psychosocial stress, the risk for subsequent co-morbid ODD and CD increases.

Many children with pervasive developmental disorders (PDDs) such as autistic disorder show behaviors that include hyperactivity, impulsivity, and inattention. The custom in DSM-III and DSM-IV has been not to diagnose ADHD in the presence of a PDD. This is based on the notion that applying the diagnosis of ADHD adds little to the management of these patients. However, a diagnosis of ADHD is allowed in the presence of mental retardation.

Assessment

ADHD is a disorder in which others experience the behavior as a problem more than the individual complains of subjective distress. Thus it is known as an externalizing disorder, and the diagnosis rests primarily on gathering information from caretakers. There are no laboratory measures or tests that are pathognomonic for the diagnosis. A careful history from the parent is usually sufficient to judge whether the presenting behavior meets the DSM-IV criteria. However, this method alone is likely to yield significant overdiagnosis. The criteria provide no standards for "developmentally inappropriate" degrees of hyperactive, distractible, or impulsive behavior. Several additional criteria have been suggested as clinically useful for identifying a core group of children with ADHD. These criteria are shown in Box 5-2.

A thorough developmental history also adds information to support a longitudinal presence for the symptoms. Parents often report that children learned to run before they walked. As toddlers, such children may have

BOX 5-2

SUGGESTED ADDITIONAL CRITERIA FOR ATTENTION-DEFICIT/ HYPERACTIVITY DISORDER

- Scores 1.5 standard deviations above the mean on standardized behavior rating scales, such as the Conners Rating Scale, completed by both parents and teachers
- Scores 1.5 standard deviations above the mean score for children of the same developmental age if the IQ is estimated to be below 80
- Symptom duration of 12 months
- Pervasiveness of behavior across multiple settings and across multiple activities within these settings

been unable to sit still for a haircut or to remain seated in a shopping cart. A parent may state that it's almost as if he needed a leash to keep up with his child at the shopping mall. Information about the child's behavior with babysitters, with relatives, and in preschool can be invaluable in documenting this early history.

Factor analytic studies on the Wechsler Intelligence Scale for Children-Revised (WISC-R) have described a freedom-from-distractibility factor consisting of the Arithmetic, Digit Span, and Coding subtests. A similar factor consisting of the Arithmetic and Digit Span subtests has been described for the more recent WISC-III. There is widespread belief that low scores on the freedom-from-distractibility factor are suggestive of ADHD. However there have been no consistent findings to support this factor as a diagnostic entity.

The continuous-performance tests are often used as diagnostic tools. They typically involve a 15- or 20-minute task during which the subject must respond or inhibit response to a specific signal. Measured variables include errors of omission, errors of commission, and response time, as well as more sophisticated statistical computations. These tests are plagued by the problem of establishing validity in the absence of a solid diagnostic benchmark. Their diagnostic utility is far from clear, and it remains difficult to establish an unequivocal national or international standard for the classification of ADHD. The continuous performance tests are more helpful in providing adjunctive information on vigilance and impulsivity, and they may have utility in monitoring treatment response.

There is a host of standardized behavioral rating scales used in the assessment of children with ADHD. Perhaps the most widely known are the Conners Rating Scales. These are symptom checklists with a 4-point rating format for symptom severity. There are two common versions: 93- and 48-item parent rating scales (PQ-93 and PQ-48), and 39- and 28-item teacher rating scales (TQ-39 and TQ-28). Several factors may be derived from the scales, but the Hyperactivity Index (HI) is most commonly used to assess and monitor hyperactive behavior. The HI score is derived by adding up and averaging the Likert ratings for all of the variables that address hyperactivity and then comparing this number with age-appropriate norms. The TQ-39 has shown high discriminant validity in differentiating children who are hyperactive from their peers. The Conners Rating Scales have also effectively discriminated between children with ADHD, specific learning disorders, and matched normal controls. The PQ-93 outperformed all other methods.

A criticism of rating scales is their tendency towards unidirectionality with regard to change, measuring only undesirable behavior. Some children can become "overfocused" on stimulants, which may not be detectable with the scales. Other scales may help determine whether improved behavior has an associated cost of reduced academic efficiency.

PEARLS & PERILS

ASSESSMENT OF ATTENTION-DEFICIT/ HYPERACTIVITY DISORDER

- It is essential that the home environment be assessed when a child has symptoms of ADHD, since a chaotic domestic setting may exacerbate these types of symptoms and increase the risk for ODD and CD.
- Low scores on the Arithmetic, Digit Span, and Coding subtests of the WISC-R are suggestive of distractibility.
- Routinely obtaining a serum lead level is not cost effective, since today it is highly unlikely to find lead ingestion as a cause of hyperactivity. A lead level should only be obtained if the child is at high risk for intoxication (for example, if the child lives in a home painted with lead-based paint).
- The prevalence of generalized resistance to thyroid hormone as a cause of ADHD symptoms is so small that routinely obtaining thyroid studies on symptomatic children is not cost effective.

There are many rating scales available. However, more important than the choice of a particular instrument is familiarity with the clinical use of some instrument to assess medication response in the home, as well as academically and behaviorally in the classroom.

The two laboratory tests commonly associated with ADHD are serum-lead-level and thyroid-stimulating-hormone assays. It is fairly well established that lead ingestion can result in hyperactivity and inattention. However, a clinical population of children with ADHD shows little if any body-lead elevations, and it is unlikely that lead is a significant cause of the disorder.

Symptoms suggestive of ADHD have also been reported in patients with generalized resistance to thyroid hormone. The presence and severity of ADHD was examined in 18 families with a history of thyroid hormone resistance. ADHD was strongly associated with generalized resistance to thyroid hormone. Subsequently a prospective screening for thyroid abnormalities in 277 children with ADHD found no generalized resistance to thyroid hormone. This study did conclude that the prevalence of thyroid abnormalities was higher (5.4%) in children with ADHD than in a general pediatric population. Finally, thyroid indexes were measured in another group of children with ADHD and in a control group. Again, none of the measures suggested thyroid resistance. One may conclude that generalized resistance to thyroid hormone is rare, and thyroid functions should not be measured routinely in individuals with nonfamilial ADHD.

Treatment

The treatment of ADHD is generally conceptualized as multimodal. Multimodal treatment has been defined as a systematic evaluation of subjects from a multidimensional viewpoint, the formulation of a treatment plan to meet the individual needs of each child and family, and the delivery of services within a single clinical setting. There are many reasons for this approach. A primary reason is the recognition that ADHD is a disorder with far-reaching consequences in all areas of a child's life. Any single intervention is unlikely to make an impact on all of the impaired areas of functioning. For example, the incidence of juvenile delinquency is greater in a group receiving only drug treatment compared with a group receiving multimodality treatment. Furthermore, improved behavior when a child is taking medication ceases when the medication is discontinued.

The major interventions have been conceptualized as pharmacologic, behavioral (including contingency management and parent training), and cognitive-behavioral therapies. It is important to add educational interventions. Unfortunately, with the exception of pharmacotherapy, the notions of treatment efficacy far outweigh the empirical data.

Parent Training

Although stimulant therapy can lead to improvements in behavior for many children with ADHD, up to 30% of the school-age population may not show a favorable response. Thus alternative treatment approaches such as parent training take on much added significance. Parent training has been used as a treatment option for those parents with antimedication preferences. Additionally, many problems exhibited by ADHD children are beyond the core symptoms and more related to the co-morbid difficulties of CD or ODD.

Parent training for ADHD has not been extensively researched. However, several studies have demonstrated efficacy in this population. Overall, parent training seems more effective in improving parent coping skills and decreasing noncompliant behavior than in improving core symptoms of ADHD.

A prototypic program has been described by Patterson. A basic premise is that positive reinforcement is a powerful agent of change. Parents are taught the principles of positive reinforcement, and how to ignore negative behaviors. A functional behavioral analysis is applied to the negative behaviors, so specific behaviors are pinpointed and their frequencies tracked. "Time out" is utilized as a basic method of consequence. In this context, parents learn to set up a reward-oriented token system as part of a contract with their child. This type of program can be taught in a group format, but it can be better individualized by working with one family at a time. The evidence that parent training improves the child's compliance is stronger than any effect it has in positively changing measures of attention.

Cognitive-Behavioral Therapy

Even when compliance with parental requests improves, children with ADHD still suffer from a myriad of difficulties involving social skills. From poor peer relations and aggression to inadequate self-regulation, these problems have been recognized as indicators of a poor prognosis. Cognitive behavioral therapy seems appropriate to target the impulsivity of the child with ADHD. It emphasizes problem solving, as well as anticipation and consequences of action. This treatment can be administered individually or in groups. It is sometimes conceptualized as social skills training, because the child is learning how to inhibit behavior, recognize social cues, and determine an appropriate social course of action. However, treatment effects have not been robust and few studies find social skills training superior to medication. But some studies have shown that cognitive behavioral therapy and social skills training supplement the effects of medication.

Educational Interventions

In 1991 the U.S. Education Department issued a policy memorandum recognizing children with ADHD as eligible for special education services on the basis of Public Law 94-142, Individuals with Disabilities Act, Part B ("other health impaired statutes"), and Section 504 of the 1973 Rehabilitation Act. Under Section 504, a person with disabilities is defined as any person who has a physical or mental impairment that substantially limits a major life activity (such as learning). It depends on the severity of ADHD whether a particular child fits the definition. However, understanding this policy is critical to ensuring that children are appropriately served in the public schools.

Teacher-administered consequences are the most commonly used classroom interventions. These usually take the form of positive teacher attention or token rewards. Negative consequences range from ignoring behavior and verbal reprimands to the use of time out. Concerns in the classroom are two-fold. There are needs for behavioral control as well as for academic achievement. A comprehensive review found that overall, behavioral interventions are superior to medication in specifically enhancing academic performance. However, combined effects are particularly powerful in modifying classroom behavior. Additionally, behavioral interventions can decrease the dose of stimulant medication required to improve classroom behavior and short-term academic performance.

Pharmacologic Treatment

Multimodal interventions may prove to be the most efficacious treatment. But there is little evidence that once they are withdrawn, they produce greater long-term benefits than medication alone. Pharmacotherapy with ADHD began in 1937 when Bradley reported the effects of benzedrine on children's behavior. Since then the role and efficacy for stimulants has been well documented. As noted, the use of medications for this condition has been fraught with controversy. A common concern is that pharmacotherapy is viewed as "making" a child behave, reinforcing a child's belief that only external events effect their behavior. Medication needs are then viewed as an excuse to avoid responsibility. However there is little to substantiate this concern.

Stimulants are the most commonly prescribed class of medication for ADHD. They have the best demonstrated efficacy in terms of treating both the motor activity and the inattention. Methylphenidate (MPH) and dextroamphetamine (DA) are the drugs most commonly used within this class.

As a class, these medications are extremely well tolerated. Despite negative publicity, they have an excellent safety record, which derives in part from the short half-lives of these drugs. But the necessity of multiple daily dosing has not gained wide acceptance because of excessive concern about toxicity and medication holidays. This concern has been so overstated that children are often under-treated when doses are omitted or treatment is discontinued for weekends and holidays. It is now better recognized that ADHD is a pervasive phenomenon that doesn't disappear in the evenings, on weekends, and during the summer. Children do homework in the evening and often require the medication to stay on task. This is also a time of family interactions when disruptive behavior is not beneficial. Similar experiences take place on the weekends. During the summer, peer relationships are a significant part of a child's development. Children who don't receive medication during the summer may be deprived of the opportunity for satisfying peer interactions. Of course the severity of ADHD symptoms should be part of the decision to medicate during these nonschool periods.

Although the stimulants are grouped as a class, their mechanisms of action may be quite different. The drugs can be subdivided on the basis of whether the drug-induced stereotypies and increased motor activity are inhibited by reserpine. DA probably enhances catecholamine activity in the CNS by facilitating norepinephrine and dopamine release and by blocking reuptake from storage pools insensitive to reserpine. MPH, although structurally similar to DA, releases neurotransmitters from pools sensitive to depletion by reserpine. Pemoline, a less commonly used stimulant, is structurally dissimilar with minimal sympathomimetic activity. MPH and pemoline have received approval from the Food and Drug Administration (FDA) for children with ADHD as young as age 6, whereas DA has approval down to age 3.

A trial of MPH commonly includes three dose ranges: 0.3 mg/kg three times a day (tid), 0.6 mg/kg tid, 1 mg/kg tid. However, it is very rare that the dose needs to exceed 20 mg tid despite a child's weight. If this occurs, it should be a signal to re-evaluate the diagnosis and treatment response. DA is generally dosed at half the MPH dose.

MPH and DA are marketed in sustained release preparations. MPH has only been available as a single 20-mg strength, but DA is available in 5-, 10-, and 15-mg strengths. These preparations make it possible to administer medication only once in the morning, with the possible addition of a regular strength dose later in the afternoon if needed. These preparations have different pharmacokinetic profiles compared with standard strengths, which is responsible for more varied absorption, clinical effect, and duration of action. There are some reports that tolerance is more common with these preparations, perhaps because of more constant receptor saturation. Most published reports show that the preparations have equal efficacy and dosage equivalency, at least for MPH.

It can be quite difficult to detect clinical change by using external ratings. Part of this problem can be alleviated through the use of placebo-controlled clinical trials. This is done easily in the case of MPH and DA because of their short half-lives. A blinded trial at each dose level should be evaluated with home and school ratings, and a side-effect profile should be collected. A continuous performance test can also be administered at each dose level. Since it is not easy to acquire matching placebos, a pharmacist has to prepare identical capsules.

Pemoline, which has a much longer duration of action, can often be administered each morning. Unlike MPH and DA, which have a same-day therapeutic effect, pemoline may take up to 3 weeks for a clinical effect. This makes it a medication that is more difficult to titrate. There is less experience with this drug's effects on preschool children. The starting dose is generally 37.5 mg/day. This is titrated up by 37.5 mg/day every week to a dose of 2 mg/kg/day but generally not over 112.5 mg/day. On occasion, a second dosage that is approximately half the strength of the morning dose can be given later in the afternoon.

Monitoring stimulant medications involves both physiologic parameters as well as behavioral indexes.

There are generally very few cardiovascular side effects from these medications. However some studies have confirmed anecdotal clinical reports of tachycardia or elevated diastolic blood pressures. It is prudent to monitor the blood pressure and heart rate at each dose change and at least every 6 months thereafter. Pemoline has been associated with elevated liver enzyme levels, which must be checked periodically. It has been our practice to monitor this within the first month of treatment, quarterly as long as there are dose changes, and then twice each year.

The major side effects from stimulants include anorexia, insomnia, stomachaches, headaches, and tics. There is a common myth that food impedes the absorption of stimulants. In fact they can be administered with meals. This may decrease anorexia and sometimes eliminates headaches. Insomnia is a more puzzling side effect. Although stimulants can induce insomnia by their very nature, some children with ADHD actually sleep better if they are given a dosage of MPH or DA at 4:00 pm, since a late dosage seems to allow better settling at night to get to sleep.

Tics are a more unusual side effect that are attributed to dopaminergic action. There is a significant rate of co-morbidity between ADHD and Tourette's disorder, and new tics may be independent of stimulant medication. However, if tics are stimulant-induced, they disappear with cessation of the medication. The stimulant-induced tics may include eye blinking, head jerking, and shoulder shrugging. They can be more difficult to detect if they take the form of sniffling or grunting. There is evidence that stimulants can be administered safely to children with tics, so the presence of tics has been considered only a relative contraindication.

A long-term side effect that has worried many physicians is the possible suppression of growth. Although weight loss tends to be minimal, this side effect is likely the result of appetite suppression that some children experience. It behooves the physician to monitor this side effect by asking specifically about anorexia and by graphing height and weight on a growth chart. In our experience, it is useful to weigh a child within 2 months of initiating stimulant treatment, because all too often parents don't recognize the subtle changes in appetite that lead to weight loss.

Behavioral rebound, also referred to as a behavioral withdrawal, is a phenomena of behavioral deterioration that occurs in the late afternoon, typically before the administration of a third dose of MPH or DA. This seems to occur in about one third of cases. It is usually avoided if the medications are given tid. Other strategies to minimize this adverse response are based on the concept that lower peak serum levels should minimize a withdrawal. Reducing the midday dosage or giving it a little later are usually effective to stop this problem.

Since the different stimulants have different effects on neurotransmitters, a side effect from one stimulant is not predictive of side effects for the class. And generally, if one stimulant is ineffective or produces side effects, the best second step is a trial with another stimulant.

Only stimulants have received FDA approval for the treatment of ADHD. However, the medications discussed in the following section have extensive support in the literature for their use with this condition.

The tricyclic antidepressants have been prescribed widely for ADHD. Their use has dropped after concerns were raised about cardiovascular toxicity. Although presumably all members of this class of medication are efficacious, an overwhelming percentage of literature has focused on imipramine and desipramine. Nortriptyline has also been used, primarily because it is available as a liquid. The general consensus is that stimulants are superior in the treatment of ADHD, but tricyclics are more effective than placebos in reducing restlessness and hyperactivity. Patients who respond better to tricyclics may also be characterized by higher levels of depression and anxiety. Both imipramine and desipramine have been prescribed in doses up to 5 mg/kg/day. In children, the half-life of these medications can be markedly shorter than the reported 24+-hour half-life in adults, necessitating twice daily (bid) or tid dosing. It has also been reported that 6.5% to 10% of the population may metabolize tricyclics slowly. Slow metabolism can lead to toxic serum levels from low doses. This finding, together with several reports of sudden death of patients taking desipramine, highlight the importance of close clinical monitoring.

After a baseline electrocardiogram (ECG) has been made, the physician should begin to treat the patient with low doses to determine tolerance to the medication. Since some children respond to doses as low as 10 mg bid, it is best to avoid dosing by weight initially. Weight assumes more importance when doses exceed 2.5 mg/kg/day because of the reported adverse experiences.

A dose-response curve has not been demonstrated for these medications. Whether a patient's failure to respond to doses up to 3 mg/kg/day should lead to further trials up to 5 mg/kg/day or to trough serum tricyclic levels that approach 200 ng/ml is therefore controversial. If a physician chooses to pursue higher doses, it is important to monitor both the ECG and the serum level. If it is demonstrated that the child is not a slow metabolizer, then dose increases should be followed up with serial ECGs.

The effect of tricyclics on cardiac conduction is like that of quinidine, and the corrected QT interval (QTc) is a critical indicator to monitor. The following ECG conduction abnormalities have been defined:

1. sinus tachycardia, heart rate (HR) ≥ 100 bpm
2. first-degree atrioventricular block, PR ≥ 200 ms
3. intraventricular conduction delay, QRS > 100 ms
4. prolonged QTc, ≥ 440 ms

Others suggest it may be wise to discontinue tricyclics if the QTc exceeds 0.425 seconds or if the heart rate exceeds 130 bpm. It is not in the child's best interest to maintain a rapid heart rate if the child is expected to require treatment for many years. In situations where the benefit from medication is great, and alternate medications are not tolerated, a continuation of tricyclics should be considered only after consultation with a cardiologist and plans for regular echocardiograms are made. The quinidine-like effect on conduction should also warrant caution when co-administering terfenadine and tricyclics.

Side effects may occur from the alpha-adrenergic and anticholinergic properties of these medications. However, they are unusual in children. When medication is discontinued, some children do experience a withdrawal associated with abdominal distress and flu-like symptoms. It can probably be minimized by a slow tapering of the medication. The most common serious adverse event is probably overdose. One of the more common limiting factors for tricyclic use is the precipitation of tachycardia.

The α_2-adrenergic agonist medications are another alternative to the stimulants. This class of medications includes clonidine and guanfacine. As antihypertensive medications, they not only pose the risk of inducing hypotension, but there is the added risk of withdrawal hypertension. Nonetheless, they have become a significant addition to the pharmacotherapy armamentarium. They are also rather unusual, in that it can take weeks for maximum clinical benefit to become apparent.

Clonidine is administered as a slow titration. The half-life is short so it needs to be administered often. It is generally given as 0.05 mg every night (qhs) for 2 to 3 nights, then increased by 0.05 mg every 2 to 3 days to a maximum of 0.1 mg four times per day (qid).

Clonidine also is available as a skin patch for transdermal administration that is changed weekly. The patch provides the additional advantage of constant serum levels, which not only decreases the risk of withdrawal hypertension, but also seems to decrease the side effect of sedation associated with the higher peak serum levels from tablets. Skin rash is a common difficulty with the patch and is a common reason for discontinuation. There is not a good conversion formula to move from pills to patch. If the patient is taking 0.05 to 0.15 mg/day a Catapres TTS-1 (Boehringer-Ingelheim) patch may be used. However, if the child is receiving a higher dose, the oral dose should be decreased by about one half when a TTS-1 patch is added. This is a conservative approach, but it minimizes any

PEARLS & PERILS

TREATMENT OF ATTENTION-DEFICIT/ HYPERACTIVITY DISORDER

- Children with ADHD may show no evidence of the disorder during a brief primary care evaluation.
- There are no laboratory tests to make a diagnosis of ADHD. Continuous performance tasks and psychometric scales are often better suited for monitoring treatment response than for making diagnoses.
- All children show a behavioral response to stimulants; a response to stimulants does not necessarily mean a child has ADHD.
- Side effects or poor response from one stimulant should not preclude a careful trial with another stimulant.
- Whenever a child shows behavioral difficulties in school, consider the presence of learning disorders.

difficulties than might ensue from erratic patch absorption and allows some time to determine whether the child tolerates the medication. Once the child tolerates the TTS-1 patch, it can be increased by one TTS-1 patch per week, up to a maximum of one TTS-3 patch. There are anecdotal reports of cutting the patch in half, but this is not recommended by the manufacturer. It is probably good practice to be certain that caregivers have patches available for use when illness precludes oral dosing, to avoid withdrawal symptoms.

The most common side effect with this medication is sedation. However, numerous other side effects are listed, including the unusual side effects of urinary retention and constipation. Because of the risks of both hypotension and rebound hypertension, children on this drug require close physiologic monitoring. Guanfacine may prove to have some advantages over clonidine. The drug has a longer half-life and is reported to have fewer side effects, particularly freedom from sedation.

It is beyond the scope of this text to explore more experimental pharmacotherapy. Bupropion has been used effectively to treat ADHD, but it is currently limited by the 75-mg nonscorable tablet size on the market. Serotoninergic agents such as fluoxetine have been cited for use in this condition. As noted, the role of serotonin in this condition is far from clear. It is much more likely that these agents are useful adjunctively in treating co-morbid anxiety and mood disorders. Sporadic reports of efficacy in treating ADHD may be the result of global behavioral improvements when anxious and depressive symptoms are improved. This would also explain the anecdotal reports regarding the efficacy of buspirone for ADHD (Table 5-2).

TABLE 5-2

PHARMACOTHERAPY OF ATTENTION DEFICIT/HYPERACTIVITY DISORDER

Medication	Dosage range	Starting dose	Common side effects	Advantages/ disadvantages	Warnings
MPH	0.3-1 mg/kg/ dose usually tid	5 mg tid	Anorexia, stomach-ache, insomnia	Safe and easy administration	Caution in the presence of tics
DA	0.15-0.5 mg/ kg/dose usually tid	2.5 mg tid	Same	Same	Same
Pemoline	Up to 2 mg/kg/day	37.5 mg/day	Same	Requires lab tests	Same
Imipramine	Up to 5 mg/kg/day	10 mg bid	Tachycardia, ACH effect	Long duration of clinical effect; must follow ECG	Caution in the presence of QTc prolongation on ECG
Clonidine	0.1-0.4 mg/day	0.05 mg qhs	Sedation	Transdermal patch available; oral dosing commonly qid	Theoretic risk of rebound hypertension

The frequency with which to monitor the behavioral response to pharmacotherapy for ADHD is not well documented in the literature. Many behavioral checklists have not been normed for repeated administration. Weekly administration of the Conners Teacher Questionnaire demonstrated a tendency for scores to drift. However, we have found that monthly monitoring of symptoms in the classroom can help detect difficulties. First, if there are missed appointments, one is never more than 2 months without a report from the teacher. This can be quite significant in terms of salvaging the remaining months of an academic year. Also, it provides information on compliance. Monthly contact can serve to reinforce the child's understanding of the role of medication.

Nontraditional Treatment

The presence of abnormalities on QEEG in children with ADHD has led to a specific treatment in which biofeedback of the EEG rhythm is used to modify and reduce specific abnormalities. The treatment is based on the hypothesis that children who have ADHD are both less able to produce beta activity and more prone to show excessive slow theta activity during periods of excitement compared to unaffected children. Although the clinical anecdotes of successful treatment have been impressive, many subjects receive multimodal interventions along with biofeedback. Despite a burgeoning practice, there have been no publications on comparisons with a control group. This technique remains an experimental intervention.

Summary

The abundant media interest in ADHD may have inadvertently led researchers to reevaluate some basic assumptions. The consideration that many children may be treated with medication for "normal" rambunctious behavior exemplifies the need for better syndromal validation.

Utilizing a categorical diagnostic scheme, many of the vagaries of the ADHD diagnosis may be better understood if clinical subtypes are well defined. This could occur along many lines, as a multitude of models have been proposed to explain attention and disordered attention. Anatomically, the symptoms of attention disorders may arise from the frontal lobes, right hemisphere, or the reticular activating system. Pharmacologic response could be predicted by neurologic subtype, which would be described on the basis of performance on neuropsychologic tests. Pharmacologic response could also be a function of receptor sensitivity. The possibility of an altered noradrenergic state in children with ADHD led to the investigation of clonidine efficacy. Rather than enhancing neurotransmitter release, this drug reduces available norepinephrine, suggesting an unusual pharmacologic effect or a subtype of children with excessive postsynaptic sensitivity.

In addition to subtyping on the basis of neurophysiology and neuropharmacology, subtypes could be based on a biologic diathesis that requires further environmental interaction. Infant temperament can be described in terms of activity level, distractibility, and attention span. Whether an infant's behavior represents an early precursor or genetic predisposition for the disorder must be determined. Infants with various combinations of these traits could have a subsyndromal appearance. This could also imply a need to reconceptualize the disorder dimensionally rather than categorically.

The difficulty distinguishing a chaotic home environment from a rambunctious child and a child with ADHD illustrates potential benefits that accrue from a valid diagnostic marker. Psychophysiologic and neuropsychologic investigations have not yet been successful in this endeavor. However, advances in neuroimaging provide promises that with this ability to link structure and function should come a better understanding and delineation of what we currently conceptualize as the unitary ADHD.

CONSIDER CONSULTATION WHEN . . .

- The physician cannot distinguish between ADHD and symptoms of a hypomanic/manic episode
- The child is aggessive, and the aggession does not respond to typical medical and behavioral interventions
- The child develops a movement disorder, such as a tic, while taking stimulant medication
- The child's symptoms do not improve despite treatment with at least two medictions at adequate dosages and over a sufficient period
- The child's symptoms worsen after pharmacologic intervention

Annotated Bibliography

Barkley RA: *Attention deficit hyperactivity disorder: a handbook for diagnosis and treatment,* New York, 1990, The Guilford Press.

This well-written, comprehensive handbook has become the most popular source for clinicians diagnosing and treating ADHD.

Weiss G, Hechtman LT: *Hyperactive children grown up,* ed 2, New York, 1993, The Guilford Press.

This is an excellent, readable overview of a longitudinal study of ADHD. It is very helpful towards understanding prognosis.

Zametkin AJ, Rapoport JL: Neurobiology of attention deficit disorder with hyperactivity: where have we come in 50 years? [published erratum appears in *J Am Acad Child Adolesc Psychiatry* 27(3):388, 1988]. *J Am Acad Child Adolesc Psychiatry* 26:676-686, 1987 [Review].

This is a well-referenced review detailing the neurobiologic contributions that have led to the current understanding of ADHD.

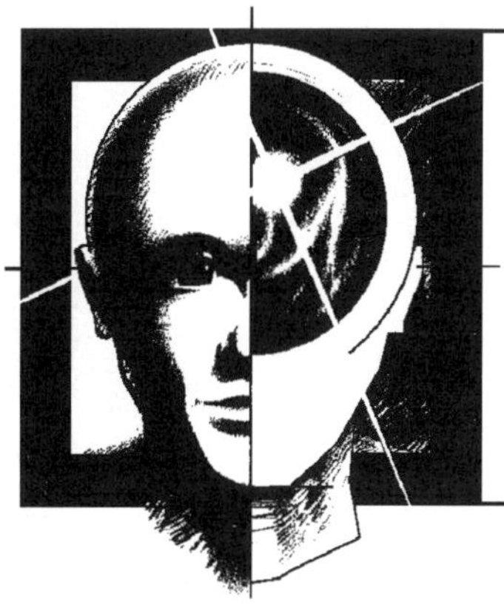

chapter 6

Conduct Disorder and Oppositional Defiant Disorder

Isaac K. Wood, MD

Diagnostic Criteria
Oppositional Defiant Disorder
Conduct Disorder
Differential Diagnosis
Assessment
Treatment
Summary

A disorder of conduct is the most common reason that a child or adolescent is referred for mental health services. In fact, disorders of conduct in children have gained such prominence that it is hard to tune into a news or talk show or to read a magazine that does not refer to behavioral difficulties in youth. The majority of children with a disturbance of conduct do not go on to develop a formal oppositional defiant disorder (ODD) or conduct disorder (CD), but for those who do, the results can be extremely challenging to physicians, parents, and educators.

CD and ODD are often linked together and are included under the umbrella of disruptive behavior disorders in DSM-IV. The basic notion of disruptive behavior disorders, or externalizing disorders, is that children with these difficulties cause more turmoil to their environments than they experience internally. For children with ODD the cardinal feature is a recurrent pattern of behavior toward authority figures that is negative, defiant, disobedient, and hostile and persists for at least 6 months. Comparatively, CD is characterized by a child behaving in a repetitive and persistent pattern that violates either the basic rights of others or major age-appropriate societal norms and rules.

At first glance, the essential features of CD and ODD raise several questions. How do ODD and CD differ from normal behavior seen in children and adolescents? After all, from toddlers to teenagers, many children are defiant and break rules. How are ODD and CD different from each other? It seems that there would be tremendous overlap between the types of problems seen in children who have ODD and those with CD.

DSM-IV DIAGNOSTIC CRITERIA

BOX 6-1 OPPOSITIONAL DEFIANT DISORDER

A. A pattern of negativistic, hostile, and defiant behavior lasting at least 6 months, during which four (or more) of the following are present:

(1) often loses temper
(2) often argues with adults
(3) often actively defies or refuses to comply with adults' requests or rules
(4) often deliberately annoys people
(5) often blames others for his or her mistakes or misbehavior
(6) is often touchy or easily annoyed by others
(7) is often angry and resentful
(8) is often spiteful and vindictive

Note: Consider a criterion met only if the behavior occurs more frequently than is typically observed in individuals of comparable age and developmental level.

B. The disturbance in behavior causes clinically significant impairment in social, academic, or occupational functioning.

C. The behaviors do not occur exclusively during the course of a Psychotic or Mood Disorder.

D. Criteria are not met for Conduct Disorder, and, if the individual is age 18 years or older, criteria are not met for Antisocial Personality Disorder.

(From American Psychiatric Association: *Diagnostic and statistical manual of mental disorders,* ed 4 [DSM-IV], Washington DC, 1994, American Psychiatry Press.)

Finally, are there different types of ODD and CD? The child who shoplifts, skips school, and lies certainly must be different from the violent, assaultive, "streetwise," delinquent youth. These questions are best answered by examining in more detail the diagnostic criteria and natural histories of ODD and CD.

Diagnostic Criteria

To fulfill the diagnostic criteria for ODD, a youth must exhibit at least four behaviors from a list of disturbances in behavior (Box 6-1, Table 6-1). These behaviors include losing one's temper often, repeatedly arguing with adults, actively defying or refusing to comply with adults' requests and rules, deliberately annoying people, blaming others for personal mistakes or misbehavior, being easily annoyed by others, or being angry, resentful, spiteful, and vindictive. Although these behaviors are common in children, the problematic behaviors must be of sufficient severity to impair social, academic, and occupational functioning, thus distinguishing ODD from normal behavior. Additionally, the behaviors cannot be attributed to another major psychiatric disorder such as a mood or psychotic disorder.

Comparatively, the behaviors necessary for the diagnosis of CD fall into four main groupings: aggressive conduct that causes or threatens physical harm to other people or animals, nonaggressive conduct that causes property loss or damage, deceitfulness or theft, and serious violation of rules. To make the diagnosis, three or more characteristic behaviors from these groupings must have been present for at least 12 months, with at least one behavior present in the 6 months preceeding the evaluation. The behavior pattern is usually seen in a variety of settings, including school, home, and the community. CD may be subclassified based on the number of diagnostic features present and whether the extent of harm to others is mild, moderate, or severe (Box 6-2, Tables 6-2 and 6-3, pp. 86-87).

CD and ODD are different from delinquency. Delinquency is a legal term used to describe the actions of any minor who has committed criminal or status offenses. A criminal offense is any act committed by an individual, regardless of age, that is considered illegal. For example, assault, burglary, and rape are considered criminal offenses regardless of whether the perpetrator is an adult or a minor. In contrast, status offenses are acts that are considered illegal for a minor but are not offenses for an adult. Status offenses include truancy, running away from home, drinking alcohol, and staying out past the legal curfew. When a youth commits a delinquent act, he does not necessarily have CD or ODD. In fact, it is estimated that as many as 90% of youth have committed a delinquent offense at some time.

To better understand the differences between CD,

DIAGNOSIS

TABLE 6-1
OPPOSITIONAL DEFIANT DISORDER

Discriminating feature

1. Negativistic, defiant, and hostile behavior in the absence of an overt violation of laws or the rights of others

Consistent features

1. Temper tantrums
2. Argumentative behavior
3. Bullying

Variable features

1. Irritability
2. Persistent lying
3. Concomitant depression or attention-deficit/hyperactivity disorder (ADHD)
4. Presence of a communication disorder
5. Physical aggression

ODD, and normal behavior, information about the natural histories, epidemiologies, and theories as to cause of these conditions is considered.

Oppositional Defiant Disorder

Symptoms of ODD typically first appear during the preschool years, when the behaviors seen may appear normal. Temper tantrums, opposition to authority, and destructiveness are common during this time of development, and it is extremely difficult, if not impossible, to differentiate what is normal from pathologic oppositionality. However, with most children, destructiveness, bullying, fighting, and defiance significantly decrease after the preschool years. Should these behaviors persist with the school-age child in a way that is disabling (that is, if the child has significant problems in school, negative peer interactions, or conflicts with parents), a diagnosis of ODD should strongly be considered. Another benchmark for ODD may be persistent lying. It has been noted that lying has a developmental pattern similar to that of ODD and correlates highly with symptoms of ODD and CD.

The prevalence of ODD has been estimated to range from 1.7% to 9.9% of the population, with a weighted average of 5.7%. In a community sample of psychiatric disorders in children, about one third of all children with an emotional or behavioral disorder are reported to have ODD, making it one of the most common behavioral conditions in youth. Additionally, reviews of community samples indicate that parents of children with ODD are more likely to use childrens' mental health services than parents of children diagnosed with CD, major depressive disorder, attention-deficit/hyperactivity disorder (ADHD), or generalized anxiety disorder (GAD). Children with ODD have also been found to repeatedly use emergency services. The prevalence of ODD symptoms in children not referred for treatment decreases with age, suggesting that many youngsters outgrow these behaviors and develop more social behaviors instead.

PEARLS & PERILS

OPPOSITIONAL DEFIANT DISORDER

- Persistent lying has a pattern similar to that of ODD.
- The best predictor that a child will progress from ODD to CD is the presence of physical aggression.
- Compared to normal children, youth with ODD actually perceive their parents as being more overprotective and less caring.
- ODD may herald the onset of CD but does not necessarily progress into CD.

Studies of children under the age of 12 reveal that ODD occurs twice as often in boys than in girls. However, with the onset of adolescence, ODD is much more prevalent in girls than boys. These ties to developmental stages suggest that at least in some cases, ODD may represent a formative aberrancy. There has been only one epidemiologic study of children with ODD that specifically examined socioeconomic status. This study found ODD to be more prevalent in groups with a lower socioeconomic status.

ODD is often associated with a number of co-morbid conditions, including ADHD and CD. Recent epidemiologic and longitudinal studies of ODD and CD reveal that 77% to 84% of youth who have CD had preexisting ODD. In contrast, 75% of boys who have "pure" ODD do not go on to become conduct disordered. This suggests that at least for some children ODD is a predictor of subsequent conduct disordered behavior or is an inherent component of CD. However, this also suggests that for other children, ODD is a singular clinical entity that does not naturally progress into CD or that some children with ODD are able to desist from the natural progression into CD. It has been postulated that the best indicator that a child will progress from ODD to CD is the presence of physical aggression.

It has been estimated that one out of every four children with ODD has concomitant ADHD, whereas about half of all children with ADHD also meet the criteria for ODD. There is also a large association between ODD, ADHD, and communication disorders. Because communication disorders are so prominent in children with

DSM-IV DIAGNOSTIC CRITERIA

BOX 6-2 CONDUCT DISORDER

A. A repetitive and persistent pattern of behavior in which the basic rights of others or major age-appropriate societal norms or rules are violated, as manifested by the presence of three (or more) of the following criteria in the past 12 months, with at least one criterion present in the past 6 months:

Aggression to people and animals

(1) often bullies, threatens, or intimidates others
(2) often initiates physical fights
(3) has used a weapon that can cause serious physical harm to others (e.g., a bat, brick, broken bottle, knife, gun)
(4) has been physically cruel to people
(5) has been physically cruel to animals
(6) has stolen while confronting a victim (e.g., mugging, purse snatching, extortion, armed robbery)
(7) has forced someone into sexual activity

Destruction of property

(8) has deliberately engaged in fire setting with the intention of causing serious damage
(9) has deliberately destroyed others' property (other than by fire setting)

Deceitfulness or theft

(10) has broken into someone else's house, building, or car
(11) often lies to obtain goods or favors or to avoid obligations (i.e., "cons" others)
(12) has stolen items of nontrivial value without confronting a victim (e.g., shoplifting, but without breaking and entering; forgery)

Serious violations of rules

(13) often stays out at night despite parental prohibitions, beginning before age 13 years
(14) has run away from home overnight at least twice while living in parental or parental surrogate home (or once without returning for a lengthy period)
(15) often truant from school, beginning before age 13 years.

B. The disturbance in behavior causes clinically significant impairment in social, academic, or occupational functioning.

C. If the individual is age 18 years or older, criteria are not met for Antisocial Personality Disorder.

Specify type based on age at onset:
Childhood-Onset Type: onset of at least one criterion characteristic of Conduct Disorder prior to age 10 years
Adolescent-Onset Type: absence of any criteria characteristic of Conduct Disorder prior to age 10 years

Specify severity:
Mild: few if any conduct problems in excess of those required to make the diagnosis **and** conduct problems cause only minor harm to others
Moderate: number of conduct problems and effect on others intermediate between "mild" and "severe"
Severe: many conduct problems in excess of those required to make the diagnosis **or** conduct problems cause considerable harm to others

(From American Psychiatric Association: *Diagnostic and statistical manual of mental disorders,* ed 4 [DSM-IV], Washington DC, 1994, American Psychiatric Press.)

ADHD, the presence of a communication disorder in a child with ODD may be more closely associated with a concomitant ADHD than ODD.

It is not unusual to find a co-morbid internalizing disorder in children with ODD. Internalizing disorders that are often seen in children with ODD are separation anxiety disorder (5% of cases), generalized anxiety disorder (5%), and major depressive disorder (11%). Symptoms of these disorders are often easily overlooked in these children because of the prominent oppositional and defiant behaviors.

Studies of the families of children with ODD reveal a higher incidence of substance abuse and antisocial personality disorder in the biologic parents of these children than those of unaffected children. However, when children who have ODD are compared with children who have CD, rates of antisocial personality disorder and substance abuse are significantly higher in the parents of youth with CD.

Compared to CD, less is known about the cause of

DIAGNOSIS

TABLE 6-2

CHILDHOOD-ONSET CONDUCT DISORDER

Discriminating feature

1. Persistent disregard for rules, law, and authority and violation of the rights of others with onset before age 10

Consistent features

1. Absence of a specific organic abnormality
2. Premorbid ODD and ADHD
3. Poor prognosis
4. Predominantly boys

Variable features

1. Physical aggression and physical harm to others
2. Concomitant substance abuse
3. Family history of CD or antisocial personality disorder
4. Lower than average intelligence
5. History of head injury and learning disorders
6. Nonspecific EEG abnormalities
7. Level of aggression increased if psychotic symptoms are present

DIAGNOSIS

TABLE 6-3

ADOLESCENT-ONSET CONDUCT DISORDER

Discriminating feature

1. Persistent disregard for rules, laws, and authority and violation of the rights of others with onset after age 10

Consistent features

1. Absence of a specific organic abnormality
2. Many more girls represented
3. Culture bound
4. Good prognosis

Variable features

1. Lack of significant violent behavior
2. Concomitant depression
3. Normal intelligence
4. Remorseful about behaviors

ODD. It has been hypothesized that ODD may occur in response to overly strict parenting. Both children with ODD and CD perceive their parents to be more overprotective and less caring than do other children. Psychodynamic theorists have postulated that ODD reflects developmental fixation at the anal stage of development. Others have suggested that ODD represents a "bad mix" between child and parent. The "difficult child" temperament appears to be closely related to oppositional behavior, and parents of children with ODD often have uncertainties about their own autonomy and issues of control.

Conduct Disorder

As noted previously, ODD may herald the onset of CD. Like ODD, a multitude of factors have been associated with CD. It is estimated that 50%-75% of children with CD have co-morbid ADHD. Additionally, at least half of youth affected by CD also have an internalizing mental illness such as depression or an anxiety disorder. Suicidality scores for children with CD and concomitant depression have been found to be higher than suicidality scores of youth with only depression. Also, there is a very high rate of self-harm without suicidal intention in this group of disturbed youth. Substance abuse is also prominent in this population. It is estimated that as many as 91% of substance-abusing juvenile offenders also have CD. There is a significant history of head and facial injuries, soft neurologic signs, psychomotor seizures, febrile seizures, and nonspecific EEG abnormalities in children with CD when they are compared with children who do not have CD. Likewise, there is a high incidence of specific developmental disorders, including problems with verbal and visuospatial-motor integration, auditory processing, and memory deficits in the population with CD. As a whole, these children tend to score lower on intelligence tests. These youth may also have vague psychotic symptoms, such as paranoia, grandiosity in the absence of hallucinations, or a formal thought disorder. Children with these types of psychotic symptoms tend to be the most violent and maladaptive of all youth with CD.

The families of youth with CD also exhibit specific characteristics. When considered as a whole, children with CD tend to come from large, urban, single-parent, and low-income families. Fathers of children with CD, who are often absent from the home, have a greater incidence of antisocial personality disorder and substance abuse than the fathers of children without CD. The mothers of children with CD have high rates of depression, antisocial personality disorder, substance abuse, and somatization disorder. Collectively, the parents of children with CD and co-morbid ADHD have the greatest history of violence, law breaking, arrests, and imprisonment when compared with children that only have CD. Parents of children with CD also tend to be violent in their disciplinary techniques, usually employing corporal punishment with a high rate of both neglect and physical abuse. Adoption and twin studies also support a familial link to CD. Adoption studies of youth with CD have demonstrated that adopted sons whose biologic parents were criminals are more likely to develop CD than adopted sons of noncriminal biologic parents. By a similar token, twin studies have revealed a higher concordance rate for criminal behavior in monozygotic than in dizygotic twins.

Overall, CD occurs more often in boys than in girls, with a rate of 6% to 16% for males and 2% to 9% for females. However, when epidemiologic studies are considered, the relative rates based on gender and type of CD differ.

Longitudinal studies of children with CD suggest that there are two primary developmental pathways, childhood-onset type and adolescent-onset type. The major differences between these two subcategories in regard to the diagnostic criteria is that in the childhood-onset type of CD there must be at least one criterion characteristic of CD present in a child before age 10, whereas for the adolescent-onset type of CD all characteristic criteria of CD must be absent before age 10. More striking differences are noted when the natural histories of these two subtypes of CD are considered.

The natural history of adolescent-onset CD is characterized by a paucity of problematic behaviors before the onset of adolescence. In fact, these youth usually fail to exhibit a history of oppositional behavior or social, academic, and community problems during the preschool and school-age years. However, during adolescence they begin to engage in oppositional and illegal activities. The illegal activities of these youth tend to occur within a group setting, are less severe than those of childhood-onset CD, and tend to be far less aggressive, particularly in regard to physical aggression directed to others. Additionally, the majority of these youth desist from their CD behaviors with the onset of adulthood, suggesting a more favorable prognosis for this group than youth with childhood-onset CD. More girls are represented within this group than in the childhood-onset group, as are more poor, urban, and minority youth. These children fail to demonstrate the severe learning problems, low intelligence, or neuropsychiatric impairments characteristic of children with CD. It is believed that this type of CD is more sociocultural in origin than childhood-onset CD.

In contrast, childhood-onset CD is characterized by a strong family history of sociopathy and violence. Symptoms of a disruptive behavior disorder emerge during early childhood, as characterized by classic ODD behaviors. There is then a progression to the early symptoms of CD, which include lying, fighting, and petty theft. Children with childhood-onset CD usually have a history of ADHD, learning disabilities, and academic underachievement. Additionally, this group is more likely to show evidence of other types of neuropsychiatric impairments, such as EEG and evoked-potential abnormalities. Overall, this group tends to be much more aggressive than the adolescent-onset CD group. There is often a history of assaultive behavior that persists into adulthood. As these children grow older, there is a progression in the severity of their offenses, with fights giving way to vandalism, torturing of animals, breaking into homes, and stealing costly items. There is also a high incidence of substance abuse within this group, with onset usually during adolescence. As young adults these individuals engage in more flagrant antisocial behavior, including forced sex. They have a chaotic employment and marital histories, and they tend to be physically abusive to their spouses and children. Diagnostically, by the age of 18 the majority of youth with CD meet the criteria for antisocial personality disorder, and it is not unusual to find these individuals imprisoned. Although the childhood-onset CD group makes up only 3% to 5% of all youth with CD, it is believed that they are responsible for at least half of the illegal offenses committed by juveniles. Additionally, this group is overwhelmingly male, and incidence is less likely to be related to a socioeconomic or ethnic group.

There is evidence to suggest that childhood-onset CD may be more constitutional or neurobiologic in origin than adolescent-onset CD. This is first gleaned from the strong intergenerational link for violent, antisocial behaviors in the families of children with childhood-onset CD. Additionally, this group is more likely to demonstrate neurochemical abnormalities. Specifically, the childhood-onset CD group has been found to have very

PEARLS & PERILS

CONDUCT DISORDER

- Rates of suicide are particularly high in children with CD who have concomitant depression.
- Children with CD who also have psychotic symptoms, even vague paranoid ideas, are the most violent and maladaptive.
- Adolescent-onset CD has a fair-to-good prognosis, with the majority of these youth desisting from antisocial behavior as an adult.
- Youth with childhood-onset CD are responsible for over half of the illegal offenses committed by juveniles.
- Although boys with childhood-onset CD have been found to have near-zero dopamine β-hydroxylase activity, abnormalities in this enzyme are not diagnostic of CD.
- Aggressive outbursts in psychomotor seizures are random, unpredictable, and usually not directed at a specific target.

low CSF serotonin levels when compared with CD youth or unaffected children. Serotonin is found widely distributed throughout the CNS, where it has a quieting and calming effect. It is not surprising that levels of serotonin would be decreased in violent, conduct disordered youth. Boys with childhood-onset CD have also been found to have abnormal activity of dopamine β-hydroxylase (DBH). DBH is an enzyme that is responsible for converting the neurotransmitter dopamine to norepinephrine. The activity of this enzyme is genetically determined, with about 4% of the normal population having near-zero activity. However, it has been repeatedly demonstrated that well over 80% of youth with childhood-onset CD have near-zero activity of DBH. It is unclear if this abnormality in DBH activity is a marker for childhood-onset CD or if it is related to the cause. The expected concomitant increase in dopamine and decrease in norepinephrine has not been demonstrated, although there is some evidence to suggest that there may be less norepinephrine available for activity outside of the neuron in boys with childhood-onset CD. There has also been a considerable amount of research that has shown that youth with childhood-onset CD have aberrant autonomic nervous system functioning, as evidenced by abnormal Galvanic skin responses, decreased sweating, decreased pulse, and lower blood pressure when compared with unaffected children or those with adolescent-onset CD.

Based on the above information, several theories have been advanced to explain the cause of CD. Within the social realm, it has been posited that these youth engage in disruptive behaviors as a product of modeling or learning from adults and siblings who are similarly disturbed. It has also been hypothesized that delinquent youth engage in illegal behaviors to attain objects they would not normally own and to gain status with their peers. Psychologic theories have emphasized abnormalities in the development of the conscience or superego. Accordingly, it has been conjectured that these youth internalize faulty values and cognitions from the experiences they have with their parents and other antisocial individuals with whom they have contact during their formative years. The consciences of these youth have been likened to Swiss cheese, with lacunae or lakes of deficits in moral values. Psychoanalytic therapists have emphasized the appearance of disruptive behavior as a manifestation of disturbed attachment during the first years of life or as a way of acting out failures in attainment in the stages of psychosexual development.

The biologic theorists have suggested that because of lower autonomic nervous system activity, these children have difficulty internalizing values. According to this theory, a child would need an intact and normally functioning autonomic nervous system to experience the sorts of peripheral responses associated with anxiety, such as a rapid heart rate, dry mouth, and tremulousness. Anxiety is thought to be necessary to develop a conscience. Fear of being harmed, being left alone, disappointing the caregiver and losing her love, and not meeting up to one's own expectations are basic steps in the development of a conscience. Normal anxiety associated with these types of experiences allows children to internalize knowledge necessary for safety, learn right from wrong, and set goals. If a child has a hypofunctioning autonomic nervous system, it has been postulated that he may not experience the normal levels of anxiety necessary to internalize these components of the conscience.

Similarly, it has been hypothesized that because of decreased autonomic functioning, these children have an extremely high thresholds for experiencing pleasure from novel situations. The typical kinds of experiences that a child finds exciting are viewed as boring to children with CD. In fact, it is not unusual to hear these children describe their baseline state as boredom. As a result, it has been theorized that these children engage in thrill seeking and illegal behaviors to experience a sense of excitement.

Finally, it has been hypothesized that there are two types of primary brain systems involved in the initiation and inhibition of behavior. The behavioral inhibition system (BIS), comprised of many of the components of the limbic system, stops or decelerates a response in the face of impending punishment by generating feelings of anxiety and frustration. It thereby functions very much like a conscience. Noradrenergic and serotoninergic neurons are believed to be the neurochemical mediators of this system. Alternatively, the reward, or behavioral activation system (BAS), is cued by signals of reward or the likelihood of nonpunishment. This system signals approach and predatory aggression. Mediated through the medial forebrain bundle and lateral hypothalamus, the principle neurotransmitter in the BAS is dopamine. Theoretically, antisocial behavior would most likely be severe and persistent in individuals with excessive BAS activity and deficient BIS control. This would be manifested by excessive dopaminergic activity and inhibited noradrenergic and serotoninergic activity. Accordingly, individuals with a predilection for the development of CD would be born with a genetically determined predisposition that would accentuate dopaminergic activity and suppress noradrenergic and serotoninergic activity. Alternatively, the early experiences of the child could influence the normal development of these pathways and lead to aberrancies. As noted previously, the expected increase in dopamine and decrease in norepinephrine has not been demonstrated, although it has been found that violent children have decreased levels of serotonin.

In reality, it appears that the factors responsible for the development of CD are probably very different for the childhood-onset and adolescent-onset types. In adolescent-onset CD, it is more likely that sociocultural factors such as the influence of poverty, delinquent peer groups, and the need to attain status in the community play a predominant role. With childhood-onset CD, it appears that a combination of biologic and psychosocial variables interplay to cause the disorder. There is evidence to suggest that children with childhood-onset CD are much more likely to have a genetic predilection toward the development of the disorder, to have a variety of neuropsychiatric impairments, and to be raised by antisocial parents. The impact of these multiple insults are most likely responsible for the resulting behaviors.

PEARLS & PERILS

DIAGNOSES OF CONDUCT DISORDER

- A youth with CD who appears dull may in fact have significant problems with language comprehension.
- When assessing the IQ of a youth with CD, the performance IQ as opposed to the verbal IQ may be the best indicator of innate intelligence.
- The physician must question youth with CD about symptoms of an internalizing disorder, since this is easily overlooked by parents and teachers.
- Laboratory testing is not likely to help evaluate youth with CD.

Differential Diagnosis

When considering a diagnosis of ODD or CD, alternative conditions should be kept in mind. There are several types of psychiatric disorders that may mimic ODD or CD. For example, a child or adolescent who is manic may engage in dangerous and disruptive behavior or act in an antisocial way that is not typical or characteristic of the youth. However, unlike the child with ODD or CD, the youth with mania will exhibit other symptoms that are specific to that illness, such as pressured speech, flight of ideas, and a decreased need for sleep. Likewise, a child, and in most cases an adolescent, may begin to manifest oppositional and conduct disordered behavior as a component of a clinical depression. Such youth often feel irritable, inadequate, isolated, and alone. They may begin to identify with, dress like, and behave as a member of a counterculture of nonconforming adolescents. A depressed adolescent may be openly defiant to parents or other adults in positions of authority, and the adolescent's behavior may include school truancy and failure, the use of alcohol or illicit drugs, sexual activity, and the appearance of delinquent behaviors. Unlike the child who is strictly conduct disordered, the depressed youth clearly shows a change in mood that predated the disturbing behavior. Likewise, as the mood disorder improves and dissipates, so will the aberrant behavior. Conduct disordered youth also often suffer from depression. However, with these children, the conduct disordered behavior clearly precedes the change in mood and a youth's actions do not significantly change with the treatment of the mood disorder.

A child may begin to exhibit oppositional or conduct disordered behavior in response to a stressful event such as starting school, parental marital conflict, or physical or sexual abuse. In such cases, the onset of the change in behavior may be clearly linked to the psychosocial stressor and should dissipate as the situation improves. If the child is suffering from an anxiety disorder, whether it be separation anxiety disorder (SAD) or GAD, the behavioral difficulties should also dissipate as the anxiety disorder is treated.

Disruptive behavior may also be a symptom of a more serious psychiatric disorder, such as a psychosis. Here, there should be a concomitant history of hallucinations, delusions, or a thought disorder.

Aggressive outbursts may be a manifestation of psychomotor seizures. However, in such cases the aggression is rarely directed at an individual or appears as if it is planned and under conscious control. Rather, the aggression is unpredictable and random. Additionally, there may be other symptoms of a seizure disorder, such as an aura, postictal confusion, and EEG changes.

Finally, disinhibited and disruptive behavior may be a manifestation of an organic personality disorder in children with a congenital or acquired CNS insult such as fetal alcohol syndrome, a closed-head injury, or an encephalopathy.

Assessment

Assessment of the child with a disturbance of behavior needs to be multifaceted. A comprehensive evaluation requires that the physician understand the child, his family, his school, and his community settings. Additionally, it is important that the physician keep an open mind when evaluating a child with a disruptive behavior disorder. These children often elicit such a negative response from the physician that important symptoms, such as the presence of a depressive or anxiety disorder may easily be overlooked.

It is best to begin by noting the age of onset of the problematic behaviors. A child who has a behavior disorder at age 3 is likely to be quite different from the adolescent who is brought to the physician with a disturbance in conduct. For this reason, and because of the natural history of the development of ODD, childhood-onset CD, and adolescent-onset CD, it is helpful to obtain a history of the symptoms from the parents within an evolutionary framework, starting with the mother's pregnancy. The physician should note any problem during the gestation, such as drug and alcohol use or fetal distress, that may be related to the behavioral disturbance. Difficulties in infancy that suggest a troublesome temperament should also be noted. Extremes of oppositionality during the preschool years and aggressive behavior suggest the possibility of childhood-onset CD. The parents need to be queried about symptoms of ADHD in the youth. Additionally, attention should be paid to problems the child may have experienced leaving the caregiver, since SAD may present with oppositional and defiant behaviors. The parents should also be questioned about any specific events that may have precipitated the disturbance in behavior and whether the child tends to exhibit the behavior when alone, which is more characteristic of childhood-onset CD, or only in the context of a group of similarly-acting youth, as is seen in adolescent-onset CD.

A medical history is also necessary. Is there any history of a head injury or encephalopathic condition? Is there any correlation between the time of onset of disruptive or disinhibited behaviors and some type of insult to the CNS?

A school history is essential. What types of behavior problems has the child exhibited in school? Is there a history of specific learning problems? How does he get along with his peers? If possible, the physician should talk directly with the child's teacher to get more objective information about the child and his family. Additionally, the physician may want to have the teacher complete some simple behavior questionnaires such as the Achenbach Child Behavior Checklist (CBCL) or the Conners Teacher Rating Scale. Using such questionnaires tends to better objectify the information obtained.

Obtaining a legal history is also imperative. Has the child been involved in the legal system? Are there charges pending at the time of examination, or is the youth on probation? A probation officer may be a knowledgeable source of information about the child and his family. The physician needs to know how the problem has been addressed before this point. Have the parents used corporal punishment? Have the parents been negligent or abusive? Has the child required special education services or been suspended or expelled from school? Has the behavior required that the child be removed from the community or detained by the police?

The physician must also obtain a good family history from the parents, including a detailed psychiatric history and a history of substance abuse. Is there a history of similar behavior problems in the parents or brothers and sisters of the youth? Has anyone else been diagnosed as having ADHD? Is there a family history of a major psychiatric illness such as a mood or psychotic disorder?

A treatment history is also essential. Has the child been on any specific types of medications? What types of treatment have and have not been helpful? Has the child's behavior necessitated hospitalization?

For the child with aggression as the primary symptom, it is important that the physician obtain a detailed history of the nature of the aggressive acts. Does the aggression seemed to be predatory and planned, or is it impulsive? Are there predictable precipitants to aggressive outbursts? Does the aggression occur in response to perceived threats when in fact the youth is quite safe, suggesting underlying paranoia? To whom or what is the child aggressive? Are there any symptoms suggestive of a seizure disorder associated with the behavior? Has the nature of the aggressive behavior changed or worsened as the child has gotten older?

The physician should also ask the parents about signs and symptoms of other psychiatric disorders. Has there been a change in energy level, sleep, or appetite suggestive of a mood disorder? Has the child been self-destructive, has he said he wishes he were dead, or has he made threats to harm himself? Are there any signs or symptoms suggestive of a psychosis? Are the parents aware of the youth abusing drugs or alcohol?

Finally, the physician needs to evaluate the child alone. A physical examination should be performed. The child may demonstrate soft neurologic signs, suggesting nonspecific CNS dysfunction. There may be physical stigmata suggestive of an organic impairment such as fetal alcohol syndrome. The physician should be alert to any physical signs indicative of abuse. The child should be questioned about any scars, bruises, or other findings that suggest he may have been harmed or harmed himself. The physician should also take note of the child's ability and willingness to cooperate for the examination. Is he unusually fidgety or restless? Is the child frankly oppositional? Additionally, the physician should be alert to the youth's ability to hear and comprehend language. Hearing may be normal, but the comprehension of language may be immature, suggesting a developmental communication disorder.

The physician should assess the child for the presence of psychiatric symptoms that may explain the behavior problems. The physician may include many questions in the general review of systems and thereby not perform a formal mental status examination. For example, the physician may ask about weight, sleep, energy level, and appetite. When questioning the child about his hearing, the physician may ask the youth if his ears ever play tricks on him. Does the child hear someone speak when no one is there? The child should be asked directly about any changes in mood. For many children with a disruptive behavior disorder, the parents are so preoccupied with the child's actions that they are not aware of an underlying depression or anxiety disorder. However, the child will be able to talk about these symptoms. Along with this, the physician should assess the child for evidence of self-harm, suicidality, and homicidality.

The physician needs to ask the child directly about a history of sexual activity, abuse, and illegal behaviors. Has the child been sexually or physically abused? Is there a history of sexual promiscuity or irresponsible sexual behavior? Children with CD may not trust the physician enough to tell the whole story. For example, when an adolescent is asked if he has ever had any types of legal problems, he may only talk about actions that have directly resulted in contact with the police. However, if the physician asks the child if he has ever done anything that would put him in trouble if his parents or the police knew about it, the physician is likely to get a broader picture. The physician also needs to ask the youth specifically about the use of drugs and alcohol.

The demeanor of the child should also be noted. The child with a tough, macho bravado or an indifferent attitude may be defending against paranoid ideas and feelings of extreme inadequacy. The physician must demonstrate tact, caring, and empathy to get beyond this armor. It is of interest to note whether the child readily "snitches" on his friends. Youth with adolescent-onset CD are often extremely loyal to their gang of delinquents, whereas a youth with childhood-onset CD has no real problem implicating others, particularly if he perceives some gain for himself.

In the face of a good history and physical examination, there should be little to no need for laboratory testing in a child with disruptive behavior. If a genetic abnormality is suspected, chromosomal studies may be useful. The EEG may be diffusely abnormal, but the likelihood of finding a specific abnormality is low. Additionally, the presence of a normal EEG does not rule out a seizure disorder, particularly a disorder with psychomotor seizures.

For the moderately to severely disturbed child, psychoeducational, psychologic, and neuropsychologic testing may prove to be extremely helpful. Such testing helps confirm the presence or absence of a major mental illness, ADHD, or a learning disability that may significantly impact treatment. Testing also helps the physician identify the child's relative strengths and weaknesses. This is important for treatment planning.

With the above information in mind, the physician should be able to determine:

1. Whether the youth has ODD or CD
2. The type of ODD or CD (that is, childhood- vs. adolescent-onset CD)
3. Whether the child has some type of psychiatric or medical disorder that is causing the behavioral changes
4. Whether the child has a co-morbid psychiatric disorder in addition to ODD or CD
5. What interventions are necessary to address the problems

Treatment

The treatment of ODD and CD is often difficult and usually multifaceted. There is little evidence that traditional talking or relationship therapies are effective with this group. However, there is considerable support for multisystemic therapy in the treatment of ODD and CD youth. Multisystemic therapy involves addressing and changing the multiple systems that encounter the youth's problematic behavior, including the child, the family, the school, and the community.

Regarding interventions with the child, there has been evidence to support the use of pharmacotherapy, cognitive-behavioral therapy, and problem-solving skills training. There is no specific pharmacotherapy for ODD or CD. If there is evidence of a co-morbid psychiatric or medical disorder such as ADHD, a mood disorder, or psychomotor seizures that respond to medication intervention, appropriate treatment should be prescribed. In some cases, this may significantly decrease the degree of oppositional and conduct-disordered behaviors. Outside of this, pharmacotherapy is usually targeted to address symptoms of rage and explosive outbursts.

A number of agents to treat rage responses have been suggested, including neuroleptics, clonidine, beta-blockers, benzodiazepines, lithium, anticonvulsants, buspirone, calcium channel blockers, and stimulants. Stimulant medication has been found to be effective in mild aggression but to be ineffective with moderate to severe aggression. Neuroleptics are the most commonly used drug in the treatment of aggressive children and adolescents, and they have been found to be very effective in curbing outbursts. However, the long-term use of neuroleptics for the treatment of nonpsychotic

PEARLS & PERILS

PHARMACOTHERAPY FOR DISRUPTIVE BEHAVIOR DISORDERS

- Stimulant medication may be effective in curbing mild aggression, but it is usually ineffective with moderate to severe aggression.
- Lithium has been found to be effective in both predatory and affective aggression.
- Carbamazepine may be effective with emotional lability, impulsivity, and aggressiveness, particularly when accompanied by an abnormal EEG.
- β-Blockers and calcium channel blockers may be useful in aggressive children with a history of head injury, particularly when there is temporal lobe involvement.

behavior disorders presents a dilemma to the physician when the possible side effects are considered. Common side effects from neuroleptic use include sedation, dystonic reactions, parkinsonian side effects, weight gain, and tardive and withdrawal-emergent dyskinesias. Haloperidol is commonly used in dosage ranges of 1.0 to 6.0 mg/day. Other neuroleptics that have been shown to be effective in treating aggressive behavior include molindone, thioridazine, and chlorpromazine. Lithium has been found to influence both predatory and affective aggression. The pharmacologic effects of lithium are believed to be mediated through the enhancement of serotoninergic activity. Dosage is based on clinical responsiveness, serum lithium levels, and the prevention of side effects or toxicity. The long-term safety of lithium use in this age group is unknown. The appearance of unexpected and unprovoked rage responses has led to the speculation that children with this behavior experience abnormal electric activity in the limbic system. Subsequently, anticonvulsants were introduced as a possible treatment for aggression. Carbamazepine, at therapeutic serum levels, has been found to be effective with symptoms of emotional lability, impulsivity, and aggressiveness. Valproic acid and diphenylhydantoin have also been used. There is little clinical experience with the use of β-blockers or calcium channel blockers for treatment of aggression in youth. There have been a few case reports using β-blockers or calcium channel blockers, and most of these have involved violent youth with head injuries who have not responded to traditional drug treatments. There are a few clinical trials of benzodiazepines, clonidine, and buspirone with aggressive children. Some children have shown improvement, but the aggressiveness worsened in others.

The mainstay of individual therapy with ODD and CD youth is cognitive-behavioral therapy. Cognitive-behavioral therapy (CBT) helps a child modify cognitive deficiencies, such as communication skills, problem-solving skills, impulse control, and anger management, that are believed to underlie antisocial behavior. For example, when the youth encounters a problematic situation, a behavior coach brainstorms with the child to think of as many responses as possible to handle the problem. The coach may be a parent, teacher, peer, or physician. All the responses generated are written down. Immediately, any responses involving aggression are crossed out, making it clear from the start that aggression is not an acceptable option. The child is then told to imagine what would happen with each of the remaining choices and to select what he thinks is the one best response. The coach and the child may then role play or practice the scenario using the selected response. The child is encouraged to try this in the real-life situation. Later, the youth reports back to the coach about how things turned out. Other cognitive-behavioral interventions actually involve teaching prosocial competencies and anger management. This often involves a step-by-step method using role playing, training in becoming sensitive to the sequence of problem development, and methods of self-soothing. At times, the training may involve the most basic interactions, such as how to give and receive a compliment.

> PEARLS & PERILS
>
> **TREATMENT OF DISRUPTIVE BEHAVIOR DISORDERS**
>
> - The cornerstone of individual treatment of youth with ODD and CD is CBT.
> - Before addressing parenting issues, the physician must assure that the home is safe and basic needs are being met.
> - Problems with auditory processing in disruptive youth must be identified and brought to the attention of teachers and parents.
> - Disposition to a correctional setting should only be considered as part of a well-planned system of treatment—not as a last alternative.

Family intervention is also imperative with ODD and CD. However, before intervening with the families of ODD and CD youth, the physician needs to make sure there is a solid foundation within the home. This means that the following conditions have been met:

- There is appropriate housing for the family, and there are adequate resources to meet basic day-to-day needs
- If a parent has a psychiatric or substance abuse disorder, he or she is receiving appropriate treatment to address the problem
- The home is safe for everyone there—the problems of spousal and child abuse have been identified and addressed
- There is adequate supervision available for all children in the home

To achieve these goals, the physician may need to make referrals to Children's Protective Services (CPS), Social Services, or mental health practitioners for appropriate intervention and assistance.

Once a solid foundation within a home has been established, the cornerstone of treatment involves working with the child's parents to improve parenting skills and to educate them about the dynamics of the situations leading up to the oppositional, defiant, or conduct-disordered behavior. The parents of children with ODD and CD often see themselves getting into battles with their children that escalate into full-scale wars. Parents often need to be made cognizant of the cycle that occurs as oppositional and conduct-disordered behavior develops, so they can change the series of actions that lead to the undesired end-product. Additionally, they need to be taught how to deal with their children in a neutral and nonemotional manner that does not involve corporal punishment. This consists of teaching parents how to offer children choices in difficult situations, how to effectively use time out, how to reward children for appropriate behavior, and how to allow natural consequences to occur. Parents often get so caught up with their child in an emotional battle of wills that they forget the true source of the problem. For example, 8-year-old Tommy says he wants pizza delivered for dinner. His mother has already prepared a meal and does not see the need to order additional food. Tommy begins to whine about the situation. He complains to his father that no one ever does what he wants and that his mother has not fixed anything he likes to eat. His father, half-heartedly, tells Tommy he needs to try to eat what his mother prepared. Tommy then throws a full scale tantrum, screaming, yelling, pounding the table, and saying he will not eat anything. At this point Father suggests that Mother relent and let him order pizza. Mother, who is determined Tommy will obey her, adamantly refuses and an argument between Mother and Father ensues. During the argument, the food Mother is preparing burns, and the family ends up ordering pizza to be delivered. Mother and Father leave the situation angry and disgruntled. Tommy is happy because he got what he wanted for dinner, and he is rewarded for his negative behavior.

How should the physician work with this situation? First, this scenario may be very typical of conflicts that occur around Tommy in this family. If so, the physician will need to identify the role of each member in creating the conflicts. In this scenario, the roles might be defined as follows:

- Tommy does not respect his mother's authority and plays his mother and father against each other to get what he wants.
- Mother has forgotten the important point in the situation, which is that she wants Tommy to eat a nutritious meal from home. Instead she has focused exclusively on Tommy being obedient.
- Father has also forgotten the important points, which are that he wants Tommy to eat a nutritious meal and to respect his mother, and that he and Mother must work together as a team to help Tommy to grow up. Instead he has focused exclusively on ending the disagreement between Tommy and his mother. In the end, he is not supportive of his wife and is enabling of his son's problematic behaviors.

Accordingly, the physician could suggest a different way of handling the situation to break the negative cycle and come to a more satisfactory ending. For example, when Tommy does not want what his mother has prepared for dinner, Mother could suggest that he fix himself something he wants to eat while firmly letting him know that ordering a pizza is not an option. (Mother's needs to have Tommy eat a nutritious meal from home and to be respectful can both be met.) If Tommy then turns to his father, Father could support Mother by underscoring her decision. (Father will prevent an altercation with Mother and teach Tommy that Mother is in a position of authority and should be respected). If Tommy begins to have a temper tantrum, he should be given time out for a prescribed amount of time (for example, 10 minutes). If he does not go to time out on his own, for each additional minute that he resists, an extra minute is added to his time out (Tommy is dealt with in a nonemotional manner by Mother and Father as a team, and he learns that he does not get what he wants through negative behavior.) If after time out, he still says he wants to order a pizza, Mother and Father should again point out his options: eat the dinner Mother prepared, fix something for himself, or go hungry (Mother and Father underscore the natural consequences of his behavior). The parents then need to stick to their guns.

The physician should inform the parents that they may need to practice these types of interventions several times with the child before they notice a change. In fact, the physician may often have to coach the parents through many difficult situations, since it is likely that the child will "up the ante" when his demands are not being met. Family members may easily fall back on familiar and more comfortable ways of responding. Additionally, the physician may need to remind the parents that they are doing what is in their child's best interest. The child's world will be more predictable, there will be less conflict between the parents and child, and the child will hopefully transfer his respect for authority into other situations, such as at school and in the community. Additionally, as the parents begin to feel more competent in their skills, they may be able to coach teachers and other adults through difficult situations with their child.

For more difficult children, it may be necessary for the physician to establish a support network for the parents in dealing with their child. This may involve respite care, in-home services, after-school care, and the use of a probation officer. In situations where the parents and youth are all overwhelmed by emotional and behavioral problems, temporary placement of the child in foster care or a group home may be helpful until the parents can rebuild the family foundation.

School is usually a frustrating source of failure for children with ODD and CD. They are disliked by their teachers and peers, and they do not fare well academically. School also becomes a source for grouping with other nonconforming youth. It is important that the physician ensure that children with ODD or CD are in the proper academic setting. The physician should be alert to any types of developmental disorders that may be interfering with the child's ability to learn. It is not unusual to find that these children have significant auditory processing difficulties. Although they hear what is said, their ability to understand may be quite limited. In school situations where the child feels confused and threatened, he is likely to resort to antisocial methods of resolving problems. These children need to be referred to appropriate academic resources, even if that means placement in a self-contained classroom or a special school. For the older adolescent with CD, the youth may be hopelessly behind in school at the time of intervention. In such cases, the school may want to focus more on teaching the youth vocational and life skills necessary for survival rather than straight academics. Teachers often need to be educated in how to deal with these students. It is not unusual to find that teachers get into many struggles with these children that could easily have been avoided. School also presents an ideal situation for learning prosocial group skills.

Interventions may also be necessary in the child's community. To "give up" and avoid conduct-disordered behavior, the child must abandon old alliances with antisocial youth and develop a new peer group. For children who lack prosocial skills, this may be quite a feat. Children may need specific instructions and practice making and keeping friends. Additionally, these youth commonly have little insight into how to fill their day so they are not tempted to get involved in antisocial behavior. It may be necessary to help these children learn new leisure skills and to get them connected with prosocial activities in the community such as boys' or girls' clubs, the YMCA, and Big Brothers or Big Sisters.

With many of these youth, there is court involvement. The court may serve as a tremendous resource for children with CD. The court may act to support parental authority, particularly if the father or another predominant male figure is absent from the home. The court may also serve as a means to attain services that would otherwise be unavailable. As a last alternative, the court may be necessary to make appropriate dispositions that involves removing children from the community and placing them in a correctional setting.

For some children with CD, more specific types of treatment may be necessary. This is particularly true for the youth who has a substance abuse problem or who is a sex offender. There is little evidence that traditional substance abuse services are effective in this group; however, when they are coupled with multisystemic therapy, results are more impressive. Sexual perpetrators may need to complete a sex offenders program geared specifically for youth with this problem.

Summary

As is evident from this chapter, ODD and CD represent a very heterogeneous group. Therefore it is difficult to address the overall prognosis in this group. It is known that there is a group of children with ODD who do not go on to become conduct disordered and that the best predictor of an unrelenting course is the appearance of aggressive behavior. In children who have CD, those with the adolescent-onset type have a very favorable outcome with many desisting from antisocial behaviors before the onset of adulthood. Overall, the most consistent factors that predict poor prognosis in CD are an early age of onset; the appearance of antisocial behavior across multiple setting such as school, home, and community; the youth exhibiting a diversity of antisocial behaviors; and the presence of hyperactivity and attention deficits. This is most consistent with childhood-onset CD. However, even with this group, there is promise, particularly if the physician is alert to the early warning signals of developing CD, aggressive intervention occurs, and treatment is multisystemic.

CONSIDER CONSULTATION WHEN . . . .

- The child's level of aggression becomes such that he cannot be safely maintained in a community setting such as home
- It is suspected that another type of psychopathologic condition, such as a psychosis or a mood disorder, may be responsible for the presenting symptoms
- The child's behavior worsens despite typical and appropriate medical, behavioral and family interventions
- There are significant co-morbid disorders, such as substance abuse or dependence

Annotated Bibliography

Egan J: *Oppositional defiant disorder.* In Wiener JM, editor: *Textbook of child and adolescent psychiatry,* Washington, 1991, American Psychiatric Press.

Hendren RI: *Conduct disorder in childhood.* In Wiener JM, editor: *Textbook of child and adolescent psychiatry:* Washington, 1991, American Psychiatric Press.

Lewis DO: *Conduct disorder.* In Lewis M, editor: *Child and adolescent psychiatry, a comprehensive textbook,* Baltimore, 1991, Williams & Wilkins.

chapter 7

Anxiety Disorders in Children and Adolescents

Craig L. Donnelly, MD, Vladimir Maletic, MD, and John S. March, MD

Generalized Anxiety Disorder
Obsessive-Compulsive Disorder
Panic Disorder
Posttraumatic Stress Disorder
Separation Anxiety Disorder
Selective Mutism
Social Phobia
Specific Phobia
Summary

Fear and anxiety are common experiences throughout childhood and adolescence. Indeed, it is in the adaptive management and development of coping strategies for these affective states that the processes of striving for mastery, skill acquisition, and cognitive maturation unfold. Thus physicians evaluating childhood anxiety disorders face the task of differentiating normal, transient, developmentally appropriate expressions of anxiety from pathologic states of anxiety.

To facilitate better continuity in clinical settings, research contexts, and treatment applications, DSM-IV has refined the diagnostic nomenclature of childhood anxiety disorders to attain greater consistency with the adult anxiety disorders. DSM-IV uses a categoric diagnostic scheme in which criteria sets, or symptom clusters, are used to define a disorder. The diagnostic thresholds, or cut-off points, are set rather sharply and stand in contrast to dimensional schemes, which allow for shadings between normal and pathologic, and hence less sharply demarcate a disorder. It is unclear which nosologic scheme best fits the actual expression of childhood anxiety disorders. This chapter employs the criteria sets used in DSM-IV to discuss the various anxiety disorders of childhood. It should be borne in mind, however, that the categoric criteria sets are guidelines, serving as models of disorder, and may not necessarily or exactly reflect the actual expressions of pathologic states of anxiety. Additionally, in assessing the criteria for a diagnostic threshold in DSM-IV, the physician is expected to exercise clinical judgment in terms of the

DSM-IV DIAGNOSTIC CRITERIA

BOX 7-1 GENERALIZED ANXIETY DISORDER

A. Excessive anxiety and worry (apprehensive expectation), occurring more days than not for at least 6 months, about a number of events or activities (such as work or school performance).

B. The person finds it difficult to control the worry.

C. The anxiety or worry are associated with three (or more) of the following six symptoms (with at least some symptoms present for more days than not for the past 6 months). Note: Only one item is required in children.

(1) restlessness or feeling keyed up or on edge
(2) being easily fatigued
(3) difficulty concentrating or mind going blank
(4) irritability
(5) muscle tension
(6) sleep disturbance (difficulty falling or staying asleep, or restless unsatisfying sleep)

D. The focus of the anxiety or worry is not confined to features of an Axis I disorder (e.g., the anxiety and worry is not about having a Panic Attack (as in Panic Disorder), being embarrassed in public (as in Social Phobia), being contaminated (as in Obsessive-Compulsive Disorder), being away from home or close relatives (as in Separation Anxiety Disorder), gaining weight (as in Anorexia Nervosa), having multiple physical complaints (as in Somatization Disorder), or having a serious illness (as in Hypochondriasis), and the anxiety and worry do not occur exclusively during Posttraumatic Stress Disorder.

E. The anxiety, worry, or physical symptoms cause clinically significant distress or impairment in social, occupational, or other important areas of functioning.

F. The disturbance is not due to the direct physiological effects of a substance (e.g., a drug of abuse, a medication) or a general medical condition (e.g., hyperthyroidism) and does not occur exclusively during a Mood Disorder, a Psychotic Disorder, or a Pervasive Developmental Disorder.

(From American Psychiatric Association: *Diagnostic and statistical manual of mental disorders,* ed 4 [DSM-IV], 1994, American Psychiatric Press.)

severity, the degree of distress, and the relative dysfunction manifested by the individual child.

The developmental course of anxiety, its appropriateness, and its boundaries are areas of intense research interest. Yet surprisingly little empiric data exists in these areas. Many of the assessment instruments used to diagnose childhood anxiety disorders are simply extrapolations of adult instruments. These may not appropriately capture the unique developmental complexities of childhood anxiety. Newer instruments are currently being developed and are undergoing validation trials. These are discussed in the diagnosis sections of the specific anxiety disorders.

Although these instruments undoubtedly help the physician make more accurate diagnoses, they are only one component in the complex process of identification, understanding, and treating childhood anxiety. To effectively engage this process, a wider perspective is necessary.

First, physicians need to maintain a high level of suspicion for anxiety disorders when evaluating children. Anxiety disorders are not rare and often mimic or are co-morbid with other childhood disorders. For example, estimates of prevalence indicate that 4% of children and young adolescents meet diagnostic criteria for separation anxiety disorder (SAD). Additionally, truancy from school may be less reflective of oppositional behavior than an underlying social phobia or panic disorder. Second, children need to be evaluated within a biopsychosocial framework. The anxiety disorder that exists in isolation, without a context, is extremely rare. Genetic vulnerability, biologic causes, life experiences, social and family contexts, and developmental phases are interwoven to a greater or lesser extent in the expression of pathologic anxiety. The role of these interdependent factors requires clarification. The physician must understand the inner experiential context and the external behavioral contingencies in which the anxious child is operating. Third, given the uniqueness of each child and the complex interplay among the internal and external variables that drive anxiety, a multimodal approach to diagnosis and treatment is the rule rather than the exception.

This chapter, which is organized in sections devoted to specific anxiety disorders, provides the basic principles for evaluating and treating childhood anxiety dis-

DIAGNOSIS

TABLE 7-1
GENERALIZED ANXIETY DISORDER

Discriminating feature

1. Excessive worry occurring in multiple settings

Consistent features

1. Absence of a physiologic disturbance that explains symptoms
2. Inability to control the degree of worrying
3. Impaired social or academic functioning
4. Periods of exacerbation and remission

Variable features

1. Irritability
2. Muscle tension and sense of fatigue or lack of energy
3. Difficulty getting to sleep and restless unsatisfying sleep
4. Excessive concern about performance and competence
5. Inattention and restlessness
6. Somatic complaints with no specific cause

PEARLS & PERILS

GENERALIZED ANXIETY DISORDER

- Fatigue, difficulty concentrating, irritability, and sleep disturbance are common symptoms of both anxiety and depressive disorders.
- Patients with GAD tend to be older and from a higher socioeconomic group than those with SAD.
- The restlessness and inattentiveness of the anxious child may be misinterpreted as symptoms of attention-deficit/hyperactivity disorder (ADHD).
- The physician should be alert to a possible anxiety disorder in the child who has unexplained and nonspecific somatic complaints.

orders. Each section presents a pragmatic definition of the disorder, the DSM-IV diagnostic criteria with current incidence and prevalence data, a discussion of the causes, and the characteristics of the disorder as it is currently conceptualized. The diagnostic presentation, considerations in the differential diagnosis, and current treatment recommendations are then discussed. When using this chapter the physician should bear in mind that the assessment and treatment of childhood anxiety is often quite complex and time consuming. The physician undertaking this task should not hesitate to consult an expert in childhood anxiety disorders if time constraints, lack of experience, or the intricacies of a particular child's situation prove problematic.

Generalized Anxiety Disorder

Diagnostic Criteria

The diagnosis of generalized anxiety disorder (GAD) in DSM-IV has subsumed the DSM-III-R diagnosis of overanxious disorder (OAD) (Box 7-1). The adult criteria, which are also used to diagnose the childhood disorder have been modified slightly: "excessive anxiety and worry" has replaced "unrealistic worries." Previously specified worries about future or past events and competence are no longer part of the criteria. Excessiveness of worries is the only required descriptor. Self-consciousness and a need for reassurance, as well as somatic complaints, are no longer required for diagnosis. The new diagnostic classification emphasizes functional impairment rather than an exhaustive list of attributes defining the disorder. Because of the significant overlap of anxiety with depressive symptoms such as fatigue, difficulty concentrating, irritability, and sleep disturbance, physicians may be more challenged to differentiate GAD from depressive disorders, especially in children. Most of the data referred to in this chapter pertains to OAD and is assumed to approximate GAD in children and adolescents (Table 7-1).

Prevalence

Since results of studies using DSM-IV criteria to evaluate GAD in children are pending, the prevalence of this disorder is estimated using epidemiologic data on OAD. The prevalence of OAD ranges from 2.7% to 4.6% of the population, according to a recent epidemiologic review. There seems to be no difference in the prevalence of GAD (OAD) between the sexes. A recent study notes that patients with GAD (OAD) tend to be older than patients with SAD (80%) and come from higher socioeconomic groups.

Etiology

Freud postulated that anxiety is a product of suppression of unacceptable libidinous or aggressive drives. Later, he described signal anxiety as a warning about approaching highly conflictual and potentially devastating repressed material.

Behavioral theories emphasize anxiety as a function of both classical and operant conditioning. For example, worries about competence that arise from a job loss might be reinforced by excessive reassurance seeking. Recent cognitive theories tend to view maladaptive cognitions as a precipitant and probably perpetuant of anxiety in children.

Other authors theorize that familial factors, such as high levels of parental expectations and an emphasis on achievement or excessive permissiveness, may facilitate the development of anxiety. Behavioral inhibition, a temperamental trait related to shyness, may also constitute a substantial risk factor for development of GAD.

Neurobiologic theories consider disturbances in the hypothalamic-pituitary-adrenal axis and the regulation of thyroid and growth hormone secretion as possible causes of anxiety. Noradrenalin, serotonin, adenosine, and γ-aminobutyric acid (GABA) dysfunction have also been implicated. These theories have yet to make a distinction between causes of different anxiety disorders (with the possible exception of obsessive-compulsive disorder [OCD]) and need further empiric substantiation.

Data from longitudinal studies of GAD in children are still pending. Thus clinical lore is the only available source of speculations about the natural course of the disorder. It appears that GAD has a variable course with exacerbations and remissions.

Assessment

Children and adolescents with GAD tend to worry excessively about their performance and competence in the absence of external scrutiny. Ruminating about past mistakes and worrying about future adversities may cause a decline in academic functioning and precipitate a referral. Parents often report apprehension about "adult issues" such as illness, old age, death, financial matters, wars, and natural disasters. Children with GAD are commonly seen as perfectionistic and self-cautious, often seeking reassurance. Because they cannot stop worrying, these children often appear inattentive, restless, tense, and irritable. Where there is a discrepancy between the high expectations and the level of achievement, depression may ensue, especially in teenagers. Co-morbid phobic or panic disorders are not uncommon. Younger children sometimes have concomitant symptoms of SAD and attention-deficit/hyperactivity disorder (ADHD). Somatic complaints, such as stomachaches and headaches, are often reported by youngsters suffering from GAD and precipitate visits to pediatricians.

The importance of an extensive and detailed history in establishing correct diagnosis and differentiating GAD from other anxiety disorders cannot be overestimated. Multiple sources of information are preferable. Structured or semistructured interviews can be used to guide data gathering. Anxiety scales, such as the Revised Children's Manifest Anxiety Scale (RCMAS), may be of assistance in confirming the diagnosis and monitoring treatment outcome. Cooperation with a family doctor or pediatrician and school authorities helps ensure a satisfactory treatment outcome.

Differential Diagnosis

GAD can be differentiated from SAD by its pervasive nature and its presence across different contexts. Panic disorder is more "phasic" compared with the more "tonic" GAD; worries in panic disorder are usually focused on the possibility of future panic attacks. In specific phobias, fears are centered on phobic objects. Obsessive thoughts can be differentiated from GAD by their intrusive nature, content, and concomitant compulsive rituals. In posttraumatic stress disorder (PTSD), anxiety stems from a previous traumatic event. Depressed mood, anhedonia, and vegetative signs set depressive episodes apart from GAD.

Finally, medical conditions often present with symptoms that may mimic GAD. The physician should be alert to possible hyperthyroidism, diabetes mellitus, pheochromocytoma, or lupus. Excessive stimulant use, including caffeinism and alcohol withdrawal, can also be manifested by anxiety.

Treatment

Traditionally, psychodynamic therapy focuses on expanding the awareness of the defensive and maladaptive nature of anxiety. Empiric validation is still pending for this technique. Cognitive and behavioral approaches show much greater empiric support. Contingency management can lead to symptom suppression through reduction of reinforcers for anxious behaviors. Relaxation, visual imagery, self-affirmative statements, and self-instruction, as well as the identification of faulty cognitions and their replacement with adaptive thoughts, have been successfully combined in various ways in different cognitive and behavioral approaches.

Antidepressants and benzodiazepines have commonly been used to treat GAD in children and adolescents. A controlled study using alprazolam to treat GAD showed a trend toward benefit, but failed to reach statistical significant Buspirone 15 to 60 mg/day split into three doses has been shown to be helpful in pilot studies.

Obsessive-Compulsive Disorder

Diagnostic Criteria

The essential features of OCD include recurrent obsessions or compulsions that are time consuming and cause marked impairment or significant distress (Box 7-2, Table 7-2).

Prevalence

OCD is more common in children and adolescents than was once thought. It is estimated that OCD occurs in 0.3% to 1.9% of all children. During adolescence, the disorder is equally common in boys and

BOX 7-2 OBSESSIVE-COMPULSIVE DISORDER

DSM-IV DIAGNOSTIC CRITERIA

A. Either obsessions or compulsions:

Obsessions as defined by (1), (2), (3), and (4):

(1) recurrent and persistent thoughts, impulses, or images that are experienced, at some time during the disturbance, as intrusive and inappropriate and that cause marked anxiety or distress
(2) the thoughts, impulses, or images are not simply excessive worries about real-life problems
(3) the person attempts to ignore or suppress such thoughts, impulses, or images, or to neutralize them with some other thought or action
(4) the person recognizes that the obsessional thoughts, impulses, or images are a product of his or her own mind (not imposed from without as in thought insertion)

Compulsions as defined by (1) and (2):

(1) repetitive behaviors (e.g., hand washing, ordering, checking) or mental acts (e.g., praying, counting, repeating words silently) that the person feels driven to perform in response to an obsession, or according to rules that must be applied rigidly
(2) the behaviors or mental acts are aimed at preventing or reducing distress or preventing some dreaded event or situation; however, these behaviors or mental acts either are not connected in a realistic way with what they are designated to neutralize or prevent or are clearly excessive

B. At some point during the course of the disorder, the person has recognized that the obsessions or compulsions are excessive or unreasonable. **Note:** This does not apply to children.

C. The obsessions or compulsions cause marked distress, are time consuming (take more than 1 hour a day), or significantly interfere with the person's normal routine, occupational (or academic) functioning, or usual social activities or relationships.

D. If another Axis I disorder is present, the content of the obsession or compulsions is not restricted to it (e.g., preoccupation with food in the presence of an Eating Disorder; hair pulling in the presence of Trichotillomania; concern with appearance in the presence of Body Dysmorphic Disorder; preoccupation with drugs in the presence of a Substance Use Disorder; preoccupation with having a serious illness in the presence of Hypochondriasis; preoccupation with sexual urges or fantasies in the presence of a Paraphilia; guilty ruminations in the presence of Major Depressive Disorder).

E. The major disturbance is not due to the direct physiological effects of a substance (e.g., a drug of abuse, a medication) or a general medical condition.

Specify if:
With Poor Insight: if, for most of the time during the current episode, the person does not recognize that the obsessions and compulsions are excessive or unreasonable.

(From American Psychiatric Association: *Diagnostic and Statistical Manual of Mental Disorders,* ed 4 [DSM-IV], Washington DC, 1994, American Psychiatric Press.)

girls; in younger children, OCD is slightly more common in boys because of the higher prevalence of comorbid Tourette's disorder.

Etiology

The recognition that the serotonin-selective reuptake inhibitors (SSRIs) were effective in treating OCD, together with challenge studies using serotonin agonists, has led to the acceptance of the serotonin hypothesis of OCD. However, several lines of evidence (for example, the association of OCD with Tourette's disorder and other basal ganglia illnesses, and the observation that OCD symptoms developed in children with ADHD who were treated with high dose stimulants) suggest that multiple neurotransmitters may be involved.

Assessment

Children with OCD tend to show evidence of both obsessions and compulsions. Patients with only obsessive behavior are rare, although patients with pure compulsive behavior are not uncommon. Girls report more

DIAGNOSIS

TABLE 7-2
OBSESSIVE-COMPULSIVE DISORDER

Discriminating feature

1. Ruminating thoughts and ritualistic, compulsive behaviors

Consistent features

1. Obsessions and compulsions cause marked distress
2. Obsessions and compulsions are time consuming
3. Impaired social or academic functioning
4. Absence of a physiologic abnormality that would explain symptoms

Variable features

1. More obsessions in girls and more compulsions in boys
2. Earlier age of onset for boys than girls
3. Stress causes a worsening of symptoms or difficulty making decisions

PEARLS & PERILS

OBSESSIVE-COMPULSIVE DISORDER

- OCD is characterized by a waxing and waning course, with symptoms worsened by stress.
- The majority of children with OCD require long-term medication treatment.
- A complex motor tic may be differentiated from a compulsion, in that tics are usually not heralded by a preceding thought or obsession and are purposeless as far as the child can interpret.
- Treatment outcome in OCD is best when medication treatment is combined with behavioral therapy.

obsessions, and boys report more compulsions. The mean age of onset is 10, with boys predisposed to both an earlier and a more likely prepubertal age of onset than girls. Younger children are distinguished by having more elaborate rituals without cognitive obsessions. The illness is characterized by a waxing and waning course, with symptoms worsened by stress.

Symptoms in children tend to follow adult patterns, with washing rituals affecting more than 85% of children with OCD, repeating rituals 51%, and checking rituals 46%. Ordering, arranging, counting, collecting, ensuring symmetry, and scrupulosity (a preoccupation with having said or done the right thing) are common. In the vast majority of patients, specific symptoms are numerous, appear and disappear, vary in intensity, and change in content over the course of illness.

Childhood onset OCD is a chronic and debilitating illness. Common co-morbid conditions such as major depressive disorder (MDD), SAD, and dysthymic disorder complicate the illness. Studies indicate that the majority of children with OCD require long-term medication treatment and that although as many as 80% experience improvement, a significant proportion (43% to 68%) continue to meet diagnostic criteria for OCD.

Developmentally, appropriate childhood rituals that usually disappear by age 8 or 9 need to be distinguished from OCD. These rituals are usually not excessive or debilitating, are discrete, and do not have the content (such as washing or counting) typical of OCD. Since children are reluctant to acknowledge and rarely volunteer information about their symptoms, a careful history taken with the help of parents or primary caregiver and semistructured interview scales are useful in making the diagnosis.

The primary instrument for assessing OCD is the interviewer-administered Yale-Brown Obsessive Compulsive Scale (YBOCS). The Leyton Obsessional Inventory-Child Version, in its modified 20-item format, is an acceptable self-report assessment instrument.

Differential Diagnosis

Because of the co-morbidity of OCD and Tourette's disorder, it is necessary to distinguish a complex motor tic from a true ritual. Tics are usually not heralded by a preceding thought or obsession.

The stereotypies and repetitive movements seen in mental retardation and pervasive developmental disorders (PDDs) tend to be more discrete and fixed than they are in OCD.

Obsessive ruminations in individuals who are depressed or have dysthymic disorder can mimic OCD symptoms, although mood symptoms predominate depression. Similarly, although obsessions or compulsions can occur in psychotic disorders, OCD is not a psychotic process. Rather, individuals with OCD are usually aware of the ridiculous or unreasonable nature of OCD symptoms. Similarly, the eating rituals of patients with anorexia nervosa or bulimia nervosa are easily distinguished from OCD on the basis of content alone. Rigid personality traits characteristic of obsessive-compulsive personality disorder (OCPD) need to be considered in the differential diagnosis of OCD, but OCPD is present in a minority of people with OCD and often improves with successful treatment.

Treatment

Cognitive behavior therapy (CBT), often in conjunction with pharmacotherapy, is currently the treatment of choice for OCD. Family therapy may provide an adjunctive role by helping families decrease the parental involvement in the child's rituals, as well as by reinforcing the behavior-based interventions.

Exposure and response prevention is the preferred behavioral treatment of OCD. After identifying all obsessions and compulsions and ranking them on a stimulus hierarchy (that is, in subjective "units of discomfort"), the patient is asked to come into contact with phobic stimuli (exposure) and to repress from rituals or avoidance behaviors. Repeated presentation of the anxiety-invoking stimuli, in the absence of rituals, results in true habituation.

Pharmacotherapy with the serotoninergic agents clomipramine (up to 3 mg/kg/day) and fluoxetine (5 to 40 mg/day) have demonstrated effectiveness in the treatment of children with OCD. The newer SSRIs, such as sertraline, paroxetine, and fluvoxamine, will likely be efficacious as well. Long-term maintenance therapy is indicated for the patient who is responsive to medication. Treatment outcome appears best when children have access to both CBT and an SSRI.

Panic Disorder

Diagnostic Criteria

Recent studies clearly establish the presence of panic in adolescents and, less commonly, in younger children. Many physicians believe that panic disorder and SAD are different developmental manifestations of the same underlying anxiety diathesis. Arguments in favor of this hypothesis include: (1) phenomenologic similarities, (2) family genetic studies, and (3) responsiveness to treatment. DSM-IV criteria for panic disorder in children and adolescents are, nevertheless, the same as for adults.

A panic attack is not a codable DSM-IV disorder. However, there are clear characteristics of a panic attack. A panic attack is defined as a discrete period of intense fear, discomfort, or terror accompanied by thoughts of impending doom or loss of control of reality. Four (or more) of the following symptoms develop abruptly and reach a peak within 10 minutes:

1. palpitations, pounding heart, or accelerated heart rate
2. sweating
3. trembling or shaking
4. sensations of shortness of breath or smothering
5. feeling of choking
6. chest pain or discomfort
7. nausea or abdominal distress
8. feeling dizzy, unsteady, lightheaded, or faint
9. derealization (feelings of unreality) or depersonalization (being detached from oneself)
10. fear of losing control or going crazy
11. fear of dying
12. paresthesias (numbness or tingling sensations)
13. chills or hot flashes

DSM-IV emphasizes the difference between a panic attack and panic disorder by stating that a panic attack may occur in a variety of other anxiety disorders. The diagnosis of panic disorder requires recurrent and unexpected attacks followed by persistent fears and worries about future attacks and their consequences.

According to DSM-IV, an individual may be diagnosed as having a panic disorder with or without agoraphobia (Boxes 7-3 and 7-4, Table 7-3). Agoraphobia is anxiety about being in places or situations from which escape might be difficult (or embarrassing) or in which help may not be available in the event of an unexpected or situationally predisposed panic attack or panic-like symptoms. Agoraphobia typically involves clusters of situations that include being outside the home alone, being in a crowd or standing in a line, being on a bridge, and travelling in a bus, train, or automobile. The situations are avoided, endured with marked distress or anxiety about having a panic attack or panic-like symptoms, or require the presence of a companion. In DSM-IV, agoraphobia can occur in the absence of panic attacks (Box 7-5).

Prevalence

Epidemiologic studies of panic disorder in children and adolescents using new DSM-IV criteria have not been completed. In the absence of current data, a good estimate of the prevalence of panic disorder in the high school population is 0.6%. As in adults, there is a higher prevalence in girls than in boys. It appears that onset after puberty is much more common than onset earlier in childhood. The peak onset of panic disorder is between ages 15 and 19.

Etiology

Multiple causes have been suggested for panic attacks, including early affective conditioning, early childhood loss, biologic vulnerability, and familial influence. A recent review finds no proof of early loss as a determinant of panic attacks. Chemical induction (sodium lactate, cholecystokinin [CCK], carbon dioxide, adrenergic agents, and serotoninergic agents), blunted thyroid-stimulating hormone (TSH) response to thyrotropin-releasing hormone (TRH), and growth hormone response to challenges have all been noted in adults with panic disorder.

Neurotransmitter dysfunction (caused by GABA, noradrenalin, and serotonin) has also been implicated in the genesis of panic disorder. A relatively good response to pharmacologic interventions supports biologic mediation as a casual factor. Interesting attempts to combine biologic diathesis with familial and dy-

DSM-IV DIAGNOSTIC CRITERIA

BOX 7-3 PANIC DISORDER WITHOUT AGORAPHOBIA

A. Both (1) and (2):

(1) recurrent unexpected Panic Attacks
(2) at least one of the attacks has been followed by 1 month (or more) of one (or more) of the following:

(a) persistent concern about having additional attacks
(b) worry about the implications of the attack or its consequences (e.g., losing control, having a heart attack, "going crazy")
(c) a significant change in behavior related to the attacks

B. Absence of Agoraphobia.

C. The Panic Attacks are not due to the direct physiological effects of a substance (e.g., a drug of abuse, a medication) or a general medical condition (e.g., hyperthyroidism).

D. The panic attacks are not better accounted for by another mental disorder, such as Social Phobia (e.g., occurring on exposure to feared social situations), Specific Phobia (e.g., on exposure to a specific phobic situation), Obsessive-Compulsive Disorder (e.g., on exposure to dirt in someone with an obsession about contamination), Posttraumatic Stress Disorder (e.g., in response to stimuli associated with a severe stressor), or Separation Anxiety Disorder (e.g., in response to being away from home or close relatives).

(From American Psychiatric Association: *Diagnostic and statistical manual of mental disorders,* ed 4 [DSM-IV], Washington DC, 1994, American Psychiatric Press.)

DSM-IV DIAGNOSTIC CRITERIA

BOX 7-4 PANIC DISORDER WITH AGORAPHOBIA

A. Both (1) and (2):

(1) recurrent unexpected Panic Attacks
(2) at least one of the attacks has been followed by 1 month (or more) of one (or more) of the following:

(a) persistent concern about having additional attacks
(b) worry about the implications of the attack or its consequences (e.g., losing control, having a heart attack, "going crazy")
(c) a significant change in behavior related to the attacks

B. The presence of Agoraphobia.

C. The Panic Attacks are not due to the direct physiological effects of a substance (e.g., a drug of abuse, a medication) or a general medical condition (e.g., hyperthyroidism).

D. The Panic Attacks are not better accounted for by another mental disorder, such as Social Phobia (e.g., occurring on exposure to feared social situations), Specific Phobia (e.g., on exposure to a specific phobic situation), Obsessive-Compulsive Disorder (e.g., on exposure to dirt in someone with an obsession about contamination), Posttraumatic Stress Disorder (e.g., in response to stimuli associated with a severe stressor), or Separation Anxiety Disorder (e.g., in response to being away from home or close relatives).

(From American Psychiatric Association: *Diagnostic and statistical manual of mental disorders,* ed 4 [DSM-IV], Washington DC, 1994, American Psychiatric Press.

namic factors have recently been published. Other authors emphasize the importance of learning in the acquisition of panic attacks.

It appears that the onset of panic disorder before age 17 carries a greater risk of substance abuse, suicidal thoughts and attempts, and a consequent higher frequency of emergency room visits than adult-onset panic disorder. Increased risk of severe morbidity should mandate additional attention in the treatment of young patients with panic disorder.

BOX 7-5 AGORAPHOBIA WITHOUT HISTORY OF PANIC DISORDER

DSM-IV DIAGNOSTIC CRITERIA

A. The presence of Agoraphobia related to fear of developing panic-like symptoms (e.g., dizziness or diarrhea).

B. Criteria have never been met for Panic Disorder.

C. The disturbance is not due to direct physiological effects of a substance (e.g., a drug of abuse, a medication) or a general medical condition.

D. If an associated general medical condition is present, the fear described in criterion A is clearly in excess of that usually associated with the condition.

(From American Psychiatric Association: *Diagnostic and statistical manual of mental disorders,* ed 4 [DSM-IV], Washington DC, 1994, American Psychiatric Press.)

DIAGNOSIS

TABLE 7-3
PANIC DISORDER

Discriminating features

1. Unexpected, abrupt bursts of anxiety, with somatic symptoms and sense of terror or impending doom
2. Excessive fear of future episodes

Consistent features

1. Absence of a physiologic condition that may explain symptoms
2. Fear of dying, going crazy, or losing control

Variable features

1. Recent stressful event
2. Mitral valve prolapse
3. Agoraphobia
4. Depersonalization
5. Derealization
6. Attacks occur specific to a given situation

PEARLS & PERILS

PANIC DISORDER

- Panic attacks may occur as a manifestation of many types of anxiety disorders, including panic disorder.
- Agoraphobia may occur singularly or as a component of panic disorder. Likewise, panic disorder may occur with or without agoraphobia.
- Onset of panic disorder before age 17 heralds a greater risk for substance abuse, suicidal thoughts and attempts, and more frequent emergency room visits than adult-onset panic disorder.
- Mitral valve prolapse often occurs concomitantly with panic disorder.

Assessment

Children, and to some degree adolescents, tend to focus on somatic sensations in their early reports of panic disorder. Trembling, palpitations, shortness of breath, sweating, dizziness, and chest discomfort are often reported. Children, more readily than adolescents, report fears of dying, loss of control, or going crazy. Adolescents often complain of derealization or depersonalization, whereas these complaints are conspicuously absent in children.

Primary care physicians are advised to think of panic disorder when a patient has multiple somatic complaints in the absence of diagnosable organic causes. Mitral valve prolapse, an often cited concurrent finding, may diminish in some cases of successfully treated panic disorder. This raises the question of whether it exists as a co-morbidity or as a consequence of panic disorder.

Panic attacks may occur concurrently with depression and SAD, creating a diagnostic challenge. As in SAD, a history of a recent stressful events is often elicited, but the disorder may begin insidiously. Agoraphobia usually sets in within a year after the emergence of panic attacks.

Three different types of panic attacks can be identified: unexpected attacks with no recognizable precipitant, cognitive or interoceptive attacks triggered by cues, and situationally predisposed panic, which occurs when circumstances are likely to cause a panic attack. Situationally bound panic attacks are sometimes difficult to distinguish from phobias.

A detailed history obtained from the patient, family members, teachers, and other professionals acquainted with the child is invaluable. In some instances, pediatric and neurologic examinations may help elucidate the origin of somatic complaints or unusual sensations.

Semistructured diagnostic interviews, or their segments dealing with anxiety disorders, may be a useful adjunct. Anxiety rating scales provide useful diagnostic information and later assist in evaluating progress in treatment.

Differential Diagnosis

It is essential to differentiate panic disorder from medical conditions such as hyperthyroidism, hyperparathyroidism, pheochromocytoma, diabetes, asthma, seizures, vestibular dysfunction, or cardiac problems. Intoxication with stimulants or withdrawal from sedatives can produce symptoms that mimic panic attacks. Differentiating panic disorder from other anxiety disorders may be challenging.

Fear and anxiety that occur only when a child is separated from an attachment figure point to SAD rather than panic attacks. If the discomfort is experienced only in situations when the child is subjected to scrutiny, social phobia is a more likely diagnosis. In the specific phobias, fear and anxiety are an expected response to confrontation of the phobic object. Recollection of past trauma usually precedes emotional and autonomic distress in PTSD. Obsessions and compulsive rituals help differentiate panic disorder from OCD. The symptoms of the problem with the generic descriptor *school phobia* must be precisely defined to determine whether refusal to attend school is anxiety related (phobic or separation) or has another cause (for example, truancy). The absence of other panic-like symptoms distinguishes panic disorder from dissociative disorders manifested by depersonalization and derealization. Although some psychotic disorders may have panic as an associated feature, patients with panic disorder do not have thought disorders.

Treatment

Behavioral, cognitive, and pharmacologic treatments of panic disorder in young people have for the most part been adapted from the adult literature, with developmentally necessary modifications. There are no controlled studies of pharmacologic treatment of panic disorder in children or adolescents. Benzodiazepines, such as clonazepam and alprazolam, and tricyclic antidepressants, such as nortriptyline, are effective in the treatment of panic disorder. SSRIs also provide symptom relief (although somewhat more slowly), have fewer side effects than tricyclic antidepressants, and are the initial treatment of choice. Buspirone may be a helpful adjunct in patients with pronounced anxiety between the attacks.

No controlled studies evaluating the efficacy of behavioral and cognitive approaches to panic in young people have yet been undertaken. Anecdotal data suggest that systemic desensitization may be helpful in the treatment of agoraphobia, whereas cognitive approaches focused on relaxation and diminishing "catastrophic thinking" may be beneficial during the attack. Exposure techniques may be particularly helpful in situationally bound and cognitively or interoceptively driven panic attacks.

Posttraumatic Stress Disorder

Diagnostic Criteria

A severe trauma, such as witnessing a murder, being kidnapped, or living through a natural disaster, commonly induces long-lasting posttraumatic symptoms. The syndrome known as posttraumatic stress disorder (PTSD) entered the diagnostic nomenclature in DSM-III, although it was not specifically applied to children and adolescents at that time. Subsequent research demonstrated that the diagnostic criteria set for PTSD is consistent in both adults and children, and that children may in fact be more sensitive to the effects of severe trauma than adults (Box 7-6, Table 7-4).

Prevalence

Lacking epidemiologic studies, the incidence and prevalence of PTSD in children and adolescents is difficult to specify with precision. Adult current and lifetime prevalence rates are 0.4% and 1.3% in the epidemiologic catchment area (ECA) studies, but a specific prevalence rate for children and adolescents is unknown.

Etiology

Exposure to a traumatic event, whether directly, by observation as a witness, in a near-miss experience, or vicariously (for example, learning about a traumatic event affecting a loved one) is the necessary prerequisite to the development of PTSD. A distinction has been made between chronic, expected, repeated trauma (type II) and sudden, unexpected, single-incident trauma (type I). Type II trauma, as experienced in chronic physical or sexual abuse, may lead to a symptoms far different from those typical of PTSD, although there can be significant overlap. Although severity, duration, and proximity to the trauma are the most important predictors for development of PTSD, little is known about the potential risk and protective factors that affect PTSD.

Several models have been advanced for PTSD, including psychoanalytic, social learning, and neurobiologic models. In the psychoanalytic interpretation, the overwhelming experience of trauma breaches ego-coping mechanisms and mobilizes a complex array of psychologic defenses, including repetition compulsion, disso-

DSM-IV DIAGNOSTIC CRITERIA

BOX 7-6 POSTTRAUMATIC STRESS DISORDER

A. The person has been exposed to a traumatic event in which both of the following were present:

(1) the person experienced, witnessed, or was confronted with an event or events that involved actual or threatened death or serious injury, or a threat to the physical integrity of self or others
(2) the person's response involved intense fear, helplessness, or horror. **Note:** In children, this may be expressed by disorganized or agitated behavior

B. The traumatic event is persistently reexperienced in one (or more) of the following ways:

(1) recurrent and intrusive distressing recollections of the event, including images, thoughts, or perceptions. **Note:** In young children, repetitive play may occur in which themes or aspects of the trauma are expressed.
(2) recurrent distressing dreams of the event. **Note:** In children there may be frightening dreams without recognizable content.
(3) acting or feeling as if the traumatic event were recurring (includes a sense of reliving the experience, illusions, hallucinations, and dissociative flashback episodes, including those that occur on awakening or when intoxicated). **Note:** In young children, trauma-specific reenactment may occur.
(4) intense psychological distress at exposure to internal or external cues that symbolize or resemble an aspect of the traumatic event
(5) physiological reactivity on exposure to internal or external cues that symbolize or resemble an aspect of the traumatic event

C. Persistent avoidance of stimuli associated with the trauma and numbing of general responsiveness (not present before the trauma), as indicated by three (or more) of the following:

(1) efforts to avoid thoughts, feelings, or conversations associated with the trauma
(2) efforts to avoid activities, places, or people that arouse recollections of the trauma
(3) inability to recall an important aspect of the trauma
(4) markedly diminished interest or participation in significant activities
(5) feeling of detachment or estrangement from others
(6) restricted range of affect (e.g., unable to have loving feelings)
(7) sense of foreshortened future (e.g., does not expect to have a career, marriage, children, or a normal life span)

D. Persistent symptoms of increased arousal (not present before the trauma), as indicated by two (or more) of the following:

(1) difficulty falling or staying asleep
(2) irritability or outbursts of anger
(3) difficulty concentrating
(4) hypervigilance
(5) exaggerated startle response

E. Duration of the disturbance (symptoms in Criteria B, C, and D) is more than 1 month.

F. The disturbance causes clinically significant distress or impairment in social, occupational, or other important areas of functioning.

Specify if:
Acute: if duration of symptoms is less than 3 months
Chronic: if duration of symptoms is 3 months or more

Specify if:
With Delayed Onset: if onset of symptoms is at least 6 months after the stressor

(From American Psychiatric Association: *Diagnostic and statistical manual of mental disorders,* ed 4 [DSM-IV], Washington DC, 1994, American Psychiatric Press.)

DIAGNOSIS

TABLE 7-4
POSTTRAUMATIC STRESS DISORDER

Discriminating feature

1. Exposure to trauma followed by reexperiencing, avoidance, and hyperarousal

Consistent features

1. Recurrent, intrusive recollections of the trauma
2. Intense psychologic distress when exposed to cues of the trauma
3. Impaired social and academic functioning

Variable features

1. Emotional numbing
2. Nightmares
3. Irritability and depression
4. Attempts to avoid anything associated with the trauma
5. Aggressiveness
6. Unexplained somatic complaints
7. Sleep disturbance

PEARLS & PERILS

POSTTRAUMATIC STRESS DISORDER

- Type I PTSD is preceded by a sudden, unexpected, single incident of trauma, whereas in type II the child is chronically exposed to repeated trauma.
- PTSD may develop any time after a child experiences trauma. Although it is more rare, the physician should be alert to delayed-onset PTSD, where symptoms may not appear until 6 months after the traumatic event.
- The earlier the intervention after a traumatic event, the less likely it is that symptoms of PTSD will develop.
- The impetus of therapy in PTSD is allowing the child reexposure to the traumatic cues under safe conditions where reworking and mastery may occur.

ciation, denial, projection, and identification with the aggressor. The social learning theory, including both classical and instrumental conditioning, is responsible for the physiologic, cognitive, and complex behavioral manifestations of PTSD. Neurobiologic models of PTSD are exceedingly complex, and data is limited in children and adolescents.

Although delayed PTSD is uncommon, children may develop PTSD any time after they experience trauma. The relative predominance of reexperiencing, avoidance, and hyperarousal, as well as the duration of symptoms, varies. Symptoms remit within 3 months in one half of all cases, but symptoms may persist for years in others. Children with PTSD may have a bewildering array of symptoms and co-morbid conditions, including sleep disturbances, irritability, aggressiveness, physical complaints, disruptive behavior, depression, and other anxiety disorders.

Assessment

Because of the extensive co-morbidity and complex symptoms of PTSD, maintaining a high clinical suspicion and using a multimodal evaluation are crucial to accurate diagnosis. No single physiologic measure or clinical scale specific for the diagnosis of PTSD is available. Diagnosis involves obtaining a thorough history from multiple sources, documenting exposure to a severe trauma, evidence of persistent reexperiencing of the trauma, avoidance and numbing of responsiveness, and increased physiologic arousal. Parent and teacher reports are useful to assess external symptoms and changes in behavior. Family interviews may detect PTSD "contagion," or related symptoms, among those close to the child. A clinical interview with the child, in conjunction with a general anxiety scale such as the RCMAS, is essential in assessing internal symptoms (such as cognitive and affective anxiety). A developmental history may identify sources of vulnerability and previous coping styles. Finally, physical and neurologic examination may rule out organicity.

Differential Diagnosis

Anxiety and affective spectrum disorders are common considerations in the differential diagnoses and often accompany PTSD. Children often show increased separation anxiety and generalized anxiety after trauma exposure. Traumatic specific phobias are distinguishable from PTSD because they are more circumscribed and lack the tonic arousal and extensive symptom cluster of PTSD. Children with PTSD sometimes exhibit compulsive anxiety-reducing behaviors that mimic OCD. However, in OCD intrusive thoughts are unrelated to a severe traumatic precipitant. Symptoms of depression are the most common co-morbid feature of PTSD. They may range from simple demoralization to a full-blown major depressive episode.

The psychotic spectrum disorders and deliria are readily distinguished from PTSD on the basis of intact reality testing, the real nature of the intrusive thoughts, and the maintenance of a clear nonfluctuating sensorium.

Disruptive behavior disorders such as ODD, CD, and ADHD, as well as aggression, irritability, substance abuse, and deteriorating school performance may be derivatives of underlying PTSD.

Acute stress disorder has symptoms consistent with PTSD, although the duration of its onset (occurring within 4 weeks of the traumatic exposure) and resolution (occurring within 4 weeks) is shorter. An adjustment disorder may be diagnosed when the symptoms are subthreshold or when the stressor is of insufficient magnitude to meet PTSD criteria. Target symptoms may be identified that warrant treatment even in cases where symptoms do not meet the diagnostic threshold for the disorder. This is especially important soon after trauma exposure, since there is evidence that early intervention may prevent the subsequent formation of symptoms.

Treatment

Well-controlled treatment outcome data are lacking for PTSD in children and adolescents. Current approaches emphasize rapid triage and debriefing, followed by a multimodal approach that includes pharmacologic therapy, CBT, and supportive psychotherapy, as well as group and family therapy interventions when appropriate. Treatment is tailored to the nature of the trauma, the particular cluster and duration of symptoms, and the developmental stage of the child. Reexposure to the traumatic cues under safe conditions where reworking and mastery can occur are the cornerstones of treatment.

When symptoms are debilitating, medication may provide sufficient relief to support other concurrent treatment modalities. Tricyclic antidepressants may help reduce the sleep-related disturbances of PTSD. Fluoxetine and the other SSRIs show promise and may help reduce the depressive sequelae of the disorder. Clonazepam may reduce anxiety, and clonidine has been shown to diminish the startle responses of PTSD. Other medications that have been used include lithium and carbamazepine to reduce affective liability and propranolol to decrease arousal. Neuroleptics appear to have limited, if any, use in PTSD except in cases where dissociative or psychotic symptoms complicate the disorder.

A "prevention-intervention" model of treatment has been outlined; it includes initial triage for acute exposure, followed by support and enhancement of coping skills for anticipated grief and trauma responses. After the first two steps, brief, focused psychotherapy for chronic PTSD symptoms is "pulsed" in accordance with the needs of the patient. Treatment of other disorders is provided if they emerge in the context of PTSD. Family therapy and group therapy (for example, in a situation where numerous children have been exposed to trauma) may provide additional opportunities for triage, ventilation, psychoeducational support, and halting the spread of traumatic contagion. Early intervention, before symptoms have become established, may be crucial in the treatment of PTSD.

Separation Anxiety Disorder

Diagnostic Criteria

The cardinal feature of SAD is excessive anxiety engendered by separation from major attachment figures or the home environment. DSM-IV requires 4 weeks duration (as opposed to 2 weeks in DSM-III-R) and clinically significant or subjectively distressful impairment in social, academic, or occupational functioning. Since avoidant disorder of childhood and OAD are omitted in DSM-IV, SAD is the only anxiety disorder in the category of disorders first diagnosed in childhood and adolescence (Box 7-7, Table 7-5).

Prevalence

A prevalence rate of 4% is cited in DSM-IV. With recent changes in criteria, this figure is best viewed as an estimate. About one half of the children seeking psychiatric attention for anxiety have SAD. Thus it is one of the more common childhood disorders. Epidemiologic studies show that separation anxiety occurs more often in girls than in boys. Not surprisingly, SAD occurs more commonly in younger children, whereas similar "panic" symptomology in adolescents eventuates in agoraphobia, manifested as school refusal.

Etiology

Attempts have been made to attribute the onset of SAD to inadequately resolved separation and individuation conflicts, vulnerability determined by temperament, or behavioral contingencies. Genetic and environmental factors have also been evoked as causes. Decisive empiric or epidemiologic proof supporting any single cause is still lacking. Recent views suggesting multiple and interactive causes seem plausible.

Assessment

SAD is typically a disorder of middle childhood (ages 7 to 9), although it has also been described in adolescents. DSM-IV has a specifier for SAD occurring before age 6 (early onset). If the disorder develops acutely, a precipitating stressor can often be identified (such as a move, a change of school, the loss of a loved one, an illness in the family, or a prolonged absence from school). Sometimes the symptoms develop more insidiously. SAD waxes and wanes. Whereas some children recover fully after a single episode, others experience a more protracted and chronic course. Later onset, comorbidities, and familial psychopathologic conditions seem to be associated with a greater risk of chronicity.

Approximately one half of the children diagnosed with SAD have a concomitant anxiety disorder, and one third have co-morbid depression. Typically, SAD precedes depression, raising the question of whether the

DSM-IV DIAGNOSTIC CRITERIA

BOX 7-7 SEPARATION ANXIETY DISORDER

A. Developmentally inappropriate and excessive anxiety concerning separation from home or from those to whom the individual is attached, as evidenced by three (or more) or the following:

(1) recurrent excessive distress when separation from home or major attachment figure occurs or is anticipated
(2) persistent or excessive worry about losing, or about possible harm befalling, major attachment figures
(3) persistent and excessive worry that an untoward event will lead to separation from a major attachment figure (e.g., getting lost or being kidnapped)
(4) persistent reluctance or refusal to go to school or elsewhere because of fear of separation
(5) persistently and excessively fearful or reluctant to be alone or without major attachment figures at home or without significant adults in other settings
(6) persistent reluctance or refusal to go to sleep without being near a major attachment figure or to sleep away from home
(7) repeated nightmares involving the theme of separation
(8) repeated complaints of physical symptoms (such as headaches, stomachaches, nausea, or vomiting) when separation from major attachment figures occurs or is anticipated

B. The duration of the disturbance is at least 4 weeks.

C. The onset is before age 18 years.

D. The disturbance causes clinically significant distress or impairment in social, academic (occupational), or other important areas of functioning.

E. The disturbance does not occur exclusively during the course of a Pervasive Developmental Disorder, Schizophrenia, or other Psychotic Disorder, and in adolescents and adults, is not better accounted for by Panic Disorder with Agoraphobia.

Specify if:
Early Onset: if onset occurs before age 6

(From American Psychiatric Association: *Diagnostic and statistical manual of mental disorders,* ed 4 [DSM-IV], Washington DC, 1994, American Psychiatric Press.)

mood disorder is partly a consequence of enduring functional impairment. Anxiety disorders and depression are commonly found in the immediate families of children with SAD. Conversely, parental depression and anxiety is associated with a greater risk of SAD in the offspring.

Children suffering from SAD often come to the physician's attention when problems with school attendance develop. These difficulties range from great reluctance to refusal and temper tantrums if parents insist on taking the child to school. Separation from loved ones is often an issue around sleep time, and the child with SAD often ends up in the parents' bed. Increasing anxiety often interferes with spending the night at a friend's house or going to camp. Once separation takes place, these children worry about the misfortunes that might befall their loved ones. Nightmares with prominent themes of separation are sometimes reported. Fears of being lost and never reunited with their families often beset these children. In the face of growing distress after separation, children may plead to be returned home, attempt to run away, or even cause enough commotion that teachers are forced to contact parents. Typically the "storm" is resolved once the child is returned home. Somatic complaints, such as morning stomachaches, headaches, nausea, and vomiting, are more often seen in younger children, although older ones may also complain of palpitations and feeling faint.

A detailed history is the most helpful diagnostic resource. Accounts from the child are usually more telling than reports from the parent and teachers. Descriptions of the events preceding the separation, response to the parent's departure, ensuing behavior (usually in school), and the consequences help the physician understand the pattern of distress and identify possible perpetuants. Physicians will find that a well-taken history goes a long way toward planning successful therapeutic interventions.

Relevant portions of structured and semistructured interviews are used to assist in the systematic gathering of information. Anxiety rating scales and general psychiatric symptom rating scales may be used diagnostically as measures of treatment outcome. Routinely

DIAGNOSIS

TABLE 7-5
SEPARATION ANXIETY DISORDER

Discriminating feature

1. Excessive fear, worry, and clinging behavior on being separated from the parent

Consistent features

1. Impaired social or academic functioning
2. Waxing and waning course

Variable features

1. More common in girls than boys
2. Onset between ages 7 and 9
3. School refusal or poor school attendance
4. Nightmares and refusal to sleep alone
5. Fears that harm will come to loved ones while separated
6. Unexplained somatic complaints

available laboratory studies do not increase the accuracy of the diagnosis.

Differential Diagnosis

The physician must differentiate SAD from developmentally appropriate fears accompanying separation from loved ones. These occur earlier in childhood, have milder symptoms, and tend to be transient and self-limited. Functional impairment is not a typical feature of fears accompanying normal development.

Delineation of SAD from other disorders that have been classified as school phobia or school refusal is sometimes a challenging task. After CD and ODD have been ruled out, the physician should carefully evaluate evidence of other anxiety disorders. GAD has more varied symptoms, and the fears involved tend to stem from matters other than separation. Both SAD and panic disorder involve panic, but the latter lacks the intense focus on major attachment figures that characterizes SAD. Relative comfort in social settings differentiates SAD from social phobia. Specific phobias are characterized by well-defined and usually singular phobic objects; distress can occur even in the presence of an attachment figure. Pervasiveness of a mood disorder, especially if it precedes the onset of SAD, demands a separate diagnosis. Teasing apart MDD from SAD is not always easy, since the two disorders often occur concomitantly. Psychotic disorders, PTSD, pervasive developmental disorders (PDDs), and learning disorders should also be addressed. Finally, familial dysfunction, substance abuse, medical problems (especially ones causing abdominal distress), and iatrogenically caused syndromes (for example, neuroleptic-induced SAD) need to be ruled out.

PEARLS & PERILS

SEPARATION ANXIETY DISORDER

- Later age of onset, co-morbid psychiatric diagnoses, and familial psychopathologic conditions predict a more chronic and protracted course of SAD.
- One out of every three children with SAD has co-morbid depression with anxiety symptoms predating the onset of depressive symptoms.
- The development of somatic symptoms when the child must be apart from a loved one should alert the physician to possible SAD.
- SAD and panic disorder may represent different age presentations of the same form of psychopathologic condition.

Treatment

In uncomplicated cases where school refusal has not lasted more than 2 weeks, treatment is fairly straightforward. After informing the parents about the nature of the disorder and eliciting their cooperation, as well as that of school authorities, the child is encouraged to return to school as soon as possible. Parents are instructed to show empathy and understanding for the child's distress, but to insist in a firm and consistent manner on regular school attendance. The child is supported to master the fears and worries incumbent in the separation. Reward and praise should accompany the desired behavior.

If school refusal has become entrenched, especially in older adolescents, therapy is much more difficult. Behavior and cognitive approaches have reportedly been successful and are recommended in spite of a lack of controlled studies. Shaping the desired behavior through contingency management—positively reinforcing nonfearful behavior and withdrawing rewards for anxious behavior—may yield results. Modeling and exposure-based treatments have also been reported to be effective.

Cognitive interventions focus on the maladaptiveness of catastrophic thoughts and their replacement by more adaptive cognitions. In combination with self-instruction and teaching realistic appraisal of fear-producing circumstances, such interventions can be fruitful. Some somatic complaints can be countered by instruction in deep muscle relaxation. Group and family therapies can be valuable adjunctive treatments.

Psychopharmacologic approaches may be useful in selected cases, especially when combined with psychosocial interventions. Imipramine, in spite of controversial findings, should be considered as a therapeutic agent. Scarce controlled studies suggest that benzodiazepines such as alprazolam and clonazepam may be useful in ameliorating anticipatory symptoms of anxiety, panic, and SAD. SSRIs have been used successfully to treat anxiety disorders in adults and may be the treatment of choice in children. Teaching realistic appraisal of fear-producing circumstances can be fruitful. Psychotropic agents should be reserved for more refractory and complicated cases. In these cases, the physician should begin treatment with an SSRI and add clonazepam. It should be borne in mind that CBT is the most powerful augmenter of treatment. Preliminary results with combined therapies in children (mostly anecdotal) are encouraging.

Selective Mutism

Diagnostic Criteria

The term *selective mutism* was coined by Tramer to describe a population of children who speak only in certain situations or to certain people. Historically the disorder has been attributed to psychologic trauma, a manifestation of family dynamics involving an enmeshed mother and an oppositional child, and the communication of hostility through passive-aggression or defiant refusal to speak. Recently a multifactorial view of selective mutism has emerged that focuses on anxiety as the underlying driving force of the disorder (Box 7-8, Table 7-6).

Prevalence

Selective mutism is a rare disorder. Most cases do not come to medical attention and resolve with age. Prevalence estimates range from 0.08% to 0.7% of all children in large community samples.

The onset is usually between ages 3 and 6. Seventy percent of referrals occur during the kindergarten years, with boys being referred an average of 2.3 years earlier than girls. The disorder is more common in girls than in boys, with a reported ratio of about 3 : 1, and in children with articulation disorders or where English is a second language.

Etiology

Children with selective mutism have been described as excessively shy, sensitive, and novelty avoidant, and familial shyness has been reported in families of children with the disorder. There is the suggestion that selective mutism may be related to either social phobia or panic disorder. Co-morbidity rates are unknown, but associated diagnoses have included depression, enuresis or encopresis, and OCD. Co-morbid anxiety disorders are probably also common. Co-morbidity with speech and language disorders is unknown.

The majority of children with selective mutism outgrow their disorder, although it is not uncommon for the disorder to persist for several years in elementary school. Some evidence indicates that children who do not improve by the age of 10 have an intractable form of the disorder.

Assessment

Diagnosis is based on clinical history. The physician should take a complete medical history and conduct a thorough physical examination of a child with selective mutism. The neurologic examination and the developmental history should focus on motor, cognitive, language, and social milestones. The quality of temperament, social interactions, and the precise contexts in which speech occurs should be assessed. Formal speech and language assessment (sometimes using the child's audio-recorded speech) may be necessary.

BOX 7-8 SELECTIVE MUTISM

DSM-IV DIAGNOSTIC CRITERIA

A. Consistent failure to speak in specific social situations (in which there is an expectation for speaking, e.g., at school) despite speaking in other situations.

B. The disturbance interferes with educational or occupational achievement or with social communication.

C. The duration of the disturbance is at least 1 month (not limited to the first month of school).

D. The failure to speak is not due to a lack of knowledge of, or comfort with, the spoken language required in the social situation.

E. The disturbance is not better accounted for by a Communication Disorder (e.g., Stuttering) and does not occur exclusively during the course of a Pervasive Developmental Disorder, Schizophrenia, or other Psychotic Disorder.

(From American Psychiatric Association: *Diagnostic and statistical manual of mental disorders,* ed 4 [DSM-IV], Washington DC, 1994, American Psychiatric Press.)

DIAGNOSIS

TABLE 7-6

SELECTIVE MUTISM

Discriminating feature

1. Failure to speak in certain social situations despite being physically able to speak

Consistent features

1. Sufficient knowledge of the language spoken
2. Impaired social or academic functioning
3. Absence of a physical condition that would prevent speech

Variable features

1. Onset between ages 3 and 6
2. Earlier age of onset in boys than girls
3. Occurs more often in girls than boys
4. Presence of an articulation disorder
5. Excessive shyness and familial shyness

Differential Diagnosis

Shyness, unfamiliarity with the language, or the presence of a communication disorder may be mistaken for selective mutism. Children with disorders such as schizophrenia, mental retardation, or a PDD may be unable to speak in social situations. However, selective mutism should only be diagnosed in a child with an established capacity to speak in some social situations (such as at home). The presence of a co-morbid anxiety disorder (for example, social phobia), communication disorder (such as stuttering), or other disorder should be diagnosed when appropriate. Finally, the presence of selective mutism does not imply that a child has been abused.

Treatment

Historically, treatments for selective mutism have included a range of individual, family, behavioral, and psychodynamic modalities. Psychodynamic treatments by themselves have generally fared poorly, though they may provide a supportive role, facilitate social interaction, and facilitate understanding of family issues unique to the child.

A multimodal approach with or without pharmacotherapy is the treatment of choice. CBT is the primary intervention aimed at reducing the anxiety that inhibits the child's speech and at positively reinforcing the child for speaking. Successful, graded exposure to public speaking is the key to habituating the child's anxiety. An attitude of expectation for normal speech and reinforcement for efforts to speak are important. Behavioral treatments are time consuming and require persistence, as well as the cooperation of parents, teachers, and other professionals. The child should not be removed from the mainstream classroom setting during treatment.

PEARLS & PERILS

SELECTIVE MUTISM

- Selective mutism occurs much more often in children with a preexisting articulation disorder or where English is a second language.
- Most children outgrow selective mutism, although continuation after age 10 suggests an intractable form of the disorder.
- During the treatment of selective mutism, the child should be kept in the mainstream classroom.

Psychosocial interventions that use modeling and peer pressure may reinforce incremental or successive approximations of speech (for example, hand raising) in the context of small groups of adults or peers. Family therapy may provide a powerful context for support, an understanding of the dynamics of the mutism, and an opportunity for application of cognitive and behavioral interventions.

Pharmacotherapy for selective mutism consists primarily of the use of SSRIs such as fluoxetine and sertraline and rarely, a supplemental low-dose, high-potency benzodiazepine such as clonazepam. Evidence is preliminary at present, but a trial of an SSRI (or phenelzine) should be considered when the symptoms of selective mutism are debilitating, of long duration, or refractory to other interventions.

Social Phobia

Diagnostic Criteria

Sociability, the preference for companionship and affiliation with others, and shyness, a form of social withdrawal accompanied by distress and inhibited behaviors, are enduring personality features, detectable at an early age and stable across development. Children who show a desire for affiliation with other children but who experience significant distress in social settings may meet criteria for social phobia (Box 7-9, Table 7-7).

Prevalence

Social phobia has a lifetime prevalence rate of 3% to 13% and affects approximately 1% of children and adolescents. Girls are affected more commonly than boys.

BOX 7-9 SOCIAL PHOBIA

DSM-IV DIAGNOSTIC CRITERIA

A. A marked and persistent fear of one or more social or performance situations in which the person is exposed to unfamiliar people or to possible scrutiny by others. The individual fears that he or she will act in a way (or show anxiety symptoms) that will be humiliating or embarrassing. **Note:** In children, there must be evidence of the capacity for age-appropriate social relationships with familiar people and the anxiety must occur in peer settings, not just in interactions with adults.

B. Exposure to the feared social situation almost invariably provokes anxiety, which may take the form of a situationally bound or situationally predisposed Panic Attack. **Note:** In children, the anxiety may be expressed by crying, tantrums, freezing, or shrinking from social situations with unfamiliar people.

C. The person recognizes that the fear is excessive or unreasonable. **Note:** In children, this feature may be absent.

D. The feared social or performance situations are avoided or else are endured with intense anxiety or distress.

E. The avoidance, anxious anticipation, or distress in the feared social or performance situation(s) interferes significantly with the person's normal routine, occupational (academic) functioning, or social activities or relationships, or there is marked distress about having the phobia.

F. In individuals under age 18 years, the duration is at least 6 months.

G. The fear or avoidance is not due to the direct physiological effects of a substance (e.g., a drug of abuse, a medication) or a general medical condition and is not better accounted for by another mental disorder (e.g., Panic Disorder With or Without Agoraphobia, Separation Anxiety Disorder, Body Dysmorphic Disorder, a Pervasive Developmental Disorder, or Schizoid Personality Disorder).

H. If a general medical condition or another mental disorder is present, the fear in Criterion A is unrelated to it, e.g., the fear is not of stuttering, trembling in Parkinson's disease, or exhibiting abnormal eating behavior in Anorexia Nervosa or Bulimia Nervosa.

Specify if:
Generalized: if the fears include most social situations (also consider the additional diagnosis of Avoidant Personality Disorder)

(From American Psychiatric Association: *Diagnostic and statistical manual of mental disorders,* ed 4 [DSM-IV], Washington DC, 1994, American Psychiatric Press.)

Etiology

Etiologic data is lacking for social phobia in children and adolescents. The onset of social phobia is typically in the mid-teens and is usually insidious, but it may follow a traumatic social event. Onset in early childhood is not rare. A childhood history of social inhibition or shyness is common, as is the presence of anxiety disorders in parents or siblings.

The course of social phobia is often lifelong with exacerbations and remissions fluctuating in relation to life stressors. The course of the illness also appears to be related to the age of onset and the presence of co-morbid symptoms. Based on a retrospective analysis of ECA data, it has been noted that onset of social phobia before age 11 is predictive of nonrecovery in adulthood. Co-morbidity with conduct problems (such as oppositionality or school refusal), depression, or substance abuse often complicates the course of illness.

Assessment

Children with social phobia typically do not spontaneously report or seek treatment for their disorder. Symptoms such as school refusal, inability to speak in class or to peers, test anxiety, shyness, poor peer relationships, and shrinking from social settings should alert the physician to the need for a more systematic evaluation of social phobia. A thorough clinical evaluation should include interviews with both the child and the parents or primary caretakers, with a focus on physical symptoms, specific worries, and distressful situations characteristic of social phobia. Physicians often have to identify the specific fears and situations with the child, since children are less adept at articulating their symptoms and often report complaints in vague terms, such as stomachaches, hating school, and so forth.

There are no laboratory tests or physiologic probes that

DIAGNOSIS

TABLE 7-7

SOCIAL PHOBIA

Discriminating feature

1. Anxiety specific to strangers or group settings

Consistent features

1. Feared situation is avoided or endured with significant distress
2. Absence of a physiologic condition that may explain symptoms
3. Anxiety occurs in setting with peers, not just with adults

Variable features

1. Onset in mid-teens
2. Insidious onset
3. Family history of an anxiety disorder
4. Premorbid shyness
5. Test anxiety
6. Child recognizes that fear is excessive and unreasonable

have been demonstrated to be pathognomonic for social phobia. The diagnosis remains a clinical one.

Differential Diagnosis

Panic disorder with agoraphobia, agoraphobia, SAD, GAD, and specific phobias are chief considerations in the differential diagnosis of social phobia. Classically, social phobia is characterized by the avoidance of social situations in the absence of panic attacks. Although social avoidance may occur in panic disorder with agoraphobia, it is the specific fear of having a panic attack or of being seen while having a panic attack that discriminates the two disorders. Fears in individuals with agoraphobia may or may not include the fear of scrutiny by others. Unlike children with social phobia, individuals who have agoraphobia may be reassured in social situations by the presence of a companion.

In SAD the greatest fear is of separation from the primary caregiver. Individuals with SAD are usually comfortable in social settings in the home, whereas socially phobic individuals are distressed in social situations, even at home.

Fear of embarrassment or humiliation in social settings may occur in children with GAD and specific phobia, but it is not the main focus of their anxiety. These children experience fear and anxiety apart from social contexts.

Social anxiety and avoidance are common in many disorders (for example, MDD, general medical disorders, and personality disorders), and the diagnosis should not be made if another disorder better accounts for the social anxiety or if its occurrence is limited to the occurrence of the other disorder.

Finally, school refusal is a descriptive term for behavior that may indicate the presence of a specific phobia, SAD, truancy, social phobia, or other disorders.

Treatment

Precise treatment outcome data for children meeting diagnostic criteria of social phobia are lacking, although much has been written about the treatment of children with social fears and social isolation. Cognitive and behavior-based treatments aimed at modifying maladaptive self-statements, affects, or behaviors are the mainstay in treating social phobia in children and adolescents. Exposure-based treatments attempt to reduce anxiety by pairing anxiety-inducing stimuli with incompatible stimuli (for example, relaxation) or by facilitating the extinction of conditioned anxiety through repeated exposure. Systematic desensitization consists of training in deep muscle relaxation, constructing a hierarchy of fearful situations from lowest to highest, and gradually presenting the stimulus hierarchy when the child is in a relaxed state. Graduated exposure is essentially systematic desensitization without relaxation training. Reinforced practice combines graduated exposure with structured positive reinforcement for the completion of progressively longer exposure tasks.

Operant and contingency management procedures involve a detailed behavioral analysis of the antecedents and consequences maintaining social phobic behavior in its various contexts. Once these are identified, reinforcement contingencies are arranged to diminish avoidance and facilitate social interaction.

Modeling procedures based on social learning theory have proven effective in diminishing anxious and socially avoidant behavior. In these procedures, children observe filmed or live models engaging in anxiety-provoking target behaviors and then are asked to imitate the model's performance. Participant modeling procedures involve the therapist or a peer physically guiding the child through anxiety-arousing situations. Peer-mediated approaches are a further variant of modeling in which "popular status" peer partners interact with socially withdrawn children to model prosocial behavior and enhance peer acceptance.

Social skills training (SST) may be used to teach basic social skills (such as eye contact, smiling, or conversation initiation) to children lacking the requisite skills to conduct successful peer interactions. SST may thus serve as a prelude to, or an element within, the more formal exposure-based anxiety management techniques.

Data from controlled medication trials are lacking on

the risks and effectiveness of pharmacologic treatment of social phobia in this population. Several medications have shown promise in children who are overanxious, separation anxious, and school phobic or avoidant and in adults who are socially phobic. These medications include benzodiazepines, tricyclic antidepressants (TCAs), SSRIs, beta blockers, and buspirone. The rationale for use of these agents is based on either downward extrapolation from adult studies or from the hypothesized role of specific neurotransmitters (such as GABA, norepinephrine, and serotonin) in anxiety states. The SSRIs (for example, fluoxetine, sertraline), and benzodiazepines (clonazepam) appear to hold the most promise in the treatment of social phobia. There is recent data to suggest that fluoxetine is effective for childhood anxiety disorders other than OCD and panic disorder.

PEARLS & PERILS

SOCIAL AND SPECIFIC PHOBIAS

- Social phobia usually begins in adolescence in a youth who is premorbidly described as shy.
- The course of social phobia is usually lifelong, with exacerbations and remissions paralleling life stressors.
- The physician should be sensitive to the child's cultural and ethnic background and beliefs before diagnosing a phobia.
- In the majority of children, phobic behavior subsides spontaneously without treatment.

Specific Phobia

Diagnostic Criteria

Specific phobia has replaced the diagnosis of simple phobia that was found in previous diagnostic classifications. The disorder has also been substantially redefined. Phobia is now characterized as an unreasonable, excessive, and persistent fear in response to actual or anticipated exposure to a specific object or situation. Common phobias include needles, animals, and public speaking. It is noteworthy that DSM-IV provides subtypes that better define the focus of the fear (Box 7-10, Table 7-8).

Prevalence

Specific phobias are relatively common anxiety disorders. A greater number of girls suffer from specific phobias than boys. Content of the phobias may be influenced by cultural and ethnic background.

Etiology

Decisive empiric proof for any single factor or combination of theoretic factors is still lacking. Psychoanalytic theory, largely unsupported by empiric evidence, viewed phobias as an attempt to master anxiety and fear stemming from repressed conflictual libidinal and aggressive urges. Fear disconnected from repressed material is then displaced onto a phobic object, allowing the child a degree of control through the act of phobic avoidance.

Behavioral theories look for an explanation of phobic behavior in classical conditioning, theorizing that fear is associated to conditioned stimuli. In an operant paradigm, the hypothesis is that positive consequences inadvertently reinforce phobic avoidance. An intriguing proposition is that phobic behavior can be acquired through social learning or modeling by parents or caretakers. Cognitive theories look for a cause of phobias in faulty cognitions. Familial aggregation of phobias cannot be fully attributed to social learning and fear acquisition through instruction. Genetic factors likely play a substantial role in propagating specific phobias.

Although phobic symptoms tend to vacillate over time and in the majority of the children gradually subside without treatment, authors of a recent review caution against hasty dismissal of a child's fears. A portion of children do not recover from their phobias, and their normal development and functioning are eventually hampered.

Assessment

Children are usually brought to the physician because of excessive fear related to a well-circumscribed situation or object. Parents often complain that the child is preoccupied with the object and that her fear or her attempts to avoid the object interfere with family life. The child's play, relationships with peers and family members, and school performance can be negatively influenced by the avoidance of a feared situation or even by incapacitating anticipatory anxiety. If the child is forced to endure the presence of a phobic object, it is often with dread.

Exposure to the phobic object elicits a response that has cognitive, emotional, behavioral, motoric, and physiologic components. The terrified child believes that great harm will befall her and experiences profound fear and autonomic activation. The usual response is to flee the fear producing the situation at all costs. The intensity of fear is usually proportional to the temporal and spatial proximity of the phobic object. Adolescents usually recognize the fear as being excessive and unreasonable, but younger children may lack this awareness.

The path to correct diagnosis lies in a detailed history with accurate descriptions of the sequence of events, the fear-producing situation, its consequences, and the intensity of the fear. An analog scale (a "fear

DSM-IV DIAGNOSTIC CRITERIA

BOX 7-10 SPECIFIC PHOBIA

A. Marked and persistent fear that is excessive or unreasonable, cued by the presence or anticipation of a specific object or situation (e.g., flying, heights, animals, receiving an injection, seeing blood).

B. Exposure to the phobic stimulus almost invariably provokes an immediate anxiety response, which may take the form of a situationally bound or situationally predisposed Panic Attack. **Note:** In children, the anxiety may be expressed by crying, tantrums, freezing, or clinging.

C. The person recognizes that the fear is excessive or unreasonable. **Note:** In children this feature may be absent.

D. The phobic situation(s) is avoided or else is endured with intense anxiety or distress.

E. The avoidance, anxious anticipation, or distress in the feared situation(s) interferes significantly with the person's normal routine, occupational (or academic) functioning, or social activities or relationships, or there is a marked distress about having the phobia.

F. In individuals under age 18 years, the duration is at least 6 months.

G. The anxiety, Panic Attacks, or phobic avoidance associated with the specific object or situation are not better accounted for by another mental disorder, such as Obsessive-Compulsive Disorder (e.g., fear of dirt in someone with an obsession about contamination), Posttraumatic Stress Disorder (e.g., avoidance of stimuli associated with a severe stressor), Separation Anxiety Disorder (e.g., avoidance of school), Social Phobia (e.g., avoidance of social situations because of fear of embarrassment), Panic Disorder With Agoraphobia, or Agoraphobia Without History of Panic Disorder.

Specify Type:
Animal Type
Natural Environment Type (e.g., heights, storms, water)
Blood-Injection-Injury Type
Situational Type (e.g., airplanes, elevators, enclosed places)
Other Type (e.g., phobic avoidance of situations that may lead to choking, vomiting, or contracting an illness; in children, avoidance of loud sounds or costumed characters)

(From American Psychiatric Association: *Diagnostic and statistical manual of mental disorders,* ed 4 [DSM-IV], Washington DC, 1994, American Psychiatric Press.)

DIAGNOSIS

TABLE 7-8 SPECIFIC PHOBIA

Discriminating feature

1. Excessive anxiety and avoidance specific to an object, environment, or circumstance

Consistent features

1. Situationally predisposed panic attacks
2. Child recognizes that the fear is unreasonable and excessive
3. Impaired social or academic functioning

Variable features

1. Occurs more often in girls
2. Preoccupation with the feared event

thermometer") can help children quantify their fears. The behavioral component is usually measured indirectly by measuring the distance from the phobic object at which a child experiences distress. Heart rate is a quantifiable correlate of physiologic response.

Differential Diagnosis

One of the initial tasks is differentiating developmentally appropriate fears from specific phobias. Good lists of common childhood fears can be found in child and adolescent psychiatry manuals. In social phobia, fears are confined to social situations, especially if a child's performance is subject to scrutiny. Fears in panic disorder are related to the anticipation or experience of the attack. Anxiety peaks during separation from loved ones in SAD. In GAD, fears and worries tend not to be confined to a specific object or situation. PTSD is characterized by fear and avoidance of memories related to past traumatic experiences. In anorexia nervosa, obsessions with food and its avoidance can have the appear-

TABLE 7-9

PRIMARY TREATMENT OF ANXIETY DISORDERS

DSM-IV diagnosis	Primary treatment	Pharmacologic treatment: Primary	Pharmacologic treatment: Secondary
Generalized anxiety disorder	CBT	SSRI	Benzodiazepine
	Medication	Buspirone	TCA
Obsessive-compulsive disorder	Medication	SSRI	
	Exposure-response prevention	Clomipramine	
Panic disorder	Medication	SSRI	TCA
	CBT	Benzodiazepine	
	Family therapy		
Posttraumatic stress disorder	CBT	TCA	Lithium
	Psychotherapy	SSRI	Propranolol
	Medication	Benzodiazepine	Carbamazepine
			Clonidine
			MAOI
Separation anxiety disorder	Behavior management	SSRI	Benzodiazepine
	CBT		Buspirone
	Medication		
	Family therapy		
Selective mutism	CBT	SSRI	SSRI
	Medication		Benzodiazepine
Social phobia	CBT	SSRI	Benzodiazepine
	Medication		
Specific phobia	CBT	Not indicated	

ance of a phobia. Bizarre fears are often a part of psychotic disorder, although a thought disorder is an obvious differentiating feature.

Treatment

Cognitive behavioral approaches show the most empiric support. Graded exposure, systematic desensitization, modeling, contingency management, and self-instruction are the approaches most often used, either individually or in combination. Graded exposure requires gradual presentation of the phobic stimulus. If there are several phobic objects, the object that produces the least fear is approached first. If in vivo exposure is not possible, it can be substituted by imagined exposure. Systematic desensitization combines exposure with previously rehearsed deep muscle relaxation and is then practiced in the presence of a phobic stimulus. These approaches can be employed with younger children once their trust is obtained. The presence of the parent is usually helpful. Modeling is often combined with exposure, especially in the early phase of treatment. The observation of a caregiver or therapist handling the phobic stimulus with no dire outcome instills trust and helps the child engage in exposure tasks.

Contingency management, based on principles of operant conditioning, can be combined with previously mentioned techniques to enhance their efficacy, or it may be used as a sole intervention. Modeling and contingency management have the advantage of requiring minimal cooperation; therefore they can be used if the child's compliance cannot be secured. Self-instruction is a cognitive approach that is usually reserved for motivated adolescents.

Psychodynamic treatment of phobias is detailed in numerous case studies; empiric support, however, is scarce. Family therapy is a useful adjunct. It can be fruitful when dealing with disturbed family relationships, whether they contribute to the onset of the child's phobia or serve as its perpetuant.

Psychosocial treatments are efficacious and tend to be the standard of care. Medications are generally not helpful.

Summary

The field of childhood anxiety disorders is currently in a state of flux. Burgeoning research in this area has provoked a reexamination of the developmental course of anxiety, including the boundaries between normal and pathologic anxiety, continuity with adult disorders, and the various biologic, psychologic and social determinants that both protect against and lead to the development of pathologic anxiety. High priority is being given to the development of precise, reliable, valid, and user-friendly assessment instruments. Cognitive, behavioral, pharmacologic, and multimodal treatment interventions are under investigation—individually and packaged in various combinations—to assess which treatments under what circumstances in which children are most effective.

Currently, empirically driven theories and effective treatments are emerging for specific anxiety disorders (Table 7-9). Simultaneously, time honored though unsubstantiated treatments and old notions about the source of anxiety are being dropped from the therapeutic and theoretic armamentaria. This process of intensive empiric investigation will continue to narrow the gap between experimental data and clinical practice. Clearer, better articulated questions will result in a more complete understanding and ultimately in more effective treatments for childhood anxiety disorders.

CONSIDER CONSULTATION WHEN . . .

- It is unclear if the child's symptoms are attributable to an anxiety disorder or representative of some other psychopathologic condition
- The child's symptoms do not improve or worsen despite trials of appropriate medications for sufficient periods in combination with behavioral therapy
- It is believed the child or family needs more in-depth forms of psychotherapeutic intervention
- The child's symptoms become so disabling that she cannot attend school, leave home, or complete age-appropriate activities despite treatment

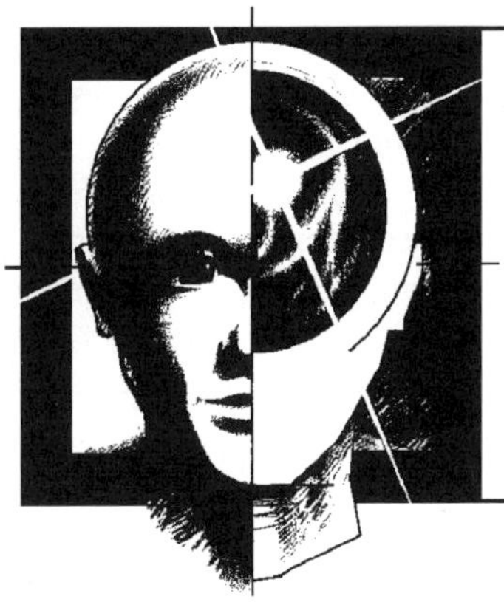

chapter 8

Mood Disorders

Robert A. Kowatch, MD, Graham J. Emslie, MD, and Betsy D. Kennard, PsyD

Depressive Disorders
Diagnostic Criteria
Assessment
Differential Diagnosis
Treatment
Summary
Bipolar Disorders
Diagnostic Criteria
Assessment
Differential Diagnosis
Treatment
Summary

Mood disorders are prevalent and serious disorders in children and adolescents. Major depressive disorder (MDD) among children and adolescents has an estimated incidence of between 1% and 2%, dysthymia occurs in an estimated 10% to 14% of children, and bipolar disorders have an estimated incidence of 0.24% to 1.2% in children. Affected children and adolescents show major impairments in their psychosocial and academic functioning, and they have overall poorer prognoses when compared with an unaffected peer group. There is some evidence that children and adolescents with MDD have specific biologic abnormalities similar to those found in adult MDD (for example, nocturnal growth hormone secretion and a shortened REM latency on their sleep EEGs). A depressed child or adolescent is also at much higher risk for both attempting and completing suicide.

Children with mood disorders are most often referred to physicians because of their behavior. The most common types of children referred are:

- children who are irritable, oppositional, and negative; refuse to do work in school; and have severe emotional outbursts at home and school
- children with unexplained physical complaints, headaches, or stomachaches and whose degrees of disability are in excess of any clear medical cause
- hyperactive, impulsive, motor-driven children who

tear up the world around them, often with severe aggression, and deny all along that anything is wrong

None of these children fit the lay person's perception of the mood of a depressed child; yet the first two are typical descriptions of children who suffer from depression, and the third describes a child with bipolar disorder. This chapter discusses the clinical characteristics of both depressive disorders and bipolar disorders, as well as treatment recommendations for them.

Depressive Disorders

Although the manifestation of depression in children and adolescents is variable, the three most common depressive disorders in children are MDD, dysthymia, and depressive disorder not otherwise specified (NOS). Regardless of the symptoms of a child or adolescent, it is necessary to characterize depression by both its severity (that is, the number of symptoms) and its temporal course.

Major Depressive Disorder

According to DSM-IV, a child with MDD must have a disturbance of mood (sadness or irritability) nearly every day for most of the day that affects feelings and behavior, or there must be loss of interest or pleasure in all (or almost all) activities nearly every day for most of the day. In addition to a disturbance of mood or loss of interest, five or more of the seven other associated symptoms must be present (see Box 8-1, p. 123). The symptom complex must be present for at least 2 weeks. MDD tends to be episodic, with either full or partial recovery between episodes (a cyclical disorder). Episodes of MDD cause significant failure and maladaptation in the child's usual functioning, as evidenced by declining school performance, withdrawal from peers, and increased conflict with peers or siblings.

Depressive Disorder NOS

In depressive disorder NOS, also called minor depression, the disorder is episodic, but the episodes are below the criteria for MDD. There are either fewer symptoms, or there is a shorter duration of symptoms. Episodes of minor depression may be precursors to MDD episodes, or they may occur independently. These episodes cause less dysfunction than an episode of MDD.

Dysthymic Disorder

Dysthymic disorder refers to a chronically dysphoric, or depressed, mood that is less intense than MDD but has no prolonged well states. The duration of the illness is at least 1 year in children (see Box 8-2, p. 124). Children with dysthymic disorder characteristically have good and bad days, or they may have many "mixed" days, but they do not have good weeks. Often these children have had symptoms since their preschool years. As they grow older, MDD may also develop. This is termed *double depression.*

Studies of the reported rates of childhood and adolescent depression have yielded varying ranges. These discrepancies are largely the result of the different age groups studied (children vs. adolescents), the use of different measures (self-reports vs. structured interviews), and the focus on depressive symptoms vs. depressive syndromes. In the general child and adolescent population, the incidence of depression ranges from 1% to 2%.

In a study of prevalence of depressive symptoms in two large high school populations (both urban and rural), 12% to 14% of students demonstrated substantial depressive symptoms on self-report measures. Three percent of the two populations related suicidal thoughts ("I think a lot about killing myself"). Some studies have indicated that in the adolescent population, there are differences across ethnic and gender

PEARLS & PERILS

MAJOR DEPRESSIVE DISORDER

- Children and adolescents only need to be symptomatic for 1 year to make a diagnosis of dysthymic disorder.
- The presence of MDD during the course of a dysthymic disorder is termed *double depression.*
- Children with MDD come from families with high rates of depression, alcoholism, and anxiety disorders in first- and second-degree relatives. The physician should assess for and treat psychopathologic conditions in relatives that may be influencing the mood disorder in the child.
- Irritability is a common manifestation of MDD in children and adolescents.
- Feelings of low self-esteem may be reflected in persecutory comments about peers, siblings, or parents.
- Terminal insomnia occurs less often in depressed children and adolescents than in adults.
- For adolescents, changing to a less socially desirable peer group may be a reflection of an underlying depression.
- Somatic complaints are common symptoms of depression in children and adolescents.
- There is a high rate of relapse for children and adolescents who have had an episode of MDD.

groups. Studies using self-report measures have reported more depressive symptoms in African-American students and girls, and especially in Hispanic girls.

The prevalence is quite high in clinical populations, with incidence reported as high as 60% in a psychiatric inpatient population and in outpatient groups of children referred to educational diagnostic centers.

There is no one specific cause of MDD. Most believe that factors leading to a depressive disorder are multiple and interact to cause the disorder. The factors include a genetic predisposition (that is, a positive family history), environmental stressors (such as trauma, loss, or school pressure), and biologic concomitants (low levels of catecholamines or indolamines; neuroendocrine abnormalities). It is important for the physician to systematically assess the child's family psychiatric history. Children with MDD have high familial rates of depression, alcoholism, and anxiety in first- and second-degree relatives.

Diagnostic Criteria

In general, DSM-IV criteria are used to diagnose depression in children and adolescents (Boxes 8-1 and 8-2, Tables 8-1 and 8-2). Whereas symptoms of depression in this age group are similar to those in adults, the manifestation of these symptoms is often quite different. Therefore criteria established for depression in chil-

BOX 8-1 MAJOR DEPRESSIVE EPISODE

DSM-IV DIAGNOSTIC CRITERIA

A. Five (or more) of the following symptoms have been present during the same 2-week period and represent a change from previous functioning; at least one of the symptoms is either (1) depressed mood or (2) loss of interest or pleasure.

Note: Do not include symptoms that are clearly due to a general medical condition, or mood-incongruent delusions or hallucinations.

(1) depressed mood most of the day, nearly every day, as indicated by either subjective report (e.g., feels sad or empty) or observation made by others (e.g., appears tearful). **Note:** In children and adolescents, can be irritable mood.
(2) markedly diminished interest or pleasure in all, or almost all, activities most of the day, nearly every day (as indicated by either subjective account or observation made by others)
(3) significant weight loss when not dieting or weight gain (e.g., a change of more than 5% of body weight in a month), or decrease or increase in appetite nearly every day. **Note:** In children, consider failure to make expected weight gains.
(4) insomnia or hypersomnia nearly every day
(5) psychomotor agitation or retardation nearly every day (observable by others, not merely subjective feelings of restlessness or being slowed down)
(6) fatigue or loss of energy nearly every day
(7) feelings of worthlessness or excessive or inappropriate guilt (which may be delusional) nearly every day (not merely self-reproach or guilt about being sick)
(8) diminished ability to think or concentrate, or indecisiveness, nearly every day (either by subjective account or as observed by others)
(9) recurrent thoughts of death (not just fear of dying), recurrent suicidal ideation without a specific plan, or a suicide attempt or a specific plan for committing suicide

B. The symptoms do not meet criteria for a Mixed Episode.

C. The symptoms cause clinically significant distress or impairment in social, occupational, or other important areas of functioning.

D. The symptoms are not due to the direct physiological effects of a substance (e.g., a drug of abuse, a medication) or a general medical condition (e.g., hypothyroidism).

E. The symptoms are not better accounted for by Bereavement, i.e., after the loss of a loved one, the symptoms persist for longer than 2 months or are characterized by marked functional impairment, morbid preoccupation with worthlessness, suicidal ideation, psychotic symptoms, or psychomotor retardation.

(From American Psychiatric Association: *Diagnostic and statistical manual of mental disorders,* ed 4 [DSM-IV], Washington DC, 1994, American Psychiatric Press.)

BOX 8-2 DYSTHYMIC DISORDER

A. Depressed mood for most of the day, for more days than not, as indicated either by subjective account or observation by others, for at least 2 years. **Note:** In children and adolescents, mood can be irritable and duration must be at least 1 year.

B. Presence, while depressed, of two (or more) of the following:

(1) poor appetite or overeating
(2) insomnia or hypersomnia
(3) low energy or fatigue
(4) low self-esteem
(5) poor concentration or difficulty making decisions
(6) feelings of hopelessness

C. During the 2-year period (1 year for children or adolescents) of the disturbance, the person has never been without the symptoms in Criteria A and B for more than 2 months at a time.

D. No Major Depressive Episode has been present during the first 2 years of the disturbance (1 year for children and adolescents); i.e., the disturbance is not better accounted for by chronic Major Depressive Disorder, or Major Depressive Disorder, In Partial Remission.

Note: There may have been a previous Major Depressive Episode provided there was a full remission (no significant signs or symptoms for 2 months) before development of the Dysthymic Disorder. In addition, after the initial 2 years (1 year in children or adolescents) of Dysthymic Disorder, there may be superimposed episodes of Major Depressive Disorder, in which case both diagnoses may be given when the criteria are met for a Major Depressive Episode.

E. There has never been a Manic Episode, a Mixed Episode, or a Hypomanic Episode, and criteria have never been met for Cyclothymic Disorder.

F. The disturbance does not occur exclusively during the course of a chronic Psychotic Disorder, such as Schizophrenia or Delusional Disorder.

G. The symptoms are not due to the direct physiological effects of a substance (e.g., a drug of abuse, a medication) or a general medical condition (e.g., hypothyroidism).

H. The symptoms cause clinically significant distress or impairment in social, occupational, or other important areas of functioning.

Specify if:
Early Onset: if onset is before age 21 years
Late Onset: if onset is age 21 years or older

Specify (for most recent 2 years of Dysthymic Disorder): **With Atypical Features**

(From American Psychiatric Association: *Diagnostic and statistical manual of mental disorders,* ed 4 [DSM-IV], Washington DC, 1994, American Psychiatric Press.)

dren and adolescents have the advantage of specifically delineating the manifestation of symptoms more appropriate for this age group. Weinberg et al. have modified the original research diagnostic criteria for major depression in adults to be more applicable to children and adolescents. Signs and symptoms of depression in children and adolescents are discussed in the following list. The DSM-IV criteria that differing signs and symptoms correspond to are included in parenthesis after each criterion from Weinberg et al.

- **Depressed Mood**—Dysphoric moods and feelings are characterized by statements and the appearance of sadness, loneliness, unhappiness, hopelessness, mood swings, irritability, hypersensitivity, a negative attitude, and being difficult to please. Children tend to be more sensitive to their

DIAGNOSIS

TABLE 8-1
MAJOR DEPRESSIVE EPISODE

Discriminating feature

1. Depressed mood or loss of interest or pleasure during the same 2-week period

Consistent features

1. Appetite and sleep disturbance
2. Impaired social or academic functioning
3. Absence of use of a mood altering substance
4. Absence of a physical condition that alters mood

Variable features

1. Irritability
2. Weight loss or weight gain
3. Insomnia or hypersomnia
4. Psychomotor agitation or retardation
5. Fatigue or loss of energy
6. Feelings of worthlessness and inappropriate guilt
7. Impaired concentration and change in school performance
8. Suicidal ideation
9. Diurnal variation with worsening of symptoms in the morning
10. Unexplained somatic complaints
11. Family history of depression
12. Sleep-wake pattern reversal

DIAGNOSIS

TABLE 8-2
DYSTHYMIC DISORDER

Discriminating feature

1. Dysphoric mood for at least 1 year

Consistent features

1. Symptoms not severe enough to diagnose a major depression
2. Absence of a psychotic illness
3. Absence of use of a mood altering drug
4. Absence of a physiologic, mood altering condition
5. Impaired social and academic functioning

Variable features

1. Poor appetite or overeating
2. Insomnia or hypersomnia
3. Low energy or fatigue
4. Low self-esteem
5. Poor concentration or difficulty making decisions
6. Feelings of hopelessness
7. Irritable mood
8. Difficulty getting along with others
9. Unexplained somatic complaints
10. Family history of a depressive disorder

environment, and they have more reactive moods than adults. They may not verbalize their dysphoria or consistently appear sad. Thus their mood disturbances are often expressed in mixed days, with days consisting of normal moods, feelings, and behaviors interspersed with periods of depressed feelings and irritability. Irritability is common in this age group, with irritable moods commonly resulting from sad feelings.

- **Self-deprecatory ideation**—Self-deprecatory ideation is manifest by feelings of being worthless, stupid, ugly, or guilty and by beliefs of persecution, death wishes, and suicidal ideation. In this age group, it is common to project feelings of lowered self-esteem into beliefs of persecution (such as, "Everyone hates me" or, "I am not a good kid"). Cognitively, it may be difficult for children to express guilt, but feelings of worthlessness and self-blame are evident in their behavior and often in their statements. This self-deprecatory ideation common to depressed children and adolescents corresponds to the DSM-IV symptoms of feelings of worthlessness or inappropriate guilt.
- **Agitation**—Agitation corresponds to the DSM-IV symptom of irritability and is evident in the way a child gets along with others. Common behaviors include fighting, disrespect for authority, quarreling, and excessive hostility. The increased conflict with others as a result of agitation is what often leads to the referral of a child. This symptom is also similar to the psychomotor agitation seen in adult patients. The presence of agitation and oppositional behavior can result in the misidentification of the problem as oppositional defiant disorder (ODD). However, the oppositional behavior usually subsides with the resolution of depression.
- **Sleep Disturbance**—In DSM-IV this symptom is characterized as insomnia or hypersomnia. Sleep problems include initial, middle, and terminal insomnia; difficulty awakening in the morning; excessive sleepiness; and hypersomnia. Depressed children often experience the subjective experience of initial insomnia, which is not always objectively confirmed. Middle insomnia (awakening after sleep onset) is not uncommon in small chil-

dren. Terminal insomnia is less common in depressed children and adolescents than in depressed adults.

- **Change in school performance**—The DSM-IV symptom of poor concentration often appears in children as a change in school performance. Teachers may complain about daydreaming, poor concentration and attention, poor motivation, loss of interest in school activities, incomplete school work and homework, and lowered grades. Children often have problems completing work in class, which results in increased homework (typically another source of parent-child conflict).
- **Diminished socialization**—Children and adolescents who have a depressive disorder often show a decline in group participation and social interests, and they are less likely to seek out friends. In adolescents, this may be manifested by changing to a less socially desirable peer group. Loss of social interest by parent report is consistent with loss of outside interests by child report. Diminished socialization in children corresponds to the DSM-IV symptom of loss of interest or pleasure.
- **Change in attitude toward school**—A changed attitude toward school also reflects the DSM-IV symptom of loss of interest or pleasure. A phobic reaction toward school (fear of going to school) is often symptomatic of depression. Children and adolescents with depression may have school refusal listed as the primary reason for referral. Whereas for some of these children, school refusal may be related to separation anxiety disorder (SAD), many children with a depressive disorder lose interest and pleasure in school and its activities. This symptom may also be a manifestation of diurnal mood variation, since some children feel able to attend school by afternoon but not when they first wake up in the morning and are most depressed.
- **Somatic complaints**—Somatic complaints are not a DSM-IV symptom of depression primarily because they are a nonspecific symptom in adults. However, in children they are a common symptom of depression. Children with depression often appear before pediatricians or family physicians with vague somatic complaints that include headaches, stomachaches, or other physical symptoms for which the physician can find no cause. It is not uncommon for this to be the only significant symptom reported, and therefore it may result in extensive medical evaluation for a physical disorder.
- **Loss of usual energy**—The depressed young person commonly complains of mental and physical fatigue and becomes less active in her usual sport or other activities. A child who is talented or active in a given area may begin to complain of tiredness, easy fatigue, less energy, and even boredom during that activity, resulting in diminished participation. There is often a substantial overlap in the vegetative symptoms of energy and sleepiness and the psychologic symptom of loss of interest. In DSM-IV, this symptom is classified as fatigue.
- **Change in appetite or weight**—Children often become "picky" eaters, craving sweets or snack foods. In some instances, they become voracious overeaters. The absence of usual weight gain rather than weight loss is common in children who are depressed. Excessive weight gain is seen in some children and adolescents, but adolescents commonly lose weight. Failure to gain weight where developmentally appropriate is symptomatic of depression.

For many children and adolescents, depression continues to be a problem for many years. Poznanski et al. report that 50% of a sample of adolescent outpatients with depression were depressed when contacted 6.5 years later. Eastgate and Gilmour recontacted 19 of 36 child inpatients with depression after 7 to 8 years. Of those patients, 42% (8) were psychiatrically ill and 21% had major depression.

Since depression tends to be an episodic condition, not only overall outcome but also the course of depressive symptoms over the intervening period is of particular interest. Remission or recovery rates have been studied in different populations of children and adolescents. In a study of 42 child outpatients with MDD, Kovacs et al. found that 59% had recovered (they were asymptomatic for 2 months) after 1 year and 92% had recovered after 18 months. Strober et al. found that 81% of 58 adolescent inpatients with MDD had recovered by 1 year and 98% had recovered by 2 years from the time of admission. The average recovery time was 27.5 weeks from admission. They also reported that 28% of those with psychotic depression developed their first manic episodes during this 2-year follow up period. Both of these studies are similar to McCauley et al.'s report of 65 children and adolescents with depression who were predominantly outpatients. McCauley found that 80% had recovered after 1 year.

However, once recovered, children and adolescents have high rates of relapse of their depression. In Kovacs et al.'s study of depressed children with MDD, there was a cumulative rate of 72% for a new episode of depression within 5 years. Asarnow et al. reported rehospitalization in 45% of inpatients with MDD within 2 years. Within McCauley's sample of children and adolescents, 54% experienced another major depressive episode within 3 years.

It appears that depression in adolescents continues and turns into adult depressive conditions. That is, many adolescents with depression become adults with depression. Kendal and Davies describe poor adult outcomes in a large group of people who as adolescents were identified by a self-report scale as having depressive symptoms. However, it is not possible from this study to determine whether the outcome was specific to the depression. Harrington et al., in a follow-up study of 80 depressed and 80 nondepressed adolescent outpatients, showed that depressive disorders were more common in the group of adults who were depressed as adolescents.

Assessment

The diagnosis of depression is based on clinical interviews that use established criteria for depression in children and adolescents. The interviews have a semistructured format for both parents and children. During an interview, questions that relate to mood symptoms are asked in a way that allows the interviewer to explore significant areas related to those symptoms. Occasionally, information is obtained from teachers and peers. Both children and their parents must be interviewed, since a parent's report alone is not sufficient. Whereas parents are important sources of information regarding the behavioral manifestations of psychiatric symptoms and the temporal course of an illness, children are more able to report subjective symptoms and some vegetative symptoms, such as sleep disturbance.

Although the diagnosis of depression in children and adolescents is best made through a clinical interview, self-report measures can be useful as screening instruments. They are also useful for detecting and monitoring symptoms in the clinical setting. Common self-report measures for children are the Children's Depression Inventory (CDI), the Beck Depression Inventory (BDI) (for adolescents), and The Weinberg Screening Affective Scale (WSAS). However, a diagnosis of depression must be confirmed through a diagnostic interview by a physician who is able to recognize the subtle signs and symptoms of a depressive illness. No evaluation of children and adolescents with affective disorders is complete without a detailed biologic history of the family that includes first-, second-, and third-degree relatives. The offspring of adults with an affective illness show high rates of depression and bipolar disorder. Conversely, children with MDD have high familial ratings of depression, alcoholism, anxiety, and other psychiatric diagnoses in first- and second-degree relatives. It is expected that children and adolescents with MDD will have a positive family history of mood disorders in 50% to 80% of cases, depending on whether first- or second-degree relatives are evaluated and depending on the criteria used (that is, treated or untreated with antidepressants, definite vs. possible by the family history). When compiling a family history, it is preferable to interview both parents of the patient, even if one parent appears to know the family history of the other.

Children and adolescents who are depressed often perform poorly in school, and psychologic testing can be useful to determine the influence of mood on cognition. Although verbal intelligence is not generally impaired in this population, academic achievement can be adversely impacted by affective illness. Additionally, recent studies have suggested that the longer a child has a depressive illness, the greater the negative impact is on academic and social functioning.

Children with mood disorders tend to demonstrate particular performance patterns on intellectual tests. In general, two areas of cognitive functioning may be affected. Children with depression tend to demonstrate performance deficits on intellectual measures (which may improve with symptom remission), and they tend to have learning disabilities. Additionally, many of these children have thinking patterns that are characterized by cognitive errors or distortions in their interpretation of daily events. Both of these areas are important to understand when assisting children with mood disorders.

Although some studies have suggested improved functioning on cognitive measures once the symptoms remit, some skill areas, including academic skills and social abilities, continue to suffer impairment. Kovacs and Goldston conclude that there are both temporary (performance deficits) and long-term negative correlates of affective illness (academic underachievement and impaired social functioning).

Differential Diagnosis

Most children and adolescents who meet criteria for depression also have symptoms that fulfill criteria for other diagnostic categories in DSM-IV. In a recent epidemiologic study, concurrent diagnoses were found in almost 50% of children and adolescents who met criteria for psychiatric disorders. In this study a high rate of co-morbidity was found among the four diagnostic domains from DSM-III (mood disorders, disruptive behavior disorders, attention-deficit/hyperactivity disorder [ADHD], and anxiety disorders). In subjects with affective disorder, 24% also had a disruptive behavior disorder, 17% had ADHD, and 17% had an anxiety disorder. Kovacs et al. found the second most common diagnosis in children with affective illness to be CD. In another study, Weinberg and Emslie found that 33% of children diagnosed with MDD according to DSM-III criteria also met criteria for ADHD.

Whether the high rate of co-morbidity in children and adolescents is the result of the lack of a well-

DIAGNOSES OF DEPRESSIVE DISORDERS

PEARLS & PERILS

- In suspected depression, psychologic testing may help determine whether poor academic performance is caused by the impact of mood on cognition.
- The second most common diagnosis in affectively ill children is conduct disorder (CD).
- A large percentage of youth with MDD also have attention deficit hyperactivity disorder (ADHD). Both conditions must be considered when providing treatment.
- In the adolescent who is depressed, the physician should carefully check for the use of drugs and alcohol that may be influencing mood state.
- Children are extremely reactive to their environments. Therefore the child who is depressed may not complain of a continuously dysphoric mood as would be expected in an adult.

developed exclusionary criteria in this age group or whether it represents true co-morbid disorders is unclear. Further clarification of this issues is underway in prospective studies.

Treatment

The treatment of children and adolescents who have depressive disorders is ideally multimodal, involving medications, psychologic therapies, and psychosocial interventions. Obviously, a careful evaluation is necessary, and the mood disorder must be persistent and cause a disability. Up to 30% of children improve with evaluation alone or with minimal intervention. The psychosocial management of children and adolescents should be multifocal. Because of their ability to influence mood and treatment outcome in this age group, family, school, and environmental stressors are assessed and included in treatment. Additionally, the type of mood disorder, the incidence of co-morbidity, and the developmental level of the patient should be considered when developing a treatment plan for a child or adolescent with a mood disorder. The primary aim of treatment is to shorten the period of the mood disorder and to decrease the negative consequences of episodes of depression. To achieve this goal, the physician must consider several important areas of intervention that may assist the child with depression. These areas include behavioral, familial, psychotherapeutic, and environmental interventions.

The patient should be encouraged to resume as normal a level of functioning as possible. Schedules and setting up positive reinforcement may be used to motivate the patient to become active and involved in daily routines. Increasing the amount of structure in the patient's daily routine often helps stabilize the patient's mood. This can be achieved through a daily schedule that uses rewards for performing routine activities such as arising with no problems, getting dressed for school, attending school, completing homework assignments, and preparing for bed. Rather than receiving punishment for unacceptable behavior, the child is encouraged through reassurance and support to spend as much of the day functioning independently of how he may feel inside. The parents should avoid removing positive reinforcers from the child or developing a program that perpetuates the child's feelings of defeat and despair. Activities helpful to the patient's mood, such as social activities or recreational events, should not be made contingent on performance, because the child needs these activities to improve his mood. It is increasingly clear that for a depressed child to talk about his bad feelings continuously does little to improve the situation but in fact worsens the depression.

TREATMENT OF DEPRESSIVE DISORDERS IN CHILDREN

PEARLS & PERILS

- The child with depression should be rewarded for performing routine activities that encourage a return to a normal level of functioning. Punishment for unacceptable behavior may perpetuate the child's feelings of defeat and despair.
- In the behavioral treatment of the child who is depressed, social and recreational activities should not be made contingent upon performance, since these events help to improve the child's mood.
- In the therapy of the child who is depressed, continuous focus on the dysphoric mood state only serves to worsen it.
- Up to one half of all children who are depressed have an affectively ill parent at the time of treatment.
- Developing a positive school environment is essential as a component of a systematic treatment of children and adolescents who have depressive disorders.

Because of a decline in interest and activity level, children typically drop out of their usual activities and withdraw from opportunities for social interaction. This further compounds the depression and hampers recovery. Daily attendance at school and the continuation of activities must be encouraged.

Parents need to be educated about what is known and not known about mood disorders. Parents who have the facts regarding affective illness are less likely to engage in self-blame or in blaming others. It is not uncommon for schools to blame parents or for parents to blame schools for the child's deteriorating behavior. Such misappropriation may lead to inappropriate solutions for the problem, such as changing schools. Physicians should emphasize to parents that mood disorders are biologic conditions and not personality flaws.

A family assessment should be conducted to evaluate the premorbid level of family functioning, the parents' marital relationship (if applicable), and the impact of the illness on the family, as well as the family's understanding of the disorder and their attempts to manage it. The family should assist in the development of a treatment plan, including the identification of problem areas to be changed. Thirty to fifty percent of depressed adolescents have a parent who has a mood disorder at the time of treatment. Thus the appropriate identification of parents who need treatment is important in the management of these patients.

Adult treatment studies have determined several types of psychotherapy (such as CBT and interpersonal psychotherapy) that effectively treat depression; comparable treatment studies in children and adolescents with mood disorder are ongoing. Recent literature has supported the use of cognitive therapy in adolescents. Several studies have also found evidence for the efficacy of cognitive-behavioral methods in group treatment studies with children and adolescents.

Cognitive therapy in adolescents applies the same principles and many of the same techniques that are used in the treatment of adults. These techniques include collaborating with the therapist to determine whether there is supporting evidence for negative thoughts, identifying and labeling distortions, providing alternative ways of understanding situations, problem-solving, role-playing, assigning homework tasks, and recording moods and thoughts. When comparing the cognitive treatment of adolescents with that of adults, some important variables that must be considered are the therapeutic alliance, the developmental level of the patient, and the involvement of the family. Cognitive therapy with adolescents places more emphasis on the delicate nature of the therapeutic alliance (acknowledging the narcissism that is normal in adolescent development). Additionally, the therapist must adapt techniques and language to the adolescent's developmental level; for example, a patient functioning at a low level may benefit from more use of behavioral methods and less use of metaphor. Finally, family assessment (of beliefs, rules, and expectations) and routine scheduling of family treatment sessions must always be included in the treatment of adolescents.

Because of the child and adolescent's greater vulnerability to environmental stressors, it is important to involve the patient's social system in the treatment plan and to include significant others such as extended family, caregivers, and school personnel. To increase the chances that gains made in individual and family modalities will generalize to other settings, other people and systems must be involved in the treatment plan. This may range from providing family members with education and information about the illness to developing a behavior plan that involves participation of school personnel.

Adapting the patient's school setting to reduce stress is also important. This could range from shortening the school day, limiting the amount of school work, developing assignment completion checklists, or arranging for a more structured classroom setting. For the depressed child, continuous focus on deficits can lead to worsening mood symptoms. Developing a positive school environment is essential for these children.

Patients often have problems relating to their peer groups as a result of social deficits. These deficits compound their depression and contribute to their feelings of worthlessness, hopelessness, and alienation. It is important for therapists, parents, and teachers to help these children clarify reality and identify behaviors that contribute to conflictual situations. Group therapy can be a helpful modality to build social skills through such techniques as role-play, problem-solving, and communication and assertiveness training, as well as through teaching methods of self-control and conflict resolution or psychosocial adjustments.

Before starting antidepressant treatment in children and adolescents with depression, there are several general issues to consider. The initial examination should include a medical evaluation to rule out disorders that can cause mood disturbances (for example, thyroid disease, infectious mononucleosis, or systemic lupus). Box 8-3 lists medical causes of depression in children and adolescents that should be ruled out before assuming

BOX 8-3

MEDICAL CAUSES OF DEPRESSION IN CHILDREN AND ADOLESCENTS

Infectious mononucleosis
Influenza
Hepatitis
Acquired Immunodefiency Syndrome (AIDS)
Cushing's disease
Hypothyroidism
Hyperparathyroidism
β-Blockers
Corticosteroids
Cimetidine
Lupus
Porphyria
Uremia

PEARLS & PERILS

ANTIDEPRESSANT TREATMENT OF MOOD DISORDERS

- Children and adolescents are particularly sensitive to the cardiac side effects of antidepressants, necessitating monitoring of serial ECGs. The PR interval should not exceed 30% of the baseline.
- Selection of an antidepressant should take into consideration the side effects that may be helpful or harmful to the child.
- There are slow and fast metabolizers of antidepressants, and substantial individual variation that influences blood levels.
- The patient taking an MAOI must adhere to a tyramine-restricted diet to prevent a hypertensive crisis.
- If a child does not respond to adequate trials of two classes of antidepressants, the physician should consider adding lithium.
- For the child or adolescent who is psychotically depressed, an antipsychotic medication may need to be added to the drug regimen.
- There is limited information on the use of electroconvulsive therapy with children and adolescents, but for the treatment-resistant or severely ill adolescent, this may be an alternative.

a primary psychiatric cause for a patient's depression. Adolescents should also be examined for possible substance abuse, with drug screens used when appropriate. Before starting tricyclic antidepressants (TCAs), routine laboratory work should include a complete blood count (CBC) and an ECG. There have been reports of sudden deaths of children taking desipramine, two of whom had family histories of cardiac abnormalities.

Attempts should be made to obtain assent from the child in addition to consent from the parents before initiating treatment. This is practical because it may improve compliance, and it is ethically important because the child is the patient—not the parents or the school. Older children who are uncomfortable about taking medications (because to them medications imply that they are sick) often agree to a time-limited trial. Once medication is initiated, systematic rating of symptoms is helpful. Either self-report questionnaires or clinical rating scales are available. Finally, the physician, child, and parent must assess the possible risk-benefit ratio, since no treatment is free of risk. Treatment should only be initiated for a disorder that causes significant dysfunction at home, play, or school.

The efficacy of TCAs for MDD in adults is well established; however only a handful of double-blind, placebo-controlled studies using current criteria for depression are available for children. Puig-Antich et al. studied 38 children with MDD. Fifty-six percent of the children taking active medication responded, compared with 68% of the children taking placebo. Geller et al. studied 50 severely depressed children who were taking nortriptyline, and 30% responded to active medication as opposed to 17% who responded to placebo. Several other studies with amitriptyline and desipramine, are ongoing but they have not been conclusive. There are more extensive open studies, but the research data is generally limited to small numbers of select subjects. Therefore the physician has to rely on clinical experience to make judgments about treatment. It is probably safest to use medications that are familiar to the physician.

Depressed children are often initially treated with TCAs such as amitriptyline, imipramine, desipramine, or doxepin. The choice of antidepressant is often selected based on side-effect profiles. A child who is not sleeping may benefit from the sedative effects of amitriptyline, whereas an overweight child will do better with imipramine or desipramine because amitriptyline tends to cause weight gain. There are no studies involving either adults or children that show any single TCA to be more effective than any other. However, children may respond better to those antidepressants that inhibit serotonin reuptake more than those inhibiting norepinephrine uptake.

SSRIs such as fluoxetine, paroxetine, and sertraline are newer antidepressants that are highly selective reuptake inhibitors of serotonin. They are well tolerated in children and adolescents, and they appear to have fewer side effects. There have been several open studies and one controlled study in depressed adolescents, with mixed results. Fluoxetine has been shown to be effective for obsessive-compulsive disorder (OCD) in children. Some children become disinhibited with fluoxetine, which can be a problem for those who are already impulsive.

Dosage for antidepressants has to take into account two factors. First, children are given proportionally more antidepressants for their size because of their faster metabolic rate, which leads to a shorter serum high-life. Secondly, there is substantial individual variation in blood levels (6 to 10 times) in similar children of similar sizes receiving the same dose. Approximately 10% of the population metabolizes slowly and can obtain high serum levels on low dosage, whereas others may require very high dosages to achieve a therapeu-

TABLE 8-3

ANTIDEPRESSANT AGENTS

Medication	Therapeutic dosage range (mg/kg qd)	Side effect*					
		Anti-cholinergic	Drowsiness	Insomnia/ agitation	Cardiac arrhythmia	Gastro-intestinal distress	Weight gain (over 3 kg)
Amitriptyline	2-5	4+	4+	0	3+	0	3+
Desipramine	2-5	1+	1+	1+	2+	0	1+
Doxepin	2-5	3+	4+	0	2+	0	2+
Imipramine	2-5	3+	3+	1+	3+	1+	2+
Nortriptyline	1.25-2.5	1+	1+	0	2+	0	1+
Trazodone	1.25-5.0	0	4+	0	1+	1+	1+
Bupropion	1.25-5.0	0	0	2+	1+	1+	0
Fluoxetine	0.16-1.0	0	0	2+	0	3+	0
Paroxetine	0.16-0.70	0	0	2+	0	3+	0
Sertraline	0.41-4.0	0	0	2+	0	3+	0
Fluvoxamine	0.41-4.5	0	1+	2+	0	3+	0
Venlafaxine	0.41-3.0	0	2+	0	2+	3+	0
Nefazadone	2-5	0	2+	0	0	2+	0

*0 = absent or rare; 4+ = relatively common

tic level. See Table 8-3 for dose guidelines and possible side effects in children and adolescents of currently available antidepressant agents.

It will be necessary for the physician to monitor the ECG throughout treatment when using a TCA. Prolongation of the PR interval should not exceed 30% of the baseline. Children and adolescents should be started at low doses, with dosages being increased every week to 2 weeks as side effects are tolerated and as clinical condition indicates. As with adults, it may take 4 weeks at therapeutic levels before there is a clinically significant improvement in the level of depression. Plasma levels of the antidepressant are helpful when titrating the dose for patients who metabolize medication fast or slowly and when determining medication compliance. Additionally, if the patient is successfully treated for depression and later has a recurrence, it is helpful to know the individual's previously effective plasma level when planning new treatment.

Little has been written about the use of MAOIs with depressed children and adolescents. There are single-case reports of the successful use of an MAOI in children and adolescents who have not responded to TCAs. It is imperative that individuals be restricted to a tyramine-restricted diet while they are taking MAOIs, to avoid the possibility of a hypertensive crisis.

When patients do not respond to antidepressants, the physician should consider the addition of lithium. Studies of adolescents (who did not have bipolar disorders) not responding to TCAs alone reveal a good response when lithium was added. Lithium may be particularly useful for children and adolescents who are considered at high risk for bipolarity. This includes patients with family histories of manic-depressive illness, patients with hypersomnia and hyperphagia during an episode of depression, and patients who are psychotic and depressed.

For children and adolescents who have psychotic disorders with their depression (that is, they have hallucinations and delusions corresponding with the onset of the mood disorder), it may be necessary to use an antipsychotic agent with the antidepressant medication. Considering the possible cumulative side effects from both agents, the physician should select the antipsychotic agent that will be the least bothersome with the smallest dose possible. As the depression remits, so should the psychotic symptoms.

Because of the limited number of studies on the use of antidepressants in children and adolescents, little is known regarding the length of time needed for treatment. Generally, physicians follow adult guidelines, maintaining the antidepressant at the acute phase dose for 6 months after remission and then slowly tapering the medication until it is discontinued.

Although substantial work is needed to identify patients who will respond to medication, antidepressants remain an important therapeutic tool in this age group for the relief of MDD.

Summary

The recognition and treatment of depressive disorders in children and adolescents remain major concerns for physicians, educators, and parents. The morbidity and mortality associated with these disorders among children and adolescents can be decreased by increasing the public's awareness of the seriousness of these disorders. In the future we will hopefully see research studies that guide physicians in the effective treatment of both acute and recurrent episodes of depression. The effective treatment of dysthymic disorder in children and adolescents is another area where there are no studies to guide physicians. Cognitive, behavioral, and interpersonal therapies hold great promise for the treatment of depressive disorders in children and adolescents. Ultimately, depression in children and adolescents may be best treated with a combination of individual therapy, family therapy, and pharmacotherapy.

Bipolar Disorders

In the section on mood disorders in DSM-IV, symptoms that occur during various episodes of a bipolar mood disorder are described and the various criteria for each specific mood disorder are given. According to DSM-IV, a manic episode is a period of an abnormally and persistently elevated, expansive, or irritable mood that lasts at least 1 week or has any duration if hospitalization is necessary. During the episode of mania there must also be marked impairment in occupational (school) functioning, in social activities, or in relationships with others, or hospitalization must be necessary to prevent the patient from harming himself or others. The diagnosis of a manic episode in a child or an adolescent requires both a significant change in mood and a variety of manic symptoms that must impair the patient's functioning. The criteria for both manic and hypomanic episodes in DSM-IV differ from previous criteria in DSM-III-R, which did not require an exact duration for manic symptoms or an impairment criteria. DSM-IV requires a duration criteria of 1 week, and a functional impairment criteria must be met for mania to be diagnosed.

Bipolar mood episodes in DSM-IV include: (1) manic episodes, (2) hypomanic episodes, and (3) mixed episodes. A child or an adolescent who has a single manic episode that lasts 1 week or more is classified as having a bipolar I disorder, single manic episode in DSM-IV (see Box 8-4, p. 134). A child or adolescent who has had one or more episodes of major depression, no episodes of mania, and at least one episode of hypomania is classified in DSM-IV as having a bipolar II disorder (see Box 8-5, p. 135). A mixed episode is characterized by both manic and depressive symptoms for at least 1 week (see Box 8-6, p. 135). A child or adolescent who is experiencing a mixed episode and who has had an episode of mania or major depression in the past, is classified as having a bipolar I disorder, most recent episode mixed.

Bipolar II disorder, during which an episode of hypomania occurs, is more common in children and adolescents than Bipolar I disorder. A hypomanic episode is characterized in DSM-IV as an abnormally and persistently elevated, expansive, or irritable mood that lasts at least 4 days. In contrast to a bipolar I disorder the illness caused by bipolar II disorder is not severe enough to cause marked impairment in occupational functioning (school functioning in children and adolescents), to interfere with social activities or relationships with others, or to necessitate hospitalization, and there are no psychotic features.

Cyclothymia is a disorder in which there are both numerous periods of hypomania and depression within 1 year that do not meet criteria for mania or major depression. During the period of cyclothymia, the child or adolescent is not without symptoms for more than 2 months at a time. Retrospective studies of adults with cyclothymia have shown that adolescence is the most common age of onset for cyclothymia. A significant proportion of adolescents with cyclothymia also progress to either mania or hypomania. In a study by Akiskal et al. of the offspring of adults with bipolar disorder, 7 out of 10 adolescents with cyclothymia progressed to mania or hypomania within 3 years of diagnosis.

Using DSM-III-R criteria, which required no duration for manic symptoms, Kashani et al. found that in a community sample of 150, nonreferred adolescents, 0.7% met criteria for mania. This estimate approximates the findings of the Epidemiologic Catchment Area study, which found a lifetime incidence of 0.24% to 1.2% for bipolar I disorder among adults. Using a structured interview, Carlson and Kashani reported finding 20 out of 150 randomly selected, nonreferred adolescents (13% of the sample) who had experienced four or more manic symptoms for at least 2 days and thus met DSM-

PEARLS & PERILS

BIPOLAR DISORDERS

- Hypomania is differentiated from mania by the severity of the symptoms present.
- If a child has had at least one manic episode, he is diagnosed with a bipolar I disorder. If he has only had hypomania, a bipolar II disorder is diagnosed.
- Adolescent-onset mania is characterized by greater severity and superior outcome when compared with adult-onset mania.
- It is estimated that as many as 70% of adolescents with cyclothymia progress to mania or hypomania within 3 years of diagnosis.
- Many children with a bipolar disorder are erroneously diagnosed with CD or ADHD.

III-R criteria for hypomania but not mania. The adolescents in this group with manic symptoms but not full mania also had higher rates of ADHD, CD, anxiety disorders, and psychotic symptoms. Carlson and Kashani suggested that although adolescents with hypomania might not always develop mania, they are part of a high-risk group whose members may show signs of incipient bipolar I disorder and may be in need of treatment.

In selected settings, bipolar disorders are more prevalent and can cause a child or an adolescent to have great difficulty. Isaacs reported that out of a class of 50 adolescents enrolled in a special education school, 8 adolescents fulfilled DSM-III-R criteria for a bipolar disorder (either manic or hypomanic). These adolescents often required crisis intervention because of their disruptive behavior and were at high risk for being removed from the program. Isaacs suggests that bipolar disorder is common in problematic adolescents, but that it is often misdiagnosed as CD, ADHD, or another disorder. In a similar study of prepubertal children enrolled in a special education class, Isaacs found five children with atypical forms of mania or hypomania. Many of these students also had periods of dysphoria or depression that lasted a few days but did not meet criteria for MDD. During these depressed periods, the children complained of feeling dizzy, dumb, or weird and of not being able to think. This clinical picture of mania interspersed with periods of dysphoria is characteristic of *dysphoric mania* in adults with bipolar disorder. It is a misconception that patients with bipolar disorder only have symptoms of manic or hypomanic states. Some children, adolescents, and adults have periods of dysphoria and anxiety as components of their dysphoric mania.

The cause of bipolar disorders in children and adolescents is unknown, but similar to depressive disorders, it is thought that both genetic and psychosocial factors are involved. Numerous studies have shown that there is a strong genetic component to bipolar illness in children and adolescents. There are several reasons why there are so few studies of the causes of bipolar disorder in children and adolescents. The low prevalence of this disorder makes it difficult to recruit adequate sample sizes for studies. Additionally, these children and adolescents are often misdiagnosed as having CD or ADHD and are subsequently excluded from appropriate studies. The cyclic and labile nature of this disorder makes it difficult to study and characterize unless expensive longitudinal study methods are employed. When these patients become symptomatic, they often require immediate treatment with both mood agents and antipsychotics, which obviates inclusion in many medication studies that routinely require a medication-free period.

PEARLS & PERILS

DIAGNOSES OF BIPOLAR DISORDERS

- In any child with anger outbursts, inappropriate sexual activity, or thrill seeking behavior, bipolar illness should be considered.
- The most common concurrent diagnosis in bipolar disorder is ADHD.
- Schizophrenia and schizoaffective disorder may be differentiated from bipolar illness in that the onset of mania is usually sudden, whereas the onset of a psychotic disorder is usually insidious.
- A thorough neurologic evaluation should be completed on any child with mania to rule out a space-occupying lesion or seizure disorder.

Diagnostic Criteria

Boxes 8-4 through 8-7 show the DSM-IV diagnostic criteria for episodes of bipolar disorders, and Tables 8-4 and 8-5 list distinguishing features of mania and cyclothymic disorder. Examples of manic behaviors in children and adolescents that correspond to DSM-IV diagnostic criteria are discussed in the following list:

- **Elevated or expansive mood**—The child may seem inappropriately giddy and silly, sing constantly, and generally be much happier than the situation warrants. Manic adolescents can also become overly silly or unrealistically optimistic. During a manic phase, these patients often have no insight about the inappropriateness of their moods.
- **Irritable mood**—The child may become markedly belligerent and highly irritable with many intense outbursts of anger. An adolescent may appear extremely oppositional, belligerent, short, curt, or hostile.
- **Inflated self-esteem or grandiosity**—The child or adolescent may think they have "super powers." For example, they may make statements such as, "I am Superman; nothing can kill or stop me" or, "I can speak 12 languages and have solved the problem of world hunger."
- **Decreased need for sleep**—The child may refuse to go to bed before 1 or 2 AM and only sleep 3 or 4 hours a night. The adolescent may stay up all night and then "crash" for short periods during the day.
- **More talkative than usual**—The child or adolescent may blurt out answers during class repeatedly and appear to "know it all." A child's speech may become very rapid and pressured to the point where it is continuous and at times unintelligible or difficult to follow.

DSM-IV DIAGNOSTIC CRITERIA

BOX 8-4 MANIC EPISODE

A. A distinct period of abnormally and persistently elevated, expansive, or irritable mood, lasting at least 1 week (or any duration if hospitalization is necessary).

B. During the period of mood disturbance, three (or more) of the following symptoms have persisted (four if the mood is only irritable) and have been present to a significant degree:

(1) inflated self-esteem or grandiosity
(2) decreased need for sleep (e.g., feels rested after only 3 hours of sleep)
(3) more talkative than usual or pressure to keep talking
(4) flight of ideas or subjective experience that thoughts are racing
(5) distractibility (i.e., attention too easily drawn to unimportant or irrelevant external stimuli)
(6) increase in goal-directed activity (either socially, at work or school, or sexually) or psychomotor agitation
(7) excessive involvement in pleasurable activities that have a high potential for painful consequences (e.g., engaging in unrestrained buying sprees, sexual indiscretions, or foolish business investments)

C. The symptoms do not meet criteria for a Mixed Episode.

D. The mood disturbance is sufficiently severe to cause marked impairment in occupational functioning or in usual social activities or relationships with others, or to necessitate hospitalization to prevent harm to self or others, or there are psychotic features.

E. The symptoms are not due to the direct physiological effects of a substance (e.g., a drug of abuse, a medication, or other treatment) or a general medical condition (e.g., hyperthyroidism).

Note: Manic-like episodes that are clearly caused by somatic antidepressant treatment (e.g., medication, electroconvulsive therapy, light therapy) should not count toward a diagnosis of Bipolar I Disorder.

(From American Psychiatric Association: *Diagnostic and statistical manual of mental disorders,* ed 4 [DSM-IV], Washington DC, 1994, American Psychiatric Press.)

- **Flight of ideas or racing thoughts**—The child or adolescent may report that they have so many great ideas they can't keep them straight or get them out fast enough. Racing thoughts are sometimes evident in a child's pressured speech. A child may rhyme words together and take great pleasure in being able to think faster then others.
- **Distractibility, short attention span**—As the manic episode progresses, the child or adolescent may report that it is impossible to pay attention in class because his thoughts move along too fast.
- **Increase in goal-directed activity**—The child or adolescent appears very restless or motor driven and shifts from activity to activity rapidly. A child may appear hyperactive but may be able to complete the multiple projects he has started before moving on to another project.
- **Excessive involvement in pleasurable activities that have a high potential for painful consequences**—The child may become hypersexual and inappropriately touch peers or adults in an attempt to engage them in sex. Adolescents may display a marked increase in reckless, thrill-seeking behavior, such as promiscuous behavior, binge drinking, and shopping sprees.

Bipolar I disorder (mania) does not occur very often before puberty, but it may first occur in adolescence. McGlashen interviewed 62 adult patients who met DSM-III criteria for mania and divided them into two groups—35 with adolescent onset of mania and 31 with adult onset of mania. He reported that among the adolescent-onset group, the mean age for the onset of symptoms was 16, they were also hospitalized more often than the adult-onset group, they displayed more psychotic symptoms than the adult-onset group, and they were commonly misdiagnosed as having a schizoaffective disorder. Surprisingly, the adolescent-onset group had superior outcomes in terms of social relationships and ability to work. Akiskal et al. studied 68 referred juvenile offspring of adult bipolar patients and found that the mean age of onset of affective symptoms (usually depression or dysthymic-cyclothymic symptoms) in this group was 15.9. They concluded that mania was most often preceeded by depressive episodes and dysthymic-cyclothymic disorders. Strober et al. studied 58 adolescents who had been admitted to a psychiatric unit because of a major depressive episode and found that during the 24-month follow-up period, mania occurred only in those patients who had a psychotic depression. In this psychotically depressed

BOX 8-5 HYPOMANIC EPISODE

DSM-IV DIAGNOSTIC CRITERIA

A. A distinct period of persistently elevated, expansive, or irritable mood, lasting throughout at least 4 days, that is clearly different from the usual nondepressed mood.

B. During the period of mood disturbance, three (or more) of the following symptoms have persisted (four if the mood is only irritable) and have been present to a significant degree:

(1) inflated self-esteem or grandiosity
(2) decreased need for sleep (e.g., feels rested after only 3 hours of sleep)
(3) more talkative than usual or pressure to keep talking
(4) flight of ideas or subjective experience that thoughts are racing
(5) distractibility (i.e., attention too easily drawn to unimportant or irrelevant external stimuli)
(6) increase in goal-directed activity (either socially, at work or school, or sexually) or psychomotor agitation
(7) excessive involvement in pleasurable activities that have a high potential for painful consequences (e.g., the person engages in unrestrained buying sprees, sexual indiscretions, or foolish business investments)

C. The episode is associated with an unequivocal change in functioning that is uncharacteristic of the person when not symptomatic.

D. The disturbance in mood and the change in functioning are observable by others.

E. The episode is not severe enough to cause marked impairment in social or occupational functioning, or to necessitate hospitalization, and there are no psychotic features.

F. The symptoms are not due to the direct physiological effects of a substance (e.g., a drug of abuse, a medication, or other treatment) or a general medical condition (e.g., hyperthyroidism).

Note: Hypomanic-like episodes that are clearly caused by somatic antidepressant treatment (e.g., medication, electroconvulsive therapy, light therapy) should not count toward a diagnosis of Bipolar II Disorder.

(From American Psychiatric Association: *Diagnostic and statistical manual of mental disorders,* ed 4 [DSM-IV], Washington DC, 1994, American Psychiatric Press.)

BOX 8-6 MIXED EPISODE

DSM-IV DIAGNOSTIC CRITERIA

A. The criteria are met both for a Manic Episode and for a Major Depressive Episode (except for duration) nearly every day during at least a 1-week period.

B. The mood disturbance is sufficiently severe to cause marked impairment in occupational functioning or in usual social activities or relationships with others, or to necessitate hospitalization to prevent harm to self or others, or there are psychotic features.

C. The symptoms are not due to the direct physiological effects of a substance (e.g., a drug of abuse, a medication, or other treatment) or a general medical condition (e.g., hyperthyroidism).

Note: Mixed-like episodes that are clearly caused by somatic antidepressant treatment (e.g., medication, electroconvulsive therapy, light therapy) should not count toward a diagnosis of Bipolar I Disorder.

(From American Psychiatric Association: *Diagnostic and statistical manual of mental disorders,* ed 4 [DSM-IV], Washington DC, 1994, American Psychiatric Press.)

group, 28% went on to develop bipolar I disorder. In a similar follow-up study of prepubertal children with depression, Geller et al. reported that bipolarity was predicted by a family history of major mood disorders such as mania, major depressive disorder, and schizoaffective disorder. These studies show that bipolar I disorder often first occurs in adolescence, may present with schizophrenic-like symptoms, may be predicted by a past history of psychotic depression, and is associated with a family history of major mood disorders.

DSM-IV DIAGNOSTIC CRITERIA

BOX 8-7 CYCLOTHYMIC DISORDER

A. For at least 2 years, the presence of numerous periods with hypomanic symptoms and numerous periods with depressive symptoms that do not meet criteria for a Major Depressive Episode. **Note:** In children and adolescents, the duration must be at least 1 year.

B. During the above 2-year period (1 year in children and adolescents), the person has not been without the symptoms in Criterion A for more than 2 months at a time.

C. No Major Depressive Episode, Manic Episode, or Mixed Episode has been present during the first 2 years of the disturbance.

Note: After the initial 2 years (1 year in children and adolescents) of Cyclothymic Disorder, there may be superimposed Manic or Mixed Episodes (in which case both Bipolar I Disorder and Cyclothymic Disorder may be diagnosed) or Major Depressive Episodes (in which case both Bipolar II Disorder and Cyclothymic Disorder may be diagnosed).

D. The symptoms in Criterion A are not better accounted for by Schizoaffective Disorder and are not superimposed on Schizophrenia, Schizophreniform Disorder, Delusional Disorder, or Psychotic Disorder Not Otherwise Specified.

E. The symptoms are not due to the direct physiological effects of a substance (e.g., a drug of abuse, a medication) or a general medical condition (e.g., hyperthyroidism).

F. The symptoms cause clinically significant distress or impairment in social, occupational, or other important areas of functioning.

(From American Psychiatric Association: *Diagnostic and statistical manual for mental disorders,* ed 4 [DSM-IV], Washington DC, 1994, American Psychiatric Press.)

DIAGNOSIS

TABLE 8-4 MANIA

Discriminating feature

1. A period with a persistently elevated, expansive or irritable mood in the absence of a known physiologic cause

Consistent features

1. Impaired social and academic functioning
2. Psychomotor agitation
3. Flight of ideas or subjective sense that thoughts are racing

Variable features

1. Grandiose or religious delusions or hallucinations
2. Excessive participation in activities that are potentially dangerous
3. Decreased need for sleep
4. Family history of mania
5. Lack of insight about the inappropriateness of behavior
6. Anger outbursts
7. Sudden onset of symptoms

DIAGNOSIS

TABLE 8-5 CYCLOTHYMIC DISORDER

Discriminating feature

1. Multiple episodes of hypomania and depressive symptoms for at least 1 year

Consistent features

1. There is no freedom from symptoms for over a 2-month period
2. Absence of a physiologic condition that may explain symptoms
3. Impaired social or academic functioning
4. Absence of a psychotic illness
5. Hypomanic episodes are present for at least 4 days

Variable features

1. Irritable mood
2. Change in mood is observable to others
3. Appearance of mania within 3 years of symptom onset
4. Family history of bipolar disorder

Assessment

Bowring and Kovacs have delineated the following four reasons that bipolar I disorder (mania) is difficult to diagnose in children and adolescents: (1) a low base rate of the disorder (mania < 1%); (2) the clinical presentation of these disorders is variable and inherently cyclic and labile; (3) the symptoms of mania may overlap with other more common childhood disorders, including ADHD and CD; and (4) a child's age and developmental level influences symptom expression. It is only by taking a careful clinical history that includes both a family history of mood disorders and the course of the patient's illness (including past episodes of depression) and by surveying the patient's range of signs and symptoms during the current and past episodes of mood disturbance that bipolar disorders may be differentiated from other more common disorders. When trying to determine whether a child or adolescent has a bipolar disorder, particular attention must be paid to changes in mood or activity level, a change in the amount of sleep they are getting, involvement in a excessive number of activities, reckless behaviors, and grandiose thinking.

Differential Diagnosis

The most common concurrent diagnosis in this population is ADHD. West et al. reported that out of 14 adolescent bipolar patients with mania, eight (57%) also met DSM-III-R criteria for ADHD. However, with careful delineation of specific symptoms, these disorders can be separated. Fristad et al. recently evaluated the adult Mania Rating Scale in a group of prepubertal children with either mania or ADHD. They found this scale to be useful in differentiating children with mania from the children with ADHD. Children who had mania reported an elevated mood, increased motor activity or energy, decreased need for sleep, increased irritability, pressured speech, flight of ideas, disruptive behavior, thought disorders, and a lack of insight. Many times during a manic or hypomanic episode, an adolescent may engage in reckless behavior and may be diagnosed as having CD when in fact the disorder is bipolar. Similarly, many times a child or adolescent with a bipolar disorder may appear very oppositional during a manic or hypomanic episode and be diagnosed as having ODD, which limits treatment options. Box 8-8 shows possible medical causes of bipolar I disorder in children and adolescents.

BOX 8-8

MEDICAL CAUSES OF MANIA IN CHILDREN AND ADOLESCENTS

Psychostimulants such as methylphenidate (Ritalin) and dextroamphetamine (Dexedrine)
Cocaine
Corticosteroids
Isoniazid
Hyperthyroidism
Head trauma
Multiple sclerosis
Cerebral vascular accidents (particularly lesions of the right hemisphere and thalamus)
Seizure disorders (particularly with a left temporal focus)
Thalamic tumors

Treatment

The pharmacologic treatment of bipolar I disorder in children and adolescents is best conceptualized to consist of two phases: treatment during the manic episode and subsequent maintenance-phase treatment. The treatment of a manic episode in a child or adolescent is based on the same medication guidelines used for adults with bipolar I disorder, since there are no well-designed, double-blind, placebo-controlled studies of the efficacy of any mood agents for the treatment of bipolar disorders in children and adolescents. However, there are numerous open studies and case series using lithium and carbamazepine to treat manic episodes in children and adolescents. And there have recently been two open studies of the efficacy of valproate in the treatment of adolescents with bipolar I disorder. The American Psychiatric Association has recently issued their *Practice Guideline for the Treatment of Patients With Bipolar Disorder*, in which the treatment of bipolar disorder in children and adolescents is also reviewed. These practice guidelines are extremely useful for any physician who treats bipolar disorders, and the interested reader should consult these guidelines because they cover numerous issues that are beyond the scope of this chapter.

Some children and adolescents become psychotic during a manic episode and may require inpatient treatment for several weeks. During this time, their mania is brought under control with a mood stabilizing agent and an antipsychotic agent such as haloperidol or thiothixene. Table 8-6 lists the three mood stabilizing agents most often used to treat mania and their dosages, half-lives, serum levels, side effects, and idiosyncratic effects. Figure 8-1 shows a treatment algorithm for the treatment of manic episodes in children and adolescents. It is recommended to start the patient on lithium, achieve therapeutic levels, and then add carbamazepine if there is no improvement in the patient's symptoms after 4 to 6 weeks of treatment. It may also be necessary to add an antipsychotic agent if a patient is psychotic. Once the manic psychosis has cleared (which may take

TABLE 8-6

MOOD AGENTS

Medication	Half-life (hrs)	Approximate therapeutic range	Dose (mg/kg qd)	Side effects	Idiosyncratic effects (rare but serious)
Lithium	17.9	0.8-1.4 mEq/liter	30	Nausea, weight gain, excessive sedation, tremor, headache, thirst	Acne, hypothyroidism, ECG changes, polyuria-polydipsia
Carbamazepine	9-15	8-11 μg/ml	10-20	Sedation, ataxia, dizziness, blurred vision, nausea	Aplastic anemia/ agranulocytosis, thrombocytopenia, elevated SGOT, SGPT, alkaline phosphatase
Valproate	8-15	60-100 μg/ml	15-60	Nausea, sedation, tremor, weight gain	Elevated SGOT, SGPT, alkaline phosphatase, hepatotoxicity

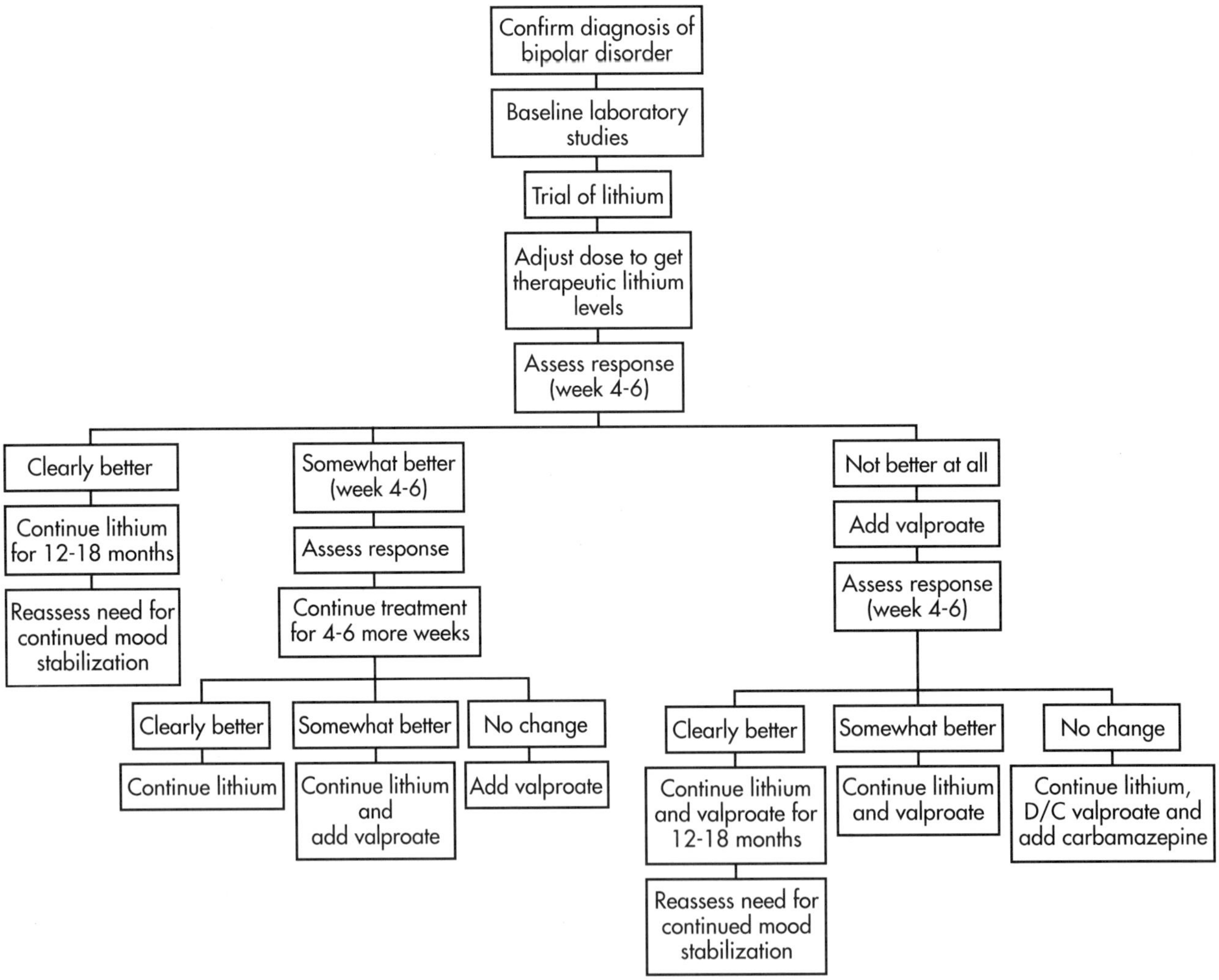

FIGURE 8-1 Treatment algorithm for a manic episode in children and adolescents.

PEARLS & PERILS

TREATMENT OF BIPOLAR DISORDERS

- For the child or adolescent who is to take lithium, renal and thyroid functioning should be assessed before initiating medication and periodically during the course of treatment.
- If a child does not show improvement on lithium alone, carbamazepine or valproate should be added.
- For the child or adolescent who is psychotic with a manic episode, an antipsychotic agent should be used with the lithium.
- After mood stabilization, the child who becomes depressed may require a course of treatment with an antidepressant.
- Lithium should be administered with food to decrease the chances of gastric distress. Slow-release forms of lithium may also help reduce side effects.
- Children taking carbamazepine should be carefully monitored for potentially fatal bone marrow suppression.
- Although there are limited studies, electroconvulsive therapy should be considered in a child who is treatment resistant or in a child who is so ill that waiting for a medication to stabilize is not prudent.
- The treatment of bipolar II disorder and cyclothymia is similar to that of bipolar I disorder, although lower plasma levels of medication may often be sufficient.

days to weeks), it is usually possible and desirable to taper the antipsychotic medication and have the patient keep taking a mood stabilizing agent such as lithium or valproate.

Research among adults with bipolar disorder has shown that approximately 60% of all patients who are manic and acutely ill benefit from lithium. Baseline studies that take place before initiating treatment with lithium should include the following components: a general medical history and physical examination; blood urea nitrogen (BUN) and creatinine levels; a pregnancy test if appropriate; thyroid function tests; an ECG; and a complete blood count with differential. Weller et al. devised a lithium dosage guide for children and adolescents based on body weight that is very useful and accurate. According to these guidelines, in a 6 to 12-year-old child, a dose of 30 mg/kg/day in three dosages produces a lithium level of 0.6 to 1.2 mEq/L within 5 days. Serum lithium levels in the range of 0.8 to 1.4 mEq/L are necessary for mood stabilization in the treatment of manic children and adolescents. Possible common side effects of lithium in children and adolescents include sedation, tremor, polyuria, and weight gain.

Among adult bipolar patients, lithium has been shown to be equally effective preventing episodes of mania and episodes of depression. Strober et al. demonstrated a threefold increase in relapse rates among adolescents with bipolar disorder who discontinued lithium after hospital discharge. Based on this study and studies of adults with bipolar disorder, it is reasonable to maintain a child or adolescent who has had a single manic episode on a mood stabilizing agent for 12 to 18 months. If a child is euthymic and asymptomatic the mood stabilizing agent may be gradually reduced over 2 to 3 months. If manic symptoms recur, the mood stabilizing agent should be reintroduced. Renal function should be tested every 2 to 3 months during the first 6 months of treatment with lithium, and thyroid function should be tested during the first 6 months of treatment. Thereafter, renal and thyroid functions should be checked every 6 months or as clinically indicated.

Some children and adolescents with bipolar disorder who are maintained on a mood stabilizing agent may develop a depressive episode after an acute manic episode while they are taking medication. These patients require the addition of an antidepressant agent to whatever mood stabilizing agent they are already taking. Adding a low dose of fluoxetine (5 to 10 mg/day) or buproprion in these situations is often an effective treatment for a depressive episode. When using an antidepressant agent with a child who has a bipolar disorder, it is important to monitor the patient's mood and behavior carefully for any signs of mania, since these agents can sometimes precipitate a manic episode.

The treatment of hypomania (bipolar II disorder) and cyclothymia in children and adolescents is an area where there are no studies to guide the physician in treatment. If the patient's hypomania or cyclothymia is causing them significant psychosocial dysfunction or academic difficulties, then it is reasonable to treat with a mood stabilizing agent. Either lithium or valproic acid can effectively treat these disorders. As with a bipolar I disorder, it is best to first give the patient a mood stabilizing agent and if periods of depression still occur, to add an antidepressant agent and monitor the patient's moods carefully.

The psychosocial strategies for the treatment of depression in children and adolescents can be very useful in the management of bipolar disorders. It is helpful to first confirm the diagnosis with the patient and his parents and then to educate them about the known causes of bipolar illness. It is important to reinforce with them the necessity of compliance with medication. A common cause of relapse among patients with bipolar disorder is noncompliance with mood agents. Patients and their parents must also be educated about the necessity of taking regular measurements of serum lithium, carbamazepine, valproate, and other laboratory values. It is also critical to ask patients and parents to contact their physician at the first signs of either mania or depression.

Summary

The recognition of bipolar disorder among children, and particularly adolescents, remains a challenge for physicians. There is a large amount of work yet to be done in the area of effective treatments for bipolar disorders among children and adolescents. Unlike MDD, where we are starting to see that psychologic therapies like cognitive therapy are helpful, we have yet to see any specific psychologic therapies for this disorder.

CONSIDER CONSULTATION WHEN . . .

- The child is actively suicidal
- The child has psychotic symptoms with the mood disorder
- The child's depression does not improve despite adequate treatment with an antidepressant over a sufficient period
- The child's symptoms worsen, particularly if mania is suspected, when traditional medical and behavioral interventions are attempted
- The child develops intolerable side effects caused by medication

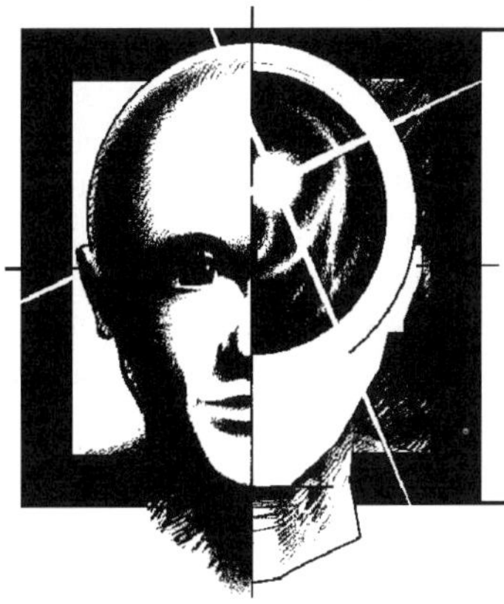

chapter 9

Eating Disorders

David Waller, MD

Feeding Disorder of Infancy or Early Childhood
Rumination Disorder
Pica
Anorexia Nervosa
Bulimia Nervosa
Summary

The term *eating disorder* is a deceptively simple phrase that refers to an extremely complex group of psychiatric disorders with prominent physical, psychologic, and social implications. The physician should be familiar with the diagnostic criteria for each of these disorders and comfortable eliciting them. Differential diagnosis is important, both to distinguish one eating disorder from another and to rule out concomitant medical illnesses. For each patient, a decision must be made as to whether inpatient or outpatient treatment is indicated. Then a treatment program must be planned that addresses each of the following important dimensions: (1) nutritional state, (2) abnormal eating behaviors and attitudes, and (3) the psychologic meaning of the eating disorder for that particular patient. The above process is made more difficult by the fact that patients with these disorders and their families may deny their existence (or at least their severity), setting the stage for a series of control struggles between the patient and the health-care team. All too often the patient does not get better, the physician becomes increasingly frustrated, and the understandable conclusion is drawn that these patients are best avoided. The purpose of this chapter is to provide the necessary information to allow the physician to proceed without undue consternation along these diagnostic and therapeutic paths.

A useful approach to these patients and their families involves a developmental perspective. This should be a familiar frame of reference for pediatricians, child and adolescent psychiatrists, and other health professionals who work with children. Eating disorders are generally the outward expression of underlying problems in psychosocial development. It is therefore important in the course of evaluating and treating the eating disorder to assess where the child or adolescent is in terms of accomplishing age-appropriate psychosocial developmental tasks. An important part of treatment constitutes helping the child and his family move along the appropriate developmental path. Erikson's stages of psychosocial development may be especially useful guideposts and are referred to in the course of discussing particular eating disorders (Table 9-1).

Another general principle is that the physician should maintain a good alliance with the patient and family, as well as act as a health care provider. The atmosphere should be one of mutual respect and team-

TABLE 9-1

ERIKSONIAN STAGES

Age	Psychosocial developmental challenge	Ideal outcome
Infant	Basic trust vs. mistrust	Hope
Toddler	Autonomy vs. shame and doubt	Will
Preschool age	Initiative vs. guilt	Purpose
School age	Industry vs. inferiority	Competence
Adolescence	Identity vs. role confusion	Fidelity
Young adulthood	Intimacy vs. isolation	Love
Adulthood	Generativity vs. stagnation	Caring
Old age	Integrity vs. despair	Reflection

work, with an unhurried pace befitting the slow-going that sometimes characterizes developmental progress. For example, at the very beginning of contact with the patient and family in the waiting room, it is useful to allow the patient and family to have input into the decision of whom the doctor first interviews. In the waiting room, the physician may also wish to find out whose idea it was to come for help and the reasons they have for wanting help. Subsequently each person's views can be elicited, and they may be compared and contrasted. The process of evaluation thereby becomes therapeutic in the sense that individuality is encouraged, and control struggles are avoided.

In DSM-IV, eating disorders are described in two separate places for the first time. Feeding and eating disorders of infancy and early childhood are discussed with other disorders commonly beginning in childhood, whereas anorexia nervosa and bulimia nervosa appear in a separate section later in the text. Nevertheless the latter two disorders commonly begin in adolescence or young adulthood. Criteria for a proposed new eating disorder, called binge-eating disorder, appear in Appendix B of DSM-IV.

Feeding Disorder of Infancy or Early Childhood

Diagnostic Criteria

From a developmental standpoint, feeding disorder of infancy or early childhood is a logical place to begin. It is a newly defined eating disorder in DSM-IV (Box 9-1). The key finding in this condition is that the child, typically an infant, fails to gain weight or loses a significant amount of weight because of not eating adequately. There must be no medical illness present to account for the feeding difficulty, and there must be adequate food available. Included under this rubric are children described by pediatricians as having "nonorganic failure to thrive." Different subcategories correspond to the position on the psychosocial developmental line that the problem first occurs.

Erikson suggests that basic trust is the first psychosocial developmental accomplishment and that it occurs when there is an appropriate relationship between a parent and an infant. The apathetic, passive type of failure to eat and gain weight that occurs with problems in this earliest relationship can be viewed as reflecting a fundamental problem in the attachment process. In contrast, if the feeding problem occurs when the child is entering the toddler phase, in which the goal is for the child to begin to establish some autonomy, the eating disorder may take a form of more active food refusal. Because the control struggle that ensues resembles that of anorexia nervosa, this disorder has been called anorexia of infancy.

Differential Diagnosis

Differential diagnosis of feeding disorder of infancy or early childhood includes a large number of chronic medical conditions that could interfere with an infant's or a child's ability to eat and grow normally. It would seem prudent to involve a pediatrician in the initial evaluation of such a child, to be certain that no medical condition (especially one that is specifically treatable) is missed. If large amounts of weight have been lost, or if the infant is substantially below expected growth parameters, then hospitalization may be indicated. This affords the opportunity to observe the child being fed by parents and other family members as well as by members of the hospital nursing staff. Infants who have been diagnosed with failure to thrive often begin to eat well when they are fed by nurses in the hospital, whereas children with the food-refusal form of the disorder may refuse to eat no matter who feeds them.

Treatment

Treatment of this disorder, as in eating disorders of all types, needs to be concerned with the child's nutritional status. A dietician may help decide what would be an appropriate intake for the child. It is essential that an adequate nutritional state be established as soon as possible, so the child's growth, including brain and mental growth, is not further compromised. Usually with careful attention to the interaction between the child and the adult feeding the child, normal eating patterns and a normal nutritional state can be restored. Parents need to be evaluated for conditions that might impede efforts to feed the child appropriately; an example

DSM-IV DIAGNOSTIC CRITERIA

BOX 9-1 FEEDING DISORDER OF INFANCY OR EARLY CHILDHOOD

A. Feeding disturbance as manifested by persistent failure to eat adequately with significant failure to gain weight or significant loss of weight over at least 1 month.

B. The disturbance is not due to an associated gastrointestinal or other general medical condition (e.g., esophageal reflux).

C. The disturbance is not better accounted for by another mental disorder (e.g., Rumination Disorder) or by lack of available food.

D. The onset is before age 6 years.

(From American Psychiatric Association: *Diagnostic and statistical manual of mental disorders,* ed 4 [DSM-IV], Washington DC, 1994, American Psychiatric Press.)

PEARLS & PERILS

FEEDING AND EATING DISORDERS OF INFANCY OR EARLY CHILDHOOD

- The nature of a child's eating disorder may be consistent with the child's stage of psychosocial development.
- An eating disorder during infancy may reflect a significant attachment problem between the baby and the caregiver.
- An eating disorder in the toddler phase may reflect issues regarding autonomy for the child and the caregiver.
- First and foremost, in treating eating disorders of infancy and childhood, the child's nutritional state must be normalized as soon as reasonably possible.
- In active food refusal, meals need to be offered on a regular schedule with no snacks between meals.
- Anatomic and physiologic reasons for an eating disorder in infancy and childhood must be ruled out.
- In pica, specific nutritional deficiencies may cause the bizarre eating habits.
- The physician should be alert to medical problems directly related to the ingestion of nonnutritive items.

might be serious maternal depression. Sometimes parenting skills such as appropriate feeding behaviors need to be taught. Cases of active food refusal are often more complicated and difficult to treat. Useful strategies include making an appropriate amount of food available to the child at a meal, deciding ahead of time on a fixed amount of time for the food to be offered, allowing the child free rein to participate (or not) in the eating process, and removing the food, making food available again at the next meal time. Snacks are not offered between meals, so natural hunger can build before the next meal. There are no material rewards for eating or punishments for not eating, because the goal is to restore the normal, self-regulating process of appetite and satiety. It is remarkable how difficult it may be for some families to refrain from the fights about food that typically occur; for some families, control issues supersede natural concern with food and nutrition. Often the parents themselves experienced problems having to do with feeding and eating as children or they have difficulty parenting in general. It is important to elicit this information, because it may provide an understanding of the parents' behavior with their children.

Rumination Disorder

Diagnostic Criteria

Rumination disorder is probably another form of developmental conflict, but it is defined separately because of the highly specific abnormal eating behavior that occurs. The name of the disorder derives from the term for animals with multiple stomachs that regurgitate their food and chew the cud (ruminate) as part of the digestion process. Infants with this eating disorder work at bringing partially digested food back into their mouths, and then, seemingly highly satisfied with having accomplished this, they mouth the food and often allow large portions of it to leak from the mouth. Thus malnutrition and even starvation may occur (Box 9-2).

The behavior appears self-stimulating and self-soothing, and in this regard perhaps could be termed a kind of "bulimia of infancy." It seems to reflect inappropriate or inadequate interaction between the parent and the child. Interestingly, when eye contact is made with these children, the rumination behavior usually ceases.

BOX 9-2 RUMINATION DISORDER

DSM-IV DIAGNOSTIC CRITERIA

A. Repeated regurgitation and rechewing of food for a period of at least 1 month following a period of normal functioning.

B. The behavior is not due to an associated gastrointestinal or other general medical condition (e.g., esophageal reflux).

C. The behavior does not occur exclusively during the course of Anorexia Nervosa or Bulimia Nervosa. If the symptoms occur exclusively during the course of Mental Retardation or a Pervasive Developmental Disorder, they are sufficiently severe to warrant independent clinical attention.

(From American Psychiatric Association: *Diagnostic and statistical manual of mental disorders,* ed 4 [DSM-IV], Washington DC, 1994, American Psychiatric Press.)

BOX 9-3 PICA

DSM-IV DIAGNOSTIC CRITERIA

A. Persistent eating of nonnutritive substances for a period of at least 1 month.

B. The eating of nonnutritive substances is inappropriate to the developmental level.

C. The eating behavior is not part of a culturally sanctioned practice.

D. If the eating behavior occurs exclusively during the course of another mental disorder (e.g., Mental Retardation, Pervasive Developmental Disorder, Schizophrenia), it is sufficiently severe to warrant independent clinical attention.

(From American Psychiatric Association: *Diagnostic and statistical manual of mental disorders,* ed 4, [DSM-IV], Washington DC, 1994, American Psychiatric Press.)

Treatment

Treatment requires helping parents and other caregivers interact more actively and meaningfully with the child and teaching them to respect the child's needs and wishes. Initially, it may be necessary to divert the child's attention away from rumination behaviors to more appropriate activities. It is important to be certain that no anatomic or physiologic abnormality, such as hiatal hernia or gastroesophageal reflux, exists that might predispose the child to this behavior.

Pica

Diagnostic Criteria

The final eating disorder of infancy and early childhood to be considered is pica (Box 9-3). Derived from the Latin word for magpie, a bird notorious for its indiscriminate eating habits, pica refers to the habitual consumption of nonnutritive substances by children old enough to be expected to know better (that is, above age 2). Additionally, children with pica are not responding to a cultural phenomenon. (In some societies, clay or starch may be routinely ingested, for example, by women during pregnancy.)

Like the disorders described earlier, pica may indicate that the normal process of child care has gone awry. Children who engage in this behavior seem to be attempting to gratify unmet psychosocial needs by substituting inappropriate eating.

Differential Diagnosis

An additional question to be asked in this situation is whether there exists a specific nutritional deficiency of some type that is driving the craving for nonedible substances. By far the most common imbalance in children with this disorder is iron deficiency anemia. For reasons that are not known, eating ice (pagophagia) has been specifically associated with iron deficiency anemia, but other types of pica may occur with this deficiency as well. Deficiencies of other minerals (such as zinc) have also been associated with bizarre cravings. Typically if a specific deficiency is identified and treated, the abnormal craving disappears. However, in many instances of pica no specific deficiency emerges.

Treatment

In addition to efforts to interrupt the abnormal eating behaviors, as well as to correct parenting problems, attention must focus on possible medical complica-

DSM-IV DIAGNOSTIC CRITERIA

BOX 9-4 ANOREXIA NERVOSA

A. Refusal to maintain body weight at or above a minimally normal weight for age and height (e.g., weight loss leading to maintenance of body weight less than 85% of that expected; or failure to make expected weight gain during period of growth, leading to body weight less than 85% of that expected).

B. Intense fear of gaining weight or becoming fat, even though underweight.

C. Disturbance in the way in which one's body weight or shape is experienced, undue influence of body weight or shape on self-evaluation, or denial of the seriousness of the current low body weight.

D. In postmenarcheal females, amenorrhea, i.e., the absence of at least three consecutive menstrual cycles. (A woman is considered to have amenorrhea if her periods occur only following hormone, e.g., estrogen, administration.)

Specify type:

Restrictive Type: during the current episode of Anorexia Nervosa, the person has not regularly engaged in binge-eating or purging behavior (i.e., self-induced vomiting or the misuse of laxatives, diuretics or enemas)

Binge-Eating/Purging Type: during the current episode of Anorexia Nervosa, the person has regularly engaged in binge-eating or purging behavior (i.e., self-induced vomiting or the misuse of laxatives, diuretics, or enemas).

(From American Psychiatric Association: *Diagnostic and statistical manual of mental disorders,* ed 4 [DSM-IV], Washington DC, 1994, American Psychiatric Press.)

DIAGNOSIS

TABLE 9-2
ANOREXIA NERVOSA

Discriminating features

1. Refusal to maintain body weight at a minimally normal weight
2. Disturbed perception of body image

Consistent features

1. Intense fear of gaining weight
2. Amenorrhea
3. Absence of a physiologic condition that explains weight loss

Variable features

1. Occurs more often in girls
2. Reduction in vital signs
3. Electrolyte imbalances
4. Mild anemia
5. Hypoglycemia
6. Low calcium and magnesium
7. Reduced T3 hormone

tions. One of the most common complications is chronic lead poisoning, which results from a child's eating plaster chips in old houses with lead-containing paint. Children who eat dirt are subject to parasite infection, commonly with dog worms (*Toxocara canis*). Chronic hair ingestion such as may occur with compulsive hair-pulling (trichotillomania) can lead to large obstructive hair balls (trichobezoars). These are but a few examples on a list of complications that is limited only by the list of possible substances that can be ingested. A 14-year-old boy with a strange pattern of gastric ulcers recently confessed to our pediatric staff that he had been consuming Ajax bathroom cleanser since the third grade!

Anorexia Nervosa

Diagnostic Criteria

Anorexia nervosa occurs in 0.5% to 1% of adolescent females in middle to upper socioeconomic classes in industrialized countries (Box 9-4, Table 9-2). About 1 in 20 cases is male, and the disorder is being increasingly diagnosed in individuals outside the usual population with greatest incidence. It may be that early recognition and treatment reduces the likelihood of a chronic, even life-threatening course, and it is important to be able to recognize early signs and symptoms of the disorder. Physicians should be alert to children and adolescents who are losing weight but who do not seem to have the appropriate concern about undue thinness. Anorexia nervosa is defined by weight loss of at least 15% of the expected weight for a person's height, age, and gender or by failure to gain weight so as to be within 85% of the expected weight. Together with low weight is the attitude that there is still danger of being too fat, which is based on an apparent misconception regarding body size. A child's weight and height should be monitored in primary care settings, even in adolescence. If persistent weight loss in the absence of medical illness is occurring, the child should be asked how

PEARLS & PERILS

ANOREXIA NERVOSA

- Early recognition and treatment of anorexia nervosa decreases the likelihood of a chronic, life-threatening course.
- Primary care physicians should carefully question the eating habits of children and adolescents who are losing weight but do not seem concerned about their thinness.
- A key question for primary care physicians to ask a child who is losing weight is if there is greater fear about continued weight loss or about weight gain. The child with anorexia nervosa fears weight gain, not weight loss.
- In anorexia nervosa, amenorrhea may occur before the loss of substantial weight and may persist despite return of weight to normal.
- Anorexia nervosa is not a diagnosis of exclusion; the physician must ask about specific symptoms of the disorder.
- Electrolyte and pH imbalances occur primarily in the purging type of anorexia nervosa.
- The mortality rate for anorexia nervosa is higher than that for any other psychiatric illness, including depression.

she feels about her body size (about right? too fat? too thin?) and whether she is more afraid of gaining weight or of losing weight. Patients with anorexia nervosa are always more afraid of gaining weight.

If the patient is a girl and expected to have menstrual periods, an additional criterion for diagnosis is that she has missed at least three consecutive cycles. Boys with the disorder have an analogous suppression of reproductive endocrine function. A decrease in gonadotropins leads to decreased output of testosterone, a lack of sexual interest, and a diminution of sexual functioning. Amenorrhea is obviously related to weight loss, but it is not totally a function of it. In a small number of women it begins before substantial weight has been lost, and it may persist after weight has returned to a normal level, especially if abnormal attitudes toward body size persist.

Physical findings include a reduction in vital signs; temperature, blood pressure, pulse, and respiration all reflect the body's attempt to conserve energy in the face of starvation. Otherwise the patient may appear remarkably (and misleadingly) healthy, especially if weight has been lost gradually.

Differential Diagnosis

There are a number of important issues related to a differential diagnosis. First, anorexia nervosa is not a diagnosis of exclusion. The patient who has lost a lot of weight for no apparent medical reason needs to be asked questions that specifically address the characteristic attitudes of anorexia nervosa. Other psychologic causes of weight loss include severe depression, in which appetite is truly lost, and failure to eat because of some other delusion, such as the paranoid fear of being poisoned (as opposed to the irrational fear of fatness in anorexia nervosa). Addison's disease, in which anorexia and weight loss may be accompanied by apathy and negativism, may be mistaken for a primary eating disorder. Even if the patient meets strict criteria for anorexia nervosa, it is still possible that some other medical illness might be present concomitantly. Crohn's disease (regional enteritis) is sometimes accompanied by typical symptoms of anorexia nervosa, and brain tumors in the region of the hypothalamus have also occasionally been associated with anorexia nervosa. An indication of Crohn's disease might be an elevated sedimentation rate (since in anorexia nervosa this value is often less than 10); patients with brain tumors often have headaches and visual field cuts suggestive of increased intracranial pressure. Gonadal dysgenesis in women (Turner's syndrome) has been associated with anorexia nervosa. Close collaboration with the pediatrician, family physician, or internist is recommended when sorting through these difficult diagnostic issues.

Laboratory abnormalities, if any, may depend to some extent on which subtype of anorexia nervosa the patient has. Patients with the restrictive type, who limit their food intake, may have different symptoms from those who binge eat and purge by inducing vomiting or by abusing laxatives or diuretics. The latter group may be more prone to electrolyte imbalances. Low potassium is especially dangerous, since it may predispose the patient to cardiac arrhythmias. Low calcium, together with the characteristic estrogen deficiency, may result in severe bone thinning, and even with subsequent weight gain the patient may still be prone to stress fractures. Low magnesium may be associated with cognitive difficulties. Severe hypoglycemia, when glycogen stores are depleted, can result in coma and death. Low phosphorus is an especially ominous finding, because if carbohydrates are given too freely during the refeeding process, remaining phosphorus stores can be quickly depleted, and death can ensue rapidly. Mild anemia is not uncommon; presumably it is caused by iron deficiency that accompanies malnutrition. Similarly, albumin may be lowered. The change in thyroid hormones that is found (reduced T3; elevated reverse T3) probably reflects an adjustment to reduced calories and should not be treated (other than by attempts to improve the patient's caloric intake).

Treatment

Treatment of anorexia nervosa needs to be nutritionally and psychologically directed. To date, no specific medication has been identified in a placebo-controlled study that targets the irrational fear of weight gain. In some respects, nutrition may have to be approached differently from the way psychologic issues are addressed. Dividing the treatment team into those concerned with nutrition and those concerned with psychotherapy has certain advantages, provided that there is good communication among members of the treatment team.

The goals of nutritional treatment are first to keep the patient from starving to death and then to help the patient slowly gain weight until she reaches the normal weight range. In the typical case, a trial of outpatient treatment is warranted. With the help of a dietician, an eating plan is worked out that brings weight loss to a halt and provides for a slow weight gain—no more than ¼ to ½ pound per day. For some patients, dietary supplements such as Ensure are more easily tolerated than other foods. Parents are encouraged to make food available but not get into struggles with their child about eating.

Weight must be monitored closely (that is, at least once each week), and the treatment team must take care not to be deceived by the patient. For example, a patient may consume large amounts of water or conceal heavy items in clothing before being weighed. If the patient continues to lose weight, then hospitalization is indicated. More intense supervision of eating is then possible, and a behavior modification program may be implemented if necessary. Rewards such as visiting privileges, time out of bed, or field trips can be made contingent on weight gain. Occasionally, the patient is so terrified of eating that nutrition has to be given with a nasogastric tube. This should be done sympathetically and with an emphasis on necessary nurturance. If the patient's condition has been allowed to deteriorate to the point that life is threatened, parenteral alimentation may be necessary. However, this carries risks not only of sepsis, but also of catastrophes related to too rapid refeeding (such as the depletion of phosphorus stores and heart failure). Although the goal is for the patient to be back in control of eating as soon as possible, responsibility for adequate nutrition initially has to rest with the treatment team.

In contrast to nutritional treatment, the focus of psychotherapy is on encouraging identity formation and the patient's comfort with an age-appropriate role. Identity is the Eriksonian goal for patients at the age that anorexia nervosa is typically contracted. One often senses that these patients are uncomfortable with the role of an adolescent or young adult, and the disorder results in a regression to a prepubertal state. The patient may feel out of control of matters in general, and that the only remaining way to feel effective in the environment is to control eating and weight. Anorexia nervosa thus becomes the patient's identity.

Families may unwittingly discourage identity formation by failing to validate the patient's ideas and feelings. Family therapy may be especially important in helping the patient carve out an effective role. There may also be other important family issues, such as a marital conflict, from which the child's anorexia nervosa is deflecting attention. Throughout individual sessions with the patient, the goal is for the patient to be assertive; the patient's feelings and ideas should provide the focus, guide the sessions, and hopefully give the patient a more clearly defined sense of who she really is as a person. Thus whereas nutritional responsibility rests initially with the treatment team, the direction of psychotherapy should come from the patient.

There has been considerable interest recently in possible relationships between anorexia nervosa and depression. Although more depression occurs in patients with anorexia nervosa and in their family members, anorexia nervosa, once contracted, appears to have a course of its own that is distinctive and not convincingly influenced by antidepressant medications. Trials are currently underway with the newer serotonin-specific, low side-effect profile agents such as fluoxetine and paroxetine, and one of these can probably be used safely as an adjunct to treatment if depression seems especially severe. However, a patient's mood often improves as weight gain occurs. Antipsychotic medications do not target the specific body image delusion, but they may have a limited role to play in instances of enormous anxiety related to this type of thinking. The best somatic treatment for anorexia nervosa is food.

Prognosis

The prognosis for this disorder is quite variable. For patients who come to medical attention, about half seem to do well; weight is recovered, menstrual cycles resume, and there is not undue concern with weight. However, some patients relapse under stress, and some are never able to emerge from a totally consuming preoccupation with food and body concerns. In these patients, weight often hovers around 80 pounds, and social relationships are severely limited. A few patients still die from the disease, and of those patients with a chronic course the mortality rate continues to rise through the years, with deaths attributable to suicide or malnutrition. Thus the mortality rate for anorexia nervosa is probably higher than for any other psychiatric illness, including depression.

BOX 9-5 BULIMIA NERVOSA

DSM-IV DIAGNOSTIC CRITERIA

A. Recurrent episodes of binge eating. An episode of binge eating is characterized by both of the following:

(1) eating in a discrete period of time (e.g., within any 2-hour period), an amount of food that is definitely larger than most people would eat during a similar period of time and under similar circumstances.
(2) a sense of lack of control over eating during the episode (e.g., a feeling that one cannot stop eating or control what or how much one is eating).

B. Recurrent inappropriate compensatory behavior in order to prevent weight gain, such as self-induced vomiting, misuse of laxatives, diuretics, enemas, or other medications; fasting; or excessive exercise.

C. The binge eating and inappropriate compensatory behaviors both occur, on average, at least twice a week for 3 months.

D. Self-evaluation is unduly influenced by body shape and weight.

E. The disturbance does not occur exclusively during episodes of Anorexia Nervosa.

Specify type:
Purging Type: During the current episode of Bulimia Nervosa, the person has regularly engaged in self-induced vomiting or the misuse of laxatives, diuretics, or enemas.
Nonpurging Type: During the current episode of Bulimia Nervosa, the person has used other inappropriate compensatory behaviors, such as fasting or excessive exercise, but has not regularly engaged in self-induced vomiting or the misuse of laxatives, diuretics, or enemas.

(From American Psychiatric Association: *Diagnostic and statistical manual of mental disorders,* ed 4 [DSM-IV], Washington DC, 1994, American Psychiatric Press.)

Bulimia Nervosa

Diagnostic Criteria

Bulimia nervosa is more common than anorexia nervosa. It affects about 3% to 4% of young women in the middle-to-upper socioeconomic class, but it is also seen in adolescents, in some males, and in women in lower socioeconomic classes. The defining feature is recurring episodes of binge eating followed by compensatory behaviors to offset the effects of the large amount of food that has been consumed, so the net effect is that the patient is usually of normal weight (Box 9-5, Table 9-3). There are two sub-types that are differentiated by the type of compensatory behavior employed by the patient. Most research studies of treatment have focused on patients with the purging subtype, in which episodes of binge-eating are followed by self-induced vomiting, often together with laxative or diuretic abuse to get rid of some of the calories. The other, nonpurging subtype is characterized by the patient's fasting, possibly in conjunction with exercise, to compensate for the binges. A binge episode is defined by the consumption of a large amount of food in a discrete time, during which the patient feels out of control of her eating behavior. There is also a frequency criterion; the episodes of binge eating and compensatory behaviors must have occurred at least twice a week for at least 3 months. Appendix B of DSM-IV contains criteria for binge-eating disorder, which differs from bulimia nervosa in that there are no compensatory behaviors (Box 9-6). This condition, if validated as a disorder, may account for a substantial number of patients seen in weight control clinics and may respond to some of the same therapeutic interventions as bulimia nervosa.

It seems helpful to conceptualize bulimia as an addiction in which food is the abused substance. Patients can often recall the exact time that the abnormal behaviors were no longer in their control but rather had assumed a life of their own. The abnormal behavior is craved, and the patient may in severe cases spend all day focused on the next indulgence in this activity. The behavior is often followed by a terrible sense of remorse and a firm intention to do better next time, and the patient experiences a sense of total failure when the behavior recurs. Since there may be few outward physical signs, it is incumbent on the primary caregiver to ask about problems in the area of eating if this disorder is to be diagnosed before it is firmly entrenched. Even then, the patient may be inclined to be secretive about the matter, sometimes foregoing treatment because of concern that it might not be possible to get along without the disorder.

DSM-IV RESEARCH CRITERIA

BOX 9-6 BINGE-EATING DISORDER

A. Recurrent episodes of binge eating. An episode of binge eating is characterized by both of the following:

(1) eating, in a discrete period of time (e.g., within any 2-hour period), an amount of food that is definitely larger than most people would eat in a similar period of time under similar circumstances
(2) a sense of lack of control of eating during the episode (e.g., a feeling that one cannot stop eating or control how much one is eating)

B. The binge-eating episodes are associated with three (or more) of the following:

(1) eating much more rapidly than normal
(2) eating until feeling uncomfortably full
(3) eating large amounts of food when not feeling physically hungry
(4) eating alone because of being embarrassed by how much one is eating
(5) feeling disgusted with oneself, depressed, or very guilty after overeating

C. Marked distress regarding binge eating is present.

D. The binge eating occurs, on average, at least 2 days a week for 6 months.

Note: The method of determining frequency differs from that used for Bulimia Nervosa; future research should address whether the preferred method of setting a frequency threshold is counting the number of days on which binges occur or counting the number of episodes of binge eating.

E. The binge eating is not associated with the regular use of inappropriate compensatory behaviors (e.g., purging, fasting, excessive exercise) and does not occur exclusively during the course of Anorexia Nervosa or Bulimia Nervosa.

(From American Psychiatric Association: *Diagnostic and statistical manual of mental disorders,* ed 4 [DSM-IV], Washington DC, 1994, American Psychiatric Press.)

DIAGNOSIS

TABLE 9-3
BULIMIA NERVOSA

Discriminating feature

1. Recurrent episodes of binge eating with compensatory behavior to prevent weight gain

Consistent features

1. A sense of lack of control over eating
2. Absence of anorexia nervosa
3. Food craving
4. Absence of a physiologic condition that explains symptoms (e.g., Kleine-Levin syndrome)

Variable features

1. Erosion of dental enamel
2. Electrolyte disturbances
3. Esophageal or gastric tears
4. Callous marks on back of hand (Russell's sign)
5. Salivary gland enlargement

The most common physical finding is erosion of dental enamel. This results from the presence of stomach acid in the mouth and particularly affects upper teeth, since the tongue protects the lower teeth during vomiting. Thousands of dollars of reparative work may be needed. If diuretics or laxatives are used to assist with purgation, electrolyte disturbances may occur. A particularly noxious form of purgation is the abuse of ipecac; emetine toxicity can result in heart failure and death. Occasionally, violent vomiting can result in esophageal or gastric tears. Enlargement of salivary glands, giving a "chipmunk cheek" appearance, probably results from recurrent vomiting and is mainly of cosmetic rather than clinical significance. A telltale sign of bulimia is Russell's sign, the presence of callous marks on the back of the hand produced by the upper teeth when the hand is pushed down the mouth to induce vomiting.

Differential Diagnosis

Differential diagnosis is more straightforward than with other eating disorders because of the stereotypical behaviors that occur. Binge-eating and vomiting in

PEARLS & PERILS

BULIMIA NERVOSA

- Patients with bulimia nervosa are usually of normal weight. This disorder is easily missed unless the physician specifically asks about eating habits and body image.
- Bulimia nervosa may be likened to an addiction, with food being the abused substance. Food is craved, the behavior is kept a secret, and the disorder affects the individual's life in multiple areas.
- Russell's sign (callous marks on the back of the hand) is a telltale sign of bulimia nervosa.
- The most common physical finding is erosion of the dental enamel.
- In children with insulin-dependent diabetes mellitus, anorexia nervosa, and bulimia nervosa may appear in the form of recurrent and unexplained episodes of diabetic ketoacidosis. In these instances, the patients purge by not giving themselves their insulin.
- As many as 50% of patients with bulimia nervosa respond to antidepressants, even in the absence of signs and symptoms of clinical depression.
- Bupropion has been associated with seizures when given to patients with bulimia nervosa.

bulimia nervosa are conscious, voluntary activities. Perhaps the most important medical condition to be excluded is a brain tumor that would essentially have different symptoms: vomiting would be in response to nausea, the compulsive eating would not be so episodic, and it might be accompanied by other neurologic or personality changes. Other examples of organic binge-eating disorders include the following syndromes: (1) Kleine-Levin syndrome, typically found in adolescent boys, in which episodes of uncontrolled eating and hypersexuality are associated with periodic hypersomnolence, presumably a result of hypothalamic insult; (2) Prader-Willi syndrome, a genetic condition in which binge eating and obesity apparently result from a deletion (or absence of paternal contribution) of the long arm of chromosome 15; and (3) Klüver-Bucy syndrome, in which binge-eating is associated with visual disturbances and sexual behavioral alterations, and which may have diverse causes (some reversible). Achalasia, in which the esophagogastric sphincter fails to relax with swallowing, has been mistaken for bulimia, and the metabolic alterations in endocrine disorders such as insulin-dependent diabetes mellitus and hyperthyroidism may predispose an adolescent to contracting bulimia.

Treatment

Although bulimia nervosa was not codified as a distinct psychiatric illness until 1980, considerable insight into treatment has been gained as a result of carefully conducted research studies. Two types of intervention have emerged as being effective. One is CBT; an example that typifies this approach is that of Fairburn. The program of treatment is divided into three stages. The first stage aims to substitute a pattern of regular eating in place of the patient's habitual binge eating, self-induced vomiting, and laxative abuse. After a period of self-monitoring is instituted, the patient is provided with specific behavioral strategies that prevent overeating. The second stage is more cognitively oriented and involves identifying and challenging thoughts, beliefs, and values that are perpetuating the eating problem. The third stage aims to maintain progress and anticipate future difficulties.

Another approach in young women is the use of antidepressants. Original trials were prompted by the observation that patients with bulimia had increased incidences of past personal history of depression and of family history of depression, and that they sometimes met criteria for depression at the time of diagnosis of bulimia. Surprisingly, it was subsequently found that the presence of depression or depressive symptoms does not affect the response a patient with bulimia has to antidepressants. Many patients—perhaps 50% or more—do respond, although a considerably smaller percentage has a total remission of binge-purge episodes. For some the improvement may be short-lived. Nevertheless, when these medications work, the results can be dramatic—almost miraculous in some patients' views. There is much less preoccupation with food and eating, and there is a newfound sense of control over decisions about food. The newer serotonin-specific agents, with their low side-effect profile and tendency to promote weight loss rather than weight gain, may be especially useful as a first line of attack. However, patients who do not respond to one of these medications should probably be given a noradrenergic medication such as desipramine. Dose appears to be very important. For example, in a large research study of young women with bulimia, 60 mg/day of fluoxetine was required for a response clearly superior to a placebo. In one study of desipramine, it was important to document blood levels and increase dosages until they reached levels associated with treatment response in depression. For the young adult patient, it is reasonable to begin with a low but possibly effective dose (20 mg/day of fluoxetine or 25 to 50 mg/day of desipramine) and then increase the dose if there is not an adequate response and there are no significant side effects. MAOIs may be used if other antidepressants are ineffective and if the patient can adhere to the MAOI diet and over-the-counter medication limitations. Bupropion should not be used because it has been found to be associated with seizures when administered to patients with bulimia. There is some evidence to suggest that a combination of antidepressant medication and CBT may be especially beneficial. However, long-term studies are required to determine the true significance of these interventions. At the present time the long-term prognosis of bulimia nervosa is not known.

Whichever of these interventions is employed, it seems important to view the patient who has bulimia within a psychosocial developmental context. The developmental task identified by Erikson for the young adult is the successful achievement of intimacy in relationships. For many patients with this severe eating disorder, bulimia is identified as a "best friend." As in other addictive disorders, a substance is turned to for self-soothing and support, failing the successful achievement of supportive interactions with other people. Often this deficit is part of a larger picture of ego deficiencies that characterize individuals with borderline personality disorder. Food is consumed in an attempt to fill up psychologic loneliness and emptiness that is destined to be futile.

Adolescents with this eating disorder who are brought for help by their parents may be especially challenging, because they may be extremely ambivalent about acknowledging their eating problem and working toward its resolution. Typically there are other disagreements between the parents and the child in addition to conflicting views about the bulimia. It may be more productive to start with other differences that can be addressed in family meetings that do not focus solely on the child's behavior. Once the child is feeling more secure as an individual and has an alliance with health care providers, she may be more comfortable addressing her bulimic behaviors and the feelings that seem to prompt them.

Summary

By now the reader should have a healthy respect for the complexity of eating disorders and the challenges inherent in treating children and adolescents who are afflicted with them. A treatment team may be especially helpful, in terms of providing the different kinds of expertise that the treatment of these children requires and in providing support among those giving help. With patience and persistence, progress can often be made. The eventual resolution of abnormal eating behaviors, improved nutrition, and meaningful psychosocial development can be as gratifying as any health care triumphs.

CONSIDER CONSULTATION WHEN . . .

- The child's weight loss is such that tube feeding or parenteral nutrition is required
- The child continues to lose weight despite appropriate behavioral interventions
- It is suspected that family issues are significantly contributing to or worsening the disorder
- A co-morbid psychopathologic condition such as a mood disorder, is also present
- Hospitalization is required.

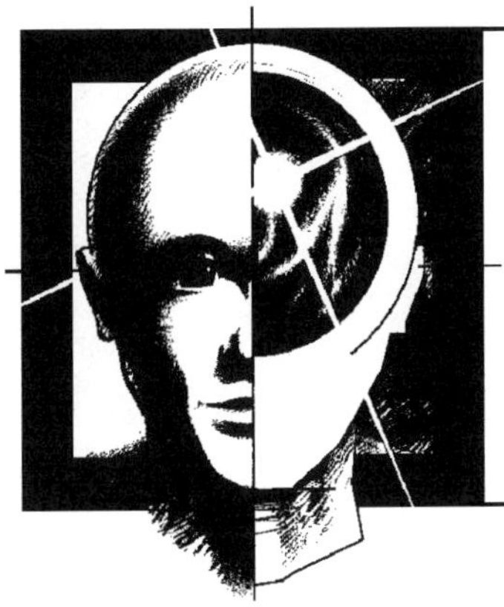

chapter 10

Schizophrenia in Children and Adolescents

Mae S. Sokol, MD

Diagnostic Criteria
Etiology
Assessment
Differential Diagnosis
Treatment
Prognosis
Summary

Psychotic disorders are among the most severe psychiatric illnesses in children and adolescents. These disorders can cause more damage to patients and their families than most physical illnesses. Besides the stigma attached to these conditions and the impairment in level of functioning, psychotic symptoms in children can hinder the process of normal development, sometimes irreversibly.

Although the importance of better understanding psychotic disorders in children is clear, there is presently little objective data available. Much of the early literature in this area is ambiguous because of numerous changes in nomenclature, diagnostic confusion, and methodologic flaws. Until recently, all psychoses in children without a specifically known organic cause were referred to as *childhood schizophrenia*. In this chapter, schizophrenia and other psychotic disorders are defined by the criteria of DSM-IV, which are basically the same for all age groups. Childhood schizophrenia refers to schizophrenia that meets DSM-IV criteria in children less than 12 years old. Pubertal status is not specified, since its role in this disorder has not been demonstrated.

The discriminating feature of schizophrenia is the presence of psychotic symptoms. Psychosis may be defined in a variety of ways, none of which is universally accepted. In this chapter, the term *psychosis* is used as it is in DSM-IV. Psychosis refers to hallucinations, delusions, disorganized speech, and disorganized or catatonic behavior as seen in schizophrenia, schizophreniform disorder, schizoaffective disorder, and brief psychotic disorder. Psychotic symptoms may be present in other disorders (such as affective conditions and substance-induced psychotic disorders) but not as defining characteristics.

Diagnostic Criteria

Criteria for the diagnosis of schizophrenia are the same for all age groups. The essential features are psy-

DSM-IV DIAGNOSTIC CRITERIA

BOX 10-1 SCHIZOPHRENIA

A. *Characteristic symptoms:* Two (or more) of the following, each present for a significant portion of time during a 1-month period (or less if successfully treated):

(1) delusions
(2) hallucinations
(3) disorganized speech (e.g., frequent derailment or incoherence)
(4) grossly disorganized or catatonic behavior
(5) negative symptoms, i.e., affective flattening, alogia, or avolition

Note: Only one Criterion A symptom is required if delusions are bizarre or hallucinations consist of a voice keeping up a running commentary on the person's behavior or thoughts, or two or more voices conversing with each other.

B. *Social/occupational dysfunction:* For a significant portion of the time since the onset of the disturbance, one or more major areas of functioning such as work, interpersonal relations, or self-care are markedly below the level achieved prior to the onset (or when the onset is in childhood or adolescence, failure to achieve expected level of interpersonal, academic, or occupational achievement).

C. *Duration:* Continuous signs of the disturbance persist for at least 6 months. This 6-month period must include at least 1 month of symptoms (or less if successfully treated) that meet Criterion A (i.e., active-phase symptoms) and may include period of prodromal or residual symptoms. During these prodromal or residual periods, the signs of the disturbance may be manifested by only negative symptoms or two or more symptoms listed in Criterion A present in an attenuated form (e.g., odd beliefs, unusual perceptual experiences).

D. *Schizoaffective and Mood Disorder exclusion:* Schizoaffective Disorder and Mood Disorder With Psychotic Features have been ruled out because either (1) no Major Depressive, Manic, or Mixed Episodes have occurred concurrently with the active-phase symptoms; or (2) if mood episodes have occurred during active-phase symptoms, their total duration has been brief relative to the duration of the active and residual periods.

E. *Substance/general medical condition exclusion:* The disturbance is not due to the direct physiological effects of a substance (e.g., a drug of abuse, a medication) or a general medical condition.

F. *Relationship to a Pervasive Developmental Disorder:* If there is a history of Autistic Disorder or another Pervasive Developmental Disorder, the additional diagnosis of Schizophrenia is made only if prominent delusions or hallucinations are also present for at least a month (or less if successfully treated).

Classification of longitudinal course (can be applied only after at least 1 year has elapsed since the initial onset of active-phase symptoms):
Episodic With Interepisode Residual Symptoms (episodes are defined by the reemergence of prominent psychotic symptoms); *also specify if:* **With Prominent Negative Symptoms**
Episodic With No Interepisode Residual Symptoms
Continuous (prominent psychotic symptoms are present throughout the period of observation); *also specify if:* **With Prominent Negative Symptoms**
Single Episode in Partial Remission; *also specify if:* **With Prominent Negative Symptoms**
Single Episode In Full Remission
Other or Unspecified Pattern

(From American Psychiatric Association: *Diagnostic and statistical manual of mental disorders,* ed 4 [DSM-IV] Washington DC, 1994, American Psychiatric Press.)

chotic symptoms, deterioration in adaptive functioning, no identifiable physical cause or marked affective symptoms, and duration of at least 6 months (Box 10-1, Table 10-1). Adults with schizophrenia display deterioration in functioning, whereas children and adolescents fail to achieve expected levels of social, self-care, vocational, and academic development.

The term childhood schizophrenia was believed to have been used too widely in the past. In DSM-III, childhood schizophrenia no longer appeared as a diagnostic entity separate from the general diagnosis of schizophrenia, and infantile autism was recognized as a sepa-

PEARLS & PERILS

SCHIZOPHRENIA

- With schizophrenia in children and adolescents, failure to achieve expected levels of social, self-care, vocational, and academic development are more likely to occur than a deterioration in functioning.
- It is difficult to define a psychosis in a very young child because of the normal lack of logical conceptualization of reality and the inability to abstract seen in this age group.
- Positive symptoms of schizophrenia include hallucinations, delusions, thought disorder, and bizarre behaviors. Positive symptoms are most likely to respond to antipsychotic medication and are most common in children with higher cognitive development.
- Negative symptoms of schizophrenia include social withdrawal, emotional blunting, and paucity of thought and speech. Negative symptoms are more common in children with brain damage and are less likely to improve with antipsychotic medication than positive symptoms.

DIAGNOSIS

TABLE 10-1

SCHIZOPHRENIA

Discriminating feature

1. Psychotic symptoms in the absence of a mood disorder or known organic cause

Consistent features

1. Deterioration from a normal level of functioning
2. Onset during late teens to mid-twenties
3. Failure to achieve expected levels of psychosocial functioning

Variable features

1. Onset rarely before age 9
2. Schizoid characteristics precede active illness
3. Negative symptoms such as apathy, social withdrawal, and paucity of thought and speech
4. Age of onset younger in boys than in girls
5. Slightly lower than normal intelligence in childhood onset
6. Family history of schizophrenic illness

rate disorder. Although pragmatic, the absence of childhood schizophrenia can obfuscate the possible differences in symptoms, prognosis, pathogenesis, and natural course between the adult and childhood-onset forms. These differences are described throughout this chapter.

The definition of schizophrenia in children remains confusing. It is difficult to clearly define psychosis, particularly schizophrenia, in children. Many of the principal symptoms are difficult to differentiate from normal developmental variations, especially when they occur in the very young child. Psychotic symptoms can be similar to age-appropriate fantasies such as imaginary friends and belief in magic or monsters. A logical conceptualization of reality and the ability to abstract are only achieved in adolescence. Developmental disorders such as mental retardation or language difficulties also complicate assessment.

Different authors have defined early-onset schizophrenia as schizophrenia that begins between the ages of 3 and 16. Schizophrenic symptoms were described in children as early as 1857. Children as young as 3 years old can manifest psychotic symptoms and have schizophrenia. Clinical symptoms do vary with age. Hallucinations and delusions may be less prominent in young children as compared with adults. Additionally, a number of childhood psychiatric disorders have disorganized behavior (for example, attention-deficit/hyperactivity disorder [ADHD]) or disorganized speech (such as pervasive developmental disorders [PDDs] or communication disorders). Schizophrenia also shares a number of symptoms with other severe psychiatric disorders in childhood.

It is rare for schizophrenia to begin before adolescence. Onset is usually between the late teens and midthirties. The most common age of onset is age 21 or 22 in both sexes. Women and men are probably equally affected. Men generally have an earlier onset, worse prognosis, and less of an affective component.

Schizophrenia is very rare in children below age 9. It is about 50 times more prevalent in the general population than in children under 12 years old. At the beginning of adolescence, there is a sharp increase in the onset of cases, and the number of new cases increases throughout the teenage years. Childhood schizophrenia is probably less common than autistic disorder. The estimated incidences of schizophrenia and autistic disorder in children under 12 years are 3:10,000 and 4 or 5:10,000, respectively.

The lifetime prevalence of schizophrenia is approximately 0.5% to 1%. This means that 1 or 2 in every 200 individuals will develop a schizophrenic condition at some point in their lives. About 1 in 10,000 individuals develop a schizophrenic condition each year. The incidence is lower than the prevalence in schizophrenia because it is a chronic condition.

In children with schizophrenia under age 16, intelligence level is slightly lower than in the general population. Boys have a younger age of onset than girls, and are 1.5 to 2 times as likely to have the disorder. Schizophrenia in this age group is more common in the lower socioeconomic classes, although symptoms are the same across social and economic strata.

Schizophrenic symptoms are quite similar in children, adolescents, and adults, except for developmental differences. Schizophrenia is a disorder that lasts for at least 6 months. The characteristic symptoms, including hallucinations, delusions, disorganized speech, disorganized or catatonic behavior, and negative symptoms, must last for at least 1 month. A failure to achieve the developmentally expected level of psychosocial functioning occurs in children and adolescents with the disturbance.

Schizophrenia is divided into subtypes mainly based on the relative predominance of positive and negative symptoms (Box 10-2). These can be assessed in children with the Scale for the Assessment of Positive Symptoms and the Scale for the Assessment of Negative Symptoms. Positive symptoms include hallucinations, delusions, thought disorders, and bizarre behavior. These symptoms are more common in children with higher cognitive development. Negative symptoms include social withdrawal, emotional blunting, and paucity of thought and speech. Negative symptoms are more common in children with brain damage. Predominant negative symptoms in adults with schizophrenia often indicate impaired cognitive abilities, poor psychosocial functioning, chronicity, and organicity.

Subtypes of schizophrenia are distinguished by the principal symptoms at the time of assessment. Therefore a patient's subtype may change with time. There are five subtypes of schizophrenia denoted in DSM-IV. In the *paranoid type* the salient features are auditory hallucinations and delusions of a persecutory nature. Affect and cognition are relatively unimpaired. The *disorganized type* is also known as the hebephrenic type. Speech and behavior are disorganized. Affect is flat or inappropriate. There may be silliness unrelated to the content of the patient's speech. If hallucinations and delusions are present, they have no coherent theme. Oddities of behavior, such as grimacing or mannerisms may be present. Cognitive functioning is also often impaired. There is marked disturbance of psychomotor activity seen in the *catatonic type*. Immobility, increased motor activity, extreme negativism, peculiar voluntary movement, waxy flexibility (the tendency to keep the body or a part of the body in one position until it is moved by an observer), echolalia (repetition of what was just said by another person), or echopraxia (imitation of another person's movements) may be exhibited. In the *undifferentiated type* the characteristic symptoms of schizophrenia are present, but criteria for the other three subtypes are not met. Finally, in the *residual type* there are no prominent positive symptoms. Negative symptoms, or at least two attenuated positive symptoms are present.

Hallucinations, formal thought disorder, and poor ability to test reality are common in schizophrenic children. Flat affect, delusions, poverty of thinking, and catatonia are rarer. Children do not usually develop the difficulties with social relatedness that adults with schizophrenia have. Auditory hallucinations are the symptoms reported most often by patients with schizophrenia who are under age 16. They are present in approximately 80% of patients in most studies. Children tend to have command or persecutory hallucinations, or they report hearing conversing voices or voices making a running commentary about their behavior. Visual, somatic, olfactory, and gustatory hallucinations are less common in this age group. Delusions are rarer in children under age 16 than they are in adults. About one half of all children with schizophrenia have delusions. Children may have persecutory, somatic, and grandiose delusions and ideas of reference. Religious delusions and thought control are much rarer in this age group. Systematized, persistent, complex, and abstract delusions are more common in developmentally advanced youngsters who are usually over age 12.

Formal thought disorder is a disturbance in the way thoughts are communicated. Loosening of associations, illogical thinking, neologisms (words made up by the patient), and poverty of speech content are examples of these difficulties in abstract or conceptual thinking. Studies in this age group show thought disorders to be present in 40% to 100% of children with schizophrenia. Loosening of associations and illogical thinking often occur in children who have had schizophrenia for a considerable length of time. It has been postulated that the presence or absence of loosening of associations might be as clinically significant in childhood schizophrenia as the concept of positive and negative symptoms in adults. Incoherence and poverty of speech content are rare in childhood schizophrenia, although they are quite common in the adult illness. Patients of all age groups with schizophrenia have more incoherent speech and produce less speech than unaffected individuals.

A wide variety of other symptoms occurs in association with schizophrenia. Affective symptoms are present in more than one half of the subjects in several studies. There may be an affective component to the illness, or children can be appropriately sad about their illness. Children with psychosis often show unmodulated and intense affective states. Aggressive be-

BOX 10-2 SCHIZOPHRENIC SUBTYPES

DSM-IV DIAGNOSTIC CRITERIA

A. Paranoid Type

A type of Schizophrenia in which the following criteria are met:

(1) Preoccupation with one or more delusions or frequent auditory hallucinations.
(2) None of the following is prominent: disorganized speech, disorganized or catatonic behavior, or flat or inappropriate affect.

B. Disorganized Type

A type of Schizophrenia in which the following criteria are met:

(1) All of the following are prominent:
 a. disorganized speech
 b. disorganized behavior
 c. flat or inappropriate affect
(2) The criteria are not met for Catatonic Type.

C. Catatonic Type

A type of Schizophrenia in which the clinical picture is dominated by at least two of the following:

(1) motoric immobility as evidenced by catalepsy (including waxy flexibility) or stupor
(2) excessive motor activity (that is apparently purposeless and not influenced by external stimuli)
(3) extreme negativism (an apparently motiveless resistance to all instruction or maintenance of a rigid posture against attempts to be moved) or mutism
(4) peculiarities of voluntary movement as evidenced by posturing (voluntary assumption of inappropriate or bizarre postures), stereotyped movements, prominent mannerisms, or prominent grimacing
(5) echolalia or echopraxia

D. Undifferentiated Type

A type of Schizophrenia in which the symptoms that meet Criterion A are present, but the criteria are not met for the Paranoid, Disorganized, or Catatonic Type.

E. Residual Type

A type of Schizophrenia in which the following criteria are met:

(1) Absence of prominent delusions, hallucinations, disorganized speech, and grossly disorganized or catatonic behavior.
(2) There is continuing evidence of the disturbance, as indicated by the presence of negative symptoms or two more symptoms listed in Criterion A for Schizophrenia, present in an attenuated form (e.g., odd beliefs, unusual perceptual experiences).

(Modified from American Psychiatric Association: *Diagnostic and statistical manual of mental disorders,* ed 4 [DSM-IV], Washington DC, 1994, American Psychiatric Press.)

havior often results and maladaptively protects the child from feelings of isolation.

The behavior and grooming of children who have schizophrenia may be bizarre. Skewed development occurs in motor, sensory, cognitive, and social functioning. Alterations in psychomotor activity, as well as ritualistic and stereotypic movements are common. Thinking tends to be concrete, although normal cognitive immaturity can make evaluation especially difficult in this age group. Depersonalization (a subjective sense of being unreal, strange, or unfamiliar to oneself), derealization (a subjective sense that the environment is strange or unreal) and hypochondriasis may occur. Certain physical characteristics seem to occur more often in children with schizophrenia; among these features are hypotonia, brachycephaly, decreased muscle strength and mass, a prominent nasal bridge, and lordosis.

Peer relationships are poor in psychotic children. These children are usually preoccupied by their symptoms and display a narcissistic, selfish attitude toward others. They ignore peers, see them only as rivals for the caregiver's attention, or relate to them as toys. Unaffected children are usually quite sensitive to the strangeness of children who are psychotic and avoid them.

Psychosis adversely affects any interaction with the environment, including a child's ability to play. The play of children who are psychotic tends to be repetitive and more difficult to interrupt. These children tend to use toys in an idiosyncratic and less symbolic manner. They might hit themselves with dolls in a ritualistic manner, rather than using them as representations of transference figures such as parents. Children with psychosis who are capable of symbolic play often exhibit extraordinary imaginations.

Etiology

Many researchers believe schizophrenia to be a diathesis-stress disorder; the clinical condition manifests in genetically predisposed individuals when aggravated by psychosocial or physical stressors. Studies in adults implicate genetics as a causative factor of schizophrenia, but this has not yet been demonstrated in children. Additionally, the elements that influence a child's chances of developing the clinical syndrome have not been elucidated.

In adult-onset schizophrenia, genetic involvement is supported by twin, adoption, and segregation studies. No specific biologic marker for the disorder has yet been identified. Reports of a chromosomal region responsible for the adult-onset disorder have also not been substantiated.

Studies of childhood schizophrenia also suggest a genetic basis to the disorder and a genetic association between the childhood and adult disorders. The prevalence of schizophrenia is increased in children whose parents or siblings have the disorder. About 10% of children with schizophrenia have a parent with schizophrenia. People with adult-onset schizophrenia have comparably elevated rates of the illness in their families. Studies of patients with schizophrenia whose illness began before age 15 have found a concordance rate for developing the illness before age 15 of 71% in monozygotic twins, and only 17% in dizygotic twins. If cases in which the second twin developed schizophrenia after age 15 are included, the concordance rate rises to 88% for monozygotic twins and 23% for dizygotic twins.

Concordance rates for twins with adult-onset schizophrenia are not usually so high. This may be because of the greater severity usually seen in the childhood-onset disorder, since seriously ill adult twins seem to have a higher concordance rate. It has been proposed that pandysmaturation, a neurointegrative defect in infants, may be the manifestation of a genotype that later predisposes a person to schizophrenia. Various environmental factors also appear to either lead to an unexpressed genotype or to the schizophrenic disorder. The best substantiation of this is the fact that monozygotic twin studies have never shown 100% concordance for any psychiatric conditions.

Whereas most children with psychosis do not have parents with psychosis, studies indicate that children of schizophrenic parents are more likely to develop psychosis and particularly schizophrenia. Factors that increase this risk include pregnancy complications, perinatal problems (including trauma), developmental delays, cognitive deficits (particularly when IQ scores are discrepant, with verbal scores lower than performance scores), soft neurologic signs, attentional deficits, and conduct problems.

No laboratory findings are diagnostic for schizophrenia. However, several laboratory findings are abnormal in patients with schizophrenia, compared with the results of subjects who do not have schizophrenia. Enlarged cerebral ventricles, signifying the loss of brain tissue or the absence of its development, have been shown to be more common in schizophrenic adults in CT, MRI, and autopsy studies. One published study of CT scans in children showed significantly enlarged ventricles in 5- to 15-year-old children with a range of psychiatric diagnoses, including schizophrenia, many of whom had concomitant neurologic abnormalities.

MRI and PET studies in adults with schizophrenia reveal functional abnormalities that suggest the localization of psychotic processes in the limbic system, especially the hippocampus. Structural imaging techniques have also shown prominent cortical sulci, decreased temporal and hippocampal size, enlarged basal ganglia, and decreased cerebral size.

Electrophysiologic studies yield nonspecific and inconclusive results. Electrophysiologic abnormalities, however, may indicate neurologic dysfunction in children who are behaviorally disturbed and particularly in children who have schizophrenia. EEG studies in adults with schizophrenia yielded no significant findings. Computer analyzed EEGs (CEEGs) of adults with schizophrenia were significant in that they showed desynchronized fast activity with slow waves and decreased alpha activity. EEG brain potential studies related to cognitive events suggest attentional and information-processing problems in children at risk for schizophrenia.

Only a few neurotransmitter studies have been done in schizophrenia, and the results are equivocal. Neuropsychologic testing shows deficits in attention and information processing, changing response set, and abstraction.

Autoimmune mechanisms may be implicated in the pathogenesis of schizophrenia. Increased B lymphocytes expressing the CD5 (Leu-1) surface antigen are present in several autoimmune conditions, as well as in a subgroup of adults with schizophrenia.

Children who are psychotic have no particular personality type or premorbid set of symptoms. Some common characteristics include academic and behavioral problems, shyness, withdrawn behavior, relational difficulties, magical thinking, and impulsive aggression.

Certain environmental stressors appear to be factors in the development of psychotic symptoms in children, including abuse and neglect by caregivers, traumatic events, sensory deprivation, and prolonged isolation. Further investigation is needed into the pathogenetic roles of the family and interpersonal dynamics in schizophrenia. A number of studies, mostly in adults, have looked at patterns of communication, or "expressed emotion," in the families of individuals with schizophrenia. These studies show that inconsistencies or high levels of affective expression seem to correlate with the development of schizophrenia in family members. Culture and religious beliefs may be salient as well, although the number of cases of schizophrenia is consistent among diverse societies.

Assessment

Clinical evaluation remains the fundamental diagnostic tool in schizophrenia, with laboratory tests and imaging techniques mainly useful for identifying organic psychoses. The diagnosis of schizophrenia (and psychosis in general) should be made cautiously. A physiologic cause for the symptoms, such as seizure disorder or substance abuse, must be ruled out. Misdiagnosis can lead to stigmatization and inappropriate treatment with potentially adverse effects.

A careful history must be obtained from as many informants as possible: the child, parents, other family members, teachers, the pediatrician, and others. A premorbid history that includes information about the following items should be taken: prenatal and perinatal complications; cognitive, motor, sensory, or social developmental problems; premorbid personality characteristics; and documentation of the highest level of functioning before the onset of active symptoms. To be adequate, a mental status examination that covers an extended period should be performed. DSM-IV target symptoms should be documented, as should the course of the illness, the speed of onset, and evidence of cyclical patterns. Careful attention should be given to any specific precipitating stressors and associated or compounding symptoms, such as mood disturbances, substance abuse, and organic factors. It is not unusual for substance abuse disorders or developmental delays, including mental retardation, to occur co-morbidly with schizophrenia. Semistructured assessments, such as the Schedule for Affective Disorders and Schizophrenia for School-Age Children—Epidemiologic Version (K-SADS-E) can help provide a diagnostic framework.

Developmental considerations are necessary when evaluating psychotic symptoms in children. Children must cognitively be able to differentiate between external and internal reality before they can actually be said to be hallucinating. Children of average intelligence can make this distinction by age 3 or 4. Suspected deficits in intellectual functioning, communication abilities, and motor skills should be evaluated, and referral should be considered for psychologic testing (IQ, projective, adaptive functioning, or academic tests), speech and language assessment, and an occupational or physical therapy evaluation.

Vocabulary limitations, differences in attention and memory, and the tendency to be oppositional or compliant with the interviewer are some factors that make assessment difficult. Young children may not spontaneously report that what they saw was in a dream. Because of age-appropriate egocentricity, they may assume it to be understood that what they describe is not real.

Children may not talk about psychotic phenomena for fear of being labelled "crazy" or being hospitalized. Other children may use the concept of psychosis to get what they want. Children who say, "The voices told me not to do my homework," may exemplify this. Understanding the meaning of a child's experiences and their impact on the child's functioning can often be more important than being absolutely sure if the symptoms were psychotic or not.

PEARLS & PERILS

ASSESSMENT OF SCHIZOPHRENIA

- A child who appears unconcerned about psychotic symptoms may have hysterical symptoms or be malingering, or the symptoms may be of such a chronic nature that they are dismissed.
- There are no laboratory tests that are diagnostic for schizophrenia.
- A sustained period of abstinence is the best way to determine if a psychosis is the result of substance ingestion.
- The best predictors of positive outcome are good premorbid psychosocial functioning, acute onset, later age of onset, and well-differentiated symptoms.

Hallucinations can be particularly difficult to evaluate in children, especially because of the increased incidence of *parahallucinatory phenomena* in this age group. It is normal for children, especially when they are lonely, to have *imaginary companions* that they do not confuse with real friends. *Eidetic imagery* involves the recall of vivid visual images that are easily distinguished from reality. *Hypnopompic* and *hypnogogic hallucinations* are normal physiologic events involving perceptual phenomena that occur when the child is awakening and falling asleep, respectively. They are associated with rapid eye movement (REM) sleep.

Hallucinations and parahallucinatory phenomena may be differentiated by examining certain characteristics, including vividness, credence, origin, and volitional quality. Questions related to each characteristic, such as those on the following list, may help the physician determine whether a child is experiencing hallucinations:

- **Vividness**—Does the person you see look like a real live person, like a person in the movies, or like make believe when you close your eyes? Do you hear the voice like you hear me?
- **Credence**—Do you think the person you see is really there? Can you touch the person? Do you have to do what the voices tell you to do? How do you feel about what the voices say?
- **Origin**—Where are the voices coming from? (Voices originating from outside the child's head and making ego-dystonic statements are likely to be hallucinations.)
- **Volitional Quality**—Can you make the voices say what you want them to say? Can you make the voices appear and disappear? Can you make the voices nicer or scarier? (Perceptions that can be manipulated are more likely to be eidetic phenomena than hallucinations.)

The most reliable way to diagnose hallucinations is to directly observe the child hallucinating. This is rare. The physician must usually rely on reports from the child and family. Spontaneous reports can be more credible than answers to questions, since children tend to be suggestible.

It is essential to make children feel comfortable when talking about psychotic symptoms. These experiences can be frightening and difficult to talk about. It is also important to note the child's anxiety level when these issues are discussed. Children are more likely to be anxious when the symptom is of recent onset. Relative disconcern is more common with chronic or hysteric symptoms.

Family emotional, communicative, interactional, and coping styles should also be noted. It is important to understand the family's explanation of the problems the child has been having. It is not unusual to have parents believe that the symptoms are entirely volitional or to blame themselves for the difficulties the child is experiencing. Additionally, a thorough family history of psychotic disorders, mood disorders, suicidal behaviors, neurologic conditions, and substance abuse should be obtained.

A thorough physical examination should be conducted, and it should include a neurologic examination, consideration of a pediatric neurologic consultation, an EEG, and a head CT or MRI. Although there are no laboratory tests that are specifically diagnostic for schizophrenia, structural imaging techniques such as CT and MRI may show enlarged ventricular systems and prominent cortical sulci in certain individuals with schizophrenia. Functional imaging techniques such as PET scans demonstrate abnormal glucose metabolism and cerebral blood flow, especially in the prefrontal cortex of some people with schizophrenia.

Medical conditions that mimic schizophrenia, such as metabolic, endocrine, or infectious disorders and acute intoxication, need to be evaluated as indicated, with laboratory tests such as blood counts, serum chemistries, thyroid functions, syphilis serology, testing for human immunodeficiency virus (HIV), drug screens, and urinalysis performed when appropriate.

Neuropsychologic and neurophysiologic testing should also be considered. Neuropsychologic tests may show disturbances in abstract thinking, attention, and ability to change response set. Neurophysiologic studies may indicate slowed reaction time, abnormal eye tracking, or impaired sensory gaiting.

Differential Diagnosis

Recent changes in nomenclature make differentiating between PDDs and schizophrenia particularly difficult (Table 10-2). PDDs and schizophrenia are now considered to be distinct entities. In PDDs, there are severe and skewed difficulties in a number of areas of development. Qualitatively odd communication, impaired social skills, stereotypic behavior, and unusual interests are the main symptoms. Individuals with a PDD are given the additional diagnosis of schizophrenia in the rare case where pronounced hallucinations or delusions develop for at least 1 month.

Autistic disorder is a type of PDD characterized by qualitatively abnormal interpersonal interactions and a narrow set of interests and activities. Intellectual functioning is more impaired than in childhood schizophrenia, with about 75% of children who have autistic disorder in the mentally retarded range. Socioeconomic status is usually higher in the families of children with autistic disorder. Children who have autistic disorder are less likely than children with schizophrenia to have

TABLE 10-2

COMPARISON OF SCHIZOPHRENIA AND AUTISTIC DISORDER

Characteristic	Schizophrenia	Autistic disorder
Age of onset	Rarely before age 5	Usually before age 3
Prevalence (cases per 100,000 individuals)	14-35	20-50
Male:female ratio	1.5-2:1	4-5:1
Intellectual functioning	Low average IQ	75% In mentally retarded range
Hallucinations and delusions	Yes	No
Clinical course	Progressive deterioration from a relatively normal level of functioning	More delayed and deviant functioning from the onset of illness

parents with psychiatric illness (especially schizophrenia). Abnormalities on EEGs and perinatal complications are more common in autistic disorder. Autistic disorder is also more common than childhood schizophrenia. The prevalence for autistic disorder is about 2 to 5 cases per 10,000 individuals. There are about 70% as many cases of childhood schizophrenia. Whereas schizophrenia seldom begins before adolescence, and childhood cases usually appear after years of relatively normal development, a PDD is usually diagnosed in infancy or early childhood.

The differentiation of schizophrenia from major affective disorders is particularly important with regard to treatment and outcome considerations. This is often difficult because mood disturbance is common in schizophrenia, and depressed children often have psychotic symptoms, especially hallucinations. The clinical course of the disorder is often the best indicator for a diagnosis. The nature of the psychotic symptoms is often different; schizophrenic hallucinations and delusions tend to be bizarre, whereas they are generally mood-congruent in affective disorders. A positive family history for one of these disorders increases the likelihood of its presence in a child.

A manic episode can be difficult to differentiate from schizophrenia because of the irritability, distractibility, loosening of associations, and other psychotic symptoms that are often present in both. An elevated and expansive mood, as well as mood-congruent psychotic symptoms are specifically characteristic of mania. In fact, manic disorders are probably underdiagnosed in children.

Schizophrenia is only diagnosed when physiologic effects of a general medical condition have been ruled out. Symptoms resembling schizophrenia can occur in children with physical illness or substance use. In DSM-IV, a diagnosis of psychotic disorder caused by a general medical condition, dementia, or delirium is made when data (from the history, the physical examination, the laboratory, or ancillary tests) demonstrate that hallucinations or delusions are the physiologic consequence of a general medical condition (Box 10-3). These include metabolic disorders (for example, thyrotoxicosis, Cushing's syndrome), infectious diseases (AIDS), and neurologic disorders (brain tumors, seizure disorders). A psychotic disorder caused by a general medical condition with predominant delusions can have symptoms that are indistinguishable from schizophrenia. An interictal schizophrenic-like picture can develop in seizure disorder, particularly if there is left temporal lobe involvement. In DSM-IV, this would be called psychotic disorder related to seizure disorder.

BOX 10-3

MEDICAL CONDITIONS THAT MAY MIMIC SCHIZOPHRENIA

- Delirium
- Toxic encephalopathies
  - Toxic psychoses related to substance abuse (amphetamines, cocaine, phencyclidine, and solvents)
  - Toxic psychoses related to prescribed medications, such as stimulants, corticosteroids, or anticholinergic agents
- Other toxins, such as heavy metals
- Neurologic conditions
- Seizure disorders, especially with temporal lobe focus
- CNS tumors
- CNS anatomic defects
- Degenerative disorders such as Wilson's disease or Huntington's chorea
- Infectious diseases such as encephalitis, meningitis, and HIV-related syndromes
- Metabolic disorders such as endocrinopathies

Symptoms similar to schizophrenia can be caused by a variety of substance-related disorders, such as substance intoxication or substance withdrawal. Abuse of psychomimetic agents such as lysergic acid diethylamide (LSD), phencyclidine (PCP), marijuana, or cocaine produce episodes indistinguishable from schizophrenia. Psychosis can be a side effect of prescribed medications such as corticosteroids and psychostimulants.

Substance-induced psychotic disorder, substance-induced delirium, or substance-induced persisting dementia is diagnosed when a substance (medication, toxin, or abused drug) causes prominent hallucinations or delusions that are severe enough to warrant medical attention, and when there are more hallucinations or delusions than are usually associated with withdrawal or intoxication. A sustained period of abstinence is the best way to determine whether the psychotic symptoms have been caused by the substance. If this is not practical, information about the symptoms associated with a specific substance, as well as the relationship between the amount of substance use and the severity of symptoms, can help the physician make a differential diagnosis.

Paranoid, schizoid, and schizotypal personality disorders have the following characteristics in common with schizophrenia: paranoid ideation, social avoidance, magical thinking, and odd speech. These three personality disorders may be present before the onset of schizophrenia. However, these personality disorders are not characterized by the presence of positive symptoms as seen in schizophrenia.

Children with schizotypal personality disorder do not have the period of persistent psychotic symptoms that is present in children with schizophrenia. They also have less severe peculiarities of speech, thought, and behavior than children with schizophrenia. Diagnostic criteria are the same as for adults with schizotypal personality disorder. However, to fulfill one of the possible diagnostic criteria of strange beliefs or magical thinking, children may exhibit bizarre fantasies or preoccupations, whereas adults may be superstitious or involved with paranormal phenomena outside their cultural norms. Children with borderline personality disorder may also have transient mild psychotic symptoms, but this psychosis does not exist to the extent or nature of the psychosis of schizophrenia.

Schizoaffective disorder is difficult to differentiate from schizophrenia because mood symptoms can be present in both disorders. In schizoaffective disorder, the mood disorder must occur at the same time as the active-phase symptoms of schizophrenia, psychotic symptoms must be present for at least 2 weeks when prominent mood disturbance is absent, and disturbance of mood must be part of a large portion of the disturbance's total duration.

Schizophreniform disorder, brief psychotic disorder, and psychotic disorder not otherwise specified (NOS) appear similar to schizophrenia. In schizophreniform disorder, the duration must be at least 1 month but less than 6 months. The diagnosis of schizophreniform disorder does not require the decrease in functioning, or the failure to achieve expected developmental advances, as in schizophrenia. Brief psychotic disorder is defined as 1 day to 1 month of psychotic symptoms such as hallucinations, delusions, disorganized speech or behavior, or catatonic behavior. Psychotic disorder NOS is diagnosed when insufficient information is available to diagnose schizophrenia or another specific psychotic disorder. This diagnosis is especially common early in the disorder's course, and when a substance-induced or medical condition is suspected.

There is a group of children who are transiently psychotic and have developmental impairment but are clearly not schizophrenic; however, these children are often mistakenly diagnosed as having schizophrenia. These children have mood instability, learning and language disorders, impulsivity, and poor social skills despite eagerness to make friends. They have recently been referred to as children who are multidimensionally impaired (Box 10-4). The early behavioral and learning problems of children who are multidimensionally impaired differentiate these children from those with borderline personality disorder. Additionally, most patients with multidimensional impairments are male, whereas adult borderline personality disorder is more common in females. Children who are multidimensionally impaired do not respond to neuroleptics, and no effective medication has yet been determined. It is particularly important to make this diagnosis, so the adverse effects of neuroleptics can be avoided.

Children with obsessive-compulsive disorder (OCD) sometimes have ideas that are difficult to differentiate from delusions. Schizophrenia's bizarre behavior and delusions are different from compulsions and obsessions because they are not ego-dystonic and not subject to reality testing. Both diagnoses should be given if the two disorders are present in the same individual.

Conduct disorder (CD) and sociopathic behavior may be early manifestations of what formerly was known as pseudopsychopathic schizophrenia. Dissociative disorders such as dissociative identity disorder (formerly multiple personality disorder) can also be confused with the delusions, hallucinations, and illogical thought processes of schizophrenia.

Mental retardation and communication disorders can be confused with psychosis because they affect language and cognitive abilities. Children who are mentally retarded or developmentally disabled (for example, deaf or blind) can lack adequate stimulation, which leads to behaviors that may appear similar to psychosis. Children who are mentally retarded can appear to have a formal thought disorder because of their low mental age. In fact, children under age 7 with no psychopathologic disorder may have speech patterns similar in certain respects to those of a formal thought disorder.

Childhood schizophrenia must also be differentiated

BOX 10-4

MULTIDIMENSIONALLY IMPAIRED SYNDROME

A. Hallucinatory experiences that do not meet DSM-III-R criteria for schizophrenia (such as brief hallucinations lasting only a few minutes or distorted perceptions such as seeing one's face change in the mirror).

B. Affective instability as evidenced by nearly daily outbursts of tantrums, aggression, and mood swings, often associated with impulsivity.

C. Poor social skills in spite of eagerness to relate to peers.

D. Excessive age-inappropriate fantasy, magical thinking, or poor ability to distinguish fantasy from reality but not clearly delusional (for example, a 14-year old challenges a bully because he believes a superhero will assist him).

OR

Moderate to severe neuropsychologic deficits such as memory impairment; visual-spatial difficulties as demonstrated on testing or apparent in interview.

Additionally, all children must have been identified as seriously disturbed by age 7, although not all symptoms may have been present at that time. At time of diagnosis all children meet above criteria. Exclusionary criteria include the presence of any group of co-morbid diagnoses that could better account for the child's symptoms.

(From McKenna et al, *J Am Acad Child Adolesc Psychiatry* 33:616-635, 1994.)

from a combination of a communication disorder with disorganized speech and ADHD with disorganized behavior. Hallucinations are present in otherwise healthy children when traumatic events, sensory deprivation, or a "shamanistic altered state" is induced. In the latter case, it is important to rule out the administration of psychotomimetic agents. Finally, normal children do not master the adult concept of reality until at least adolescence, making the concept of psychosis especially difficult to apply to children. It is also normal for children of all ages to regress in times of stress to the magical thinking typical of the preschool preoperational stage of cognitive development.

PEARLS & PERILS

TREATMENT OF SCHIZOPHRENIA

- The presence of abnormal involuntary movements should be documented before starting and during the course of administration of antipsychotic medication.
- Clozapine and risperidone are two newer antipsychotic drugs that tend to have fewer side effects than traditional antipsychotics. Agranulocytosis is a side effect specific to clozapine that requires weekly blood monitoring.
- The symptoms of neuroleptic malignant syndrome include severe muscular rigidity (lead-pipe rigidity), stupor, catatonia, hyperpyrexia, and labile pulse and blood pressure. Myoglobinemia, myoglobinuria, and an elevated serum creatine phosphokinase (CPK) may also occur with the syndrome.
- When discontinuing antipsychotic agents, gradual tapering reduces the likelihood of withdrawal dyskinesias. However, if neuroleptic malignant syndrome occurs, the antipsychotic agent should be abruptly discontinued.

Treatment

No definitive intervention has been established for this severe psychiatric disorder. Treatment needs to be individualized to meet the needs of the specific child and family. The goal of treatment must be not only to decrease symptoms, but to enhance development. A multidisciplinary team approach with multimodal treatment is optimal.

When a child is first brought to the physician with psychotic symptoms, hospitalization may be necessary, depending on the severity and potential dangerousness of the symptoms and on the social supports of the family. Hospitalization may also be necessary given the extensive array of psychiatric and neurologic evaluation resources required to complete the initial assessment.

There is substantial scientific evidence in the literature about adults to suggest that the treatment of schizophrenia involves the use of antipsychotic medications in conjunction with multimodal psychotherapeutic interventions. Specialized psychoeducational programs for patients and families, when used to augment medication therapy, have been shown to decrease relapses. The phase of the illness needs to be considered when making decisions about medication therapy (Table 10-3).

TABLE 10-3

TREATMENT PHASES OF SCHIZOPHRENIA

Phase	Characteristics
Acute	Active psychotic symptoms such as hallucinations, delusions, thought disorder, and confusion are present. Antipsychotic medication is needed to eliminate active symptoms.
Recovery	Acute psychotic symptoms are stabilized; the patient may still have difficulties with confusion, disorganization, amotivation, and possible dysphoria. Antipsychotics should be maintained to prevent acute exacerbations. The goal of treatment is to reintegrate the patient back to his home and school, if possible.
Remission or residual	Patient is clinically stable. Active psychotic symptoms have significantly diminished. Negative symptoms may persist. The patient should be maintained on the lowest effective dose of the antipsychotic medication. The dose should be reassessed every 6 months. Many patients are chronically impaired and need to be maintained on long-term antipsychotic agents. The goal is to prevent relapse and recurrence.

During the acute phase before antipsychotic therapy is initiated, preexisting abnormal movements should be noted, so they can later be differentiated from tardive diskinesia. Informed consent for a medication trial should be obtained from parents and adolescent patients, and assent should be obtained from preadolescent patients. The choice of antipsychotic medication should be made based on the agent's relative potency, the spectrum of side effects, and the history of medication response in the patient and his family. Other factors to consider are the physician's familiarity with the medication, cost, and administration route. Children tend to respond to antipsychotic medication, but usually not as well as adults.

Clinical trials in the treatment of children with schizophrenia are limited as a result of the relative rarity of this illness. Spencer et al.'s study of haloperidol administration in a double-blind crossover trial suggests haloperidol's efficacy in treating children with schizophrenia. Sixteen hospitalized subjects with schizophrenia and a mean age of 8.86 (ranging from ages 5.5 to 11.75) responded better to active medication than placebos. Optimal doses of haloperidol were 0.5 to 3 mg/day, or 0.02 to 0.12 mg/kg/day. After completion of the study, all 16 subjects continued to receive the medication with positive effects. Green et al. administered various conventional neuroleptics to 35 children who had schizophrenia in an open clinical trial. Subjects ranged in age from 5.7 to 11.11. Symptoms were not totally alleviated in any patient. Modest to moderate improvement occurred in 21 of the children. Seven improved minimally. Six did not have a positive response. One dropped out of the study.

Adverse effects of conventional neuroleptic treatment are a concern throughout treatment. These effects include extrapyramidal effects, akathisia, hypotension, cognitive impairment, and especially tardive dyskinesia. Neuroleptic malignant syndrome is also of concern. When using antipsychotics, antiparkinsonian agents such as diphenhydramine (Benadryl), benztropine mesylate (Cogentin), and trihexyphenidyl (Artane) may be needed for the treatment of extrapyramidal side effects. The types of antipsychotic medications used and other pertinent information about these drugs are outlined in Table 10-4.

Neuroleptic-induced dyskinesias occur in 8% to 51% of children. Benign withdrawal dyskinesia appears to be the most common form, occurring in about one third of children after neuroleptic withdrawal. Persistent tardive dyskinesia seems to be less of a concern than originally thought. The Abnormal Involuntary Movement Scale (AIMS) can be used to monitor for this adverse effect throughout the treatment course (Table 10-5).

Clozapine, a newer and atypical neuroleptic, is a dibenzodiazepine. Whereas conventional neuroleptics apparently act through dopamine antagonism, clozapine is a serotonin antagonist. Clozapine causes fewer extrapyramidal effects, and it is beneficial to adolescents who do not respond to conventional antipsychotic agents. However, clozapine can cause a potentially life-threatening adverse effect: agranulocytosis.

Risperidone, another new atypical neuroleptic, is a benzisoxazole derivative that is both a dopamine and a serotonin antagonist. It has potent antipsychotic effects and fewer side effects than conventional neuroleptics when used in adults. It decreases positive and negative symptoms, has a rapid onset of action, and causes fewer extrapyramidal effects. The most common adverse effects, noted in order of decreasing frequency are agitation, anxiety, insomnia, extrapyramidal symptoms, headache, and nausea. Risperidone administration to two 15-year-old adolescents in open trials lead to significant improvement within 1 week.

To determine whether or not an antipsychotic medication is effective, it must be used for at least 4 to 6 weeks at adequate dosages. If no effects are seen at that point, consideration should be given to changing to a different class of antipsychotic medication. Before it is

TABLE 10-4

ANTIPSYCHOTIC MEDICATION

Drug	Chemical classification	Therapeutically equivalent dose (mg)	Sedation	Autonomic	Extrapyramidal reaction	Approved ages for use	Usual optimal dose/ maintenance dose range*
Chlorpromazine (Thorazine)	Aliphatic Phenothiazine	100	+++	+++	++	Over 6 months	Ages 3-12 years; 0.5 mg/kg every 4-6 hours; titrate up gradually
Thioridazine (Mellaril)	Piperidine Phenothiazine	100	+++	+++	+	2 years	Ages 2-12 years; 10 mg/day up to 3 mg/kg/day
Loxapine (Loxitane)	Dibenzoxazepine	15	++	+/++	++/+++	16 years	As per adults
Molindone (Moban)	Dihydroindolone	10	++	+	+	12 years	No specific doses for children
Perphenazine (Trilafon)	Piperazine Phenothiazine	10	++	+	++/+++	12 years	No specific doses for children
Trifluoperazine (Stelazine)	Piperazine Phenothiazine	5	++	+	+++	6 years	Ages 6-12 years; 1 mg qd or bid up to 15 mg/day
Thiothixene (Navane)	Thioxanthene	5	+	+	+++	12 years	No specific doses for children
Fluphenazine (Prolixin)	Piperazine Phenothiazine	2	+	+	+++	Not recommended for children	Not recommended for children
Haloperidol (Haldol)	Butyrophenone	2	+	+	+++	3 years	Ages 3-12 years; 0.5 mg qd up to 0.05-0.075 mg/kg/day
Pimozide (Orap)	Diphenylbutylpiperidine	10	+	+	+++	Over 12 years	0.2 mg/kg/day or maximum, 10 mg/day

*In general, adult doses may be used with adolescents, depending upon body size.
(Modified from Lewis M, editor: *Child and adolescent psychiatry: a comprehensive textbook,* Williams and Wilkins, 1991.)

decided that a patient will not respond, the patient must receive at least two adequate trials of different antipsychotic agents. In adults, there are reports of successfully augmenting antipsychotic therapy with lithium, anticonvulsants, benzodiazepines, and fluoxetine. However, these reports are yet unproven, and the combinations have not been studied in children and adolescents.

During the residual or remission phase the patient should receive the lowest effective dose of antipsychotic medication. Once the patient is clinically stable, the dosage should be reassessed approximately every 6 months. Many patients are chronically impaired and need to take long-term antipsychotic agents.

When the physician is discontinuing antipsychotic drugs, gradual tapering is best, given the increased risk

TABLE 10-5

ABNORMAL INVOLUNTARY MOVEMENT SCALE (AIMS)

NAME: ____________________ DATE: __________

INSTRUCTIONS: Complete examination procedure before making ratings.

MOVEMENT RATINGS: Rate highest severity observed. Rate movements that occur upon activation one *less* than those observed spontaneously.

CODE: 0 = None
1 = Minimal
2 = Mild
3 = Moderate
4 = Severe

Facial and oral movements	
1. Muscles of Facial Expression (forehead, eyebrows, periorbital area, cheeks, frowning, blinking, smiling)	0 1 2 3 4
2. Lips and Perioral Area (puckering, pouting, smacking)	0 1 2 3 4
3. Jaw (biting, clenching, chewing, mouth opening, lateral movement)	0 1 2 3 4
4. Tongue (rate only increase in movement both in and out of mouth, not inability to sustain movement)	0 1 2 3 4
Extremity movements	
5. Upper (arms, wrists, hands, fingers) Include choreic movements (i.e., rapid, objectively purposeless, irregular, spontaneous) and athetoid movements, (i.e., slow, irregular, complex, serpentine) but do not include tremor, (i.e., repetitive, regular, rhythmic)	0 1 2 3 4
6. Lower (legs, knees, ankles, toes) Lateral knee movement, foot tapping, heel dropping, foot squirming, inversion and eversion of foot)	0 1 2 3 4
Trunk movements	
7. Neck, shoulders, hips (rocking, twisting, squirming, pelvic gyrations)	0 1 2 3 4
Global judgement	
8. *Severity* of abnormal movements	0 1 2 3 4
9. *Incapacitation* due to abnormal movements	0 1 2 3 4
10. *Awareness* of abnormal movements Rate only patient's report: 0 = No awareness 1 = Aware, no distress 2 = Aware, mild distress 3 = Aware, moderate distress 4 = Aware, severe distress	0 1 2 3 4

(From Guy W: Abnormal involuntary movement scale (AIMS), *ECDEU Assessment Manual for Psychopharmacology,* Rockville, Md. 1976, NIMH Psychopharmacology Research Branch.)

in children for withdrawal dyskinesias. However, if neuroleptic malignant syndrome occurs, the antipsychotic agent should be abruptly discontinued. Careful monitoring is needed during times in which the dosage is being changed to assess for symptoms of relapse.

If a patient relapses, it should first be determined whether or not the patient was compliant with the antipsychotic medications. If not, the medication should be restarted. If the patient was compliant and previously tolerated and responded to the agent, an increase in dose may stabilize the psychotic symptoms. If the patient does not adequately respond to the current antipsychotic agent (at adequate dosage and for a sufficient length of time), a different antipsychotic trial should be undertaken.

Patients who relapse may require acute hospitalization. This decision should be based on the severity of psychotic symptoms, the potential danger to self or others, the degree of impairment in the patient's ability to maintain basic self-care, and the availability of supportive services in the community.

Although medication is important, it is only an important adjunct to the rest of the treatment plan. Individual supportive therapy is believed to be valuable. Behavior modification can be employed to decrease maladaptive behaviors. Parent counseling and family therapy are also important therapeutic modalities. Support groups are beneficial to many families. An example is the National Alliance for the Mentally Ill-Children and Adolescents Network (NAMI-CAN). Specialized educa-

TABLE 10-5

ABNORMAL INVOLUNTARY MOVEMENT SCALE (AIMS)—cont'd

Dental status (0 = No 1 = Yes)

11. Current problems with teeth and/or dentures	0	1
12. Does patient usually wear dentures?	0	1

Examination procedure

Either before or after completing the Examination Procedure, observe the patient unobtrusively at rest (e.g., in waiting room).

The chair to be used in this examination should be a hard, firm one without arms.

1. Ask patient whether there is anything in his/her mouth (i.e., gum, candy, etc.) and if there is, remove it.
2. Ask patient about the **current** condition of his/her teeth. Ask patient if he/she wears dentures. Do teeth or dentures bother patient **now?**
3. Ask patient whether he/she notices any movements in mouth, face, hands or feet. If yes, ask to describe and to what extent they **currently** bother patient or interfere with his/her activities.
4. Have patient sit in chair with hands on knees, legs slightly apart and feet flat on floor. Look at entire body for movement while in this position.
5. Ask patient to sit with hands hanging unsupported. If male, between legs. If female and wearing a dress, hanging over knees. Observe hands and other body areas.
6. Ask patient to open mouth. Observe tongue at rest within mouth. Do this twice.
7. Ask patient to protrude tongue. Observe abnormalities of tongue movement. Do this twice.
8. *Ask patient to tap thumb; with each finger, as rapidly as possible for 10-15 seconds; separately with right hand, then with left hand. Observe facial and leg movements.*
9. Flex and extend patient's left and right arms (one at a time). Note any rigidity and rate on DOTES.
10. Ask patient to stand up. Observe profile. Observe all body areas again hips included.
11. *Ask patient to extend both arms outstretched in front with palms down. Observe trunk, legs and mouth.*
12. *Have patient walk a few paces, turn, and walk back to chair. Observe hands and gait. Do this twice.*

Italics = activated movements

tion to enhance academic, social, adaptive, and vocational abilities is essential for schizophrenic children. Day hospital treatment or residential placement can provide educational and psychiatric interventions together. There is a shift towards community-based interventions, but acute hospitalization is often indicated for evaluation and initial treatment of children with schizophrenia. Residential placement or chronic hospitalization may also be necessary.

Prognosis

Conclusive data regarding the prognosis and treatment outcome in children with schizophrenia are lacking. The few available studies indicate a more guarded prognosis and poorer medication response than in adults. The illness is usually chronic with subtle onset. The best predictors of positive outcome are good premorbid psychosocial functioning, acute onset, later age of onset, and well-differentiated symptoms.

The progression of schizophrenia in adults usually involves increasing deterioration after acute psychotic breaks, followed by a recuperation phase and leading to remission or a residual state that lasts months to years. There are characteristically multiple cycles with increasing deterioration of functioning after each cycle. About 10 years after onset, positive symptoms diminish, leaving a residual state with poor psychosocial functioning and a predominance of negative symptoms.

Evidence exists that prognosis improves when neuroleptic treatment is promptly instituted in the first episode of adult schizophrenia. Conclusive studies in the younger age groups are lacking. However, it appears that adolescents, more than children, are responsive to psychotropic medications. Just as in adults, psychotropic medications are particularly beneficial for positive symptoms, and less helpful for negative symptoms.

Summary

Studies of childhood schizophrenia will increase knowledge about the disorder in all age groups. The variations in symptoms at different stages of life may elucidate protective factors in the younger age group. Research is needed in many areas, especially in the fields of treatment, outcome, and cause. Because of the disorder's rarity, pooling of data across studies would be desirable.

CONSIDER CONSULTATION WHEN . . .

- This is the child's first episode of psychotic symptoms, and the physician is unsure of the diagnosis
- The child does not respond to the use of antipsychotic medications, or his symptoms worsen after taking antipsychotic medication
- The physician is unsure if the child's symptoms may be the result of a specific and treatable medical problem
- The child develops intolerable side effects caused by medication
- The child develops a movement disorder during the course of medication

Annotated Bibliography

Cantor S: *Childhood Schizophrenia,* New York, 1988, Guilford Press.
This is an excellent textbook chapter about the disorder.

Lombroso PJ, Pauls DL, Leckman JF: Genetic mechanisms in childhood psychiatric disorders, *J Am Acad Child Adolesc Psychiatry,* 33:921-938, 1994.
This is a timely review of the current state of research on the genetics of the major childhood psychiatric disorders.

McClellan J, Werry J: Practice parameters for the assessment and treatment of children and adolescents with schizophrenia, *J Am Acad Child Adolesc Psychiatry,* 33:616-635, 1994.
This article summarizes the American Acadamy of Child Psychiatry's recommended practice standards for children and adolescents with schizophrenia.

Pilowsky D, Chambers W, editors: *Hallucinations in children,* Washington DC, 1986, American Psychiatric Press.
This book provides an excellent discussion of hallucinations in children and the various special considerations necessary in this age group.

Rubin TI: *Jordi,* New York, 1960, Macmillan Publishing Company.
The life of a psychotic youngster is depicted in this fictional book. It is written by a psychiatrist who is also the author of *David and Lisa*.

chapter 11

Learning Disorders

Debora L. Scheffel, PhD

Diagnostic Criteria
Features
Etiology
Natural History
Associated Disorders
Assessment
Treatment
Summary

The diagnostic classification of child and adolescent disorders from a psychiatric perspective had its formal beginning with the publication by Leo Kanner of the first English text of child psychiatry. In the third edition (1957) of his textbook (originally published in 1935), a section called *Problems of Behavior* constituted the final and largest grouping in his diagnostic classifications. This grouping included learning disorders of scholastic performance. Similarly, when the first edition of the DSM was published in 1952, learning disturbances in children and adolescents were listed as specific conditions, in spite of the prevalent influence of psychoanalytic theory and a low priority given to childhood and adolescent disorders. Over the years, as the theoretic orientation within psychiatry has shifted from a psychoanalytic to a biologic perspective, there has been a substantial change in the number and specificity of diagnostic categories applicable to children and adolescents. Whereas DSM-I included four such categories, DSM-IV includes at least 55 categories, one of which is concerned with developmental disorders of learning in childhood and adolescence. With this progression has come the belief that learning disorders must be understood from many perspectives.

A comprehensive approach to learning disorders must take into account the complex relationship between organic and emotional factors. Effective participation of the primary care physician on multidisciplinary diagnostic and treatment teams requires familiarity with definitional and etiologic issues, characteristic features, treatment approaches, and associated disorders as they are viewed by a variety of disciplines, including child psychiatry, pediatric neurology, neuropsychology, cognitive psychology, speech and language pathology, and special education. It is imperative that the physician be well informed and able to communicate and coordinate efforts with the family and school.

Diagnostic Criteria

Learning disorders are a subset of childhood developmental disorders that can be classified according to

DSM-IV criteria. The term *developmental* implies persistence of the disorder in spite of advancing chronologic age. According to DSM-IV there must be deviance in the developmental profile such that there is unevenness and maladaptation in the emergence of developmental competency.

Learning disorders, as recognized within the DSM-IV diagnostic scheme, include disorders of reading, mathematics, and written expression. These three types of learning disorders are defined according to several major diagnostic criteria (Boxes 11-1, 11-2, and 11-3). These include the presence of a significant aptitude-achievement discrepancy in the relevant academic area; a statement about the impact of co-morbidity, and exclusionary criteria.

According to the first criteria in each category, a learning disorder may be diagnosed when an individual's achievement on individually administered standardized tests in reading, mathematics, or written expression is below that expected for age, school experience, and intelligence (Tables 11-1, 11-2, and 11-3). Care should be taken to ensure that tests used for diagnosis are consistent with the individual's cultural or ethnic background and that the examiner is familiar with the individual, so responses can be interpreted responsibly.

The discrepancy between aptitude and achievement must result in a significant decrement in academic achievement or in difficulty with application of the academic skill in functional, everyday situations. The use of the term *significant* suggests that there must be sufficient severity to merit educational intervention. A variety of statistical approaches can be used to establish that a discrepancy is significant; a common guideline is two or more standard deviations of difference between achievement scores and an intelligence measure.

Since learning disorders are commonly found in association with other conditions, the diagnostic criteria specify that a learning disorder may be present when achievement is compromised more than what is typically expected from the usual impact of the co-morbid condition. Sensory deficits are specifically mentioned as conditions that may be associated with decreased

BOX 11-1 READING DISORDER

DSM-IV DIAGNOSTIC CRITERIA

A. Reading achievement, as measured by individually administered standardized tests of reading accuracy or comprehension, is substantially below that expected given the person's chronological age, measured intelligence, and age-appropriate education.

B. The disturbance in Criterion A significantly interferes with academic achievement or activities of daily living that require reading skills.

C. If a sensory deficit is present, the reading difficulties are in excess of those usually associated with it.

Coding note: If a general medical (e.g., neurological) condition or sensory deficit is present, code the condition on Axis III.

(From American Psychiatric Association: *Diagnostic and statistical manual of mental disorders,* ed 4 [DSM-IV], Washington DC, 1994, American Psychiatric Press.)

BOX 11-2 MATHEMATICS DISORDER

DSM-IV DIAGNOSTIC CRITERIA

A. Mathematical ability, as measured by individually administered standardized tests, is substantially below that expected given the person's chronological age, measured intelligence, and age-appropriate education.

B. The disturbance in Criterion A significantly interferes with academic achievement or activities of daily living that require mathematical ability.

C. If a sensory deficit is present, the difficulties in mathematical ability are in excess of those usually associated with it.

Coding note: If a general medical (e.g., neurological) condition or sensory deficit is present, code the condition on Axis III.

(From American Psychiatric Association: *Diagnostic and statistical manual of mental disorders,* ed 4 [DSM-IV], Washington DC, 1994, American Psychiatric Press.)

BOX 11-3 DISORDER OF WRITTEN EXPRESSION

DSM-IV DIAGNOSTIC CRITERIA

A. Writing skills, as measured by individually administered standardized tests (or functional assessments of writing skills), are substantially below those expected given the person's chronological age, measured intelligence, and age-appropriate education.

B. The disturbance in Criterion A significantly interferes with academic achievement or activities of daily living that require the composition of written texts (e.g., writing grammatically correct sentences and organized paragraphs).

C. If a sensory deficit is present, the difficulties in writing skills are in excess of those usually associated with it.

Coding note: If a general medical (e.g., neurological) condition or sensory deficit is present, code the condition on Axis III.

(From American Psychiatric Association: *Diagnostic and statistical manual of mental disorders,* ed 4 [DSM-IV], Washington DC, 1994, American Psychiatric Press.)

TABLE 11-1 READING DISORDER

DIAGNOSIS

Discriminating features

1. At least average verbal or nonverbal intellectual potential
2. Significant discrepancy between intellectual potential and performance on measures of reading

Consistent features

1. Not a unitary disorder; heterogeneous population demonstrating a variety of levels of functioning in facets of reading performance
2. May cooccur with language disorders
3. May cooccur with writing disorders
4. Deficient functioning in any one or a combination of: reading silently or orally, individual words or words in context, decoding or comprehension, or rate

Variable features

1. May occur concomitantly with other handicapping conditions or extrinsic influences (but not primarily attributed to either)
2. Deficient performance in skills representing either disrupted visual processes (for example, poor sight vocabulary, or reversals), disrupted lexical processes or semantic access (for example, poor decoding of multisyllabic words), or combinations thereof
3. 35% to 45% heritable
4. Neurodevelopmental motor soft signs
5. Neurologic signs of abnormality (asymmetries of associated movements and reflexes, choreiform movements, diffuse EEG abnormalities)

TABLE 11-2 MATHEMATICS DISORDER

DIAGNOSIS

Discriminating features

1. At least average verbal or nonverbal intellectual potential
2. Significant discrepancy between intellectual potential and performance on measures of mathematics achievement

Consistent features

1. Not a unitary disorder; heterogeneous population demonstrating a variety of levels of functioning in facets of mathematics performance
2. Deficient functioning in any one or combination of: performing written and oral mathematic calculations or understanding and applying mathematic concepts

Variable features

1. May occur concomitantly with other handicapping conditions or extrinsic influences (but are not primarily attributed to either)
2. Deficient performance in skills representing either a language-based disorder (for example, poor comprehension of instructional vocabulary), disrupted visual-nonverbal processing (for example, inaccurate reading of operational signs), or a combination thereof
3. Associated with slow eye-hand coordination, poor tactile form recognition, finger agnosia, cognitive inflexibility, gross motor incoordination, and poor socio-emotional adjustment, if nonlanguage based

DIAGNOSIS

TABLE 11-3
DISORDER OF WRITTEN EXPRESSION

Discriminating features

1. At least average verbal or nonverbal intellectual potential
2. Significant discrepancy between potential and performance on measures of writing

Consistent features

1. Not a unitary disorder; heterogeneous population demonstrating a variety of levels of functioning in facets of writing performance
2. May cooccur with reading and language disorders
3. Deficient functioning in any one or combination of: motor control or planning affecting legibility, spelling, syntax and grammaticality, ideation, or formulation

Variable features

1. May occur concomitantly with handicapping conditions or extrinsic influences (but are not primarily attributed to either)
2. Deficient performance in skills representing either disrupted visuomotor, audioverbal (for example, syntax or dysphonetic spelling errors), visuoverbal (for example, over-phoneticized spellings or capitalization omissions), or combined processing deficits

PEARLS & PERILS

LEARNING DISORDERS

- A learning disorder may be based on difficulty applying the academic skill in a functional, everyday situation as opposed to strictly within school.
- The physician must be familiar with the guidelines used by a state to quantify a severe discrepancy between aptitude and achievement.
- The basis of a disorder in learning cannot be primarily attributed to an emotional or behavior factor.
- Learning disorders based on deficits of early emerging skills have an excellent prognosis compared with those based on deficits of late emerging skills that tend to worsen as the child ages.

academic ability and that may co-occur with a learning disorder. The exclusionary criteria suggest that learning disorders must be differentiated from scholastic difficulties caused by lack of opportunity, poor teaching, cultural factors, or normal variations in academic attainment.

The current federal definition of a learning disorder (termed *learning disability*) is stated in the Individuals with Disabilities Education Act. According to the federal definition, a specific learning disability is a disorder in one or more of the basic psychologic processes involved in understanding or in using spoken or written language. The disorder may be evident in an imperfect ability to listen, think, speak, read, write, spell, or do mathematic calculations. Conditions such as perceptual handicaps, brain injury, minimal brain dysfunction, dyslexia, and developmental aphasia are included. However, the term does not include learning problems that are primarily the result of visual, hearing, or motor handicaps; of mental retardation; of emotional disturbance; or of environmental, cultural, or economic disadvantage. Approximately one half of the states use the federal definition of learning disabilities. State definitions can be broader than the intent of the federal law, but they may not be more restrictive.

Two of the central components of the federal definition of learning disabilities overlap with the definition of learning disorders used in DSM-IV. These include aptitude-achievement discrepancy and exclusionary criteria. All states include the discrepancy component in their definitions, and three fourths of states provide guidelines as to how to quantify a severe discrepancy. The exclusion clause in the federal definition suggests that an individual's underachievement may not be primarily the result of mental retardation, emotional disturbance, sensory deficits, motor disabilities, or environmental, economic, or cultural disadvantage. Currently, 96% of the states include the exclusion clause in their regulations. Fourteen states limit the identification of learning disorders to children who have intelligence quotients in the average range, and six states and the District of Columbia require a minimum IQ above the mental retardation level.

Legislative definitions generally do not overtly recognize co-morbidity of learning disorders with other conditions; however, the use of the word *primarily* in the exclusion clause implies that whereas the learning disorder must be predominant, other conditions may coexist.

In contrast with the DSM-IV diagnostic criteria, the federal definition of learning disabilities includes receptive and expressive oral language on its list of areas of underachievement. DSM-IV categorizes oral language difficulties in the separate category of communication disorders. Additionally, the federal definition addresses the issue of cause by stating that the underachievement is the result of an intrinsic disorder in a person's basic psychologic processes. These processes refer to the ways an individual takes in information, processes it, and responds. The process component has been interpreted primarily within the three contexts of perceptual-motor, psycholinguistic, and cognitive processes of attention and memory. Finally, by allying learning disorders with terms such as *minimal brain dysfunction, brain injury,* and *dyslexia,* neurologic involvement is implied.

Generally characteristics of learning disorders can be viewed as either representative of a qualitative difference in the way the child or adolescent learns or as evidence of a maturational lag. The first view suggests that there are long-term residual effects of a learning disorder, and the second implies that an individual learns like a child of a younger age and that the disorder is likely to resolve with time. These two ways of interpreting characteristics are referred to as a *deficit* or *difference approach* and a *developmental lag* or *delay perspective,* respectively.

One long-term study found evidence of maturational lag in children with learning disorders. When test results from early childhood through young adulthood were compared, many of the subjects as adults no longer had difficulty in areas such as spatial orientation of symbols, auditory discrimination, or left-right discrimination. By comparing children's months of birth with the percentage of children referred for learning disorders in school, researchers have found that younger children (those born near the cut-off date for school entrance) are much more likely to be referred for learning disorders services than their chronologically older peers. This has been called the birthdate effect. In a large-scale study, many children were identified as having dyslexia in the first grade but no longer met the criteria by sixth grade. It has been suggested that the learning difficulties representing maturational lags in children include those in which children reach high levels of sophistication at relatively young ages. An example of such a skill is left-right letter reversals. By age 9, the reversal tendency has disappeared in most children and no longer complicates reading or writing; copying is another skill that reaches a ceiling rather early, usually by age 12 or 13. When the child's deficits are only in early emerging skills that require merely enough mastery to no longer interfere with academic progress, the prognosis for later high-level learning is excellent. However, children are unable to catch up if the disorder involves more complex, late-emerging skills that have higher thresholds for adequacy, because the educational and social demands on these abilities continue to grow as the child gets older. For example, a verbal deficit such as that associated with the ability to retrieve names rapidly from memory is not likely to be recovered. Naming is a slow-maturing skill related to the abilities to rehearse, organize, and store information, and lags often get greater through the years and persist into adulthood.

Features

Reading Disorder

Reading is one of the most prominent difficulties of children with learning disorders; some suggest it is the principal cause of failure in school (see Table 11-1, p. 171). Reading difficulties are often referred to as dyslexia. Most definitions of dyslexia consider it to be a congenital neurologic condition that persists into adulthood and has perceptual, cognitive, and language dimensions. The different dimensions result in subtypes within the larger group, and it is believed that dyslexia leads to deficits in many skill areas as the individual matures. Dyslexia is primarily a medical term; many educators prefer to use the term *severe reading disabilities.* It is estimated that 10% to 15% of the general school population exhibits reading disabilities and that 85% to 90% of all students with learning disorders have reading problems. The incidence of reading disabilities is marked by gender differences, with a male-to-female ratio of 3.8:1.

A consistent finding that has emerged from conducted research is that reading disorder is not really a single disorder; rather there are several kinds of reading disorders manifest in children and adolescents. Because the reading process is mediated by several components, a breakdown of one or a combination of these components can result in different forms of reading disabilities.

The reading process is comprised of two major components: decoding and comprehension. The dissociation between comprehension and decoding is well supported by neuropsychologic, developmental, and genetic studies. The two-component classification of reading disorders has been referred to as a dual-route model. This model postulates that words can be read through a phonologic route where the pronunciation of words is realized without intermediate semantic processing, and a semantic route where the meaning of a word can be realized without intermediate phonologi-

PEARLS & PERILS

LANGUAGE DISORDERS

- Having the child read a paragraph and then explain the content may help screen the child who cannot decode the words from the child who can decode but cannot comprehend.
- The development of written language is dependent on the successful development of oral language.
- Children with depressed math and language skills demonstrate a generalized language-based deficit whereas children with a pure math deficit evidence high scores on verbal and auditory-perceptual measures.

cal processing. The decoding difficulties of children with reading disorders are generally recognized as being caused by phonologic weakness. Phonologic weaknesses have been interpreted as insufficient awareness of the phonetic structure of spoken language, resulting in difficulty analyzing the internal structure of printed words or in matching alphabetic symbols to their phonetic counterparts. The phonologic deficit manifests itself in slow reading speed, errors in oral reading, poor spelling, errors of syntax, and excessive dependence on context for reading; together these symptoms constitute the syndrome of dyslexia.

In addition to evidence that phonologic weaknesses are responsible for decoding difficulties among children with reading disorders, there is some support for subtle disorders of eye movement or vision laterality. Impaired visuospatial function that is associated with poor binocular control caused by disordered development in the right hemisphere has been identified as a contributing factor to the poor reading-decoding abilities of some children. It has also been suggested that children with dyslexia suffer from a deficit in transient channel activity in the visual system, which plays a major role in guiding eye movements and interpreting information across fixations. This deficit results in increased retinal image blur, loss of visual direction and constancy, and instability of the visual world. Children who can read aloud well but do not comprehend constitute a small proportion of children with reading disorders. This subtype of reading disorder has been called *hyperlexia*. Since listening comprehension and reading comprehension are highly correlated and share the same cognitive mechanism, a test of listening comprehension can be used to differentiate between reading disorders resulting from decoding weaknesses and those caused by comprehension deficits alone.

The great majority of children with reading disorders have both decoding and comprehension weaknesses. In addition to decoding and spelling deficits, children belonging to this category perform poorly on tests of comprehension of vocabulary and syntax. They do not rely on context for word recognition, and their errors are often meaningless and inappropriate for the context.

There have been many notable attempts to classify the heterogeneous group of individuals with reading disorders using statistical techniques, syndrome analysis, and clinical approaches. Generally, verbal, spatial, and mixed language-spatial subtypes have emerged consistently across different analyses, the most prominent being the language-disordered subtype.

Disorder of Written Expression

Historically, the term *dysgraphia* has been used to describe disorders of written expression. It is a disorder that is symbolic in nature, in that a child cannot combine auditory and visual verbal information into the motor actions needed for writing. Most research efforts have been directed toward understanding the primary language and motor-based deficits contributing to this disorder. Because disorders of written expression have typically been considered secondary to disorders of oral language, there has been a delayed acknowledgment of the need to define a disorder of written expression as a distinct entity. Since the 1980s, writing has been conceptualized as a problem-solving process based on the writer's knowledge of the topic, knowledge of the writing process, and understanding and use of writing strategies. Neuropsychologic factors such as attention, language, memory, and neuromotor functions have also been proposed as factors that influence written expression. Current research suggests that most, if not all, children with learning disorders have difficulty with some aspects of writing, such as handwriting, spelling, written syntax, vocabulary, or written discourse (see Table 11-3, p. 172). Some studies have shown differential gender effects that are consistent with evidence about children with developmental language disorders.

The writing process is a multidimensional phenomenon. Five subtypes of writing disorders have been proposed (Box 11-4). Pure agraphia refers to writing problems without any other significant language problems; aphasic agraphia involves language-based problems that interfere with written language; agraphia with alexia involves deficits in reading and writing in the absence of aphasia; apraxic agraphia is characterized by deficits in the formation of the graphemes when writing spontaneously; and spatial agraphia involves problems writing on a horizontal line and poor use of spacing. New subtypes organized around the linguistic, visuospatial, and motor components of writing are being studied.

Empiric data identify several subgroups of children with writing disorders. The largest group has fine-motor and linguistic deficits evidenced by poor phonetic spelling, slow motor output, and problems with me-

BOX 11-4

SUBTYPES OF WRITING DISORDERS

Pure agraphia—writing problems without any other significant language problems

Aphasic agraphia—language-based problems that interfere with written language

Agraphia with alexia—deficits in reading and writing in the absence of aphasia

Apraxic agraphia—deficits in the formation of the graphemes when writing spontaneously

Spatial agraphia—problems writing on a horizontal line and poor use of spacing

chanics. A second group manifests primarily visuospatial deficits that result in poor legibility and poor spatial organization. A third group shows problems with attention and memory resulting in poor spelling with many omissions, insertions, and inconsistencies. A final group shows deficits in sequencing, and writing is characterized by poor automatization of letter production, poor mechanics, and poor legibility.

Since the 1980s, writing has also been viewed as a problem-solving process. This process is governed by at least the three interdependent phases of planning, translating, and reviewing. The planning phase involves the generation and organization of ideas and goal setting. The translating phase is the process whereby the writer puts ideas into visible language using syntactic, lexical, motoric, grammatic, and spelling knowledge. Reviewing involves reading what has been written to make modifications. Although variants of these three production components have been proposed, all those that are accepted by professionals in the field are similar in substance.

Given the multidimensional nature of writing, it is understandable that a number of cooccurring features combine in a variety of ways to result in a writing disorder. If language is mastered according to a hierarchy, with written language superimposed on oral language and developing chronologically later, the occurrence of an isolated writing disorder is relatively rare. Furthermore, given the convergence of so many cognitive processes and neuropsychologic functions in the writing process, written language disorders are often associated with academic problems that pervade a child's development and academic career.

Mathematics Disorder

Developmental dyscalculia is a cognitive disorder of childhood affecting the ability of an otherwise intelligent child to learn arithmetic. Developmental dyscalculia has been described as a structural disorder of the maturation of mathematic abilities. Federal law, in the Individuals with Disabilities Education Act, recognizes two main areas in mathematics where an individual can experience a learning disability: mathematics calculation and mathematics reasoning. Children with developmental mathematics disorders have difficulties in the areas of understanding numbers, counting skills, computational skills, and solving word problems (see Table 11-2, p. 171). It has been suggested that arithmetic function can be divided into three basic subskills: number comprehension, number production, and calculation processing. The comprehension category includes comprehension of quantities, the symbolic nature of numbers, and digit order. The number production subsystems are counting, reading, and writing numbers, and calculation processing is subdivided into comprehending operational symbols, executing arithmetic exercises, and memorizing numeric facts. Although deficits in reading and writing performance are more commonly cited as characteristics of students with learning disorders, deficits in mathematics may be just as serious for many of these students. Overall, children with learning disorders spend one third of their special education intervention time addressing mathematics difficulties. It is estimated that 6% of all children exhibit symptoms of developmental dyscalculia. Both reading and math disabilities tend to coexist, although the severity of each may vary. This coexistence occurs because the child's information-processing weaknesses affect all academic subjects, and common cognitive skills, such as language skills, attention, and reasoning, are required for both reading and mathematics.

The various types of dyscalculia reflect analysis of the perceptual, linguistic, cognitive, and functional demands of performing mathematic tasks. Neuropsychologic processes implicated in mathematics disorders include the skills and functions shown in the following list:

- perceptual skills of visuospatial organization needed for comprehension and production of written mathematics
- linguistic skills needed to name quantities, symbols, and relationships
- association and reasoning skills needed for reading and understanding word problems, math concepts, and procedures
- executive functions necessary for rapid mental calculation
- motor functions for the written aspects of math performance
- sequencing abilities for performing a series of procedures or interpreting number sentences
- verbal memory for recall of math facts and procedures

Six types of developmental dyscalculia based on processes involved in performing mathematic functions have been posited (Box 11-5). These include *verbal dyscalculia* (naming difficulties), *practognostic dyscalculia* (difficulty mathematically manipulating objects, pictured or real), *lexical dyscalculia* (difficulty reading math symbols), *graphic dyscalculia* (difficulty writing math symbols), *ideognostic dyscalculia* (disorder in understanding math concepts and performing calculations mentally), and *operational dyscalculia* (disability performing computations).

Differences have been noted between children with a pure math disorder and those with both math and language disorders. Children with only low math performance show a pattern of high scores on verbal and audioperceptual measures and low scores on visuoper-

BOX 11-5

SUBTYPES OF MATHEMATICS DISORDER

Verbal dyscalculia—naming difficulties
Practognostic dyscalculia—difficulty mathematically manipulating objects, pictured or real
Lexical dyscalculia—difficulty reading math symbols
Graphic dyscalculia—difficulty writing math symbols
Ideognostic dyscalculia—disorder in understanding math concepts and performing calculations mentally
Operational dyscalculia—disability performing computations

ceptual and visuospatial measures. Those with depressed math and language skills show a more generalized language-based deficit. Error analysis suggested that the number and type of errors were distinct and depended on whether the deficit was based on visuoperceptual and visuospatial deficits or on linguistic deficits. Despite these apparent differences, the literature on subtyping makes a strong case for the heterogeneous nature of math disorders and the different processes that can combine to result in difficulty with calculation, math applications, or related math skills.

Etiology

A consideration of the biophysic aspects of learning disorders suggests that there is evidence supporting an intrinsic cause for such disorders. Researchers working within this perspective have found that a brain dysfunction can alter the neurologic processes that affect learning and behavior. Evidence from cases of acquired trauma or injury to the CNS, structural brain differences, genetic or hereditary influences, and biochemical irregularities support the influence of biophysical factors on learning disorders. Most research has been conducted with subjects who had reading or other language-based disorders.

Injury to the CNS that results in a learning disorder is called acquired trauma and can occur during gestation, at birth, or after birth. A number of pre-, peri-, and postnatal traumas have been found to be associated with the presence of learning disorders (Box 11-6).

BOX 11-6

BIOPHYSICAL CAUSES OF LEARNING DISORDERS

Prenatal

Alcohol consumption
Cigarette smoke
Cocaine use
Malnutrition
RH factor incompatibility
Maternal diabetes
Placental insufficiency
Maternal kidney malfunction
Fetal infections

Perinatal

Prematurity
Anoxia
Prolonged labor
Premature separation of the placenta
Mechanically assisted delivery

Postnatal

Accidental head injury
Strokes
High fevers
Dehydration
Brain tumors
Meningitis
Encephalitis
Hypoglycemia
Hypothyroidism

The most common prenatal cause of CNS trauma is maternal drug consumption including alcohol, prescription and nonprescription drugs, chemicals found in cigarette smoke, and cocaine. Adverse effects vary depending on the amount of toxic exposure, the point in development of the exposure, and the general health of the fetus. A number of studies have demonstrated correlations between maternal drug consumption and the existence of learning disorders. Adverse effects of drugs in infants may include low birth weight, abnormal EEGs, irritability, and decreased social interaction. In children, academic difficulties, hyperactivity, attention problems, fine motor problems, and delayed language development may be observed.

Other factors associated with prenatal CNS damage include malnutrition (especially during the last trimester of prenatal life), RH-factor incompatibility, maternal diabetes, hypothyroidism, x-ray exposure, extremes in maternal age, placental insufficiency, maternal kidney malfunction, and fetal infections.

Perinatal events are those that affect the child during birth. Common causes of CNS dysfunction during birth include prematurity, anoxia, prolonged labor, premature separation of the placenta, and difficult delivery, which often leads to injury from medical instruments. One study showed that 96% of children with learning disorders experienced birth trauma, as opposed to 10% of children without learning disorders. Incidence of neonatal intensive care has also been associated with a high rate of special education intervention for children when they reach the elementary school years.

Postnatal causes of CNS dysfunction are those accidents and diseases occurring after birth that cause brain damage and resultant learning problems. The most common is acquired cerebral trauma resulting from an accidental head injury. It has been estimated that 31% of students have sustained a mild head injury by the time they reach high school, with unconsciousness involved in one half of the incidents. Common behaviors associated with traumatic brain injury are distractibility, impulsivity, memory deficits, and maladaptive behaviors. Other postnatal causes include malnutrition during the first year of postnatal life, strokes, high fevers, dehydration, brain tumors, or diseases such as meningitis or encephalitis.

Caution is warranted in interpreting the presence of pre-, peri-, and postnatal factors associated with brain injury. Although events related to brain injury are more common among children who later exhibit learning disorders, such events are also present in significant percentages among other learners.

Structural brain differences between individuals with and without evident learning disorders have been identified through a number of techniques, including autopsy studies, CT, and MRI. As early as 1925 it was proposed that incomplete cerebral dominance may be the major cause of developmental reading retardation. Later it was hypothesized that in children with reading disorders, the asymmetry of the temporal lobes that occurs during the development of lateralization is abnormal in both structure and sequence. This hypothesis has been supported by autopsy studies, which have demonstrated an excessive number of neurons in the subcortical white matter of individuals with reading disorders, as well as left-right hemispheric symmetry in the temporal plane and focal cortical dysgenesis with fibromyelinic plaques. The abnormal symmetry is apparently the result of an overabundance of nerve cells in the right hemisphere rather than a lack of development of neurons in the left hemisphere. Cortical dysgenesis, which has been observed in both hemispheres, but mainly in the left along the sylvian fissure is probably caused by abnormal neuron migration during the second half of fetal brain development. Finally, the fibromyelinic plaques are thought to be the result of alterations in microcirculation that occur during the last trimester of fetal development or during the period before the second postnatal year.

In addition to autopsies, structural studies using CT and MRI also point to anatomic differences between those with and without reading disorders. For example, a high proportion of subjects with dyslexia have been shown to have symmetry of the occipital widths and temporal lobe volumes. Individuals with dyslexia have also been shown to have a reversal of the typical pattern of brain structure asymmetry. Consequently, it has been hypothesized that a reduction of volume in the left hemisphere may reflect a relative risk factor for the development of language-based skills in the left hemisphere.

Historically, the use of EEG data in studies of learning disorders has not yielded reliable information. However, with the advent of QEEG, specific waveform data may be more easily read. For example, QEEG studies of individuals with dyslexia have demonstrated abnormal brain electric activity in the left temporal and parietal regions and in the medial frontal area.

The evidence for genetic influences on learning disorders is substantial. Current evidence supports the view that dyslexia is familial (35% to 40% of first-degree relatives are affected), heritable (approximately 50% of the time), and heterogeneous in its mode of transmission (both polygenic and major gene forms of the disorder). This is also supported by twin studies showing that learning disorders coexist among fraternal twins 20% to 35% of the time but are shared from 65% to 100% of the time in identical twins. Linkage analysis studies have suggested that the learning disorders in some families are linked to variations on chromosome 15, whereas other studies have traced some reading disorders to a gene located in one section of chromosome 6. Given the multiple types of learning disorders, it is likely that there is more than one genetic mode of inheritance.

Several biochemical irregularities, including abnormal neurochemical transmissions, glandular disorders, and hypoglycemia, may lead to learning disorders in children and adolescents. Biochemical imbalances are inferred from reduced numbers of neurotransmitter metabolites in the urine, blood, or cerebrospinal fluid or from observation of how drugs that alter brain chemistry impact attention, learning, and behavior. Imbalances in the production of neurotransmitters (for example, serotonin, dopamine, norepinephrine, and acetylcholine) are assumed to cause difficulties in neural impulse transmission and in consequent learning and behavior problems. The effectiveness of psychoactive drugs to improve attention and learning and to decrease hyperactivity supports the existence of a chemical imbalance in some individuals with learning disorders. In children with learning disorders and associated attentional problems, there is evidence that these individuals may use too little of the chemical needed to inhibit neural transmission. Stimulants activate the chemicals that inhibit neurotransmissions and thereby cause clinical improvement. In contrast to the hyperactive child, the CNS' inhibitory mechanisms in the hypoactive child may be overactive rather than underactive. Sedatives, which reduce the overactive inhibitory mechanisms and allow more stimuli to be attended to by the child, may be helpful.

Glandular disorders, such as thyroid deficiencies and hypothyroidism, in the young child can cause permanent damage to the brain, affecting overall intelligence, language functioning, and motor abilities. Low blood sugar compromises brain development, especially during the first 2 years of life, with one of the most common results being reduced brain size.

Cognitive psychology, a subfield within psychology, attempts to understand the psychologic processes involved in learning disorders. The study of psychologic processes suggests that learning disorders are caused by underlying intrinsic deficits in specific areas of learning, including memory, visual processing, auditory processing, attention, and executive functions.

The study of memory in children and adolescents with learning disorders has typically been approached from an information processing perspective. Information processing, broadly defined, is the way input is transformed, reduced, elaborated, stored, retrieved, and used. Theorists working from this perspective function on the basis of a model of memory. Most models include the structural components of sensory, short-term, working, and long-term memories and an executive monitor. Sensory memory refers to the initial complete copy of information available for processing for a maximum of 3 to 5 seconds; short-term memory also has limited capacity, processes information for a maximum of 3 to 7 seconds, and is concerned with storage by way of rehearsal; working memory focuses on interpretation of new material; long-term memory is a permanent storage system with unlimited capacity; and executive functions monitor and coordinate the system.

Generally, research concerning the sensory register of the memories of children with learning disorders suggests that the sensory register is intact. In contrast, short-term memory deficits have been shown to be evident and have been attributed to control processes (that is, rehearsal) and the meaningfulness of the material. Long-term memory, that is, the permanent storage of information, is primarily a function of control processes like rehearsal. Studies have shown that children with learning disorders are less skilled than their normal peers in the use of rehearsal strategies to consolidate the target information into long-term memory. Others suggest that children with learning disorders are less adept than their peers at retrieving information once it has been stored in long-term memory. Some studies indicate that working memory, integration of existing information with new information, is deficient in readers who have learning disorders, compared with the working memory of readers with no learning disorder. Finally, a number of studies have found that children with learning disorders have difficulty in executive functions involving checking, planning, and monitoring control processes.

PEARLS & PERILS

COGNITIVE PROCESSES

- The verbal IQ score is more predictive of school functioning than the nonverbal IQ score.
- Children with learning disorders have problems with the use of both short- and long-term memory, particularly the visual memory. Visual processing deficits are more prominent in young children with respect to the reading process but auditory deficits are more debilitating overall.
- Children with learning disorders have particular problems with selective attention.

Visual processes involved in reading and writing include visual perception, visual analysis (extraction of relevant visual features), visual memory for patterns, and visuospatial ability (left-to-right scanning). A number of studies indicate that young children with learning disorders have underlying difficulties in visual perception and analysis, in that they differ from their unaffected peers in how quickly they can perceive and extract information from a visual stimulus. It has been suggested that the brains of individuals with dyslexia may process visual information, which is fast and transient and which has high contrast sensitivity and low spatial selectivity, more slowly than control subjects because of atypical development of the two major neural pathways that connect the retinae to the two lateral geniculate nuclei of the thalamus and to the two primary visual cortices.

Most studies designed to investigate visual memory differences between average children and those with learning disorders have employed recognition memory, reproduction memory, paired associate learning, or serial learning tasks. The pattern of results from these studies suggests that young learners with disorders make more errors and are slower at responding to visual memory tasks in the initial stages of processing than other learners. Few differences have been found with children older than age 8 in the later stages of processing. Studies using tasks that measure visuospatial abilities have been inconsistent, partially because of the age of the subjects. Some have found no differences, whereas others have suggested differences between young children with and without learning disorders on visuospatial processing tasks. In conclusion, it appears that younger children have difficulty with visual perception and memory related to visual learning tasks, whereas children older than age 8 do not show consistent visual processing deficits.

Whereas there is less general consensus as to the role of visual processing deficits in learning disorders, there is relative agreement as to the impact of language abilities and auditory processing on learning disorders, particularly reading disorders. It has been observed that children deficient in visuoperceptual or visual motor skills do not encounter reading difficulty any more often than matched controls, whereas children with deficits in speech and language encounter reading problems at least 6 times more often than the controls.

Reading requires language processing skills at several different levels, including speech perception, vocabulary skills, linguistic short-term memory, information about syntactic and semantic structure, and phonemic awareness. A number of studies suggest that speech perception, the ability to identify target words from among nontarget words, is difficult for children with learning disorders in reading, particularly in a noisy condition. Similarly, there are numerous indications that reading ability is related to oral vocabulary skills. For example, children who are poor readers need more time to name a series than good readers. It has been found that on a test of letter-naming ability, kindergarten children who take more time to name a randomized array of capital letters are more likely to perform poorly on word decoding and comprehension tests in first grade than children who can name the letters quickly.

Research has supported the hypothesis that short-term memory difficulties are associated with reading disorders. For example, when recalling letter strings, word strings, and sentences, poor readers are much less successful than good readers. Problems with the syntax and semantics of oral language also appear to interfere with the processing of reading information among poor readers. It has been demonstrated that poor readers do not comprehend sentences as well as good readers and that good and poor readers differ in the ability both to repeat and comprehend spoken sentences that contain relative clauses. Some interpret differential performance on syntactic and semantic tasks predominantly as a memory deficit and not as a comprehension deficit. Finally, research has shown a strong positive correlation between lack of awareness about phonemes and problems in learning to read. For example, one study found that 85% of a population of kindergarten children who went on to become good readers in first grade correctly counted the number of syllables in spoken words, whereas only 17% of the future poor readers could do so. It has been suggested that phoneme awareness accounts for 66% of the variance in children's first-grade reading ability. In short, there is an extensive research base that links reading disorders to deficits in auditory processing.

Learning disorders and attention disorders are generally assumed to be different entities; whereas learning disorders are characterized by the specificity of dysfunction, attention disorders are more diffuse and affect functioning in a wide range of contexts. However, in an estimated 40% of children with learning disorders, symptoms of attentional disorders are also present. In regards to learning disorders, attention has been studied according to theories of attention and subcomponents of the attention process identified by each theory, such as selective attention, sustained attention, or focus of attention. Studies from this perspective compare the performance of children with and without learning disorders on measures of these subprocesses of attention.

Studies of selective attention, the ability to maintain attention to target stimuli when distractors are present, suggest that children without learning disorders retain more central items than do children with learning disorders, and that the latter retain more of the incidental items than their peers without learning disorders. Thus it has been concluded that children with learning disorders are deficient in selective attention.

Sustained attention, or time on task, refers to vigilance or maintenance of attention for an extended period. Some research indicates that children with learning disorders are on task generally from 30% to 60% of the time, compared with 60% to 85% of the time for their peers without learning disorders. Most studies involving continuous performance tasks with children, in which the child is asked to monitor visually or auditorily presented letters or numbers for target stimuli, use trial durations of at least 10 minutes to assess sustained attention. On these relatively content-neutral tasks, children with learning disorders generally perform similar to their nondisabled peers. However, it has been suggested that students with learning disorders have difficulty maintaining the intense degree of attention required for conscious effort on complex tasks.

Executive functions are functions that allow an individual to engage in self-monitoring and self-appraisal during learning tasks. They are often referred to as metacognitive skills. Metacognition refers to a person's own knowledge about his own cognitive processes and products of them and includes both knowledge about cognition and regulation of cognition. Awareness of one's learning and how to monitor and maximize it is a developmental process. It is not until children are 10 to 14 years old that many learning strategies become highly developed.

In a number of studies, children with learning disorders have been found to possess faulty or ineffectual strategies for learning. For example, it has been found that poor readers use a word-by-word approach in which they do not integrate known textual information across sentences. Children with learning disorders, though they may possess strategies for learning, do not spontaneously activate their use and require external prompting. Some suggest these children have difficulty choosing appropriate problem solving devices across a number of tasks. Students with learning disorders are generally less mature in their repertoire of memory strategies and in their awareness and use of these strategies than their unaffected peers. Furthermore, they may not allocate study time according to task difficulty and do not consistently monitor their level of understanding of incoming information. One body of research focused on faulty or ineffective strategy use during learning as a basis for learning disorders and assumed that children with learning disorders do not exhibit intrinsic competence deficits. Rather, the study implied that they exhibit performance deficits as a result of a lack of executive control or self-regulation in learning. Some hypothesize that these performance deficits result from poor motivation, nonbelief in the value of effortful strategic learning (because of poor past learning outcomes), and low self-concept. Another body of research relates poor executive control to function of the prefrontal area of the brain.

Natural History

The majority of research on learning disabilities has consisted primarily of isolated investigations that compare children achieving normally to children with learning disorders. Although most research has not taken into account that learning disorders may be manifest in different ways across the age span, several notable exceptions have attempted to determine the course of learning disorders over time.

It has been demonstrated that deficits in phonologic processing and pseudoword reading that have been documented in childhood persist into adulthood and lie at the core of a reading disability. In contrast, visual deficits involving the correct recognition of the visual form of words do not persist across educational levels. This likely relates to the nature of reading acquisition, which involves a gradual shift from reading being a global, visuoprocessing task to one that analyzes and sequences sounds and attributes meaning to written language.

Written language skills are most often the greatest stumbling block for children with learning disorders because the language processes involved in reading, spelling, listening, speaking, and thinking must complement each other simultaneously. Spelling disorders are ubiquitous among individuals with learning disorders and usually coexist with disorders of oral language, reading, motor skills, and attention. Spelling is never mastered by most people with reading disabilities; they often improve their reading decoding skills but usually continue to be poor spellers. More pervasive writing problems, including errors in punctuation and capitalization and written products that are short, poorly organized, and impoverished in ideation, are characteristic and persist over time.

Finally, mathematics disorders are evident early in the schooling of children and are reported to continue through adolescence.

Learning disorders are not thought to be school-specific or the exclusive province of school-age children. There has been a proliferation of programs for secondary school students and adults, and recent federal legislation (PL 99-457) mandates special education services for handicapped children from birth to age 3.

In the Retrospective Study of Learning Disabilities, a 10-year longitudinal study, researchers found that at follow-up (mean age of 19), individuals with learning disorders were inferior to their siblings without learning disorders in educational attainment and achievement. The standards for measurement included the drop-out rate, the rate of continued postsecondary education, and the college graduation rate. Only 23% of those with learning disorders experienced high academic success in school, whereas the comparable figure for their siblings was 75%. In the social area, subjects with learning disorders had fewer friends and less adequate interpersonal relationships compared with their siblings.

The Prospective Study of Reading, another longitudinal study, concluded that over 85% of children were correctly classified as having the potential to have problems reading. The best single predictors of reading achievement were measures of language, specifically verbal subtests of the intelligence scale given at entrance to kindergarten. At eighth grade, the average reading score for the poor readers was 4.1 grade years below expectancy and 6.9 years below the group mean. False-positives, results of children who were incorrectly identified as at risk, came from families with higher socioeconomic status and without histories of learning disorders.

Findings of longitudinal studies confirm that a child's vulnerability, or risk plus environmental conditions, leads to positive or negative developmental outcomes. Significant positive experiences and opportunities early in life may compensate for the presence of at-risk biologic conditions. Therefore early identification and intervention have both preventive and ameliorative potential. Those children who were identified early in life and continued to have problems throughout development tended to be those with extreme or severe biologic-neurologic conditions, and those with multiple indicators of problems.

Associated Disorders

The field of learning disorders has been slow to recognize the reality of co-morbidity, or that a learning disorder can coexist with other disabilities. The National Joint Committee on Learning Disabilities recently modified their definition of learning disorders concerning the issue of co-morbidity, acknowledging that a learning disorder may occur concomitantly with other disabling conditions. The committee went on to state that it is not the direct result of those conditions or influences.

Attention-Deficit/Hyperactivity Disorder

Attention deficit/hyperactivity disorder (ADHD) is one of the most commonly diagnosed disorders of childhood and accounts for one half of all child referrals to outpatient mental health clinics. It has been estimated that up to 40% of children with learning disorders display symptoms of ADHD. At least some of this association may be a consequence of definitional overlap; the concepts of learning disorders and attention disorders were both derived from the concept of minimal brain dysfunction.

A robust two-way association between ADHD and dyslexia does not exist. The rate of dyslexia in children with ADHD is not necessarily greater than population expectations. The higher rate of ADHD that is commonly found in people with dyslexia suggests either that there is a subtype of dyslexia plus ADHD with a common cause or that dyslexia leads to ADHD as a secondary symptom. In a study that examined underlying neuropsychologic deficits in children with both dyslexia and ADHD and in children with either deficit alone, performance on measures of executive function and phonologic processing supported the independent existence of both syndromes, as well as the hypothesis that ADHD in dyslexia is usually a secondary symptom.

Turner's Syndrome

Turner's syndrome is a disorder in which females are missing all or part of one X chromosome as a result of nondisjunction during meiosis of the paired X chromosomes. In addition to having characteristic physical features, Turner's syndrome is associated with average verbal skills and a pattern of nonverbal learning disorders. Selective impairments in visuospatial and memory areas, as well as significant underachievement in arithmetic, particularly numeric ability, mental calculation, geometry, and reasoning, are common. In one study, girls with Turner's syndrome earned average scores on mathematics tests that were two grade levels below their grade placement in school. A detailed analysis of math deficits revealed that the conceptual and factual areas of mathematics seemed to be compromised to a greater degree than computational areas. Whereas reading and spelling abilities were within normal limits, results indicated a relative weakness in decoding ability but not reading comprehension. Some have suggested that children and adolescents with Turner's syndrome are similar to children with learning disorders in mathematics and associated weaknesses in processing nonverbal visuospatial information. Outcomes of subtyping studies of learning disorders consistently identify a group of children with deficits in nonverbal skills such as visuospatial orientation or visuomotor functions. Children with deficits in nonverbal skills have been found to make more mathematic errors, such as misaligning numbers in columns and misreading mathematic signs. The prevalence of nonverbal learning disorders within the population of people with learning disorders is estimated to be 5% to 10%.

Fragile X Syndrome

Fragile X syndrome is a recently identified condition that involves a weakened arm on the X chromosome. Detection has been possible since 1977. Most males who inherit the fragile X locus are mentally retarded, since they lack a normal second X chromosome to compensate, and thus by definition they are not found in samples of individuals with learning disorders. In contrast, the majority of females with fragile X syndrome are not mentally retarded. Several studies concerned with the cognitive and behavioral sequelae of females with fragile X syndrome have found deficits in spatial skills. Regarding academic skills, weaknesses in mathematics are more characteristic than deficits in reading and spelling. Since variation in mathematics performance has a known heritable component, it is likely that for at least some children with learning disorders in mathematics and related functions, fragile X syndrome may be an implicated cause.

Tourette's Disorder

Tourette's disorder is a disorder characterized by the early onset of chronic motor and vocal tics. The cause of this syndrome is not completely understood. A number of neurotransmitter alterations have been implicated. The response of symptoms to dopamine-receptor-blocking agents like haloperidol and pimozide suggests dopaminergic involvement. Additionally there is evidence to suggest a strong genetic contribution.

Tourette's disorder is a complex disorder that is commonly associated with other conditions related to learning difficulties, such as ADHD and learning disorders. Previous reports have suggested that approximately 50% of children with Tourette's disorder also have a learning disorder.

In one study of children with Tourette's disorder, it was found that 51% of the sample had evidence of a learning disorder in at least one subject and that 21% of the subjects had disorders in two or more areas. Some researchers have observed that the severity of the learning disorders in children with Tourette's disorder tends to lessen over time. This observation is consistent with evidence that Tourette's disorder represents a marker for improvement over other developmental conditions, such as pervasive developmental disorders (PDDs). Given the presence of learning disorders among children and adolescents with Tourette's disorder, evaluation for the presence of learning disorders is necessary.

Disorders of Social Competence

The prevalence of social dysfunction among students with learning disorders is considerable, estimated at over one third of these children. A study conducted among resource-room teachers reported a prevalence rate of 38.3% for social dysfunction among students with learning disorders in elementary through high school settings. Social competence has been described as having positive relations with others, accurate and age appropriate social cognition, the absence of maladaptive behaviors, and effective social behaviors. Children with deficits in social competence are at risk for school dropout, psychiatric difficulties, depression, suicide, juvenile delinquency, and criminality in adult life.

A hypothesized model of subtypes of social dysfunction suggests the heterogeneity in the manifestation of social skill deficits among people with learning disorders. The first subtype corresponds to conduct disorder (CD) and oppositional defiant disorder (ODD), with or without associated ADHD. Children in this group often have associated reading, spelling, and writing deficits. Some of these children also have severe language processing problems. The second subtype describes children with PDD-NOS. Other psychiatric diagnoses sometimes applied to these children include anxiety disorders, depression, obsessive-compulsive disorder (OCD), nonverbal learning disorder, or social-emotional learning disorder. The core feature involves an inability to interpret and process information of a social-emotional nature. These children tend to have deficits in visuospatial skills, attention, and arithmetic. The third subtype describes children who seem aware of the rules but have difficulty applying them and using this information to regulate their behavior. These children have deficits in executive functions and are often unintentionally disruptive and disorganized. Given the extensive literature suggesting that children with learning disorders may be particularly vulnerable to impairments in social competence, the report of the U.S. Interagency Committee on Learning Disabilities suggested that disorders of social skills be included as a type of learning disorder.

Communicative Disorders

The majority of children with learning disorders also have coexisting language disorders. Although research programs distinguish between primary developmental disorders of language and developmental disorders of school-acquired learning, these conceptual divisions are more theoretic than they are real. The dependence of written language competence on oral language is well documented and suggests that other specific learning disorders are not likely to occur in the absence of oral language deficits. Early language disorders in preschool children have been known to be associated with later difficulties in learning to read and write. It is believed that 80% of school-age children identified as having learning disorders have reading disorders. Undifferentiated groups of students with reading disabilities do poorly on a variety of oral language tests when compared with control groups of children who do not have such disorders. It has been proposed that reading disorders, the largest category within the field of learning disorders, are a symptom of a broader underlying problem with the apprehension of the structural aspects of language. This theoretic view is consistent with the findings of a number of researchers who have documented deficits in oral language areas of phonology, morphology, syntax, and semantics, in children with learning disorders.

Assessment

A learning disorder should be suspected in any child who demonstrates a deficit in a specific academic area, such as reading, writing, or mathematics, relative to performance in other areas. The physician should also be alert to a possible learning disorder in the child who does not seem to be performing in school at a level commensurate with her general level of intelligence and functioning. Finally, the physician should be suspicious of a possible learning disorder in any child with ADHD or other school-related problem, such as refusal to attend school.

The assessment requires that the physician obtain a careful prenatal, birth, and developmental history. The physician should ask for information from the parents and the child's teacher regarding the current difficulties. Special emphasis should be placed on ascertaining whether there are any current emotional, social, family, or behavioral difficulties that may be causing the learning problems. Additionally, the physician should search for any environmental factors that may be impairing the child's ability to learn. For example, a child with an apparent reading disorder who is being taught to read by a whole language technique may do fine if he is switched to a phonetic approach.

A physical examination should be performed with emphasis on a thorough pediatric neurologic examination. Soft neurologic signs are not uncommon in children with learning disorders. The physician should be observant of any sensory or motor problems that may be influencing the child's ability to read, write, or perform mathematics. Vision, hearing, and speech screening may prove to be invaluable in the assessment of the child with a possible learning disorder.

If after the initial assessment, the physician believes the child probably has a learning disorder, a referral should be made to the school or an educational diagnostician for further evaluation. The course of school assessment varies from state-to-state and between school districts. Generally the school first performs a prereferral intervention. This usually involves the child's teacher determining whether there are any environmental factors affecting the child's ability to learn. At this point, the teacher may change a teaching intervention or strategy to see if the child improves. The next step involves a formal assessment. This generally involves at least a test of intelligence, such as the Wechsler Intelligence Scale for Children-III (WISC-III), and a test of academic potential and achievement, such as the Wide Range Achievement Test (WRAT). Additionally, it is not unusual for the school to perform some tests of the child's ability to attend and of his emotional state, since both may interfere with learning. The way the results of these tests are used to determine whether there is a formal learning disorder varies between states. Achievement is most commonly compared with intelligence or ability, and the tests are scrutinized for significant differences between specific levels of abilities. Based upon this, the child is deemed to have or not have a learning disorder, and an intervention occurs.

Culture may also affect the assessment, diagnosis, and treatment of learning disorders. Culture consists of a number of components, including values and behavioral styles, languages and dialects, nonverbal communication, awareness of cultural distinctiveness, world views or perspectives, and identification with a cultural group. Since a child's performance on a variety of tests determines identification of a learning disorder and since test performance is affected by cultural constraints, children from culturally diverse groups may be misdiagnosed. There is, in fact, clear evidence that there is some degree of bias in many of the assessments that are used to document eligibility for services for children with learning disorders. This has resulted in a disproportionate number of minority students identified as having learning disorders. However, this overrepresentation appears to be decreasing. Assessment in the child's primary language is a legal requirement, as stated in the Individuals with Disabilities Education Act. Evaluation of discrepancies between potential and achievement is best accomplished by comparing stronger and weaker skill areas, such as adaptive behavior and reading. A comparison of the child with peers from the same cultural background is preferable to a comparison of the child with those of the dominant culture. Nonverbal intelligence tests can be used to make decisions about intellectual potential, even though they are less predictive of school functioning than verbal measures.

Treatment

There is no specific pharmacologic treatment for learning disorders. If the child has a concomitant condition, such as a depressive disorder or ADHD, the physician may want to provide medication treatment specifically for these conditions. It is not unusual to find that the child with a learning disorder also has a mood disorder. For the school-age child, self-worth is often measured by academic achievement. It is not unusual for the child with a learning disorder to be the subject of teasing by peers, rejection by children who do not have learning disorders, and reprimands and poor understanding by parents who are uninformed about the condition.

As part of the treatment, it is imperative that the physician educate the child and the family about the nature and cause of the disorder. It often helps if the physician emphasizes that the child has a unique way of learning rather than a disordered mechanism. Family conflicts and parenting issues that have arisen around school issues need to be addressed. The parents need to be taught how to help the child learn and how to be an advocate for him in the academic arena.

The major thrust of intervention with the child who has a learning disorder is educational. In light of the heterogeneity among the population of children and adolescents with learning disorders, planning educational interventions to match specific abilities and learning styles is an individualized process. To tailor educational intervention to meet individual needs, educators need to take into account student and instructional variables. This suggests a consideration of student variables, what the student is taught, and how she is taught.

With regards to student variables, it is necessary to consider the mental processes involved in thinking and learning, including perception, memory, comprehension, attention, concept formation, and problem solving in verbal and nonverbal areas. The physician must determine which of these processes are strengths and which are weak areas for a given individual. Typically, educators try to teach through strengths to address weak areas of processing. In addition to processing, the individual must be understood in the context of stages of normal development. At times, students are not ready to try to master a given knowledge domain until they have mastered developmentally prerequisite skills. A third way to analyze student variables is to consider how the individual approaches learning, remembering, problem solving, and understanding. Some students are capable of acquiring information, but their capability is not evident because they do not know how to study, how to integrate new material, or how to monitor their progress. This "how to" approach to learning is called strategy instruction and focuses on teaching individuals techniques for acquiring information.

In addition to considering student variables, an understanding of curricular content and instructional techniques is necessary. Curricular content may be understood by analyzing the sequence of skills needed to master a concept or procedure. Called task analysis by some, this way of understanding curricular content assumes that a student must acquire each specific subskill to learn a task or subject. Finally, regarding how an individual is approached instructionally, there are a number of specialized instructional techniques. One such technique is called multisensory methods and was developed to teach individuals with learning disorders based on a variety of theories of the disorder's origin.

Although empiric research on the efficacy of teaching approaches and methods is limited, some conclusions are warranted. For example, it is well documented that students with learning disorders respond favorably to instruction that focuses on specific strategic approaches to completing tasks. Among many researchers in the area of reading, the consensus is that the student who does not naturally crack the code with exposure to print requires systematic, explicit, skill-by-skill phonics instruction to become a fluent reader. Phonemic awareness training that draws attention to parts of words for young children with reading deficits has been shown to be successful and leads to better reading performance. Some research has supported the efficacy of multisensory approaches to reading instruction. Examples of this approach are the Orton-Gillingham-based programs and their use of tracing to commit words to memory. The effectiveness of spelling training to facilitate word recognition in reading has also been supported through research. Additionally, computer assisted instruction has been shown to enhance word recognition skills in children with reading disorders. Techniques that provide an individual with experiences related to reading material or that help an individual identify personal knowledge related to the material, such as brainstorming, also help foster better reading comprehension. Techniques that have children say letter names as they write words appear to accelerate spelling progress. Additionally, arranging words by their common spelling patterns has been found to be a beneficial instructional method.

In the area of math, the use of concrete materials has been supported by research, since students benefit from seeing and manipulating the quantities and algorithms they are studying. Fleischner, Nazum, and Marzola, as well as others, have demonstrated the efficacy of teaching students problem solving strategies such as identifying given information, examining the mechanics of the problem, and identifying the question.

Summary

Learning disorders are a varied group of disturbances in learning that significantly impact the lives of children and adolescents who evidence them. Given the interaction between emotional factors and academic difficulties, physicians are well served by an understanding of definitional and etiologic aspects, characteristics, co-morbid conditions, and educational treatment approaches. Because of this relationship, a thorough understanding of the child or adolescent's learning skills should augment information gained from a psychiatric evaluation. Therefore treatment planning should address not only psychosocial functioning but also deficits in learning and academic skills. Helping a child or adolescent gain greater academic success is likely to foster the success of therapeutic efforts in other areas of psychosocial adaptation.

CONSIDER CONSULTATION WHEN . . .

- There is a co-morbid pathologic condition with the learning disorder
- The child's disorder does not improve after appropriate school interventions
- Results of psychoeducational testing do not adequately explain the disorder of learning

Annotated Bibliography

Ceci E, editor: *Handbook of cognitive, social, and neuropsychological aspects of learning disabilities,* vols I and II, Hillsdale, N.J., 1986 and 1987, Lawrence Erlbaum.

Dr. Ceci's two-volume handbook provides a comprehensive discussion of characteristics of learning disorders from a cognitive, social, and neuropsychological perspective and is an excellent resource for the clinician.

Lyon GR, editor: *Frames of reference for the assessment of learning disabilities,* Baltimore, 1994, Brookes.

Dr. Lyon's volume presents a thorough discussion of identification and assessment issues and techniques across a variety of areas, including oral language, reading, written language, mathematics, learning strategies, and social competence and skills.

Obrzut J, Hynd G, editors: *Neuropsychological foundations of learning disabilities,* San Diego, 1991, Academic Press.

Drs. Obrzut and Hynd present an excellent volume addressing theoretic issues related to the neuropsychology of learning disabilities, assessment techniques, and syndromes and practice in aspects of learning disorders, including oral language, reading, mathematics, and nonverbal learning disorders.

Wong B, editor: *Learning about learning disabilities,* San Diego, 1991, Harcourt Brace Jovanovich.

Dr. Wong's volume presents an excellent treatment of conceptual and historical aspects of learning disorders, assessment, and instructional aspects, as well as lifespan issues related to learning disorders.

section three

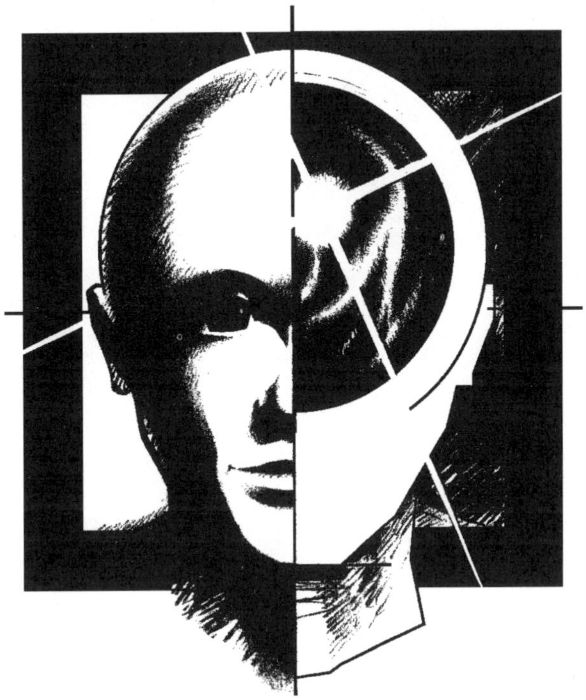

Clinical Conditions and Situations

Cheryl Al-Mateen, MD and Richard R. Brookman, MD

chapter 12

The At-Risk Infant

Joan Plotkin, MD

- History of Infant Psychiatry
- Epidemiology
- Infant Assessment
- Assessment History
- Clinical Assessment
- Physical Examination
- Screening Tests
- Laboratory Assessment
- Diagnostic Classification
- Treatment and Prevention
- Special Concerns in Infant Psychiatry
- When to Refer
- Summary

Infant psychiatrists work with children age 36 months and younger, and consider infants, toddlers, and early preschoolers within their treatment group. When they speak about infants at risk, they are not focusing simply on their tiny patients' particular vulnerabilities. In infant psychiatry, more than in any other medical discipline, physicians must focus on a patient's sociocultural environment. The infant, by virtue of developmental incompetence, is completely dependent on this environment. The vicissitudes of a child's life are determined to a high degree by the context of her being.

An infant's developmental risk derives from the complex interaction of biologic endowment and the sociocultural milieu, which greatly influences the expression of that biologic potential. An infant may be born at risk as a result of congenital or birth-related factors that do not allow full development of her social potential. Conversely, a healthy newborn is placed at risk in a suboptimal or deprived environment. The truly unfortunate, but not uncommon, child is multiply afflicted by biology and society.

The interplay between each child's unique temperament and biologic predisposition and the baby's environment determines later functional and developmental capacity. The immense potential for shaping the baby's environment to positively influence the child's current and ultimate potential compels those who build careers in human birth and development.

History of Infant Psychiatry

Psychiatric focus on infancy began with the dawn of psychiatry itself. Early analytic theorists looked to infant development to find clues to understanding adult personality, defenses, and adaptive capability. Sigmund Freud based much of his theoretic framework on the early relationship of the infant and preschooler to his parents. Anna Freud, Margaret Mahler, and D.W. Winnecott all based much of their theory on the very early relationship between the infant and the mother. Attachment studies by the developmental theorist John Bowlby emphasized the importance of physical contact between the mother and the infant to the emotional and cognitive development of the child. By the early 1960s, we had access to a wealth of literature richly describing the quintessential mother-child relationship. However, we had few resources to guide our approach to the assessment and treatment of this dyad.

True infant psychiatry, offering diagnostic and therapeutic modalities to the clinician, emerged in the 1960s. In the text *Infant Psychiatry,* Eveoleen Rexford defended and promoted the concept of infant psychiatry to more actively involve child psychiatrists in the problems of infancy. She reasoned that if physicians could help at-risk mothers and babies negotiate the early basic issues between them, the infant would more easily move along the developmental lines of growth for relationships, self-differentiation, and tolerance of frustration.

At the same time Selma Fraiberg, perhaps the grandmother of infant psychiatry, presented her work with congenitally blind infants. Her work modeled the still relevant approach of clinicians who work with infants, be they educators, psychologists, primary care physicians, nurses, social workers, or psychiatrists. She emphasized the clinician's role as an advocate to reclaim the infant's human rights for the family, as well as the clinician's imperative to establish a common language for communication between a mother and her infant. Perspectives on infant assessment and intervention were catapulted to the forefront of clinical expertise by the 1970s.

Even so, it was generally felt that psychiatric clinicians, especially those who specialized in treating infants, still struggled to unite the fields of biology and psychology. At-risk babies of the 1960s and 1970s were premature (generally greater than 1500 gm), congenitally infected with rubella, blind, autistic, or mentally retarded.

The past two decades have brought a flourish of research and thinking on the mental health of infants. Besides the vast array of articles published yearly in multidisciplinary journals, there are now several journals and newsletters devoted specifically to infant mental health. Psychiatry programs designed for infants are blossoming across the United States and abroad. In the field of infant psychiatry biologic, social, and psychologic forces are still intertwined, but this specialty is becoming increasingly well known and secure. The physician is part of a multidisciplinary team that is eager to tackle complex vectors and assist in the healthful development of the child and family.

Recent texts offer comprehensive techniques for physicians who work with children 36 months and younger in areas of diagnosis, treatment, and prevention. Charles H. Zeanah emphasizes the need to gain better insight into infant development so we can better appreciate individual risk, vulnerability, and protective factors related to the development of psychopathologic conditions. Our responsibility, too, is to apply knowledge gained from our research and clinical efforts to revise social policy affecting our young families.

In the past few decades the problems facing our children have intensified. Some of the risks we increasingly face are widespread poverty, extreme prematurity, adolescent parents, and parents absent because of substance abuse, incarceration, or emotional unavailability. We continue to address classic disorders of infancy such as mental retardation; attachment and autistic disorders; sleep, feeding, and regulatory disorders; and post traumatic stress disorders.

New and widespread challenges to America's babies are cocaine-dependent parents, congenital HIV infections, and increasing neighborhood violence, as well as the dissolution of the nuclear and extended families. As sociocultural issues facing infants have changed over the decades, the physician's role has evolved as well. The fundamental principles governing the physician's work have not changed. We must be advocates for the child and nurture the infant's development within the sociocultural milieu by using careful assessment and intervention through education, prevention, support, psychotherapy, and medical treatment.

Epidemiology

Estimating the number of infants at risk in the United States is virtually impossible. This number would include all infants facing physical, social, or emotional hardship. Physical disabilities can be tabulated and projected based on scrutiny of medical records. Social statistics are measured via the U.S. Census and governmental investigations. Estimating the extent of psychopathologic conditions in the 0-to-3 age group is fraught with difficulty. Criteria for deviance from normal behavior and emotional constitution are not clearly delineated in this group. Psychiatric interviews and rating scales are costly, cumbersome, and unreliable for young children. A tenuous estimate of emotional disorders in the young would be about 5% to 10% of the population.

In 1990, just over 4 million babies were born in the

TABLE 12-1

1990-1994 APPROXIMATE ANNUAL STATISTICS OF AT-RISK INFANTS

Type	Number of U.S. newborns affected yearly	Percentage of annual births
Congenital defects	150,000	4%
Teenage mothers	500,000	12.8%
Low birth weight	300,000	8%
Very low birth weight	50,000	1.3%
Late/no prenatal care	250,000	6.4%
Prenatal cocaine exposure	100,000	2.6%
Fetal alcohol syndrome	1600	0.04%
Prenatal HIV exposure	6000	0.15%
Poverty	1,000,000	25%

United States. Of these, 150,000 were afflicted with congenital defects (Table 12-1). Over 500,000 (12.8%) were born to teenage mothers. About 300,000 had low birth weights (less than 2500 gm), and 50,000 had very low birth weights (less than 1500 gm). About 250,000 mothers received late or no prenatal care.

Each year, approximately 100,000 infants are prenatally exposed to cocaine. 1600 babies are born with fetal alcohol syndrome, representing a small fraction of babies exposed to varying levels of alcohol in utero.

Approximately 6000 babies are born yearly to the 110,000 HIV-infected women in the United States. Of these babies, up to 2000 become HIV positive. Nearly 50,000 American children and adolescents were orphaned by the HIV/AIDS epidemic by the end of 1995. About one fourth of American babies are born into poverty, and 1.75 million children under age 2 live in poverty in America.

Infant Assessment

Infants must be assessed in the context of their environments. A data base that allows diagnostic understanding of the patient and caregivers also allows appropriate planning of intervention and treatment strategy.

Imperative to infant assessment is a comfortable understanding of normal infant development. From this base and allowing for variation in temperament, personality, and diurnal variation, the physician can begin to appreciate pathologic conditions.

In this field, as in most others, it behooves the physician to use a "wellness" model. The physician should look for and emphasize strengths in infant and family functioning and attempt to remediate deficiencies. A more cooperative and encouraging approach, rather than a judgmental and punitive one, is much more apt to promote gains within the family system.

Interviewing an infant and family mandates a two-pronged approach. The first and most crucial approach is experiential. It is based on the encounter at hand and is designed to foster the alliance between the family and the physician. Completeness and accuracy in the collection of historical information, honesty in personal divulgence, and ultimate compliance with treatment are all contingent on the degree of trust the physician is able to engender in the infant's primary caregivers.

The family's trust is based on perceived respect of the family, empathy, and appreciation of their competencies. It is essential that the physician convince the family that their thoughts and feelings are important and that the physician cares and is invested in a good outcome for them. The physician must expect and accept diverse family structures. Often the traditional mother-father-baby unit is not the family unit that arrives at the office. Family members or other caregivers, such as the mother, grandmother, foster mother, social worker, or aunt may bring the child for an examination. The physician's positive or negative countertransference (prejudicial reactions based on the family's appearance and lifestyle) must be thoroughly monitored when building an effective therapeutic relationship.

The second approach is structured and geared toward amassing specific and objective data about the child and family. The physician must be a good listener and a skillful investigator. Adhering to principles of open-ended inquiry, the physician must form a complete understanding of the child by continually forming, testing, and redesigning hypotheses on the child's and the family's behavior and affective experience. Data collection should fulfill requirements of a basic psychiatric assessment and be tapered to reflect the infant patient. This assessment should include identifying data, information sources, the reason and source of referral, the history of symptoms, the medical history, the family history, developmental and social histories, and a systems review. The clinical assessment concerns the parent-infant dyad and should review observations of appearance, behavior, interactions, and cognition of both the infant and the primary caregiver. The dyadic relationship between parent and child is emphasized. One procedure for obtaining and recording an assessment history of an infant is shown in Box 12-1 and in the following section of this chapter.

Assessment History

Identifying Data

List the infant's name, ethnoracial heritage, and age in months. Note whether the baby was significantly premature. The caregiver's or family's name and residence, as well as the terms of custody are included.

Source of Information

List those present for the evaluation. Although the mother or father may be present, the most capable informant is often the primary caregiver, who may be a maternal grandmother or aunt. List other sources of history, such as hospital records, social services, the health department, or judicial reports. Often, no records are available and the physician may be unable to elicit a thorough history from the primary caregiver.

Reason for Referral

List the specific reason for the evaluation. Include the party initiating or enforcing the consultation. This is often not the primary caregiver, who may not perceive that a problem exists. Establish who is concerned and why.

History of Symptoms

Elaborate on the chief complaint. Write a short narrative describing the who, what, when, and where of the current symptoms, and focus on precipitating events, as well as family and infant psychosocial stressors. Mention should be made of occurrences that reduce or exacerbate symptoms.

This is a good place to describe the infant's daily functioning—temperament, feeding, sleeping, elimination routines, and relationships. A basic description and any concerns in these areas should be detailed.

Medical History

List any major or minor medical or surgical illnesses and any known allergies. Describe medications and diet, as well as vitamin and iron supplementation.

Family History

Collect data concerning medical and psychiatric or emotional disturbances in biologic relatives. Describe developmental and relationship histories of caregivers, siblings, and agencies influencing the identified infant. Include parenting and sibling relationships of caregivers, as well as cultural and personal child-rearing approaches employed through the generations. An understanding of these historical dynamics often sheds light on perceived or existing difficulties or dysfunction. Enumerate siblings, providing brief descriptions of each and focusing on their emotional health and life situations.

Developmental History

Provide extensive detail of the mother's pregnancy. It is helpful and enlightening to gain an appreciation of the context of conception—how, when, why, and by whom was this child conceived? Was the pregnancy planned? Was this time filled with happy, loving associations, or bad feelings, or hateful, even rageful, feelings? How was the news of conception received by the parents, family, and extended family? What were the family's hopes, expectations, and fantasies of the pregnancy and of their child? Again, by understanding frustrated expectations, much insight is gained into current symptoms.

Focus on the course of the pregnancy. How was the fetus perceived? What was its in-utero activity and diurnal cycling like? How involved was the father? What was the extent of prenatal obstetric care? Were prenatal classes attended? Were there any complications, and how were these handled? Were there any serious emotional stresses during the pregnancy, such as a death in the family or the father serving in military action?

Mechanics of birth should be described, and the early reactions of mother, father, newborn, and clinical staff should be reviewed. Examine the motor, cognitive, and emotional development of the infant.

Motor Development

Describe the newborn's tone. What has been her general activity level? When did the baby first raise her head and trunk, roll over, sit, crawl, walk, manage steps, or ride a tricycle?

Cognitive Development

Was the baby alert at birth? When did she coo, smile, or raspberry? When and what were her first words? When did she first put words together?

Emotional Development

The infant's emotional development can be described by her social and behavioral capacities. When did the baby first smile socially? Was she cuddly or indifferent? How has she reacted to family and strangers? When and how was she affected by stranger anxiety? How did she attach or bond with her mother? When did she see herself as separate from her? Has she individuated from the family? How does she respond to

BOX 12-1

TAKING AN ASSESSMENT HISTORY

Identifying data
Source of information
Reason for referral
History of symptoms
Medical history
Family history
Developmental history
  Motor development
  Cognitive development
  Emotional development
Social history
Review of symptoms

others? Is she clinging or independent? How does she respond to others' feelings?

Understand the baby's temperament. Has she been shy and slow to warm up, easy going, or irritable? Does she cry a lot? Is she consoled easily? Is she a self-soother, or does she need outside help? How regular has she been in diurnal activities such as feeding, sleeping, and interacting? How does she adapt to new—pleasurable or aversive—situations or stimuli?

What are her special talents or fears? Does she like books, videotapes, and music, or does she dance to television commercials and the radio? Is she especially fearful of loud noises, swings, or over-sized costumed creatures?

Social History

Describe the living arrangements of the child. What are the family's socioeconomic circumstances? What community and government services are established? If the parents are employed, what are their occupations? Who cares for the infant when the primary caregiver is away, and what is the length and quality of this relationship? Describe the infant's day-care facility. Who provides financially for the child? How easily are her expenses covered?

Review of Systems

Any concerns about physical problems or discomforts should be described. A baby's behavior is exquisitely dependent on her well-being. Is she sleepy or hungry? Is she clean and dry? Is she struggling with respiratory, gastrointestinal, or febrile illness?

Clinical Assessment

Strategies of engagement initiated during the introduction and history-taking phases should be continued during the clinical assessment of the infant and family. Whether assessment must be limited to half an hour or can be extended to three or four sessions, the process should never seem rushed. Depending on the time available and the age of the child, the physician may wish to evaluate the parents and child individually and together. Children age 2 or younger may be included with their parents during the initial session. Children over 30 months might be best included after parents have had the opportunity to fully discuss their concerns in the child's absence.

Clinical assessment should complete one's understanding of the child's developmental sophistication and emotional themes. The physician should assess the child's repertoire of fine and gross motor skills, speech and language, and cognitive abilities. The physician should also explore the quality of parental support. It is important to analyze the interaction between the parent and the child and to specifically note the quality of verbal and nonverbal communication, emotional availability, physical and emotional support, and advocacy of the child.

BOX 12-2

CLINICAL ASSESSMENT OF INFANTS

- See the parent(s) and child together.
- Fully understand the child's developmental level.
- Describe mental status of infant and caregivers.
- Observe the caregiver in play with the child.
- Identify physical factors placing infant at risk.
- Take a psychiatric history of parent figures.

In individual evaluations, the physician assesses the mental status of both infant and caregiver. The physician describes the infant's appearance, level of engagement, behavior (for example, passive, cooperative, oppositional, or aggressive), mood (separation-anxious, depressed, elated), and communication patterns. Similarly, in the adult's mental status evaluation, his appearance, behavior, relatedness, mood (depressed, anxious, paranoid, or hostile), speech, and thought patterns, and general cognition, including abstraction ability, judgment, and capacity for insight, are described.

In a parent-child session, the parent may be observed in play with the child. The physician should evaluate the way a child negotiates developmentally appropriate tasks. How does the adult respond to the child's developmentally determined demands and themes? How do the parent and child communicate? To determine whether the parent provides a secure base for the infant, the physician may look for clues suggesting that the parent is able to provide a steady, safe, and protecting foundation from which the child can tentatively venture and to which she can securely retreat. What is the quality of attachment between the parent and the child? What of the presenting concerns can be validated or seen as distortions or projections based on clinical observation (Box 12-2)?

Physical Examination

In performing a physical examination, the physician can identify factors placing the infant at risk for developmental delay. Limited or lagging height and weight suggest feeding disorders, failure to thrive, or possible neglect. Tracking head circumference reveals existing or emerging microcephaly or macrocephaly. Dysmorphic features may suggest an underlying chromosomal or genetic abnormality. Appropriate visual and auditory evaluation should be included.

Gross dermatologic review should exclude any neurocutaneous lesions, such as neurofibromas, café au lait spots, scars, or bruises. Neurologic "red flags" are failure to be alert, abnormal tone or reflexes, and asymmetry.

Screening Tests

Developmental Screening

To supplement such clinical observation, especially when mild developmental abnormalities are suspected, the physician may wish to employ one of a variety of instruments designed to assess developmental delay in infants and young children. These tests provide standardized observation of the child's performance and a safeguard to the busy physician. Table 12-2 lists several tests commonly used to screen infants for developmental delay.

The Clinical Adaptive Test/Clinical Linguistic Auditory Milestone Scale (CAT/CLAMS) is a clinically expedient, reliable, and valid test that screens cognitive and language development as well as neurologic function. It combines parental report with direct observation to assess infants with cognitive ages from 1 to 36 months. A CAT/CLAMS scoring sheet is shown in Table 12-3. Most neurodevelopmental screening instruments do not assess specific psychosocial behaviors or issues.

Psychosocial Screening

Achenbach's Child Behavior Checklist (CBCL) for ages 2 to 3 offers a carefully tested standardized rating scale to assess behavioral and emotional problems in 2- and 3-year-old children. A sample CBCL/2-3 is shown in Figure 12-1, pp. 198-199. Stanley Greenspan et al. have recently developed a clinically-based and interactive instrument, the Functional Emotional Assessment Scale for Infancy and Early Childhood (FEAS/IEC), which emphasizes the infant's emotional and social functioning in the context of his relationships and family. It has been developed and standardized for infants and young children with special needs and adds a much needed dimension to infant assessment. Greenspan's text provides a comprehensive review of this scale, as well as an appendix offering an extensive review of useful infant assessment instruments.

Newborn Screening

Table 12-4 lists newborn screening tools. Of these, the National Behavioral Assessment Scale is the most widely used. Many of these require specific training in their use and interpretation; they are most often administered by psychologists. The Newborn Individualized Developmental Care and Assessment Program (NIDCAP) allows developmental and behavioral assessment of the premature infant.

Laboratory Assessment

In addition to laboratory measures generally obtained during a well-baby visit, specific testing of a child who is possibly developmentally impaired should include lead testing. Chromosomal studies may be in order if dysmorphic features are noted. Thyroid testing and metabolic screening tests are helpful for the evaluation of motor or cognitive delay. Children with abnormal muscle tone should be screened for muscular dystrophy with CPK or aldolase. Neurologic studies, including EEGs, CT, and MRI, should generally be reserved for children with such neurologic findings as asymmetry, upper or lower extremity weakness, seizures, sensory impairment, or abnormal head growth.

Diagnostic Classification

Mental health clinicians generally refer to the DSM for diagnostic classification. The current edition, DSM-IV, contains only few diagnostic categories relevant to

TABLE 12-2

INFANT DEVELOPMENT SCREENING TESTS

Screening test	Age range	Time to administer
Batelle Developmental Inventory	0 to 8 years	30 minutes
Bayley Scales of Infant Development	1 to 30 months	45 to 90 minutes
Clinical Adaptive Test/Clinical Linguistic Auditory Milestone Scale	1 to 36 months	15 to 20 minutes
Denver Developmental Screening Test II	0 to 6 years	30 minutes
Developmental Screening Inventory Revised	1 to 18 months	20 to 30 minutes
Early Language Milestone Scale	0 to 36 months	5 minutes
Gesell Preschool Test	2.5 to 6 years	40 minutes
Infant Monitoring Questionnaire	4 to 36 months	15 to 20 minutes
Miller Assessment for Preschoolers	8 months to 5 years	20 to 30 minutes
Minnesota Child Development Inventory	1 to 6 years	10 to 15 minutes
Peabody Picture Vocabulary Test	2.5 to 4 years	10 to 20 minutes
Vineland Adaptive Behavior Scales	0 to 19 years	20 to 60 minutes

TABLE 12-3

CAT/CLAMS SCORING SHEET

CLAMS

Language skills	Yes	No
1 Month		
Is alert to sound (0.5)*		
Is soothed when picked up (0.5)		
2 Months		
Social smile (1.0)*		
3 Months		
Coos (1.0)		
4 Months		
Orients to voice (0.5)*		
Laughs aloud (0.5)		
5 Months		
Orients toward bell laterally (0.3)*		
"Ah-goo" (0.3)		
Razzing (0.3)		
6 Months		
Babbling (1.0)		
7 Months		
Orients toward bell (1.0)*		
(Upward indirectly 90 degrees*)		
8 Months		
"Dada" inappropriately (0.5)		
"Mama" inappropriately (0.5)		
9 Months		
Orients toward bell (upward directly 180 degrees) (0.5)*		
Gesture language (0.5)		
10 Months		
Understands "no" (0.3)		
Uses "dada" appropriately (0.3)		
Uses "mama" appropriately (0.3)		

CAT

Visual-motor abilities	Yes	No
1 Month		
Visually fixates momentarily on red ring (0.5)		
Chin off table, prone (0.5)		
2 Months		
Visually follows ring horizontally and vertically (0.5)		
Chest off table, prone (0.5)		
3 Months		
Visually follows ring in circle (0.3)		
Supports on forearms in prone (0.3)		
Visual threat (0.3)		
4 Months		
Unfisted (0.3)		
Manipulates fingers (0.3)		
Supports on wrists, prone (0.3)		
5 Months		
Pulls down rings (0.3)		
Transfers (0.3)		
Regards pellet (0.3)		
6 Months		
Obtains cube (0.3)		
Lifts cup (0.3)		
Radial rake (0.3)		
7 Months		
Attempts pellet (0.3)		
Pulls out peg (0.3)		
Inspects ring (0.3)		
8 Months		
Pulls ring by string (0.3)		
Secures pellet (0.3)		
Inspects bell (0.3)		
9 Months		
Three-finger scissor grasp (0.3)		
Over the edge for toy (0.3)		
Rings bell (0.3)		
10 Months		
Combines cube-cup (0.3)		
Uncovers bell (0.3)		
Fingers pegboard (0.3)		

Continued.

The numbers in parentheses refer to the score given for each correct answer. The total score is the sum of all passed items above the basal level.

*CLAMS items were done at the time of assessment.

†From Cottell picture cards.

(From Hoon AH Jr et al: Clinical Adaptive Test/Clinical Linguistic Auditory Milestone Scale in early cognitive assessment, *J Pediatr* 123:S1-S8, 1993.)

TABLE 12-3

CAT/CLAMS SCORING SHEET—CONT'D

CLAMS

Language skills	Yes	No
11 Months		
One word (other than "mama" and "dada") (1.0)	____	____
12 Months		
One-step command with gesture (0.5)	____	____
Vocabulary 2 words (0.5)	____	____
14 Months		
Vocabulary 3 words (1.0)	____	____
Immature jargoning (1.0)	____	____
16 Months		
Vocabulary 4-6 words (1.0)	____	____
One-step command without gesture (1.0)	____	____
18 Months		
Mature jargoning (0.5)	____	____
Vocabulary 7-10 words (0.5)	____	____
Points to one picture (0.5)*†	____	____
Body parts (0.5)	____	____
21 Months		
Vocabulary 20 words (1.0)	____	____
Two-word phrases (1.0)	____	____
Points to two pictures (1.0)*†	____	____
24 Months		
Vocabulary 50 words (1.0)	____	____
Two-step command (1.0)	____	____
Two-word sentences (1.0)	____	____
30 Months		
Uses pronouns appropriately (1.5)	____	____
Concept of one (1.5)*	____	____
Points to seven pictures (1.5)*†	____	____
Two digits forward (1.5)*	____	____
36 Months		
Vocabulary 250 words (1.5)	____	____
Three-word sentence (1.5)	____	____
Three digits forward (1.5)*	____	____
Follows two prepositional commands (1.5)*	____	____

CAT

Visual-motor abilities	Yes	No
11 Months		
Mature overhand pincer movement (0.5)	____	____
Solves cube under cup (0.5)	____	____
12 Months		
Release one cube/cup (0.5)	____	____
Crayon mark (0.5)	____	____
14 Months		
Solves glass frustration (0.6)	____	____
Out-in with peg (0.6)	____	____
Solves pellet-bottle with demonstration (0.6)	____	____
16 Months		
Solves pellet-bottle spontaneously (0.6)	____	____
Round block in formboard (0.6)	____	____
Scribbles in imitation (0.6)	____	____
18 Months		
Ten cubes in cup (0.5)	____	____
Solves round hole in formboard reversed (0.5)	____	____
Spontaneous scribbling with crayon (0.5)	____	____
Pegboard completed spontaneously (0.5)	____	____
21 Months		
Obtains object with stick (1.0)	____	____
Solves square in formboard (1.0)	____	____
Tower of three cubes (1.0)	____	____
24 Months		
Attempts to fold paper (0.7)	____	____
Horizontal 4-cube train (0.7)	____	____
Imitates stroke with pencil (0.7)	____	____
Completes formboard (0.7)	____	____
30 Months		
Horizontal-vertical stroke with pencil (1.5)	____	____
Form board reversed (1.5)	____	____
Folds paper with definite crease (1.5)	____	____
Train with chimney (1.5)	____	____
36 Months		
Three-cube bridge (1.5)	____	____
Draws circle (1.5)	____	____
Names one color (1.5)	____	____
Draw-a-person test with head plus one other body part (1.5)	____	____

TABLE 12-4

NEWBORN DEVELOPMENTAL SCREENING TESTS

Test	Age of Infant
Neonatal Behavioral Assessment Scale	2 days to 6 weeks
Neurological Examination of the Fullterm Newborn Infant	1 to 9 days
Newborn Individualized Developmental Care and Assessment Program (NIDCAP)	Preterm infants
Rosenblith Revision of the Graham Behavior Test for Neonates	1 to 14 days

the infant. The DSM-IV is a phenomenologic, or symptom-based guide. More meaningful for infant work is a comprehensive and narratively described diagnosis encompassing the varied symptoms and behaviors, developmental pathways, and family and community interrelationships that affect the infant.

Diagnosticians who work with infants may now turn to the Diagnostic Classification of Mental and Developmental Disorders of Infancy and Early Childhood (DC: 0-3). The DC: 0-3 is the product of 8 years' collaboration by clinicians and researchers convened by the Zero To Three/National Center for Clinical Infant Programs. It provides much needed focus and elaboration on disturbances in infancy. It identifies and describes disorders not classified elsewhere and details the earliest manifestations of those disorders that are applied to older children in other classification schemes.

Several diagnoses included in the DSM-IV are applicable to infants, toddlers, and preschoolers. Box 12-3 lists these diagnostic categories.

Most of these diagnoses may be made by the specialist who evaluates children younger than 36 months. Since many of these disorders are covered in detail elsewhere in this text, only the early feeding disorders and the reactive attachment disorders are discussed in this chapter.

BOX 12-3

DSM-IV DISORDERS DIAGNOSABLE IN INFANCY AND EARLY CHILDHOOD

- Mental retardation
- Motor skills disorder
  - Developmental coordination disorder
- Pervasive developmental disorders
  - Autistic disorder
  - Rett's disorder
  - Childhood disintegrative disorder
  - Asperger's disorder
  - Pervasive developmental disorder NOS
- Attention-deficit and disruptive behavior disorders
  - Attention-deficit/hyperactivity disorder
- Feeding and eating disorders of infancy or early childhood
  - Pica
  - Rumination disorder
  - Feeding disorder of infancy or early childhood
- Other disorders of infancy, childhood, or adolescence
  - Separation anxiety disorder, early onset
  - Reactive attachment disorder of infancy or early childhood
  - Stereotypic movement disorder
  - Disorder of infancy NOS

Feeding and Eating Disorders of Infancy or Early Childhood

The experiences of being fed and eating are fundamental to early symbiosis and attachment, and they are critical to the healthy development of the mother-child dyad. Satisfaction in this experience is crucial to affirm the mother's ability to parent and to afford the infant the pleasurable, secure, and need-fulfilling sustenance with which he can build a healthy ego and grow strong. Feeding represents the baby's first experience with socialization. A positive experience becomes basic to a future broad repertoire of socialization skills. Although nonorganic feeding and eating disorders are rarely specifically diagnosed in infancy, difficulties related to nutritional intake are common. Eating problems are common concerns discussed between mothers and pediatricians, especially during the first 2 years of a child's life. It is thought that "failure to thrive" accounts for 1% to 5% of all pediatric hospital admissions, and nonorganic causes are responsible for about one half of these cases.

These psychosocial causes of poor feeding or eating are based on and usually exacerbated by maternal-child conflicts or tension (Box 12-4). There is often poor temperamental compatibility, or "fit," between the mother and the child. These infants tend to be withdrawn and irritable. Mealtimes are anxiety-laden experiences that quickly turn into battle grounds for a chronic power struggle between the two. The baby is uncomfortable and inconsolable, and the mother feels victimized, helpless, and incompetent. Other risk factors for eating disorders or failure to thrive include maternal dysfunction resulting from mental retardation, a psychopathologic disorder, lack of information, extreme poverty, or social isolation (Box 12-5). Child abuse or neglect can also cause failure to thrive.

CHILD BEHAVIOR CHECKLIST FOR AGES 2-3

For office use only
ID #

CHILD'S NAME			PARENTS' USUAL TYPE OF WORK, even if not working now *(Please be specific—for example, auto mechanic, high school teacher, homemaker, laborer, lathe operator, shoe salesman, army sergeant.)*
SEX ☐ Boy ☐ Girl	AGE	ETHNIC GROUP OR RACE	FATHER'S TYPE OF WORK: ________
TODAY'S DATE Mo.____ Date____ Yr.____	CHILD'S BIRTHDATE Mo.____ Date____ Yr.____		MOTHER'S TYPE OF WORK: ________

THIS FORM FILLED OUT BY:

☐ Mother (name): ________

☐ Father (name): ________

☐ Other—name & relationship to child: ________

Please fill out this form to reflect *your* view of the child's behavior even if other people might not agree. Feel free to write additional comments beside each item and in the space provided on page 2.

Below is a list of items that describe children. For each item that describes the child **now or within the past 2 months**, please circle the **2** if the item is **very true** or **often true** of the child. Circle the **1** if the item is **somewhat** or **sometimes true** of the child. If the item is **not true** of the child, circle the **0**. Please answer all items as well as you can, even if some do not seem to apply to the child.

0 = Not True (as far as you know) **1 = Somewhat or Sometimes True** **2 = Very True or Often True**

0 1 2 1. Aches or pains (without medical cause)
0 1 2 2. Acts too young for age
0 1 2 3. Afraid to try new things
0 1 2 4. Avoids looking others in the eye
0 1 2 5. Can't concentrate, can't pay attention for long
0 1 2 6. Can't sit still or restless
0 1 2 7. Can't stand having things out of place
0 1 2 8. Can't stand waiting; wants everything now
0 1 2 9. Chews on things that aren't edible
0 1 2 10. Clings to adults or too dependent
0 1 2 11. Constantly seeks help
0 1 2 12. Constipated, doesn't move bowels
0 1 2 13. Cries a lot
0 1 2 14. Cruel to animals
0 1 2 15. Defiant
0 1 2 16. Demands must be met immediately
0 1 2 17. Destroys his/her own things
0 1 2 18. Destroys things belonging to his/her family or other children
0 1 2 19. Diarrhea or loose bowels when not sick
0 1 2 20. Disobedient
0 1 2 21. Disturbed by any change in routine
0 1 2 22. Doesn't want to sleep alone
0 1 2 23. Doesn't answer when people talk to him/her
0 1 2 24. Doesn't eat well (describe): ________
0 1 2 25. Doesn't get along with other children
0 1 2 26. Doesn't know how to have fun, acts like a little adult
0 1 2 27. Doesn't seem to feel guilty after misbehaving
0 1 2 28. Doesn't want to go out of home
0 1 2 29. Easily frustrated
0 1 2 30. Easily jealous
0 1 2 31. Eats or drinks things that are not food—**don't** include sweets (describe): ________
0 1 2 32. Fears certain animals, situations, or places (describe): ________
0 1 2 33. Feelings are easily hurt
0 1 2 34. Gets hurt a lot, accident-prone
0 1 2 35. Gets in many fights
0 1 2 36. Gets into everything
0 1 2 37. Gets too upset when separated from parents
0 1 2 38. Has trouble getting to sleep
0 1 2 39. Headaches (without medical cause)
0 1 2 40. Hits others
0 1 2 41. Holds his/her breath
0 1 2 42. Hurts animals or people without meaning to
0 1 2 43. Looks unhappy without good reason
0 1 2 44. Angry moods
0 1 2 45. Nausea, feels sick (without medical cause)
0 1 2 46. Nervous movements or twitching (describe): ________
0 1 2 47. Nervous, highstrung, or tense
0 1 2 48. Nightmares
0 1 2 49. Overeating
0 1 2 50. Overtired
0 1 2 51. Overweight
0 1 2 52. Painful bowel movements
0 1 2 53. Physically attacks people
0 1 2 54. Picks nose, skin, or other parts of body (describe): ________
0 1 2 55. Plays with own sex parts too much
0 1 2 56. Poorly coordinated or clumsy
0 1 2 57. Problems with eyes without medical cause (describe): ________
0 1 2 58. Punishment doesn't change his/her behavior
0 1 2 59. Quickly shifts from one activity to another
0 1 2 60. Rashes or other skin problems (without medical cause)
0 1 2 61. Refuses to eat
0 1 2 62. Refuses to play active games
0 1 2 63. Repeatedly rocks head or body
0 1 2 64. Resists going to bed at night

Please see other side

FIGURE 12-1 For legend see p. 199.

0 = Not True (as far as you know) | 1 = Somewhat or Sometimes True | 2 = Very True or Often True

0 1 2 65. Resists toilet training (describe): ____________

0 1 2 66. Screams a lot
0 1 2 67. Seems unresponsive to affection
0 1 2 68. Self-conscious or easily embarrassed
0 1 2 69. Selfish or won't share
0 1 2 70. Shows little affection toward people
0 1 2 71. Shows little interest in things around him/her
0 1 2 72. Shows too little fear of getting hurt
0 1 2 73. Shy or timid
0 1 2 74. Sleeps less than most children during day and/or night (describe): ____________

0 1 2 75. Smears or plays with bowel movements
0 1 2 76. Speech problem (describe): ____________

0 1 2 77. Stares into space or seems preoccupied
0 1 2 78. Stomachaches or cramps (without medical cause)
0 1 2 79. Stores up things he/she doesn't need (describe): ____________

0 1 2 80. Strange behavior (describe): ____________

0 1 2 81. Stubborn, sullen, or irritable
0 1 2 82. Sudden changes in mood or feelings
0 1 2 83. Sulks a lot
0 1 2 84. Talks or cries out in sleep
0 1 2 85. Temper tantrums or hot temper
0 1 2 86. Too concerned with neatness or cleanliness
0 1 2 87. Too fearful or anxious
0 1 2 88. Uncooperative
0 1 2 89. Underactive, slow moving, or lacks energy
0 1 2 90. Unhappy, sad, or depressed
0 1 2 91. Unusually loud
0 1 2 92. Upset by new people or situations (describe): ____________

0 1 2 93. Vomiting, throwing up (without medical cause)
0 1 2 94. Wakes up often at night
0 1 2 95. Wanders away from home
0 1 2 96. Wants a lot of attention
0 1 2 97. Whining
0 1 2 98. Withdrawn, doesn't get involved with others
0 1 2 99. Worrying

100. Please write in any problems your child has that were not listed above.

0 1 2 ____________
0 1 2 ____________
0 1 2 ____________

PLEASE BE SURE YOU HAVE ANSWERED ALL ITEMS. UNDERLINE ANY YOU ARE CONCERNED ABOUT.

Does your child have any illness, physical disability, or mental handicap? ☐ No ☐ Yes—Please describe

What concerns you most about your child?

Please describe the best things about your child:

FIGURE 12-1 Child behavior checklist for ages 2 to 3. (From Achenbach, TM: *Child behavior checklist for ages 2-3,* Burlington, Vt., 1988, Center for Children, Youth, & Families.)

Annie, a Child Failing to Thrive

Annie was a healthy 6-pound, 15-ounce firstborn to her 17-year-old mother. She and her mother were discharged from the hospital on postpartum day 2. By the time she was 11 days old, the routine well-baby examination revealed that she had gained 1 pound. However, 2 months later she weighed only 8 pounds, 8 ounces. After another 2 weeks she had gained only 6 ounces. Serum chemistry tests showed remarkably low serum protein. On inquiry about the infant's diet, it was learned that Annie's mother had steadfastly held to the pediatrician's initial discharge instructions to offer her baby only 2 to 3 ounces of formula per feeding. Furthermore, this young mother did not know how to mix formula and was inadvertently using too much water. During one observed feeding session, the pediatric nurse found that the nipple on the bottle was clogged. Annie was not fed overnight, because her mother was loathe to wake her out of fear of disturbing her irritable husband, who was prone to violence when angered. Annie's teenage father was apparently guided by the philosophy that babies should neither be seen nor heard. She worried that he would think she was an incompetent mother if her baby cried in the night. Fortunately, a very capable and stalwart maternal aunt availed herself to this young at-risk family. Through the pediatrician's, nurse's, and family's efforts, Annie's feeding problems were quickly resolved. She gained 17 ounces by the next 2-week follow-up appointment.

Bobby, a Child Born in Social Isolation

Bobby was conceived by his teenage mother and her uncle. He was brought for his first pediatric visit unbathed and without clothes. He wore a soiled diaper and was wrapped in a blanket. He was fed undiluted formula. The Department of Social Services was immediately called. Clinic staff bought clothes for immediate use, and nurses taught his mother bathing techniques. Social services staff were able to arrange for more clothes and a crib. Home health nurses taught basic formula mixing and feeding skills. Because of the mother's reticence to approach the local Woman Infant Child (WIC) program (perhaps because of her apparent marriage to her uncle), the pediatrician's office supplied baby formula until the mother could be cajoled into registering with WIC. Bobby was enrolled in the local Child Find high-risk tracking program and in the local health department's home visitation program, which provided weekly health checks and parenting classes. Through crisis-oriented intervention assisted by consistent follow-up care, Bobby quickly became a healthy, growing, and well-behaved baby.

BOX 12-4

PSYCHOSOCIAL CAUSES OF FAILURE TO THRIVE

- Poor temperamental fit between mother and child
- Psychopathology preventing caretaker efficacy
- Mental retardation in caregiver
- Ignorance of infant needs
- Extreme poverty
- Child abuse
- Child neglect

Reactive Attachment Disorder

Reactive attachment disorder was originally described as anaclitic depression by Rene Spitz in his work with institutionalized or hospitalized infants and toddlers. This syndrome is the result of chronic and extreme early neglect. These children have struggled to thrive in minimally responsive environments. Their cries go unregarded. Their hunger is not appeased according to their need. Smiles are not rewarded. They experience no predictable or consistent learning. Events occur randomly and often inadequately without regard for the child's physical or emotional needs. In the best of situations, the child's physical need for food and shelter are met. In a very bad situation, these too

BOX 12-5 FEEDING DISORDER OF INFANCY OR EARLY CHILDHOOD

DSM-IV DIAGNOSTIC CRITERIA

A. Feeding disturbance as manifested by persistent failure to eat adequately with significant failure to gain weight or significant loss of weight over at least 1 month.

B. The disturbance is not due to an associated gastrointestinal or other general medical condition (e.g., esophageal reflux).

C. The disturbance is not better accounted for by another mental disorder (e.g., Rumination Disorder) or by lack of available food.

D. The onset is before age 6 years.

(From American Psychiatric Association: *Diagnostic and statistical manual of mental disorders,* ed 4 [DSM-IV], Washington DC, 1994, American Psychiatric Press.)

are neglected. In the worst cases, the infant is also physically and sexually abused.

Because of the extreme neglect, the infant who has reactive attachment disorder shows severely impaired social relatedness. Some children become highly inhibited and anxious. Others become indiscriminant in terms of attachment figures. Therefore reactive attachment disorder is divided into the subtypes of inhibited or disinhibited types (Box 12-6).

Any infant with an inadequate parent is at risk for this disorder or for characteristics of this disorder. These parents are either unwilling, unable, or do not know how to parent. Reasons for this parental incapacity to offer even rudimentary care to toddlers can be lack of information, psychiatric conditions, incompetence, or severe conflicts related to the parent's own nurturing. The substance-abusing or addicted mother's needs carry a much greater urgency than her child's.

Gregory, a Child with Reactive Attachment Disorder

Gregory first arrived for psychiatric evaluation at the age of 32 months. Children's Protective Services (CPS) had been contacted by the staff of one of the community's fast food restaurants. Apparently, Gregory and his 5-year-old brother Shawn had been found sleeping and eating in the trash dumpster behind their premises. The children had often come to the restaurant counter begging for food. On investigation, CPS found the two children alone in a home without electricity or heat. There was no food, and Gregory, who was not yet potty trained, was soiled by the feces and urine that were caked on the inside of his clothes. The children were placed in emergency foster care, but 2 months later their polysubstance-dependent mother was allowed to take them back home on the grounds that she was rehabilitated. Within 1 month, the children were again found in a state of severe neglect.

Gregory was brought in by his new foster mother,

PEARLS & PERILS

REACTIVE ATTACHMENT DISORDERS

- Almost all children with reactive attachment disorder are victims of extreme abuse or neglect.

DSM-IV DIAGNOSTIC CRITERIA

BOX 12-6 REACTIVE ATTACHMENT DISORDER OF INFANCY OR EARLY CHILDHOOD

A. Markedly disturbed and developmentally inappropriate social relatedness in most contexts, beginning before age 5 years, as evidenced by either (1) or (2):

(1) persistent failure to initiate or respond in a developmentally appropriate fashion to most social interactions, as manifest by excessively inhibited, hypervigilant, or highly ambivalent and contradictory responses (e.g., the child may respond to caregivers with a mixture of approach, avoidance, and resistance to comforting, or may exhibit frozen watchfulness)

(2) diffuse attachments as manifest by indiscriminate sociability with marked inability to exhibit appropriate selective attachments (e.g., excessive familiarity with relative strangers or lack of selectivity in choice of attachment figures)

B. The disturbance in Criterion A is not accounted for solely by developmental delay (as in Mental Retardation) and does not meet criteria for a Pervasive Developmental Disorder.

C. Pathogenic care as evidenced by at least one of the following:

(1) persistent disregard of the child's basic emotional needs for comfort, stimulation, and affection

(2) persistent disregard of the child's basic physical needs

(3) repeated changes of primary caregiver that prevent formation of stable attachments (e.g., frequent changes in foster care)

D. There is a presumption that the care in Criterion C is responsible for the disturbed behavior in Criterion A (e.g., the disturbances in Criterion A began following the pathogenic care in Criterion C).

Specify type:
Inhibited Type: if Criterion A1 predominates in the clinical presentation
Disinhibited Type: if Criterion A2 predominates in the clinical presentation

(From American Psychiatric Association: *Diagnostic and statistical manual of mental disorders,* ed 4 [DSM-IV], Washington DC, 1994, American Psychiatric Association.)

who was in the second trimester of pregnancy. She was most concerned about Gregory's aberrant behaviors. He wouldn't play with her young son. He had many fears. He was terrified of baths and of water in general. He often broke into a panic during mealtimes, screaming that he saw bugs in his food. Even so, his appetite was insatiable.

The most remarkable finding in the evaluation was Gregory's extreme listlessness and lack of affect. His frail arms and legs were limp and mottled from cold exposure, which had caused a mild neuropathy. He quickly moved to sit on the therapist's lap and remained seated quietly through most of the first session, unwilling or unable to communicate. He woefully cast his big blue eyes up to the therapist toward the end of the hour and stated in a monotone, "Hungry!"

Gregory and his foster mother, brother, and foster brother attended therapy weekly, and each session was divided into a time for individual play psychotherapy and a time for family teaching and therapy. Gregory came to expect juice and crackers during his visits, and soon he was willing to play kitchen-based games, during which he pretended to cook and serve large meals for the therapist and himself.

Within the year, and with a good bit of love, reassurance, and consistent provision of his basic needs, Gregory was transformed into a rambunctious and quite rotund little boy. He was still on the lookout for food, but he was also interacting well with peers and adults at home and in preschool, and he was quite capable of love and play.

Treatment and Prevention

In treating the disturbed infant, the best approach is team-based and holistic. The treatment team is variably comprised of pediatricians, child psychiatrists, child psychologists, social workers, educators, nurses, and nutritionists, as well as occupational, physical, and speech therapists.

The team's therapeutic goal is to promote the infant's healthy development in cognitive, social, emotional, and motor spheres, as well as to promote healthy growth and development of the infant's family. At the core of treatment is the process of enabling the family and child to move forward in a healthful, competent, and independent way.

Treatment Modalities

The vision often evoked when one first ponders the field of infant psychiatry is that of a troubled baby on a psychoanalytic couch. Though psychoanalytic theory underlies much of our understanding of infancy and infant relationships, psychoanalytic technique offers little that can be applied to therapeutic work with infants and toddlers. A baby lacks all the traits that might deem her a proper candidate for psychotherapy in the traditional sense. She has at best little verbal ability, no capacity for insight, and no ability to form a therapeutic alliance.

Much of the psychotherapeutic work with infants is done in conjunction with the collaborative efforts of parents or surrogate parents. Whether this work is done in the hospital, clinic, office, or home, the work is most effective when the baby is present. Parent counselling or training in the baby's absence is diluted and can easily become poorly aimed. The baby is included in the therapy for good reason. Though the baby is not a good therapeutic candidate in the traditional sense, she brings the richest material to the therapeutic dialogue. She brings strong emotions, such as happiness, contentment, sadness, anger, frustration, and fear. She clearly demonstrates physical integrity or ills. She reflects, in one small person, the general and specific functioning and well-being of herself and her family.

The treatment of choice is based on the clinical setting and the clinically determined needs of the family. A brief and crisis-oriented approach is often necessary when treating the at-risk infant. Problems can often be remediated through emergency provision of basic food, clothes, or shelter, or by addressing the external factors contributing to the current crisis.

Physicians who treat infants base their work on the double pillars of education and psychotherapy. Treatment, like history taking, is experiential. Through observation of the intricate relationships of the family, the physician learns about the behavioral and psychologic dynamics of the patients. With information from history and direct observation supporting the chosen methods, the physician is able to directly reach therapeutic goals.

The physician must educate or train the innocent, inexperienced, or incapable parent to recognize and respond appropriately to a child's needs. Psychotherapy is based on the understanding of psychodynamics affecting the parent-child relationship. These dynamics incorporate feelings and reactions to past and present relationships, expectations, and experience. The therapy is aimed to opening up channels of mutual love and respect between parent and child. The parent should be able to provide adequate supportive parenting and affirmation to the child and his specific, sometimes special, needs. The physician works to promote the stable and trusted bonds between parent and child. Sources of parental conflict impeding the relationship's development must be investigated and systematically relieved.

Treatment of a parent-child pair can take several forms, which are largely determined by the clinical setting and by clinically determined needs. The most urgent form of therapy, and often the most straightforward, is crisis intervention. Often the treatment team is contacted to arrange emergency services for a child or a parent-child pair. This parent-child dyad might function well enough generally, but it is in peril if it is lacking basic food, clothes, or shelter or if it is affected by other external factors (for example, the pair may be threatened by community violence). Another scenario that requires crisis intervention work is the case of an infant who is neglected or abused. In this case, the treatment team must first move to protect the child.

When the parent-child dyad is experiencing internal difficulties, psychotherapy and teaching are in order. The pair might experience difficulties stemming from maternal conflicts or impairments, from the infant's impaired innate capacities, or from both sources. The physician employs several types of intervention during visits with the parent and the child. It is important to remain supportive and empathic to the parent, to facilitate parent-child communication, and to model healthy communication and interaction. The physician should teach the parent about normal and abnormal development. Through psychotherapy, the physician focuses on the parent's past as it relates to current parenting techniques, and through behavioral intervention the physician helps the parent-child dyad engage and progress together.

The physician is free to vary techniques according to patient needs. Play involving the mother and the baby may be encouraged through direct interaction and teaching or through observation and assisted play or teaching. The physician may work directly to enable the motivated parent to work with the child. Direct work with the child may be necessary if the child has significant developmental deficiencies, significant difficulties with sensory reactivity, or behavioral modulation, especially if the parent is not yet able or motivated. The physician should never interrupt treatment of the child to first treat the incapacitated parent. Time is too precious to the rapidly developing infant and toddler. Delaying infant intervention for 6 months, or even 1 or 2 years, to help the parent overcome developmental hurdles could permanently derail a young child from normal developmental pathways.

Children with significant deficiencies in several developmental spheres mandate a more comprehensive and intensive treatment. These children and their families may require several weekly visits with multiple therapists to optimally improve their motor, communicative, and adaptive capacities. A more comprehensive, or holistic, approach to the developing infant is more likely to promote future gains in the child's human relatedness and capacity for intimacy than a "shotgun" approach aimed at isolated deficiencies.

> PEARLS & PERILS
>
> **TREATMENT OF EMOTIONALLY DISTURBED INFANTS**
>
> - Immediate intervention in emotionally disturbed infants is imperative.
> - A brief crisis-oriented approach may be needed initially.
> - The goal of treatment is to start the infant on a normal developmental path.
> - The parent-child dyad should be treated.
> - A multidisciplinary team should be used.

A parent-child therapy group allows for effective intervention in a supportive and interactive setting. A group is the best format for social and educational support for the isolated parent and for children with socialization problems. Group therapy affords the parent-child dyad an opportunity to feel its problems are shared, provides a reliable family-type structure, and gives guidance and a sense of hope to the sometimes desperate family. These groups can be quite structured in format. Generally, time is allotted for parent-child interactive activities, supervised free play for the children, and special time for parents. This parent time can be used for education, parent training, or mutual support.

Prevention

Prevention in infant mental health begins in the prenatal, perinatal, and postpartum periods. Priority strategies must encourage optimal prenatal care, positive parent-infant relationships, and positive environments for at-risk populations. Support and education about fetal development, obstetric health care, and early parenting are essential, especially for teen and low-income populations where the risk of newborns with low birth weights is highest. The premature or low birth weight baby is most likely to suffer cognitive delay, developmental delay, or retardation; to experience inadequate mother-infant relationships; to develop psychopathologic conditions or emotional disturbance; and to be the victim of child abuse or neglect. It is crucial for pediatricians and child psychiatrists to play an active part in community health planning and to foster the cause of the at-risk infant.

> PEARLS & PERILS
>
> **PREVENTION**
>
> - Parent education is the cornerstone of prevention in infant psychiatry.

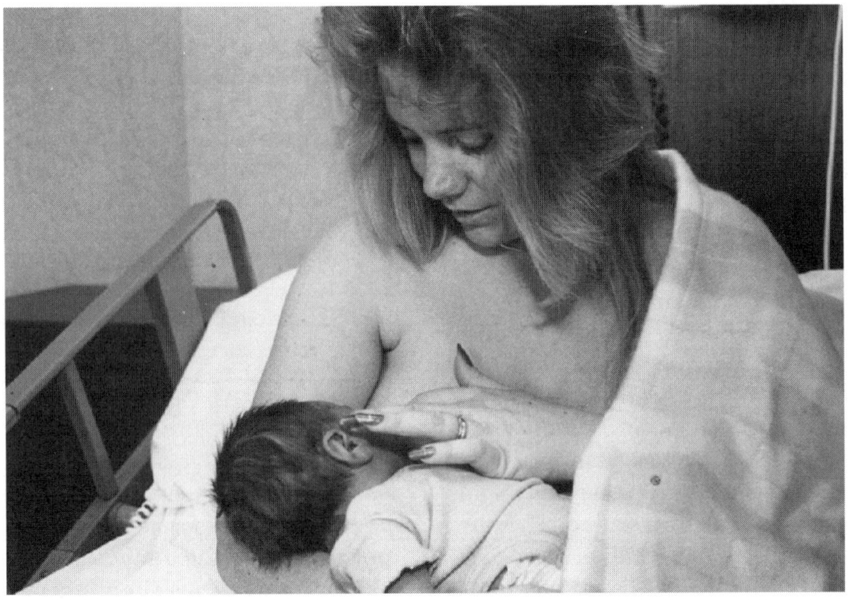

FIGURE 12-2 A mature and confident mother nurses her third child on the morning after an uneventful, spontaneous vaginal delivery at term.

Special Concerns in Infant Psychiatry

The Baby in the Neonatal Intensive Care Unit

From birth, the experiences of a baby who is dependent on a neonatal intensive care unit (NICU) are starkly different from those of a healthy, full-term newborn. Figures 12-2 and 12-3 depict the contrasts between the containing environments and initial social experiences of a NICU baby and that of a healthy newborn. In the best of circumstances, a lovely, robust newborn is swaddled, cuddled, rocked, and breast or bottle fed on demand by a confident, competent, healthy, and euphoric new mother. The experiences of a mother and an NICU baby bears little resemblance to this blissful bonding process. Perhaps as much at risk as the baby's precarious physical fortitude are the fundamental attachments of the mother and the baby.

Risk factors affecting the NICU baby and his mother are multifaceted. For several months the mother, father, and extended family have fantasized about their baby. These fantasies are generally idyllic. Their baby will be perfect—a lovely little girl or a robust little boy, affirming the parents' own worth and capability and strengthening the foundations of their egos. With the trauma of an emergency birth (that may be premature) or with the horrible news that a term baby is defective, these dreams are shattered. The birth of an imperfect baby imparts a profound psychologic injury to families. It is experienced more as a crisis than as a miracle.

Technologic advances in neonatology allow physicians to save the gravely ill patients, as well as the extremely premature babies. Most NICUs can now boast the ability to support even the 23- or 24-week infant (400 to 500 gm) to graduation from the unit. With these advances in perinatology and neonatology come fundamental psychosocial challenges. The physician must be able to support the family in crisis, to approximate the natural environment of the premature infant or full-term baby (the womb, the warm and quiet nursery where needs are met on demand, or the mother's cradling arms and body), and to support the crucial mother-child bonding process amid great obstacles (Figure 12-4).

Many babies spending their first months in the NICU were not planned. Many are delivered shortly after their first quickening or when mothers are just beginning to don maternity clothes and settle into the role of the expectant mother, which is sometimes experienced as a rite of passage. The bonding that began with the parent's first dreams is strengthened prenatally. The last few months of a normal gestation are often when parents begin communicating with their baby. They whisper and sing to the growing fetus and begin to respond to their baby's diurnal cycles. This prenatal bonding is shortened when a baby is born early (Box 12-7). Parents are often not allowed to touch their babies, and they barely see their critically ill newborns before they are hastened away for intervention. Additionally, the mothers themselves are often quite ill after delivery.

The intensive care nursery can frighten even the most devoted parents. Denial is a significant defense mechanism used by parents facing such trauma, and avoidance of their baby can effectively assist their emo-

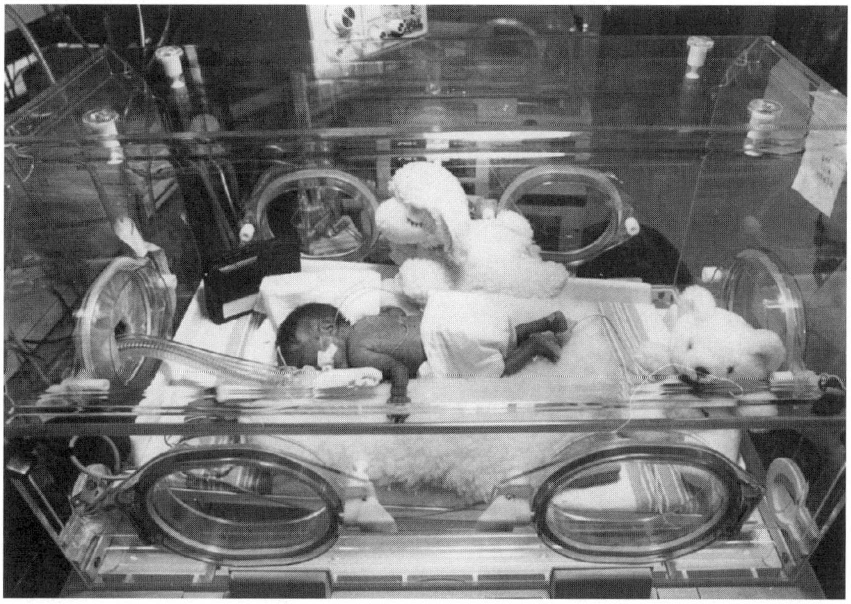

FIGURE 12-3 The early environment of the preterm baby who must stay in the NICU contrasts markedly with that of the healthy newborn in Figure 12-2.

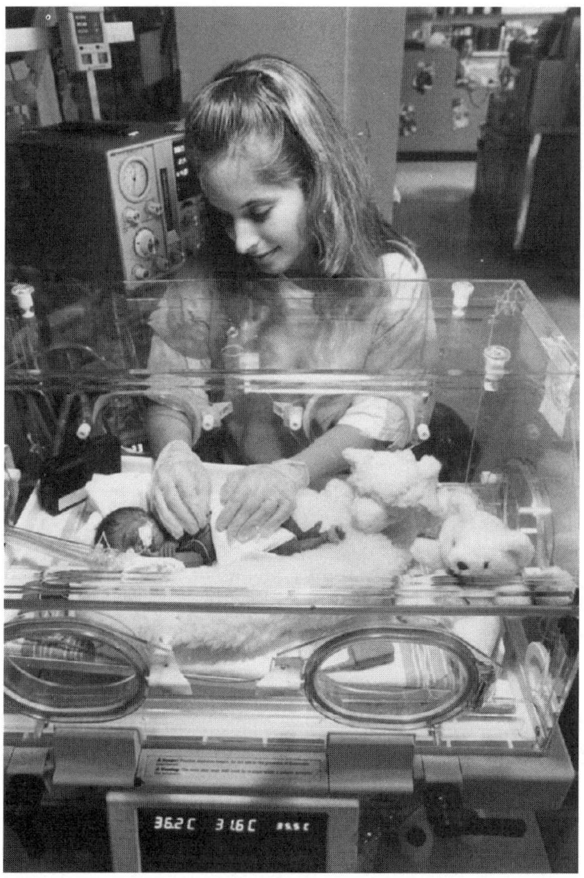

FIGURE 12-4 Staff of modern NICU attempt to normalize the newborn's early experience, which approximates as well as possible that of the fetus within the womb.

BOX 12-7

NICU BABIES

The infant shatters fantasies because of imperfection.

The parent-child bonding process is interrupted.

Parents often use denial regarding the infant's condition.

Education is needed to help parents with physical demands.

tional state. The constant flashing and high intensity lights, the beeping of alarms, and the plethora of lines invading their sick child can be a further hindrance to parental caresses. Though many neonatology units now try to afford their patients the most comfortable and secure surroundings, this is often difficult as they attempt to provide top quality medical care. The challenge is to provide a normative and nurturing an environment to the baby and the visiting parents without compromising the infant's medical stability and progress (Figure 12-5).

Adapting to their baby's special physical needs and temperamental demands are additional challenges facing the parents of the NICU baby, both in the nursery and after discharge. These demands are met with great difficulty for the most willing and capable of parents and communities, and they can be unmanageable in situations that are less than optimal. A good deal of preparation, education, and support are necessary to help these families through their first years with their NICU graduate (Figure 12-6).

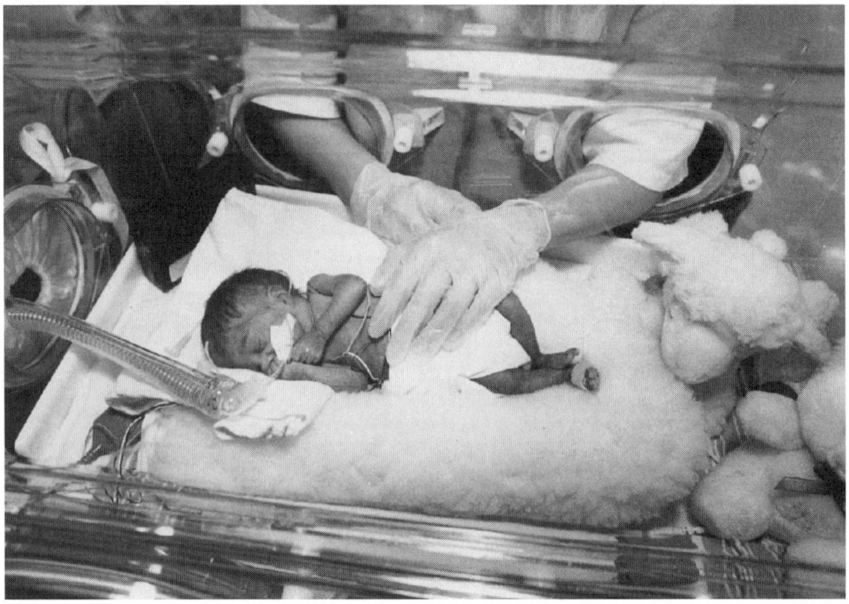

FIGURE 12-5 Attention to details relating to oral, auditory, visual, and tactile stimuli assist the premature infant's development.

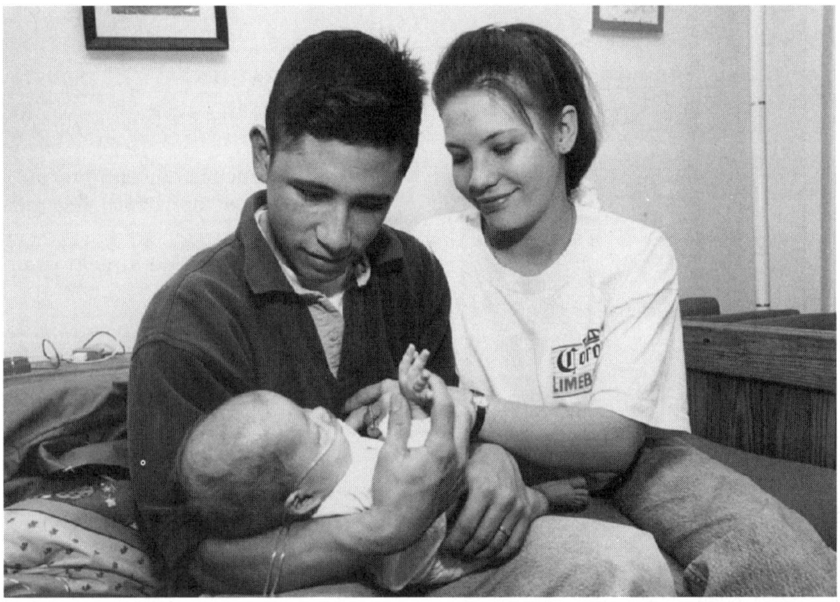

FIGURE 12-6 A young couple prepares for their baby's discharge following 5 months' stay in the NICU. They had stayed in an adjoining guest suite over weekends for the 2 months before the baby's discharge. Parent education, a form of prevention, occurs during such weekends.

Sara, an NICU Graduate

Sara was welcomed to the world via emergency cesarean section after 36 weeks' gestation because of premature placental detachment. She weighed 4 pounds. Though saddened by their inability to experience their carefully planned, Lamaze-guided birthing room delivery, Sara's parents felt fortunate that both mother and baby had survived their near disaster. Sara was allergic to formula and developed bloody diarrhea. She also experienced several episodes of apnea during her NICU stay. She was discharged after 10 days and sent home with an apnea monitor. She was to be given aminophylline, hyoscyamine (Donnatal), and evaporated milk with Karo syrup, which she was able to tolerate. Although they were adjusting to new parenthood, her parents (both health professionals) seemed to adapt well to Sara's unforeseen needs.

Sara cried constantly and had severe reflux until she

was 5 months old. By age 2, she had undergone nine ear operations because of chronic otitis, myringotomy tubes, and abscesses around the tubes. Her father was afraid to handle his tiny and frail little girl. Both parents felt insecure, incompetent, and guilty about parenting their irritable and sickly child during her first year. They were anxious, exhausted, and overwhelmed. Fortunately, Sara's health and well-being turned around in her second year, and the family reached equilibrium with few scars.

The Crack Baby

In the past few decades the extent of cocaine use, especially in inner cities, has reached and maintained crisis levels. It is estimated that there are over 2 million cocaine addicts in the United States. It is felt that approximately 20% of newborns in urban centers may have been exposed to cocaine use in utero. In the 1980s, the country was alerted to prepare for the millions of children expected to be deleteriously affected by this toxic exposure. Physicians expected hordes of cocaine-exposed children to emerge with developmental delays and broad-based disruptive behavioral problems, such as including attention-deficit/hyperactivity disorder (ADHD), aggression, and impulsivity. Fortunately, this onslaught has not occurred. Recent well-controlled studies have failed to demonstrate conclusively that cocaine is a major CNS toxin. The effects of prenatal cocaine exposure remain unclear at this time.

It is especially difficult to isolate the effects of cocaine or "crack" on infants. Cocaine-abusing or dependent pregnant women also tend to abuse alcohol, marijuana, and nicotine, all known teratogens. Mothers tend to be young, often uninvested in parenting, and commonly burdened with their own emotional, cognitive, and behavioral disturbances. These babies commonly have low birth weights and are often raised in impoverished and dysfunctional settings. They are the too often victims of abuse and neglect.

Montee, a Casualty of Cocaine

Montee weighed 9 pounds when he was delivered at term by cesarean section. He was brought to the Salvation Army Emergency Shelter for homeless mothers and children at 10 weeks by his 18-year-old mother and 27-year-old father. His mother admitted to using cocaine regularly throughout her pregnancy, and his father acknowledged an extensive history of cocaine use. Montee's mother, scared and unsure about her first baby, felt unable to manage his diet. She was alternating between milk and formula, but he was vomiting whatever was fed to him. Montee was dressed in an outfit that was entirely too small and caused his legs to be drawn up, preventing full extension. He had a severe diaper rash, his abdomen was distended, and his forehead looked big. His eyes were glossy and unfocusing. He didn't smile. He was fussy and soiled, but his parents had brought no food or diapers along for him. The Denver Developmental Screening Test was attempted but abandoned because of his extreme fretfulness.

> **PEARLS & PERILS**
>
> **PRENATAL COCAINE EXPOSURE**
>
> - Pregnant mothers who abuse cocaine often abuse other substances such as alcohol, marijuana, and nicotine.

It was apparent that Montee's mother lacked basic nurturing skills. She held him distant from herself and did not interact with him in any way. The Shelter staff put forth great effort to teach the parents to care for their child, but were repeatedly frustrated in their attempts to engage the couple. They were able to procure temporary housing for the family. At 16 weeks, the parents reported that Montee suffered crib death, or sudden infant death syndrome. After an investigation, the parents were arrested and incarcerated for using and distributing cocaine and marijuana from their apartment. Charges of child neglect entered by the Department of Social Services were also under investigation.

Babies Exposed to Human Immunodeficiency Virus

Many questions remain about maternal-fetal transmission of HIV. In the 1980s, it was thought that about 70% of fetuses exposed to HIV would contract HIV and AIDS. Given time, a more sophisticated diagnostic approach, and new pharmacologic interventions, these estimates have been shrinking yearly. It is now expected that roughly 30% of infants exposed to HIV will become infected. A recent study of a series of pregnant women who were infected with HIV and receiving antiretroviral therapy beginning with their second trimester reported an infection rate of only 8.3% in their offspring. However, the uninfected infants are far from unaffected by their mothers' HIV or AIDS.

Like crack exposure, HIV exposure tends to be "just one more problem" in a long list of foreboding risk factors. Along with the social problems wrought by poverty, drugs, and poorly supportive families, HIV and AIDS bring unique challenges to a child and family. The chronic, uncertain course of HIV with the certain outcome of significantly premature death imposes extreme emotional, financial, and social stress on a family. If multiple family members are infected, the hardships are quite overwhelming. Since HIV is increasingly transmitted through heterosexual contact, it is not unusual to encounter families where both parents and more than one child are living with HIV or AIDS.

At a time when most young families are growing together, establishing roots and relationships, and building for the future, families coping with HIV are learning to let go of relationships as they face the death of one or more family members in the not-too-distant future. A family dealing with such a depressing sentence may find it difficult to cultivate the normal bonds of familial relationships. Attachment between the mother and the baby, when one or both are infected by HIV, can be seriously impaired. Infants and children of parents who are infected face repeated illness and the separation necessitated by hospitalization. When intravenous drug use has been the route of maternal infection, children may face repeated separation from their mothers because of her continued substance abuse and the associated behaviors and consequences.

Families with members who have HIV are some of the most isolated and unsupported of beleaguered families because of the tremendous social stigma and lack of knowledge surrounding the diagnosis of HIV. This diagnosis can be an unwelcome topic for discussion in families and is commonly kept secret from other family members. Children often spend intermittent periods in foster care (often in multiple foster care settings), which further disrupts any sense of security and attachment. Ultimately, these young mothers and their children face permanent separation through death.

Ms. Johnson, Deedee, and Warren, a Family Coping With the Diagnosis of HIV

Ms. Johnson was a 38-year-old mother of three children. Her first son lived with his paternal grandparents. Her daughter Deedee was 34 months old. She was incarcerated for theft related to funding a cocaine addiction when she learned she was 5 months pregnant. At that time she also learned she was infected with HIV. Shortly after hospital-based delivery, Ms. Johnson returned to complete the remaining 3 months of her jail time. Warren, an 8-pound, 4-ounce baby that appeared healthy, joined his sister at a foster home where they awaited their mother's release.

When she returned to the community, Ms. Johnson resumed child-rearing responsibilities, a task she seemed to take seriously. Although she continued to use drugs, she insisted that she always took care of the children first. When Ms. Johnson arrived at the pediatric infectious disease clinic, she and the children were neat, clean, well-mannered, and in appropriate developmental and cognitive stages of growth. Ms. Johnson's mood was euthymic, and both children were joyful. When asked how she was coping with her new diagnosis and the possibility that baby Warren might also be infected, Ms. Johnson stated that she tried to be positive about life, tried not to worry, and tried not to think about the HIV. This sort of coping strategy was obviously workable and appropriate to this healthy family in the early stages of HIV infection.

> **PEARLS & PERILS**
>
> **HIV INFECTED BABIES**
>
> - Infants with HIV in their families may also contend with poverty, drugs, and poorly supportive families.
> - Attachment to parents can be impaired because of illness and separation.
> - The family may be isolated from external supports.
> - Children may be in multiple foster placements.

Multiple Births

The phenomenon of dizygotic twinning has roughly doubled in the past 2 decades. Such twinning is now estimated to occur in about 1 in 50 pregnancies. The frequency of triplets has increased as well. This is generally felt to be related to the increasing number of women who defer child-bearing to after their mid-30's, as well as to the widespread treatment of infertility, which often places a woman at risk for multiple births. Multiple births bring a variety of risks to each fetus or infant and its relationship to the mother. These risks are rarely appreciated in the lay literature. The physician must help the family cope with the troubling realities of twins or even triplets.

Twin gestations are commonly complicated by hyperemesis gravidarum, hypertension or preeclampsia, hydramnios, and preterm delivery. Fetuses are at risk for growth discordance, intrauterine growth retardation, and low birth weight. The usual risk of a congenital anomaly is about 3%, but it is doubled with a twin delivery. The most common association with twin births is prematurity, which in itself brings the many risks mentioned in the discussion of infants in NICU. The stress to the family is amplified, since more than one baby must often be retained for intensive care. Delivery is also complicated by multiple gestations, and obstetricians often choose to minimize risk by delivering the babies via cesarean section.

Parenting a set of twins or triplets is a daunting task. The constant task of responding to the needs of more than one demanding infant can seem beyond human possibility. The physical and emotional demands can be overwhelming. Beyond the provision of basic care, these babies and mothers need quality time too—time for cooing, kissing, and bonding of each baby with its mother. Many mothers of multiples might question whether this can truly happen. The pediatrician or infant specialist can ensure that the frantic young family finds some relief and happiness by modifying mothering techniques, referring the family to support groups (such as the National Organization of Mothers of Twins Club), and assisting in arrangements for child care relief.

A Twin Story

Drs. Jill and Jerry Smith were high-achieving young physicians. As they anticipated furthering their subspecialty training through advanced fellowships, they also decided to increase the size of their young family. After careful consideration of work demands and child care needs, the couple conceived what they thought would be their third child. The diagnosis of twins, made at the time of second trimester ultrasound, brought many unforeseen problems. Third trimester prophylactic bedrest exhausted the time planned for maternity leave, left the mother without pay, and necessitated creative management of work responsibilities. Costs of child care for the unexpected baby far exceeded the couple's fairly meager budget, and necessitated extra employment for both parents, which furthered the family's stress related to quality child rearing.

The first 6 months were described as "hell." There was little quality time for anyone at home, despite the best of intentions. Although both parents felt fortunate to have added two healthy little boys to their family, the constant demands and rambunctious nature of the twins, as well as the oppositional and quite difficult temperament of one of them, left little physical, intellectual, or emotional energy for the other arenas of the couple's lives. Mrs. Dr. Smith was close to tears daily and consulted the boys' pediatrician when they were 26 months old.

Both had mastered escaping from their cribs and graduated to toddler beds. They were now little masters of their destinies, or at least of the house. They controlled the rules now, and they decided if, when, or where to nap or go "night-night." The twins' obvious newfound confidence bolstered new exploits, and they became virtual partners in crime. When they rearranged furniture, nothing was beyond their grasp. The Smiths' nights, which had finally become fairly predictable after a year or so of largely interrupted sleep, were once again chaotic. Dr. Smith, who was comfortable in any critical care or emergency room experience, was at his wit's end. His wife was also obviously overwhelmed.

Enhancing support through involvement of the extended family and good child care providers allowed the couple to achieve the peace of mind needed to balance their family and careers. The couple learned to have more realistic expectations of themselves and their children. By maintaining limits and reestablishing structure in the childrens' routines, the twins' general level of compliance and apparent sense of security and comfort improved.

> **PEARLS & PERILS**
>
> **MULTIPLE BIRTHS**
>
> - Pregnancies have more complications.
> - Parenting more than one infant can be overwhelming.

When to Refer

When a parent-infant dyad requires more time or expertise than the physician is able to offer, a referral for further assistance is indicated. The physician should consider referring an infant and parent as early as possible, because there is no justification for lost time in a child's early years. Waiting for an infant or parent-infant pair to outgrow the problem may permit irreversible losses to the child's physical or emotional integrity.

Similar principles should be used when considering the involvement of Child Protective Services. Physicians are legally bound to involve CPS if child abuse or neglect is suspected and to file a report regardless of the parents' educational, economic, or social status. In an infant, such maltreatment could quickly devastate, if not erase, a child's future.

Summary

As American society reaches toward the 21st century, the welfare of the American baby is threatened. Modern conveniences facilitating baby care are handy, but modern times have complicated the lives of our babies. Modern conveniences do little to promote mother-child bonding, the most fundamental and old-fashioned principle underlying healthy human development. Modern times have witnessed the threat to mother-child attachment at all levels of the socioeconomic spectrum. The new mother, regardless of her financial status, is expected to be back at work 6 weeks after delivery. Few mothers have the luxury these days of entrusting their newborns to their own mothers for the crucial responsibility of caring for the child. There are few community programs set up to ensure quality or consistent care for these infants. Paternity leave is rarely endorsed in the work place. Fast-paced social demands of modern living often make the baby the last consideration, and the child is often left with multiple caregivers.

Families merge and split. Poverty, crime, and drugs are rampant. Teens, too young themselves to ponder the meaning, worth, or needs of a newborn, continue to reproduce. Costly social programs are slashed. The welfare of the baby, it seems, is taken for granted. It is up to the physician to reverse modern trends and return tradition to infant care. Families must be supported to provide consistent and reliable love and care to their young. Infants should be the focus, not the afterthought, of a progressive society.

CONSIDER CONSULTATION WHEN . . .

- There is developmental delay
- There is poor parent-child bonding
- The Department of Social Services becomes involved

Annotated Bibliography

Fraiberg S, editor: *Clinical studies in infant mental health: the first year of life,* New York, 1980, Basic Books.
This is an eloquent compilation of case studies.

Fraiberg S: *The magic years: understanding and handling the problems of early childhood,* New York, 1959, Charles Scribner's Sons.
This is required reading for all child professionals.

Greenspan SI: *Infancy and early childhood: the practice of clinical assessment and intervention with emotional and developmental challenges,* Madison, Conn., 1992, International Universities Press.
This in-depth volume has a complete description of assessment tools and techniques.

Minde K, Minde R: *Infant psychiatry: an introductory textbook,* Beverly Hills, Calif., 1986, Sage Publications.
This is a succinct, basic review of history, epidemiology, and techniques.

Rexford E, Sander L, Shapiro T, editors: *Infant psychiatry: a new synthesis,* New Haven, Conn., 1976, Yale University Press.
This is the first compilation on the topic. It is a good historical reference with "the beginning" of infant psychiatry.

Zeanah CH, Jr, editor: *Handbook of infant mental health,* New York, 1993, The Guilford Press.
This is the latest text on the topic. Special topics are covered in depth.

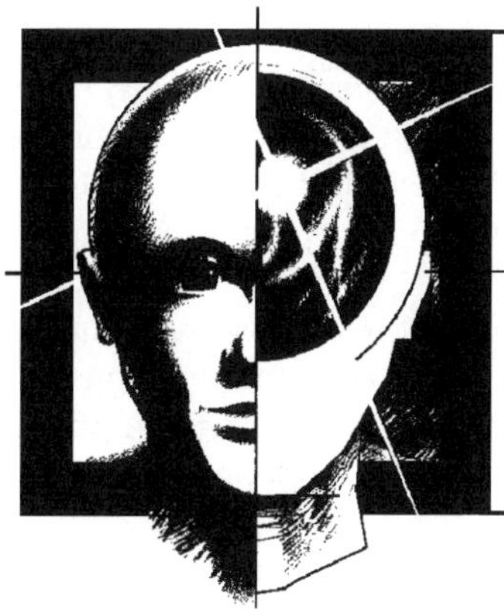

chapter 13

Aggressive Behavior

Donald P. Oswald, PhD

Assessment of Aggression in Children
Problematic Aggression
Treatment of Aggressive Behavior
Guidelines for Referral
Summary

Terry, age 8, is an active, engaging child with a quick temper. He has generally been successful in school, but recently teachers have complained of increased disruptive behavior in the classroom and on the playground. His parents have noted increased irritability at home, as well as more disagreements with neighborhood children. A number of fights at school eventually led Terry's teacher to suggest that his parents seek professional guidance regarding his behavior.

A pediatrician's interview with Terry's parents showed that he has always had a short fuse. He is prone to take offense at minimal slights and typically storms off in a rage. His developmental and family histories are unremarkable. Terry is big for his age, but a physical examination reveals no other unusual features. He is healthy, his activity level and concentration appear within normal limits, and he has no health complaints. Terry's parents want to know whether they should be concerned and what sort of treatment might be available for him.

Cases like Terry's are common in most schools and pediatric settings. Potentially problematic aggression is one of the most common behavior complaints when children are brought to the attention of professionals. What constitutes normal aggressive behavior in children? When does it become a problem? What interventions are available to treat the problem? These are the questions that parents are likely to ask when they are confronted with an aggressive child.

Assessment of Aggression in Children

Aggression is a term that has eluded a precise, universally accepted definition. In the context of child behavior, aggression is typically considered to be behavior that hurts people or destroys things or that has a high probability of hurting or destroying if it is unchecked. Efforts to elaborate on such a definition have foundered on issues such as intent to harm, physical vs. verbal aggression, level of harm resulting, awareness of the probable result, and others.

Further complicating the definition of aggression as a problem behavior is the fact that it is ubiquitous. All children and many adults display some behavior that could be labeled aggressive. Yet not all children have a problem with aggressive behavior. Thus the assessment of aggression must begin with a sense of how much aggressive behavior is typical in children.

Normal Limits of Aggressive Behavior: A Developmental Perspective

Infancy

Some parents may describe their infants as aggressive. The "difficult infant" temperament described by Thomas and Chess displays some behaviors that may be interpreted as aggression in older, stronger, better coordinated children: intense reactions, slow adaptation, unpleasant mood, and irregular rhythms.

Parents often worry that a difficult temperament in infancy foreshadows behavior problems or psychopathologic conditions in later life. Although these characteristics may be maintained into childhood, the temperament of a majority of babies changes between the first year of life and the preschool years. Thus any inclination to label an infant as aggressive should be resisted. In the absence of other developmental abnormalities, parents can be encouraged to view temperament as a feature of the baby's personality that is likely to evolve with time.

Toddlers and Preschoolers

The challenge of distinguishing problematic aggression from normal displays of independence and assertion seen throughout childhood first becomes difficult in the preschool years. At some developmental stages such displays commonly take on an aggressive quality; for example, 2- and 3-year-old children are particularly likely to display temper tantrums. Furthermore, virtually all preschoolers display some form of aggressive behavior at some point during a tantrum. They may strike out when they are disciplined or break something when they are denied their own way. Isolated incidents of such behavior during this stage are not problematic aggression. Tantrums within the normal developmental range are undoubtedly best ignored by caregivers. They tend to abate in frequency and intensity within a relatively short time, and no other intervention is required.

Preschoolers, when in a group of children, inevitably come into conflict. This conflict sometimes escalates into aggressive interchanges involving hitting, kicking, or biting others, throwing toys, or screaming and crying. Such behavior is so common in toddlers and preschoolers that it is counterproductive to call it problematic aggression, lest it be seen as indistinguishable from similar behavior in older children. All preschoolers need encouragement and help finding other ways to resolve peer conflicts, as well as clearly stated and consistently enforced rules about refraining from hurting others.

Parents and teachers are sometimes inclined to intervene too early and too often in preschoolers' conflicts, thinking they can prevent aggressive interactions. Whereas the sentiment is understandable, preschoolers need opportunities and encouragement to learn to resolve differences on their own. Caregivers can monitor conflict without taking charge of it unless the children need help negotiating a solution or restricting aggressive impulses.

Modeling effective conflict resolution without aggression is one of the most potent interventions for helping preschoolers manage aggressive impulses. Parent-parent and parent-child interactions surround the child every day and are continuously observed. Young children who are still learning alternatives to aggression in conflict resolution benefit from the example of their parents using words instead of violence, asserting themselves while retaining emotional control, and actively defusing situations that threaten to get out of hand.

Early Childhood

Aggressive play is common in the preschool and early childhood years, particularly in boys. Parents are sometime shocked to observe the level of imaginary violence in the play of young children, and may even label such play as aggression. Violent fantasy play may result from modeling the behavior of older peers and adults or from media exposure, especially television cartoons and fantasy shows. The physician can help parents by distinguishing between aggressive fantasy play, a normal developmental activity, and aggressive acts that genuinely threaten to harm.

Parents who continue to be concerned about aggressive fantasy play may be encouraged to limit and control television exposure, to be selective about their child's playmates, and to monitor the child's play more closely, encouraging alternative activities and themes. However, in the final analysis, there is little evidence to suggest that aggressive fantasy play is connected to aggressive behavior. In fact, some schools of thought maintain that such fantasy play is an alternative, socially acceptable means of expressing aggressive impulses that decreases the likelihood of real-life interpersonal violence.

General fussiness, quarreling, and increased reactivity, which sometimes escalate to aggressive behavior, are more likely when young children are tired, hungry, or bored. Parents who are questioning whether their child's periodic aggression is a problem do well to attend carefully to the circumstances surrounding the behavior to determine whether these or other routine physical states are generally associated with the child's behavior.

Middle Childhood

Middle childhood, or latency, is traditionally seen as a time of diminished problem behaviors in typical children. Intellectual, social, and emotional development have proceeded far enough to offer the child some tools for coping with emotional arousal. Aggressive impulses can be inhibited or contained so that no real damage is done; the average 9-year-old child has learned that pinching a sibling leaves no mark but that a blow to the face may produce a bloody nose and result in severe recriminations. Peer relationships are beginning to be more important, and most children have learned that aggressive interactions do not win friends. Adult relationships are still highly valued by the child of this age, who is not yet ready to overtly challenge authority; aggressive behavior threatens those relationships.

Even so, peer interactions that escalate to moderate aggression are not uncommon in middle childhood. Impulse control is imperfectly developed, and isolated incidents of aggression attest to this fact. However, by middle childhood, typical children can control the level of force used in aggressive incidents, generally ensuring that no serious harm results. Furthermore, aggression directed toward adults has largely disappeared by this time in most children.

By middle childhood, most parents have come to expect or even demand that the child demonstrate remorse following an aggressive incident. Remorse has some functional value for the child in that it tends to decrease the intensity of negative consequences. Furthermore, the absence of remorse is associated in popular thought with the amoral attitudes and behavior of people with psychopathic personalities. Parents who focus on remorse sometimes do so out of frustration and helplessness, feeling that if they cannot stop the child from behaving aggressively, at least they can insist that he subsequently demonstrate some socially approved response toward the victim. Whereas there is some apparent association between problematic aggression in children and a lack of remorse, emphasis on this association is rarely productive in individual cases. Children primarily need to learn to inhibit aggressive impulses, not to apologize sincerely after they have hurt someone.

Adolescence

By mid-adolescence, the standards for defining aggression are approaching those of adult society. Normal peer interactions in adolescence may include posturing, threatening, and ritualized aggressive behavior. Low intensity, overt aggression is not uncommon in groups of adolescents, who are generally skilled at hiding or misrepresenting both the behavior and any physical damage that ensues. However, typical adolescents are generally expected to possess the judgment and impulse control needed to limit or avoid behavior that produces harm (Box 13-1).

BOX 13-1

NORMAL AGGRESSION

Infant—Not categorized as aggressive
Toddler—Brief temper tantrums when disciplined or frustrated
Preschool—Brief altercations when in peer conflict
Early childhood—Aggressive fantasy with no genuine threats; aggressive reaction to peers or sibling agitation, especially when tired, hungry, or bored
Middle childhood—Poor impulse control
Adolescence—Same as adult

Factors Associated with Problematic Aggression

Considerable research supports transactional or biopsychosocial models for the cause of childhood aggression. Such models emphasize the complex interaction of biologic, psychologic, and social factors. Biologically based characteristics such as reactivity and impulsivity clearly put children at risk for the development of aggressive behavior (see Chapter 6 for a discussion of the biologic bases of disruptive behavior disorders).

Psychologic characteristics such as emotional relatedness and perceptual biases also play a role in the cause of aggression. Young children who fail to display the strong emotional relationship with a caregiver known as secure attachment are more likely to develop emotional or behavior problems. Deviant perception and interpretation of social interaction cues and inadequate problem solving skills are also associated with childhood aggression. Children who are unusually aggressive are more likely to interpret others' behavior as hostile, and they tend to be aware of fewer alternative responses when they feel threatened. Thus their behavior escalates relatively quickly to aggression in situations where typical children would be able to solve the problem peaceably. Although these psychologic models are not complete in themselves, they emphasize important aspects of childhood aggression and offer some directions for treatment.

Finally, social factors such as modeling, reward contingencies, and environmental stimuli also influence the likelihood of aggressive behavior. One social model with considerable empirical support tracks the development of coercive parent-child interaction cycles that serve to establish and maintain aggressive behavior. Coercion cycles occur when aggressive or disruptive behavior is rewarded by a parent giving in to a child's demands; in return, the parent is rewarded for giving in when the child temporarily stops the aggressive or disruptive behavior. However, the end result of each cycle is that the child is more likely to act out in the future.

Effective parental monitoring and discipline are two social factors that are consistently and inversely related to antisocial behavior in young children. Parents who monitor their young child's behavior appropriately and who offer firm and consistent rewards and punishments are less likely to see the child develop problematic aggression.

Another class of social influences on aggressive behavior is exposure to violence. Many children have been the victims of physical or sexual abuse or have witnessed violence in their homes or neighborhoods. Such experiences may contribute to the development of aggressive behavior, particularly if they occur repeatedly and over an extended period and if responsible adults in the child's life are unable or unwilling to protect the child.

When contributing biologic, psychologic, and social factors converge, the risk of developing problematic aggression is increased substantially. Children with difficult temperaments who are reared in stressful and violent environments with few resources to support problem solving and prosocial behavior are surrounded by a nexus of pernicious influences that markedly increase the likelihood of problematic aggressive behavior (Box 13-2).

BOX 13-2

INFLUENCES ON AGGRESSION

Biologic

Reactivity
Impulsivity

Psychologic

Emotional relatedness
Poor interpretation of social cues
Poor problem solving skills

Social

Violent behaviors of parents
Violent behaviors in the media
Parental monitoring and discipline

Stability of Aggressive Behavior

A common concern among parents of aggressive children is that the behavior portends a career of aggressive and criminal activity extending into adulthood. When children are young, this worry is often disproportional to the severity of the problem. Parents can be reassured that there are effective means of reducing aggressive behavior in childhood and that the progression to adult antisocial behavior is not inevitable.

Nevertheless, the concern is not without some basis in reality. Young children who are more aggressive do tend to continue to be more aggressive throughout childhood. In fact, aggression is one of the most stable childhood behavior syndromes identified. Although overall, the rate of aggression tends to decrease as children grow older, the level of aggression that a child shows compared with that of his peers remains much the same; the most aggressive preschoolers tend to be the most aggressive third graders and the most aggressive adolescents. Furthermore, the "early starters," the children whose early conduct problems persist through childhood, have the most negative prognosis.

The apparent contradiction regarding stability rests on the fact that although aggression can be successfully treated, the interventions are rarely simple or short-term. The conditions that tend to produce aggressive children (such as family chaos, inadequate supervision, parental psychopathologic disorders, antisocial peers, and adult modeling of aggression) also make it difficult to initiate and sustain comprehensive, stable, environmental changes. Thus parents who are concerned and who have the resources to devote to their child's treatment can expect to see positive results, but those parents who have limited resources for treatment and support, who fail to acknowledge the behavior as a problem, or who are for some other reason unable to significantly alter the environment in which the family lives have good reason to be concerned about their child's future.

Aggressive children often become aggressive adolescents. However, not all aggressive adolescents have a history of aggressive behavior in childhood. There is emerging support for a second major pathway for the development of conduct problems in youth. Although the data are less consistent, a consensus is building that a large group of youth begin to show conduct problems, including aggressive behavior, for the first time in adolescence. In such cases, association with deviant peers may play an important part in the onset of antisocial behavior. These adolescents, compared with those who have a long history of aggression, tend to display less violent behavior and are more likely to desist as they grow older, but they are far more numerous.

Understanding Current Social Influences on Aggressive Behavior

One of the most common ways of understanding aggressive behavior emphasizes the social aspect of etiologic models. Designated as functional analysis, this approach examines the environment in which aggression occurs for clues about controlling influences. Whereas an extended discussion of the functional analysis of aggressive behavior is impractical in this context, the fundamental principle of functional analysis can be stated simply. In many children, aggressive behavior is elicited by some specific event, such as peer teasing or demands by an authority figure, or it is inadvertently rewarded by naturally occurring consequences, such as getting one's way or increased parental attention. Probing the circumstances surrounding aggressive incidents often yields productive hypotheses about the function of the behavior. The goal of functional analysis is to identify the eliciting events and consequences that tend to evoke aggressive responses from a specific child. An understanding of these events and consequences and their relationship to aggression often leads to practical, common sense changes that parents can make in their behavior and in the home environment that reduce the likelihood of aggressive acts.

Problematic Aggression

Efforts to clarify problematic aggression have taken a variety of forms. However, the most common approaches are to view aggressive behavior as a failure in the child's socialization or to interpret it in the context of a psychiatric disorder. In either case, further assessment is required to determine a reasonable response.

Differential Diagnosis

Aggression is best understood as a class of behaviors, not a diagnosis. Aggressive behavior is a prominent feature of several child psychiatric disorders and is a characteristic related to many more. The chief differential diagnostic task in treating an aggressive child is to determine which disorder, if any, lies at the root of the aggression.

Child Psychiatric Disorders with Aggression as a Defining Characteristic

Two common childhood diagnoses, characterized as disruptive behavior disorders, include specific mention of aggressive behavior in their diagnostic criteria. Oppositional defiant disorder (ODD) is generally described as a pattern of negative, defiant, disobedient, and hostile behavior toward authority figures. The behavior must occur more often than is typically observed in children of the same age and developmental level. Conduct disorder (CD) is a repetitive and persistent pattern of behavior in which a child violates the basic rights of others, as well as major age-appropriate societal norms and rules. Key diagnostic criteria for these two disorders may be found in Boxes 13-3 and 13-4.

These criteria are primarily descriptions of disturbing behaviors that are likely to occur together. The descriptions offer no insight into reasons for the behaviors and do not rule out other important factors that may be exacerbating the aggression. In fact, children with CD or ODD are at a substantially increased risk for internalizing disorders, such as anxiety or depression. Children with ODD or CD should be routinely

DSM-IV DIAGNOSTIC CRITERIA

BOX 13-3 OPPOSITIONAL DEFIANT DISORDER

A. A pattern of negativistic, hostile, and defiant behavior lasting at least 6 months, during which four (or more) of the following are present:

(1) often loses temper
(2) often argues with adults
(3) often actively defies or refuses to comply with adults' requests or rules
(4) often deliberately annoys people
(5) often blames others for his or her mistakes or misbehavior
(6) is often touchy or easily annoyed by others
(7) is often angry and resentful
(8) is often spiteful or vindictive

Note: Consider a criterion met only if the behavior occurs more frequently than is typically observed in individuals of comparable age and developmental level.

B. The disturbance in behavior causes clinically significant impairment in social, academic, or occupational functioning.

C. The behaviors do not occur exclusively during the course of a Psychotic or Mood Disorder.

D. Criteria are not met for Conduct Disorder, and, if the individual is age 18 years or older, criteria are not met for Antisocial Personality Disorder.

(From American Psychiatric Association: *Diagnostic and statistical manual of mental disorders,* ed 4 [DSM-IV], Washington DC, 1994, American Psychiatric Press.)

DSM-IV DIAGNOSTIC CRITERIA

BOX 13-4 CONDUCT DISORDER

A. A repetitive and persistent pattern of behavior in which the basic rights of others or major age-appropriate societal norms or rules are violated, as manifested by the presence of three (or more) of the following criteria in the past 12 months, with at least one criterion present in the past 6 months:

Aggression to people and animals
(1) often bullies, threatens, or intimidates others
(2) often initiates physical fights
(3) has used a weapon that can cause serious physical harm to others (e.g., a bat, brick, broken bottle, knife, gun)
(4) has been physically cruel to people
(5) has been physically cruel to animals
(6) has stolen while confronting a victim (e.g., mugging, purse snatching, extortion, armed robbery)
(7) has forced someone into sexual activity

Destruction of property
(8) has deliberately engaged in fire setting with the intention of causing serious damage
(9) has deliberately destroyed others' property (other than by fire setting)

Deceitfulness or theft
(10) has broken into someone else's house, building, or car
(11) often lies to obtain goods or favors or to avoid obligations (i.e., "cons" others)
(12) has stolen items of nontrivial value without confronting a victim (e.g., shoplifting, but without breaking and entering; forgery)

Serious violations of rules
(13) often stays out at night despite parental prohibitions, beginning before age 13 years
(14) has run away from home overnight at least twice while living in parental or parental surrogate home (or once without returning for a lengthy period)
(15) is often truant from school, beginning before age 13 years

B. The disturbance in behavior causes causes clinically significant impairment in social, academic, or occupational functioning.

C. If the individual is age 18 years or older, criteria are not met for Antisocial Personality Disorder.

Specify type based on age at onset:
Childhood-Onset Type: onset of at least one criterion characteristic of Conduct Disorder prior to age 10 years
Adolescent-Onset Type: absence of any criteria characteristic of Conduct Disorder prior to age 10 years

Specify severity:
Mild: few if any conduct problems in excess of those required to make the diagnosis **and** conduct problems cause only minor harm to others
Moderate: number of conduct problems and effect on others intermediate between "mild" and "severe"
Severe: many conduct problems in excess of those required to make the diagnosis **or** conduct problems cause considerable harm to others

(From American Psychiatric Association: *Diagnostic and statistical manual of mental disorders,* ed 4 [DSM-IV], Washington DC, 1994, American Psychiatric Press.)

screened for other psychiatric symptoms.

Intermittent explosive disorder is a diagnosis given relatively seldom in childhood, and children with intermittent explosive disorder commonly display other developmental delays or abnormalities as well. This disorder also explicitly includes aggressive behavior as a defining characteristic. Key diagnostic criteria are found in Box 13-5.

Childhood Psychiatric Disorders Commonly Associated with Aggression

Other common childhood disorders do not include aggressive behavior as a diagnostic feature but may predispose children to display more aggression than is typical. A core feature of attention-deficit/hyperactivity dis-

BOX 13-5 INTERMITTENT EXPLOSIVE DISORDER (DSM-IV DIAGNOSTIC CRITERIA)

A. Several discrete episodes of failure to resist aggressive impulses that result in serious assaultive acts or destruction of property.

B. The degree of aggressiveness expressed during the episodes is grossly out of proportion to any precipitating psychosocial stressors.

C. The aggressive episodes are not better accounted for by another mental disorder (e.g., Antisocial Personality Disorder, Borderline Personality Disorder, a Psychotic Disorder, a Manic Episode, Conduct Disorder, or Attention-Deficit/Hyperactivity Disorder) and are not due to the direct physiologic effects of a substance (e.g., a drug of abuse, a medication) or a general medical condition (e.g., head trauma, Alzheimer's disease).

(From American Psychiatric Association: *Diagnostic and statistical manual of mental disease,* ed 4 [DSM-IV], Washington DC, 1994, American Psychiatric Press.)

order (ADHD) is hyperactivity-impulsivity, a characteristic that is likely to lead to potentially dangerous or harmful behavior without consideration of the consequences. Problematic aggression is common in children with ADHD.

Some children with mental retardation display aggression as an associated feature, often as a substitute for verbal communication. Children with pervasive developmental disorders (PDD), such as autistic disorder, are often aggressive, particularly if they have severe social and communication deficits. Families that display parent-child relational problems often complain of problematic aggression in their children, and aggression is sometimes a part of the symptom picture of childhood depression. Aggression may also occur during periods of delirium or in association with substance intoxication or substance withdrawal. Finally, aggressive behavior is sometimes a component of personality changes associated with a specific medical condition, such as brain injury following head trauma.

The symptom of aggression is common in many childhood psychiatric disorders and, of itself, is not associated with any single treatment of choice (Box 13-6). Differential diagnosis in the treatment of aggression involves assessing the possible sources of the aggressive behavior, including developmental features and distinguishable associated psychopathologic disorders.

The clinical interventions discussed in the following section target aggressive behavior. Physicians who are treating an aggressive behavior should concurrently assess the child for other psychiatric disorders that may be contributing to the problem. Children who display other symptoms in addition to aggression are unlikely to respond optimally to these interventions until the other disorders are also adequately treated.

BOX 13-6

DIAGNOSES ASSOCIATED WITH AGGRESSION

Aggression is often seen

Oppositional defiant disorder
Conduct disorder
Intermittent explosive disorder

Aggression may be seen

Attention-deficit/hyperactivity disorder
Mental retardation
Pervasive developmental disorders
Parent-child relational problems

BOX 13-7

STAGES IN THE TREATMENT OF AGGRESSIVE BEHAVIOR

Guidance and support for parents
Behavior management training for parents
Working with the school
Social skills training for children
Impulse control and anger management for children
Pharmacotherapy

Treatment of Aggressive Behavior

Treatment options for the aggressive child are many and varied, ranging in intensity from the single-contact consultation to inpatient, psychiatric hospitalization. In this section we describe some commonly employed treatment strategies used with children in clinical settings (Box 13-7). These methods may be used successively or in tandem.

Guidance and Support for Parents

Many parents feel a need for periodic consultation regarding their child's behavior. This may range from brief telephone consultation on an as-needed basis to a series of regular, weekly sessions with a physician. Some parents merely need to be reassured that their instincts are correct and to be encouraged to stick with a plan through a difficult time, whereas others are genuinely unprepared to face the continuous new challenges from their children.

In the context of parental guidance and support, the physician helps the parent solve problems related to the child's behavior. Issues regarding whether the child's level of aggression is abnormal, such as those addressed earlier in this chapter, are common. Also common are basic questions about discipline. Parents can be given some simple guidelines regarding discipline that cover many uncomplicated problems of aggression in young children. Some of these guidelines are detailed in the following list of suggestions:

- Develop disciplinary alternatives to spanking.

  Although few parents who use spanking pay attention to a physician's advice to abandon it entirely, most can be easily encouraged to begin using other consequences as alternatives to spanking, such as time out or removal of privileges. Many parents can accept the logic that if a behavior such as aggression is not decreased after two or three spankings, it is unlikely that more of the same will help.
- Spend scheduled, positive, child-oriented time with your child.

  Particularly if part of the parent's plan is to implement punishments more firmly and consistently, he should be encouraged to schedule specific, regular blocks of time in which the child chooses the activity and has the parent's undivided attention. Twenty minutes a day of such time may help determine whether any other rewards or punishments have any effect on the child's behavior.
- Agree on the rules about behavior and consequences, make them clear, and stick with them.

  If parents don't agree on the rules, they will never work. Children come equipped with a natural ability to detect and exploit discrepancies between parents' rules. Repeatedly bending the family rules teaches children how to manipulate parents to get what they want.
- Don't give a direction unless you are willing to make sure it is followed.

  "Nattering" (that is, repeating directions and threats without additional consequences for noncompliance) is one of the hallmarks of ineffective discipline. When given a clear direction, the child should either follow the direction or be given a time out. If a parent isn't willing to insist on this, she can turn the direction into a request or a suggestion with an incentive for complying and allow the child the choice of earning the incentive or passing it up.

BOX 13-8

GUIDANCE AND SUPPORT FOR PARENTS

guidelines for discipline

- Develop disciplinary alternatives to spanking.
- Spend scheduled, positive, child-oriented time with your child.
- Agree on the rules about behavior and consequences, make them clear, and stick with them.
- Don't give a direction unless you are willing to make sure it is followed.

Guidance for parents of latency-age children and adolescents commonly involves helping parents adjust to the normal, increasing demands for independence without abdicating their roles as heads of the family. As children grow older, parents cannot and should not try to physically control the child's behavior. Attempts to do so generally make situations worse and often result in one or both parties getting hurt. Parents often need reminders that even though they cannot absolutely control their child's behavior, they are still in charge of the consequences of that behavior; through the manipulation of consequences, they can exercise some influence over the choices the child makes regarding her behavior (Box 13-8).

Behavior Management Training for Parents

Some parents of aggressive children are unable to use the suggestions offered in a brief parental guidance context because they do not understand them or lack the skills to carry them out. Others find themselves caught in recurring negative interactions with their children that escalate to aggression by the children, the parents, or both. Such parents need more intensive support in learning these fundamental parenting skills.

Community agencies and parent groups often offer such training programs at reasonable costs. One popular curriculum is the Systematic Training for Effective Parenting (STEP) program. Such parent training programs typically emphasize providing information about child rearing and child discipline, on the assumption that the participants know how to apply the information in their own family, with the necessary modifications, and are able to demonstrate the skills involved with little direct training and supervised practice. Parents who benefit from such programs are generally bright, educated, emotionally stable, and able to work together without significant marital conflict. The children for whom such programs are effective are typically those whose aggressive behavior is less severe and less long-standing.

When these parent and child characteristics are not present, parent training may need to take a different course. Forehand and McMahon produced a structured parent training program that is intended to be presented in a series of clinician-parent sessions. Involving substantial actual practice of the requisite skills, the approach is tailored to meet the needs of parents who are unable to benefit from group or information-based training. A significant component of the program emphasizes teaching the parent to do things with the child that foster a more positive relationship. Although the management of difficult behavior is a key skill included in the program, parents are taught that reconnecting with their children as positive, nurturing caregivers comes first. Subsequent sessions teach parents how to recognize ineffective directions, how to give effective directions, and how to use time out.

Working with the School

Some children display aggressive behavior only in specific settings, such as in school or even only in a particular classroom. In such cases, the first task of treatment is to determine what features of the setting are related to the aggressive behavior. Often even young children whose aggression is setting-specific can verbally identify what it is about the setting that bothers them. Talking with the child about the problem and encouraging parents to do the same often suggests a direction for intervention. Aggression in early and middle childhood is sometimes associated with significant academic weaknesses that are making the child's school experience unusually unpleasant. Remediating the weaknesses or placing the child in an academic setting that allows her to compensate for the weakness may reduce aggression and other behavior problems.

However, aggressive children often display problem behavior across settings, including school. Guidelines for parents in this case are given in the following list:

- Communicate regularly with the classroom teacher.

  Parents can be encouraged to set up a system of daily written communication with the teacher and frequent face-to-face contacts to ensure that all of the adults in the child's life are working together.
- Get to know the other people at the school who might offer support.

  Guidance counselors, school psychologists, school nurses, principals, and assistant principals are some of the school personnel likely to come in contact with a child who has behavior problems. Parents who are personally acquainted with these people have a better chance of working out a plan that serves the best interests of their children.
- Be present in the school building. If possible, volunteer in the classroom or for other school activities.

  Children who see their parents and teachers working together find it easier to control their behavior at home and at school.
- Let the school personnel know who else in the community is involved with the child.

  Communication among teachers, counselors, and pediatricians about the child's progress allows everyone to work more effectively.
- Get to know your rights as a parent.

  Parents' rights and responsibilities are most clearly spelled out for children in special education. School personnel are required to inform these parents of their rights, but many times this information is not emphasized or is presented in a way that renders it minimally helpful. Informed parents are in a better position to be advocates for their children (Box 13-9).

Some classroom interventions have shown considerable promise reducing aggressive behavior in more severely affected children. Contingency management (behavior modification) programs can have long-term, positive effects on this group, significantly reducing their aggressive behavior. Physicians should remember, however, that the effects of such a program, at least the short-term effects, are generally limited to the setting in which the program occurs. If a child displays aggression across settings (home, school, community), a contingency management program in school may result in reduced aggression in school, but the child's behavior in other settings may remain a problem or grow even worse. Nevertheless, success with a classroom contingency management program offers valuable information about the child's ability to inhibit aggression in a context where expectations are clear, adaptive behavior is rewarded, limits are enforced, and consequences are consistently applied.

Social Skills Training for Children

Some views of aggression emphasize the aggressive child's limited repertoire of cognitive and behavioral skills related to successful peer and adult interaction. This perspective has yielded skills training programs

BOX 13-9

PARENT WORKING WITH SCHOOLS

- Communicate regularly with the classroom teacher.
- Get to know the other people at the school who might offer support.
- Be present in the school building.
- Let the school personnel know who else in the community is involved with the child.
- Get to know your rights as a parent.

that are generally implemented in small groups of children who have been identified as aggressive. One such program consists of a series of small group activities designed to teach prosocial peer interaction skills, which are reinforced by regular rehearsal in a role-play context. Stable, positive changes in behavior and in peer perceptions have resulted from this program. Such programs are most commonly implemented in school settings by a guidance counselor or similar staff person. Less often, community based clinics offer social skills training groups for children. This approach has the advantage of teaching and reinforcing children's social interaction skills and is more likely to lead to behavior changes that generalize across settings.

In the absence of ongoing groups to which a child can be referred, many physicians choose to implement social skills training in the context of individual child or family therapy. The key steps for teaching social skills are: (1) presenting the target skill by describing it to the child and discussing when it is relevant; (2) demonstrating the skill by modeling for the child exactly how it might be used; (3) asking the child to rehearse the skill and giving feedback and reward for approximations; (4) role playing example situations that call for use of the skill and giving the child feedback and reinforcement; and (5) giving the child an assignment involving practice of the skill in real-life settings outside the clinical setting.

Social skills that are often taught in this manner include initiating and sustaining social interaction with peers, paying attention to peers' words and nonverbal communication, ignoring teasing and provocation, joining an ongoing group activity, accepting positive or negative feedback, saying "no" to stay out of trouble, asking for clarification when one doesn't understand, and stopping to think before acting. Instruction and rehearsal of these skills and reinforcement for practicing them in the real world can help reduce aggressive behavior in children who are undersocialized.

Impulse Control and Anger Management for Children

Programs that emphasize impulse control and anger management are an extension of the social skills training programs described above. Typically more intensive and more focused on aggression and its precursors, such programs represent another option for treating childhood aggression.

The study of cognitive characteristics that distinguish aggressive children has yielded some valuable findings that can inform impulse control and anger management training. Moderately and severely aggressive children are known to display abnormalities in social perception and attribution; severely aggressive children are uniquely deficient in social problem solving skills. These findings suggest that moderately aggressive children may be more planned and proactive in their aggression, whereas severely aggressive children may be more reactive to social cues.

Impulse control and anger management programs typically focus on a set of cognitive and behavioral objectives in the domains of problem solving, perspective taking, means-end thinking, affect identification and awareness, and prosocial skill development. Such programs are not uncommon in some school settings, but they may also be implemented in inpatient, day-treatment, or outpatient psychiatric settings. Although these programs are often part of group therapy sessions, many physicians include components of impulse control and anger management programs in their individual work with children and in their therapy with families.

Programs such as these are most applicable to late middle childhood and adolescence. They tend to be applied to patients who demonstrate marked inability to control their behavior when aroused and angry. Some anger management training programs emphasize self-statements, or things that children can say to themselves when faced with a difficult situation. One such program teaches self-statements associated with each phase of the situation. In the following list, self-statements in parentheses correspond to the phases of a confrontation: preparing for provocation (Keep cool. Remember don't get angry.); impact and confrontation (I'm not going to let him get to me.); coping with arousal (Take it easy. Time to take a deep breath.); and reflecting on the provocation (That wasn't too hard; I stayed calm and got through it.)

Pharmacotherapy

Treating aggressive behavior with medication makes the most sense when the aggression is associated with some identifiable psychiatric diagnosis that can be effectively treated with medication. Examples include ADHD (see Chapter 5), depressive disorder (see Chapter 8), and psychosis (see Chapter 10). In such cases, appropriate pharmacotherapy for the identified diagnosis often results in a decrease in the child's aggressive behavior.

The literature on medication used to specifically target aggressive behavior in children is limited, and results are not particularly hopeful. Open studies of the use of β-blockers (for example, propranolol) for this purpose have been encouraging; 75% to 85% of the subjects have shown improvement. However, no controlled clinical trials of β-blockers have yet been conducted, so firm conclusions regarding their efficacy cannot be drawn.

Based on findings from animal studies, some researchers have hypothesized that aggression in children may be associated with defects in GABA neurotransmission in the brain. This hypothesis has led to investigation of the effects of clonidine, a drug that stimulates release of GABA in animal brains, in the treatment of aggressive behavior. Some highly aggressive children and adolescents have shown decreased aggression and minimal side effects in an open clinical trial of clonidine. The improvement was found to be associated with increased plasma GABA levels in children who were compliant with the medication directions.

Haloperidol has shown some effects in the treatment of aggressive conduct disorders in a controlled clinical trial, but children displayed some untoward effects. Other antipsychotics are also reported to be clinically effective in severely aggressive children, although there are few controlled trials of their use for this purpose. Early positive results using lithium in the treatment of aggressive behavior have not been consistently replicated, although the use of lithium in clinical settings is common. A recent double-blind study of inpatients preselected as potential lithium responders concluded that the risk and inconvenience of treatment with lithium outweighed its minimal benefits.

Psychopharmacologic treatment of aggression and other forms of disruptive behavior is covered in more detail in Chapter 6. Although the use of medication for the treatment of aggressive behavior is not uncommon in many primary care settings, many physicians prefer to refer such children to a psychiatrist, particularly if the initial response to treatment is limited or mixed.

Guidelines for Referral

Many children who display aggression are treated successfully in a pediatric primary care setting. However, there are some markers that generally clearly indicate a need to refer the child for a different or a more intensive intervention. Several of these indicators are discussed in the following paragraphs.

Evidence of Serious Emotional Disturbance

Aggressive behavior, in and of itself, does not necessarily constitute an emotional disturbance. However, aggression is commonly associated with psychiatric disorders that may respond to treatment. A comprehensive psychiatric evaluation should be among the first steps in the assessment of aggression in children. Physicians who are not comfortable conducting such an evaluation themselves should obtain a consultation or refer the child for evaluation before initiating treatment.

Intractable Aggression in Young Children

Young children who display aggressive behavior that does not respond to parental guidance and support may require more intensive treatment. Such a pattern may reflect a developmental disorder, a more serious psychiatric or emotional disturbance, or the presence of maladaptive family interaction patterns.

Parents' reports of aggression in young children should be followed up regularly until the problem is resolved. Some parents habituate to their child's behavior and do not raise the issue again unless they are specifically asked about it, even though earlier interventions have not worked. Physicians do well to maintain a fairly low threshold for referring young children with serious, intractable aggression for more intensive treatment.

Maladaptive Family Patterns of Behavior

Treating aggression in children nearly always involves work with the family at some level. However, the physician sometimes observes regular, maladaptive patterns of interaction among the family that seem to be associated with the aggression. Examples of common maladaptive patterns are excessive blaming of the aggressive child, marital conflict that places the child between fighting parents, and abdication of parental rights and responsibilities by giving them over to a child. In such cases, interventions with the child's family are seen as the primary means of dealing with aggressive behavior. Family therapists generally explore aspects of family functioning that maintain the child's aggressive behavior. The work of family therapy may involve aspects of many of the interventions described above; however, there is typically more attention given to the way each member of the family system influences, or is influenced by, the problem that brought them to therapy.

The various perspectives on family therapy emphasize different aspects of family functioning. Structural family therapy, for example, emphasizes the way the parts of the family system work together. Key concepts in structural family therapy include boundaries (who is in and who is out with regard to specific family operations such as decision making), alignment (how the members join or oppose one another in carrying out family operations such as conflict resolution), and power (the relative influence of each family member on the outcome of an activity). Therapists seek to identify and point out family patterns in each of these areas and to help the family make changes in those patterns that contribute to current problems.

Many different models exist for approaching work with families, and there are few data regarding the relative efficacy of the interventions arising from these models. Physicians who possess a general background in family therapy concepts are better equipped to recognize systemic problems in the family and to intervene effectively or refer for more intensive treatment.

Presence of Physical Abuse

Whereas aggressive behavior of itself is not a reliable indicator of physical abuse, children who are physically abused often become aggressive toward others. Furthermore, children who tend to be excessively aggressive are more likely to elicit severe punishment—punishment that can sometimes, through frustration or impulsive anger, evolve into child abuse. When an aggressive child or his parents report adult behavior that is abusive, the physician is obliged make a report to the local CPS agency. The child does not differ from any other child in this respect, and the fact that he displays aggression does not alter the mandate to report abusive behavior.

In some cases, an aggressive child who has been abused may require more intensive treatment than most primary care providers are prepared to offer. The alternatives for treating the aggressive behavior in an abused child are the same as for any child. However, a history of traumatic abuse may make the patient less responsive to some of the approaches outlined above until some resolution is achieved with regard to the thoughts, feelings, and images associated with the abuse (see Chapter 16).

Need for Special Education Services

Children whose aggressive behavior occurs mostly in school may be experiencing specific, school-related problems that indicate a need for special education services. If aggression is paired with academic failure or significant underachievement in school, a referral for a special education evaluation should be considered. Physicians can be helpful in this process by discussing with parents their rights regarding referral for evaluation, by supporting them in their efforts to work with school personnel, and, at the parents' request, by communicating directly with school staff involved in decisions about special education referral, evaluation, and placement.

Children whose aggressive behavior is seen at home and in the community, as well as in school, are also often appropriate candidates for special education services. In such cases, the physician is generally involved not only in the initial referral and evaluation process, but also in ongoing communication and collaboration with the family and the child's teachers, guidance counselors, principal, therapist, and any other professionals who are working with the child. Collaboration with educators is an essential component of effective treatment for children in special education services.

Criminal Behavior

The onset of criminal aggressive behavior clearly indicates a need for more intensive professional involvement. Whether or not the child has gotten involved with the juvenile justice system, criminal aggressive activity indicates that some aspect of the child's development has gone significantly awry. Although mental health treatment may not always be necessary, a child who is beginning to display criminal aggression is presenting the family, school, and community with a major challenge. Most families benefit from professional consultation regarding the best way to respond to the incident and welcome an opinion regarding whether the child is experiencing other psychiatric symptoms related to the aggression.

Summary

The treatment of aggression is a common demand on any physician who serves children and their families. Aggressive behavior generally elicits adult attention quickly and motivates the child's family and community system to respond. Primary care providers are commonly the first professionals called on when aggression emerges as a problem. The physician's tasks in such cases include helping the family determine whether the aggression is a problem, initial assessment and treatment, and referral for more intensive treatment as needed. Throughout this process, the physician plays a critical role by monitoring the child's progress, supporting the child's family through the challenges associated with the problem, and collaborating with the family and other professionals to ensure coordination of treatment efforts. Whether serving as the treatment provider, as a source of emotional support, or as a goad to the family and community system, the physician bears a key responsibility in ensuring that appropriate and effective interventions are provided for children's aggressive behavior.

CONSIDER CONSULTATION WHEN . . .

- There is evidence of serious emotional disturbance
- There is intractable aggression in young children
- There are maladaptive family patterns of behavior
- There is physical abuse
- Special education services are needed
- There is criminal behavior

Annotated Bibliography

Finch AJ, Nelson WM, Moss JH: *Childhood aggression: cognitive-behavioral therapy strategies and interventions.* In Finch AJ, Nelson WM, Ott ES, editors: *Cognitive-behavioral procedures with children and adolescents,* Boston, 1993, Allyn and Bacon.

This chapter offers a conceptual framework for understanding childhood aggression and suggestions for evaluation tactics, with a focus on anger assessment. The bulk of the chapter, however, consists of extensive descriptions of cognitive-behavioral interventions for aggressive children and session-by-session guidelines for one treatment protocol.

Forehand R, McMahon RJ: *Helping the noncompliant child: a clinician's guide to parent training,* New York, 1981, Guilford Press.

An older resource but still among the best of its type, this manual offers detailed instructions for a structured program of training for parents of noncompliant children. Because aggression and noncompliance are commonly linked in children, the program is highly relevant for the problem of aggression as well. *Helping the noncompliant child* helps physicians teach parents the skills that may prevent children's behavior from escalating to aggression.

Gurman AS, Kniskern DP: *Handbook of family therapy,* vol 2, New York, 1991, Brunner/Mazel.

An extension of the first volume published in 1981, this work represents a valuable resource for physicians working with families of children with aggressive behavior. Although no amount of reading can replace live supervised experience in treating families, this volume offers a broad overview of the most popular schools of thought in family therapy. Readers can gain an excellent background in the key concepts involved in a variety of approaches to working with families.

Kazdin AE, Siegel TC, Bass D: Cognitive problem-solving skills training and parent management training in the treatment of antisocial behavior in children, *J Consult Clin Psychol* 60:733-747, 1992.

A model study of clinical intervention with children, this paper demonstrates the efficacy of problem-solving training and the added impact of parent management training. Kazdin, Siegel, and Bass not only demonstrate exemplary methodology but offer substantial detail on clinical issues and implications.

Patterson GR, Reid JB, Dishion TJ: *Antisocial boys,* Eugene, Ore., 1992, Castalia.

This volume represents the latest in a series authored by Patterson and colleagues. This body of work describes the most carefully executed, long-term program of research on aggressive and other antisocial behavior in children. Patterson has moved the field forward immeasurably with conceptual and methodological innovation and a commitment to remaining grounded in the real world of clinical work with aggressive children.

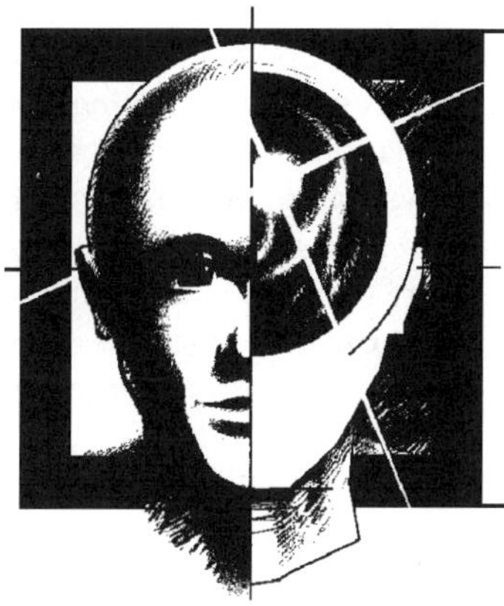

chapter 14

The Suicidal Child or Adolescent

David J. Mullen, MD and Robert L. Hendren, DO

Suicide in Children and Adolescents
Assessing Suicidal Risk
Treatment Plan and Disposition
Case Analysis
Summary

Christi, a 16-year-old girl, comes to the office of Dr. Richard Edwards, a family physician, complaining of persistent fatigue and insomnia. Dr. Edwards takes a focal history and performs a limited physical examination. Although he notes no obvious medical pathologic disorder, he notices that Christi appears distinctly sad and speaks in a low, soft voice with little emotional inflection. Her conjunctivae are slightly red, and her eyes are somewhat puffy, as if she had been crying often. He decides to inquire about her mood and says, "You know, you look like you might be feeling kind of down. How have things been going for you lately?"

Christi, who now begins to cry softly, answers that her life has been terrible since her boyfriend broke up with her about 6 weeks ago. She finds that she cries several times during the day, and at times she feels like she can't stop. She feels tired constantly but has trouble falling asleep, and she says she often wakes up in the middle of the night and can't return to sleep. During the day she has difficulty concentrating, and she feels that this is affecting her grades. She ruminates about the break-up often, wondering what she could have done to make him want to end the relationship. She feels both hopeless and helpless, and she states that sometimes she just wants to leave everything behind.

At this point, after noting multiple depressive symptoms and the reference to escape, Dr. Edwards asks about support people with whom she has been able to share her feelings. Christi now begins to cry harder and states emphatically, "No one." She reveals that she recently changed schools after a family move, and her best friend moved away unexpectedly about 3 months ago. Furthermore, she is afraid that she would just bring everybody down with her problems. She also describes herself as shy and finds it difficult to meet new people. When asked about family members, Christi says that her father—an accountant for the state government—is always busy. Her stepmother (Christi's mother died when she was 6 years old) is described as nice but remote, and their relationship has always been somewhat superficial.

Dr. Edwards then inquires directly whether she has

thought of taking her life. "Often people who are feeling very depressed think about killing themselves. I wonder if you have thought about it." Christi slowly nods yes. She reveals that she has been thinking a lot about dying over the past few days and has begun to consider specific methods, including wrist slashing and overdosing on her father's high blood pressure medication. Dr. Edwards has now become substantially concerned about Christi's potential for suicidal behavior, and he is considering a psychiatric consultation.

Suicide in Children and Adolescents

The need to evaluate the suicide potential of a child or adolescent is likely to occur at some point in the practice of any physician who works with this population. Eighty-five percent of adolescents who complete suicide expressed their suicidal thoughts to others before their attempt. Suicide is a substantial cause of mortality in the United States and ranks as the third leading cause of death in adolescents. The overall rate of suicide has increased substantially during the second half of the twentieth century and has nearly tripled since 1950.

Although completed suicide is relatively rare before age 14, even the suicide rate of young children has doubled since 1960. Suicide has been documented in every socioeconomic, racial, and ethnic group, but in the United States, white boys are the most common victims of suicide. Native American youth are also at high risk for suicide, particularly among tribes with a greater degree of acculturation. Although girls attempt suicide approximately 3 times more often than boys, boys actually kill themselves 5 times more often than girls. This discrepancy is largely because of the more lethal and violent means selected by boys (self-inflicted gunshot wounds vs. overdosing). However, there is some evidence that girls are beginning to use guns more often, particularly in geographic areas where handguns are more abundant. These sobering facts obligate any physician working with young people to be aware of the reality of suicidal behavior in the young and the corresponding need to develop skills in the assessment of child or adolescent suicide potential. In this chapter, we explore the process of such an evaluation, including specific interviewing techniques, risk factors for suicidal behavior, and patient management issues confronting the physician.

Assessing Suicidal Risk

Establishing Rapport: The Clinical Interview

The assessment of the suicidal youth involves three interrelated steps: (1) establish rapport; (2) elicit risk factors and information; and (3) determine the initial disposition and treatment plan. A good clinical interview is the most effective means of accomplishing this assessment process. The evaluation of a suicidal child or adolescent requires the physician to be familiar with developmentally appropriate interviewing techniques that establish adequate rapport with the young person. Without appropriate techniques, the physician may face considerable obstacles when gathering the information necessary to determine the degree of risk and the appropriate disposition and treatment plan (Box 14-1). To accomplish the goals of an interview, a skilled interviewer does all of the following: (1) allows the patient to tell his own story while maintaining an organized interview; (2) employs language appropriate to the patient's age and background; (3) uses tact in framing questions that relate to sensitive matters; (4) moves effectively from one area of questioning to another; (5) allows the patient to express feelings; and (6) conveys an understanding and empathy for the patients' feelings.

Allowing the patient to tell his own story helps the patient feel both understood and respected as a person, and maintaining some organization allows the coverage of all relevant domains of information. For all patients, the physician should be sensitive to the degree of verbal sophistication required to ensure that the patient is able to adequately express his feelings verbally. It is important to select an appropriate vocabulary. The use of tact is mandatory, particularly when dealing with adolescents, who are often exquisitely sensitive to potential slights. Smooth transitions between areas of questioning allow for better elaboration of the patient's story and therefore more complete information. Additionally, abrupt transitions can confuse the patient and contribute to impaired rapport. The patient's expression of feelings is an important aspect of assessing the patient's emotional status, and an interview that inhibits emotional expression is unlikely to effectively establish adequate rapport. Demonstration of accurate em-

BOX 14-1

ASSESSING THE SUICIDAL PATIENT

- Establish rapport with the young person.
- Allow patient to tell his own story.
- Use language appropriate to patient's age and background.
- Use tact in forming questions.
- Move smoothly from one topic to another.
- Allow the patient to express feelings.
- Convey empathy for the young person's feelings.
- Elicit risk factors known to be associated with suicide in young people.
- Determine the need for inpatient or outpatient treatment based on risks and protective factors.

pathy for the patient is an effective means of helping the patient feel understood. The patient may also feel much relief and support.

The skilled interviewer adjusts the interview approach according to the age and developmental level of the patient. Generally, most physicians find that beginning the interview with a few questions that cover neutral areas, such as place of residence or composition of the family, before moving to more problematic areas helps establish initial rapport, particularly with young patients. Developmentally appropriate interviewing for the young child may mean that the physician utilizes and recognizes play and fantasy as a means of communication. Drawing is also an effective means of self-expression that may at times be preferred over more verbal modes. Although verbal techniques are usually preferred for adolescent patients, the physician must maintain flexibility, since some older children may also benefit from the use of nonverbal methods.

The adolescent is best interviewed with simple, direct questions rather than vague, open-ended inquires. The teenager is likely to resist a more indirect approach to information gathering. When interviewing the adolescent, the physician must recognize the impact of adolescent conflicts in the area of dependency, which may complicate the process of seeking help from adults. These conflicts often result in a tendency to deny or minimize problems. The adolescent's autonomy must be respected, and the physician should avoid explicitly pointing out the young person's dependency needs. A closely related issue to autonomy is confidentiality. Although confidentiality is often an issue for the older child and adolescent, it is crucial that the physician not promise confidentiality when there is self-destructive intent. Once lost, the adolescent's trust is difficult to regain. It is paramount that the physician inquire directly about the presence of suicidal ideation or plans. Contrary to popular belief, asking about suicidal ideation does not give the patient the idea to kill himself. Typically, the depressed individual has already been thinking of suicide, and the patient may experience relief at the opportunity to share these thoughts and feelings with an empathic individual, thereby diminishing suicide risk. Initially, many young people may deny suicidal ideation. Therefore physicians should be prepared to reassess the topic at various points in the interview after the establishment of rapport. Because most severely depressed individuals experience at least fleeting thoughts of suicide, the patient's complete denial of such thoughts should arouse suspicion.

Along with carefully monitoring the patient's emotional responses during the interview, it is important that physicians be aware of their own emotional reactions to the patient. The suicidal individual can evoke feelings ranging from intense sympathy and desire to rescue the patient, to anger, contempt, and rage, to complete indifference. It is vital that an awareness of these reactions be maintained, so the evaluation process is not disrupted. The physician who is experiencing a strongly adverse reaction to the patient may wish to avoid the topic altogether or to prematurely close exploration with leading questions that encourage the patient to deny or minimize suicidal ideation, such as, "You don't want to kill yourself do you?" Unrealistic reassurance may also be dispensed, which leads to a lack of communication from the patient and statements such as, "Everything will turn out just fine." If the physician is feeling an excessively strong negative reaction to the patient, it is imperative that consultation be sought.

Risk and Protective Factors

The second step in the evaluation process is the collection of information to establish the risk for self-harm. This requires that the physician be familiar with the relevant risk and protective factors of suicidal behavior in children and adolescents. Most suicidal people experience a number of factors that individually increase their vulnerability to emotional pain and suffering but cumulatively may result in actual suicidal behaviors. Generally, the greater the number of risk factors and the fewer the protective factors, the higher the risk of suicidal behavior (Box 14-2).

The following classes of risk and protective factors are examined in the next sections: (1) mood and psychopathologic factors, (2) environmental stresses or supports, and (3) adaptive or coping skills. Mood or psychopathologic factors are related to specific psychologic, behavioral, genetic, or biologic characteristics of the individual that increase the probability of suicidal behaviors. Environmental stresses impinge on the individual and result in significant distress. Environmental supports are largely interpersonal resources available to the person to serve as a buffer against adversity. Adaptive or coping skills are those psychologic and behavioral strategies available to the person for dealing effectively with stress.

Common Psychiatric Diagnoses

Several psychiatric diagnoses substantially increase a child's or adolescent's risk for suicide. These include

BOX 14-2

RISK FACTORS FOR SUICIDE

High risk psychiatric diagnosis
Significant mental status findings
Historical and genetic factors
Family stresses
Peer group stresses
Social environment
Communication skills deficits
Deficits in problem solving and planning

major depressive disorder (MDD), bipolar mood disorder, substance abuse or dependence, and conduct disorder (CD). Schizophrenia and borderline personality disorder also are associated with an increased risk of suicide. Although individuals with borderline personality disorder often demonstrate repeated nonlethal suicide gestures, their actual completed suicide rate approaches 50 times that seen in the general population. Within many diagnostic categories are combinations of associated features that may significantly increase an individual's risk for suicidal behaviors. For example, psychotic features (mood congruent delusions and hallucinations) may be present in an individual with MDD, and may increase the risk of suicidal behaviors. Substance abuse is also commonly present in the suicidal young person, particularly in male patients who often also have an associated conduct disturbance.

The contribution of substance abuse to suicidality occurs on multiple levels. A person involved in substance abuse is often experiencing a significant degree of conflict with the family and others in his social support system. Fights or arguments with family are stressors that often precipitate suicidal behavior. Several substances are associated with an increased risk of secondary psychiatric symptoms, such as depressed mood, that may be directly attributable to the effect of the substance on the CNS. It is also recognized that substance abuse often represents a kind of self-medication for many people who are suffering from a preexisting psychiatric disorder such as MDD. Additionally, the intoxication syndrome that accompanies many drugs (for example, alcohol) may be associated with emotional lability and diminished impulse control; this combination may directly increase the probability of impulsive suicidal behavior. Substance abuse is also often associated with legal problems related to associated aggressive behaviors and criminal activity. The latter is particularly likely if the person is dependent on an illicit substance and becomes involved in criminal activity to maintain an uninterrupted drug supply.

CD, a common diagnosis associated with suicide, is often accompanied by legal or disciplinary action, a well-recognized stressor associated with suicidal behavior in adolescents. The young person with a chronic tendency to antisocial behavior is often the product of a chaotic social milieu and may be the victim of physical or sexual abuse. Both a dysfunctional family background and a history of abuse are found to correlate with suicidal behavior in adolescents. Antisocial behavior is associated with impulsivity, a character trait seen with other high-risk psychiatric disorders such as the major mood disorders, substance abuse, and borderline personality disorder (Box 14-3). In fact, the combination of depressive symptoms and antisocial behavior appears to be particularly dangerous. A learning disorder, another condition commonly associated with CD, also may increase the risk of suicide. Finally, people with disorders of impulse control may suffer from a dysregulation of the brain's serotonin system, a biologic characteristic that has been associated with violent suicide.

BOX 14-3

HIGH-RISK PSYCHIATRIC DIAGNOSES FOR SUICIDE

Major depressive disorder
Bipolar mood disorder
Substance abuse
Conduct disorder
Borderline personality disorder
Schizophrenia

BOX 14-4

HISTORICAL AND GENETIC FACTORS CONTRIBUTING TO SUICIDE

Previous suicide attempts
Family history of suicide
Anniversary of loss

Schizophrenia, a major mental illness resulting in a substantial degree of impairment in interpersonal and occupational functioning is also associated with a high risk of suicide. The patient with hallucinations should be asked about the specific nature of hallucinations, including whether the patient hears voices commanding him to harm himself or others. Depressive symptoms may often develop in the patient who has schizophrenia with associated suicidal ideation and behavior, resulting in a suicide rate of approximately 10%.

Another patient attribute associated with increased suicide risk includes an inhibited personality. Young people with this personality style are excessively shy, lack close friends, do not share problems with others, tend to be lonely, and are extremely sensitive. The high-achieving child belongs to another group overlooked as a potential suicide risk because of apparent success. However, these children may feel the burden of their own and others' high expectations. Finally, it is important to ask about any family history of suicide, since there may be a genetic component to suicidal behavior (Box 14-4).

Mental Status

In addition to identifying the presence of a high-risk psychiatric diagnosis, the physician should carefully evaluate the current mental status of the patient, especially the nature of the patient's suicidal ideation and plan. Common motivations for a suicide attempt include the desire to influence others, to gain attention, to communicate love or anger, or to escape from a difficult situation. Generally, the more rational the suicide attempt seems to the patient, the higher the risk. Seemingly altruistic motivations for suicide (such as, "My parents would get along much better if I weren't around") should alert the physician to a high level of risk. The intent to die is important to assess, since the patient may actually wish to alter his environment rather than die. Anticipated relief from pain through suicide is a danger signal. In young children, it is important to assess the child's conception of death. A child may believe that death is reversible, like going to sleep, and thus allows the child to avoid a painful situation and return unharmed. The child may believe that dying will allow him to be reunited with a deceased love one, such as a grandparent.

Four patterns of play in children may be associated with suicidal behavior. Themes of loss and retrieval (jumping, hiding, and throwing) may represent conflicts over separation and autonomy. The child's use of the body as a play object in the repetition of dangerous and reckless behaviors is associated with the potential for serious self-harm. The suicidal child may consistently misuse playthings by hitting or breaking them. Finally, children at high risk for suicide may act out omnipotent fantasies in a life-endangering manner. Any one of these types of play may be seen in nonsuicidal children, but if the child's play is pervasively imbued with these features or if the degree of dangerous behavior is high, the physician's suspicion should be heightened.

The young person should also be questioned in detail about any suicidal plan. The physician should inquire about the means of inflicting death, its availability, and the relative lethality of the method. Any history of suicidal behavior should be sought, because a previous attempt is strongly predictive of subsequent attempts. The degree of preparation, including precautions taken against rescue, should be examined. Has the patient given or thrown away prized possessions? Is a suicide note written, and what is its content? Profound hopelessness, particularly with high levels of chronic stress, may predispose the patient to self-destruction. How preoccupied is the patient with death? The relative disparity between the rates of suicide in young children and adolescents may be less the result of differences in the degree of suicidal ideation but more because of the greater cognitive sophistication and capacity for planning in the adolescent. The physician should be mindful of this when evaluating the intellectually precocious young child.

Although the previous discussion emphasized the evaluation of the individual child, it is important for the physician to use multiple sources of information when available. The patient's family is a valuable source of collateral information about the young child and about the adolescent (the young child because of cognitive immaturity and the older child and adolescent because of the tendency to deny or minimize problems). Contact with the family also helps establish a collaborative relationship with the physician, an important element in the development of an effective initial disposition and treatment plan. A hostile or antagonistic family can interfere with patient compliance. The family system may be mobilized to provide critically needed support to the beleaguered patient. Finally, the process of interviewing the family provides the physician with an opportunity to evaluate the family system as a source of emotional support or a source of conflict-related stress (Box 14-5).

BOX 14-5

SIGNIFICANT MENTAL STATUS FINDINGS

- Suicidal ideation or intent
- Detailed plan (especially with precautions against rescue)
- Availability and lethality of method
- Altruistic motivation
- Depressed mood (especially with psychosis)
- Intoxication with disinhibiting substance (e.g., alcohol)
- High levels of hostility
- Hopelessness

Environmental Stress and Support

The next category of risk and protective factors to evaluate is the nature of any environmental stresses and supports. The range of potential environmental stressors is quite broad but may be divided into the following categories: (1) stresses related to family conflict and dysfunction; (2) stresses related to relationships with peers, including romantic relationships; and (3) stresses related to the patient's difficulties with other individuals or institutions, including the school, law enforcement agencies, and the media (Box 14-6). The typical suicidal young person has vulnerabilities from a preexisting psychiatric disorder along with one or more of these stresses, which precipitates a crisis. The child is often compromised to the degree that suicidal behavior is envisioned as the only solution to his predicament.

Family conflict is a common suicide-related stress, and an altercation with a family member often precedes suicidal behavior. These patients may be experiencing painful effects of the conflict. The child or adolescent may feel that his relationship with the involved family member is irrevocably damaged or lost. As a result, the child may feel hurt and angry. The associated suicidal ideation may involve revenge fantasies, wherein the embroiled family member experiences great grief and guilt as a result of their presumed role in the patient's suicide. Usual causes of friction between parents and school-age children include power struggles about the performance of household chores, aggression toward siblings, school grades, or general disobedience. These issues may also occur with adolescents. However, new issues related to an adolescent's bid for increasing autonomy and his struggles with identity typically emerge. These include choice of friends, curfew timing, the ownership and use of a car, dating rules, dress styles, and music selection. The normal teen and his parents may experience conflicts around these and many other issues. However, for the young person who is psychiatrically disturbed, particularly if the adolescent is living with chronic family dysfunction, conflict with parents may be frequent, severe, and violent. The adolescent with CD is likely to become involved in conflicts with any authority. Problems with school suspensions, brushes with the juvenile justice system, defiance of multiple parental directives, and specific antisocial behaviors including theft from family members and physical aggression within the family are all fertile ground for severe discord. For the substance-abusing young person, the issue of drug use and its many associated problems (for example, truancy from school, neglect of social responsibilities, and legal problems) are all potential sources of strife. In addition to specific family conflicts, the loss of a loved one can have a particularly harsh impact on the vulnerable child or adolescent and can result in the precipitation of a suicidal crisis.

Chronic family dysfunction is a significant source of stress. The dysfunctional family may have poor communication patterns, difficulty with clear role boundaries, inconsistency in child-rearing patterns, and problems with impulse control among one or more of its members that may be related to patterns of substance abuse or violence. Such family systems are usually deficient in their ability to manage conflict and provide emotional support. These families are at high risk for sexual and physical abuse, stresses that are associated with psychopathologic disorders, including suicidal behavior. Abused young people may suffer from depression and prominent anxiety. They may experience nightmares and intrusive memories related to episodes of abuse. They may deny the impact of the abuse but demonstrate a clear pattern of emotional and behavioral deterioration. A pattern of emotional distance, or numbing and avoidance, alternating with episodes of hyperarousal that includes severe anxiety or rages may be observed. Posttraumatic stress disorder (PTSD), as well as mood, personality, or conduct disorders may be present. The victim of abuse, particularly of chronic abuse by a family member, may have immense difficulty establishing trust in adults, including the physician. The normal transition in emphasis from adult to peer relationships in adolescence may thus be intensified in the abuse victim.

BOX 14-6

ENVIRONMENTAL STRESSES

Family context

Recent altercation with family member
Recent death of loved one (especially if by suicide)
Sexual or physical abuse
Family dysfunction

Peer group

Recent termination of romantic relationship
Loss of close peer relationship
Recent humiliation
Severe conflicts with peer group

Social Environment

Academic difficulties
Legal and disciplinary problems
Chaotic environment

Discord among peers, a source of distress for the school-age child, is even more significant for the adolescent. The world of adolescent peer relationships is a venue of high drama and intense emotional engagement. This is particularly true of romantic involvements in the context of rapidly developing sexuality. For the normal adolescent, the demise of a romantic relationship may lead to intense, but typically (and mercifully) brief suffering. Hopefully, the adolescent gleans useful information from the experience about this arena of human relationships. For the disturbed adolescent, however, such a loss may result in severe depressive symptoms, loss of hope for the future, and a sense of desperation that may culminate in self-harm behaviors. It is critical that the adult not underestimate the suffering of the young person. Empty utterances such as, "You'll get over it; it's just puppy love," or "Don't worry; there are millions of girls out there" should be avoided at all costs. A problem related to peer relationships and sexuality is the acknowledgement by an adolescent that he may be homosexual. In the context of a relatively homophobic culture, this discovery may bring substantial distress and may be associated with an increased suicide risk. Problems with nonromantic relationships can also be a significant source of pain, particularly if the young person feels that he has become an outcast from the peer group. The narcissism of the adolescent, particularly that of the disturbed youth, is exquisitely tender, making him vulnerable to the experience of humiliation in a variety of social contexts. The occurrence of a humiliating event often precedes suicidal behavior.

A variety of stresses that originate from people and institutions in the wider social context of a young person may impinge on the child. Academic problems are a prominent source of distress associated with suicidal behavior. Obviously, the school expulsions, suspensions, and failing grades associated with CD may mean trouble for the young person (though he may behave as if he were completely indifferent). However, the "B" grade on an examination may be experienced as a major calamity by an introverted, sensitive, high-achieving individual, since such an event may be experienced as deeply humiliating. Disciplinary problems and involvement with the juvenile justice system are well-known risk factors for suicidal behavior, and the day before a court appearance is a period of increased risk. Here too, the young person's distress may be related to feeling humiliated. A chaotic social context with high levels of crime and the opportunity for involvement with a deviant peer group (such as a gang) may increase the risk of the development of CD and thus increase suicide risk. A problem related to criminal involvement is the greater availability of guns, a factor closely related to risk for completed suicide. Exposure to suicide first hand or through the media is also associated with an increase in suicide risk among vulnerable young people. The specific mechanism for this effect may involve a kind of social contagion. To minimize this effect, it is suggested that newspapers relegate stories involving suicide to the back pages, and televised accounts strive to deglamorize suicide. Finally, a general risk factor that may involve all three of the above domains includes the anniversary of an unhappy event.

The patient's environment may also serve as a buffer against stress occurring in the family, the peer group, and the wider social context. A supportive family may be of substantial benefit to members experiencing distress. A close friend may serve as a sounding board and source of emotional support. Trusted adults in the patient's school, church, or other civic organization may provide guidance to a troubled young person. During the evaluation, it is important to identify significant actual or potential sources of support for the patient and to mobilize these resources in support of the patient.

Coping or Adaptive Factors

The next area to assess is that of coping skills possessed by the patient. Coping skills represent those behavioral mechanisms that enable the patient to adapt to difficulty. The following abilities should be identified if present: (1) the ability to seek help and support, (2) the ability to abstain from self-destructive behavior in the face of an impulse to harm the self, (3) the ability to identify and express feelings, and (4) the ability to plan coping strategies for dealing with situations that might lead to suicidal behavior (Box 14-7). It is important to identify specific ways in which the patient adapted to specific difficult situations in the past. These skills may aid the physician in developing a less restrictive treatment plan that will maintain an acceptable degree of safety for the patient. The physician should not naively accept the youngster's promise to abstain from self-harm if his history suggests that he is unreliable, lies readily, and is impulse ridden. The patient may be entirely sincere at the time the promise is made but may quickly forget the promise in the face of an emotional storm.

BOX 14-7

COPING AND ADAPTIVE SKILLS DEFICITS

Communication skills deficits

Inability to identify and express feelings
Inability to seek help and support

Deficits in problem solving and planning

Inability to resist an impulse to harm self
Inability to plan ahead for coping with stressful situations

Treatment Plan and Disposition

At this point in the evaluation, the physician will have gathered sufficient information to develop an overall impression of the patient's risk for self-harm. Unfortunately, there is no simple formula for the calculation of risk and the determination of a corresponding degree of treatment intensity. The prediction of violence is notoriously unreliable, but such estimations of risk for harm must nonetheless be made. Figure 14-1 outlines a decision tree to help guide decision making. As a rule, immediate hospitalization is indicated if the patient is unable to promise the physician that he will not harm himself. Hospitalization may be considered despite the patient's promise not to attempt suicide if numerous risk factors for suicide are present with few environmental supports or if the patient demonstrates little coping skill, unreliability, and impaired impulse control. It is advised that the physician seek consultation with a child and adolescent psychiatrist if hospitalization is necessary or if there is a significant degree of uncertainty. This process may be facilitated by the physician's prior development of a working relationship with a psychiatric consultant. If hospitalization is indicated, a psychiatric hospital with specific space devoted to the treatment of children and adolescents is preferred. The staff of such a facility is likely to be familiar with the developmental needs of this population and should be better able to provide appropriate safety, structure, and support for the young person. If such a

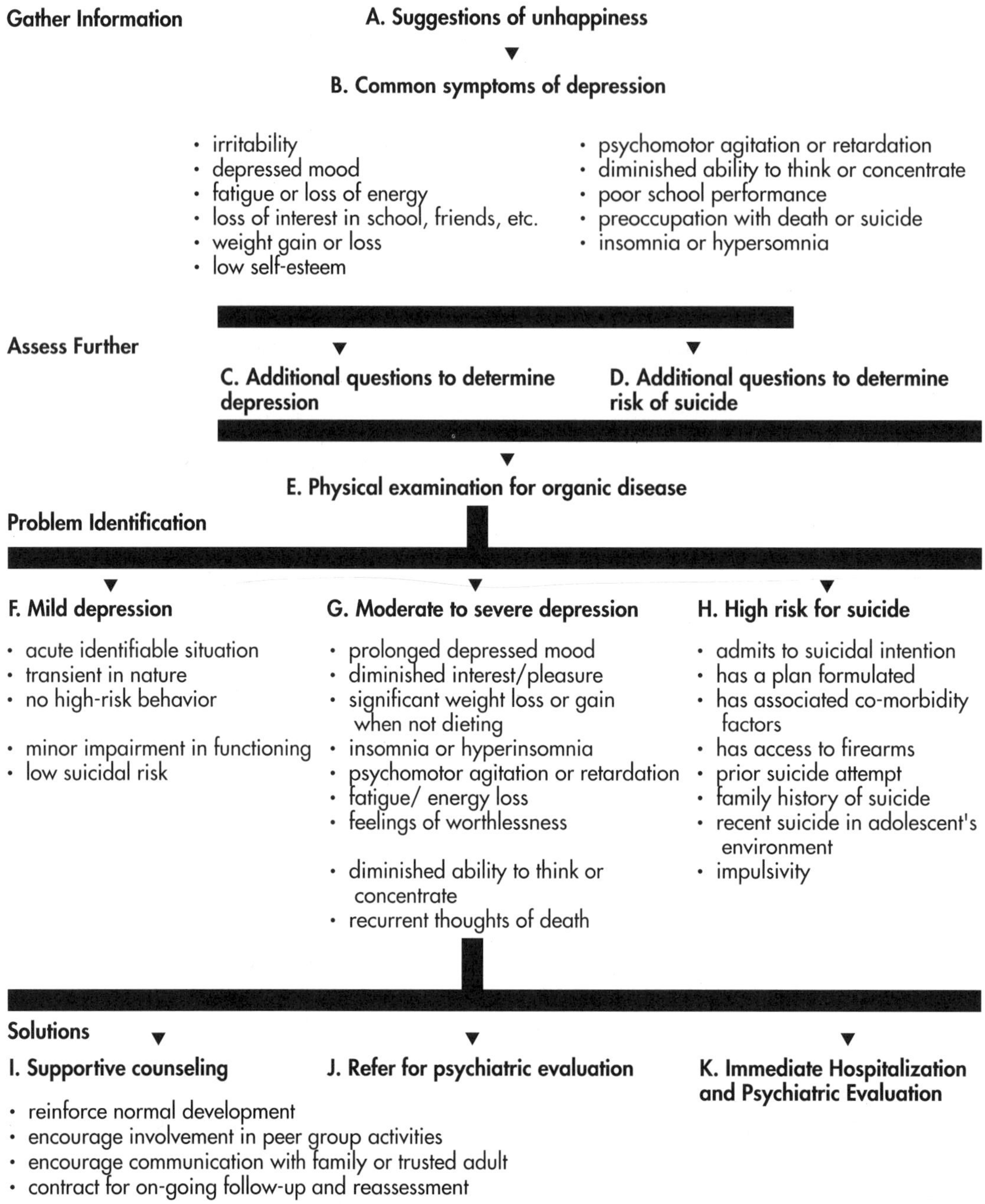

FIGURE 14-1 Decision tree for suicide risk. (Modified from American Medical Association: *GAPS: clinical evaluation and management handbook,* 1993, author.)

facility is unavailable, a general adult psychiatric hospital may be used, but the hospital staff may need additional education regarding the special needs of the child or adolescent patient. Finally, if the patient must be hospitalized on a general hospital unit, a high degree of staff education and support will probably be required to ensure the maintenance of safety (for example, one-to-one observation or removal of sharp objects) and the creation of an adequately therapeutic environment.

The communication of the need to hospitalize must be made with considerable tact and care. The family of an adolescent in crises may be sensitive and prone to defensive posturing. The recommendation for institutional intervention may suggest to the family that they have failed. The accompanying guilt feelings may be intensely painful, and the family may defend against this pain in a number of ways. They may completely deny the presence of a problem and adamantly reject the notion that there is any need for treatment by stating,

"There is nothing wrong; he is just going through a phase." This stance may be accompanied by considerable hostility, and there is a real risk of complete noncompliance. Alternatively, the family may readily accept the recommendation but may be expressing a wish to rid themselves of a difficult child, which results in a lack of family participation in the treatment process. Ideally, the family will express appropriate concern, ask reasonable questions, and indicate a willingness to comply with and participate in the treatment process. The previous establishment of a collaborative relationship with the family can greatly facilitate this process.

The manner and timing of relating a recommendation for hospitalization to the child or adolescent must be carefully considered. If the physician senses that the recommendation will be negatively received (as may be the case with an angry, defiant adolescent) and if the patient is felt to be in immediate danger of self-harm, the appropriate resources for containing the child should be in place before informing the patient of the decision to hospitalize. In addition to providing safety and support, hospitalization may remove the patient from a stressful environment and allow for intensive treatment. Multiple sophisticated methods for patient evaluation can also be used, which may optimize treatment planning. The physician's direct participation in this process (instead of the use of a consultant) depends on the physician's interest, experience, and comfort in dealing with the psychiatric emergency, as well as on the local availability of psychiatric services and support.

If the physician determines that hospitalization is not warranted, an initial outpatient treatment plan should utilize a combination of resources in the patient's home environment and community. The patient may be referred for intensive outpatient psychotherapy or a day treatment program associated with a local inpatient psychiatric facility. The physician may elect to see the patient in the office several times a week during the patient's crisis. Again, the amount of active involvement with the treatment process depends on the physician's comfort and experience managing patients in a psychiatric crisis. The nonmental-health practitioner has a number of effective therapeutic techniques that may be of benefit to the patient experiencing a crisis. These include allowing the patient to express painful feelings, discussing alternative approaches to dealing with difficult situations, examining various strategies for improving interpersonal relationships, working to reduce negative thinking patterns, helping the patient focus on the future, and encouraging hope. A variety of creative treatment plans can be developed, but regardless of the specifics of the individual plan, the following elements should be included: (1) intensive and appropriate treatment should be provided for any existing psychiatric disorders; (2) the physician, psychiatric consultant, or designated substitute should be available on a 24-hour basis; (3) available social support systems, particularly the family, should be maximally utilized if conflicts in the systems are manageable and not unduly contributing to the suicidal crisis; (4) potential methods of self-harm, such as guns, knives, and stores of medications, must be removed from the house; and (5) the patient should be called if he misses a follow-up appointment. Medication may be considered if the patient has a psychiatric diagnosis that may be responsive to pharmacotherapy. Although the efficacy of antidepressants in children and adolescents has not been clearly demonstrated in controlled trials, numerous case reports and open studies have been positive, and some controlled studies show trends in favor of an active drug over a placebo. Given the potentially catastrophic outcome of an inadequately treated major depressive illness, medication may be considered as part of a multimodal treatment plan. If medication is prescribed, the patient should be given no more than a 2- or 3-day supply and should have to call the physician for additional refills. Such precaution is particularly warranted for the tricyclic antidepressants because of the potential for severe toxicity in overdose. An SSRI might be considered, since there is much less apparent overdose toxicity. Additionally, there is some evidence of serotoninergic hypofunctionality in the CNS of people who were victims of violent suicide and generally in people who have impulse control disorders. Other medications that might be considered include lithium for the patient with bipolar disorder and antipsychotic medications if psychosis or severe dyscontrol is present. However, the suicidal patient needing these medications for acute stabilization typically requires hospitalization. Furthermore, the side-effect profiles and potential toxicity of these medications require that the physician possess considerable familiarity with them to allow safe usage. Close consultation with a child and adolescent psychiatrist is therefore strongly recommended.

Should a young person under the care of the physician actually commit suicide, it is of paramount importance that the needs of the family be taken into careful consideration during such a difficult time. For the family, coping with the death of a child is enormously difficult, and the difficulty may be greatly magnified if the death is by suicide. The grieving family member may experience tremendous feelings of guilt, which may be complicated or exacerbated by anger at the suicide victim. Family members may ruminate endlessly over their last encounters with the victim, searching for clues to the subsequent suicide. Self-recrimination is common, as are statements such as, "There must have been something I could have done," or "I should not have said or done . . ." Furthermore, the stigma associated with suicide may inhibit the family from using social supports commonly available to the bereaved. For these reasons, the physician should be available to the family for support. The physician can help normalize some of the guilt and anger experienced by the survivors. Appropriate reassurance may be provided by educating the family regarding the difficulty inherent in predicting or controlling the behavior of others, even if we know them well. During this process it is advised that the physician maintain a high degree of awareness of personal feelings. The loss for the family is also a loss for the physician and may result in similar feelings that, if not dealt with appropriately (which may involve consultation with a colleague) may lead to acting out through avoidance. Furthermore, anxiety related to legal liability may further complicate the physician's response. However, a recent study examining the reaction of the survivors to physician support revealed that such support was positively received and the overall family perception of the physician was enhanced.

Case Analysis

At this point, let us return to the opening clinical vignette that can now be analyzed according to the assessment principles outlined in this chapter. The vignette illustrates a typical clinical situation involving an adolescent girl, Christi, who is experiencing a psychosocial crisis and has a significant potential for associated suicidal behavior. The quantity and quality of the information provided to the physician suggests that he was successful in establishing an initial rapport with her. The pattern of emotional symptoms strongly suggests the presence of a major depressive episode with severe (by patient report), impairing (drop in school performance), and persistent (almost all day, every day for several weeks) depressed mood accompanied by marked fatigue, disturbance in sleep and appetite, poor attention and concentration, crying episodes, hopelessness, helplessness, and excessive guilt. Her mental status suggests a significant degree of distress. She is experiencing suicidal ideation, including specific methods of self-harm. The methods of suicide under consideration are typical of adolescent girls and are, fortunately, not often as lethal as the more violent methods preferred by boys. Her specific motivation for self-harm and associated fantasies are unclear, though escape from pain may be one of them (note her reference to leaving everything behind). The degree of planning is unknown. We do not know about previous episodes of depression or suicide attempts. Information about comorbid CD, substance abuse, and problems with impulse control would also be desirable. An inhibited personality style may be present. No family psychiatric history is known, but the death of Christi's mother when she was 6 years old is significant (particularly if the mother committed suicide). Numerous recent environmental stressors are noted, including the break-up with her boyfriend, changing schools, her best friend moving, and her family relocating. Although Christi relates that she cannot talk to anyone, this may be more the result of her inhibited personality style than the unavailability of social supports. Christi's presentation to the physician's office and her willingness to describe her plight in some detail suggest that she is willing to seek help. She has demonstrated the capacity to identify and communicate feelings well. The ability to resist harming herself in the face of self-destructive impulses should be assessed, as should her potential to plan strategies to cope with suicidal ideation. Christi's specific skills for adapting to past stressors should be examined. How has she dealt with any previous suicidal thoughts that did not lead to self-destructive behavior? Her personality style may make the use of available social supports more difficult. To fully assess Christi's current situation, collateral information should be actively sought, especially from family members. This process may elucidate additional areas of Christi's life, including a previous history of psychiatric disorders, any specific de-

PEARLS & PERILS

SUICIDE

- The physician should ask about suicidal ideation at more than one point in the interview, especially after rapport has been established. Patients often deny suicidal ideation when initially asked.
- Most severely depressed individuals have at least fleeting thoughts of suicide; therefore the complete denial of such thoughts should arouse suspicion.
- The best predictor of a future suicide attempt is a past suicide attempt.
- The physician should obtain a *detailed* description of any suicidal plan, especially the availability and lethality of the method and any precautions taken against rescue.
- It is important to avoid asking leading questions about suicidal ideation (for example, "You don't want to kill yourself do you?").
- The physician should avoid prescribing large quantities of medication to the potentially suicidal patient. Instead, only a 2- or 3-day supply should be prescribed, and the patient should have to call for refills.
- It is important for the physician not to promise confidentiality that cannot be kept. Once lost, the patient's trust is hard to regain.

velopmental problems, or behavioral problems. Additionally Dr. Edwards can assess the availability and quality of the family support system while gathering this information. How does the family react to his concern about Christi's mood disturbance and potential for self-harm? How has the family responded to Christi's episodes of distress? Does the family indicate a willingness to become involved in a treatment plan?

If the results of the patient and family interviews suggest that Christi is relatively reliable, a contract not to harm herself could be sought. If Christi agrees to such a contract, a day hospital or outpatient treatment plan could be investigated. Medication, especially an SSRI, should be considered given the diagnosis of a major depressive episode. The degree of structure required in an outpatient plan depends on Christi's previous history of self-destructive behavior, her relative reliability (beyond the minimum required to establish a meaningful contract), her demonstrated coping skills, and the quality and availability of social supports.

The family should be encouraged to be emotionally available to Christi and to assist in compliance with medication, as well as to keep follow-up appointments with Dr. Edwards or a consultant. The family should be asked to remove readily available means of suicide, such as guns and medications, from the house.

If Christi is unable or unwilling to contract not to harm herself, or if additional information suggests that she is extremely impulsive or unreliable, hospitalization is indicated. Hospitalization should also be sought if the family context is so noxious that further clinical deterioration appears inevitable despite Christi's apparent willingness to comply with a treatment contract. Dr. Edwards was appropriately considering consultation with the discovery of suicidal ideation. Consultation is also highly recommended if hospitalization is necessary.

Summary

Patients at risk for suicidal behavior are likely to consult any physician who treats young people. It is crucial that evidence of suicidality be taken seriously and thoroughly evaluated. A complete assessment requires the use of a developmentally appropriate interview technique to establish patient rapport and allow the gathering of an adequate data base for risk estimation and subsequent treatment planning. A satisfactory data base should include the identification of relevant risk and protective factors in the following areas: (1) mood and psychopathologic factors including possible psychiatric diagnoses, current mental status, and any family history of psychiatric disorder; (2) environmental stresses and supports in the immediate family or peer group, as well as in the patient's larger social milieu; and (3) coping and adaptive skills. It is important that collateral information be gathered when available, especially from the family. The physician should strive to establish a supportive alliance with family members. After the completion of the assessment phase, an initial disposition and treatment plan should be developed. Hospitalization should be considered if the patient is unable to contract with the physician to avoid self-harm, if the patient is unreliable, or if the environment is extremely toxic. If outpatient management is chosen, professional support should be readily available to the patient, and all available social supports should be optimally utilized. Medication may be considered for appropriate psychiatric diagnosis, but care should be taken to minimize any risk of overdose. Consultation is encouraged at any point in the process, particularly if hospitalization is under consideration.

The death of a young person is always a tragedy, particularly if it is by suicide. Hopefully, by maintaining a high index of suspicion, the physician can identify potentially suicidal patients. Through careful evaluation and timely intervention, the catastrophic termination of some young lives can be avoided.

CONSIDER CONSULTATION WHEN . . .

- The youth meets criteria for moderate to severe depression (see Figure 14-1)
- There is a suicide gesture or attempt
- The youth is unable to contract not to harm himself

ANNOTATED BIBLIOGRAPHY

Biederman J: *Psychopharmacology.* In Wiener JM, editor: *Textbook of child and adolescent psychiatry,* Washington DC, 1991, American Psychiatric Press.

This chapter provides a comprehensive overview of child and adolescent psychopharmacology.

Blumenthal SJ et al: Youth suicide: risk factors, assessment, and treatment of adolescent and young adult suicidal patients, *Psychiatr Clin North Am* 13:511-557, 1990.

This paper provides an excellent and detailed review of the many risk factors involved in youth suicide.

Blumenthal SJ, Kupfer DJ: An overview of early detection and treatment strategies for suicidal behavior in young people, *J Youth Adolesc* 17:1-23, 1988.

This paper is recommended for its emphasis on early detection strategies.

Brent DA: Depression and suicide in children and adolescents, *Pediatr Rev* 14:381-389, 1993.

This is a succinct paper that examines the issue of youth suicide from the perspective of the pediatrician.

Davis G, Hendren RL: What pediatricians should know about adolescent psychiatry, *Adolescent Medicine: State of the Art Reviews,* 3:131-145, 1993.

This chapter provides a thorough overview of relevant issues in adolescent development.

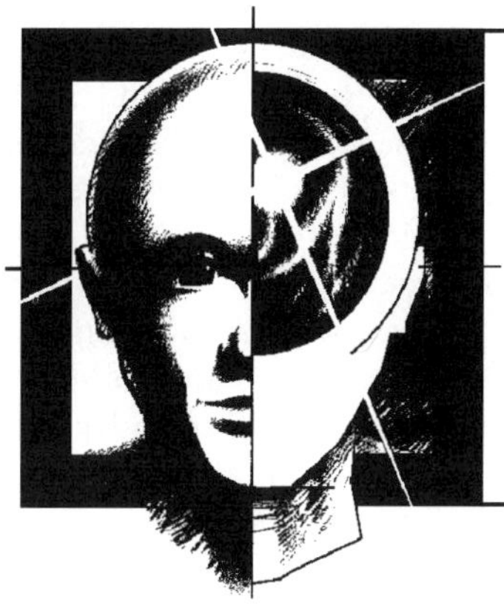

chapter 15

The Substance-Abusing Youth

Steven Jaffe, MD

Epidemiology
Diagnosis
Risk Factors
Assessment
Confidentiality
Urine Drug Screening
Determining Stage of Involvement and Treatment Strategies

Joey is a 15-year-old boy who was an excellent student until the beginning of this school year. Since then he has begun to skip school, not do his homework, break home rules, and lie to his parents about where he goes and who his friends are. He no longer seems to care about his appearance, and he has changed his peer group. He is brought to his physician by his mother, who wants to know what has happened to him.

Mark is a 12-year-old boy who attends a special class for children with learning disabilities. He has been diagnosed as having attention-deficit/hyperactivity disorder (ADHD) and receives methylphenidate (Ritalin). He is brought to his physician by his parents, who found him in the garage inhaling gasoline.

Joan is a 17-year-old girl who is brought to her physician by her parents after they found her in a state of panic, terrified that she was going to die. She told them that she had taken two hits of blotter acid an hour before.

Bill is a 17-year-old boy who had been arrested for drunk driving and assaulting a police officer. This happened 2 months before his consultation. He tells his physician that he does not have a drinking problem and that he was just unlucky to have been caught. Furthermore, he denies that he assaulted the officer, but he is not sure because he does not remember the night in question.

These clinical vignettes illustrate some of the typical ways teenagers with drug and alcohol problems come to a physician's attention.

Epidemiology

After a downward trend of alcohol and drug abuse in teenagers during the late 1980s and early 1990s, there is a recent increase in alcohol and drug abuse. This is especially alarming, since the largest increase in use is in the early adolescent population. Marijuana use peaked in 1979 and then decreased through 1991. The most recent National Institute of Drug Abuse (NIDA) survey indicates that between 1993 and 1994 there was a sharp increase in marijuana use. The survey showed that that 40% of twelfth graders had used marijuana in the past year and that 3.6% of these twelfth graders indicated daily use. The sharpest increase was among eighth graders, with 13% admitting to smoking marijuana at least once in the past year and 0.7% admitting daily use. Cocaine use peaked in 1986 and decreased until 1991, but it has shown a slight increase between 1994 and 1995.

Alcohol continues to be the illegal substance that is most abused by teenagers, and the 1993 Monitoring the Future Survey indicated that 28% of twelfth graders admitted to having five or more drinks in a row on at least one occasion in the 2 weeks before the survey.

LSD use during the 1980s was fairly constant, but there has been a sharp increase in use since 1991. Although the epidemic use of LSD during the 1960s decreased because of severe and numerous detrimental reactions, a less potent form called blotter acid has appeared on the scene during the past few years. Its use in the teenage population is sharply increasing. A single sheet of blotter paper may contain one hundred "hits" of acid and may sell for between $2.00 and $5.00 a hit. Blotter paper may be named for its color (for example, Blue Blotter, Red Blotter, or Yellow Blotter) or for a picture printed on it (such as a tulip, a happy face, or a cartoon character). Inhalants, such as glue, solvents, and aerosols, have also risen in use during the past few years. Unlike other substances, which are used more as teenagers grow older, inhalant use peaks in the eighth grade. In 1994, 11.7% of the eighth graders in the NIDA survey admitted to inhalant use in the past year, an increase from 9% in 1991. Types of inhalants include gasoline, fluorocarbons (Freon) used in air conditioners, butane, Scotchgard, and even household bleach.

Adolescents tend to use alcohol and drugs in an inverse relationship to their recognition and understanding of the risk of harm. Thus this recent increase in general use corresponds to a decreased perceived risk of harm. Many factors, such as lack of education about the risks of drugs and the glamorization of alcohol and drugs on television and in the music industry, appear to have contributed to the increase of use. Although teenagers are highly educated in the use of computers, they are poorly informed about the realistic and actual risks of alcohol and drugs. Since early use correlates directly with a later degree of use and with the use of more than one drug, the increase in use by eighth graders is an alarming trend.

In recent years, increasing the age of legal alcohol consumption has been seen as a primary method of decreasing alcohol and drug use in the teenage population. However, the trends discussed in this chapter have devastated the possibility of increased age as a significant influential factor. Suicides, homicides, and accidents account for 80% of teenage deaths, and alcohol and drugs are involved in one half of these cases. The extensive use and abuse of alcohol and drugs during the preadolescent and adolescent years, as well as the strong contribution of drugs and alcohol to emotional problems, indicate that whenever there are problems in the teenage years the physician should consider that alcohol and drugs may be a contributing factor.

Diagnosis

As with much diagnostic work, the history of the patient holds much of the diagnostic information. The physician quickly develops hypotheses when listening to and observing the patient and tests them with further inquiry. The evaluation of an adolescent who may be abusing drugs or alcohol but is not about to admit to it calls on a physician's greatest skills in relationship building, empathic confrontation, and knowledge of popular substances and patterns of abuse (Box 15-1).

BOX 15-1

SUBSTANCES OF ABUSE

Most commonly abused drugs

Inhalants
Volatile hydrocarbons, ether, amyl nitrate (poppers), nitrous oxide, glue, correction fluid, butane, carburetor cleaner, Freon, gasoline

Cannabis products
Marijuana, hashish (dope, reefer, doobie)

Alcohol*

PCP
(Angel dust)

Stimulants
Amphetamine, methamphetamine (ecstasy, MDMA, speed, crank, ice)

Hallucinogens
LSD (acid), mescaline, psilocybin, peyote

Anabolic steroids
(Roids) (usually abused by boys and men)
Oral: methandrostenolone (Dianabol), stanozolol (Winstrol)
Intramuscular: nandrolone decanoate (Deca-Durabolin)

Less commonly abused drugs

Sedative hypnotics*
Benzodiazepines, barbiturates (yellow jackets), methaqualone (ludes)

Opiates*
Heroin, codeine, oxycodone (Percocet)

Minor tranquilizers*
Librium, valium

*Physical addiction may develop with these drugs.

DSM-IV DIAGNOSTIC CRITERIA

BOX 15-2 SUBSTANCE ABUSE

A. A maladaptive pattern of substance use leading to clinically significant impairment or distress, as manifested by one (or more) of the following, occurring within a 12-month period:

(1) recurrent substance use resulting in a failure to fulfill major role obligations at work, school, or home (e.g., repeated absences or poor work performance related to substance use; substance-related absences, suspensions, or expulsions from school; neglect of children or household)
(2) recurrent substance use in situations in which it is physically hazardous (e.g., driving an automobile or operating a machine when impaired by substance use)
(3) recurrent substance-related legal problems (e.g., arrest for substance-related disorderly conduct)
(4) continued substance use despite having persistent or recurrent social or interpersonal problems caused or exacerbated by the effects of the substance (e.g., arguments with spouse about consequences of intoxication, physical fights)

B. The symptoms have never met the criteria for Substance Dependence for this class of substance.

(From American Psychiatric Association: *Diagnostic and statistical manual of mental disorders,* ed 4 [DSM-IV], Washington DC, 1994, American Psychiatric Press.)

DSM-IV DIAGNOSTIC CRITERIA

BOX 15-3 SUBSTANCE DEPENDENCE

A maladaptive pattern of substance use, leading to clinically significant impairment or distress, as manifested by three (or more) of the following, occurring at any time in the same 12-month period:

(1) tolerance, as defined by either of the following:
 (a) a need for markedly increased amounts of substance to achieve intoxication or desired effect.
 (b) markedly diminished effect with continued use of the same amount of the substance
(2) withdrawal, as manifested by either of the following:
 (a) the characteristic withdrawal syndrome for the substance
 (b) the same (or closely related) substance is taken to relieve or avoid withdrawal symptoms
(3) the substance is often taken in larger amounts or over a longer period than was intended
(4) there is a persistent desire or unsuccessful efforts to cut down or control substance use
(5) a great deal of time is spent in activities necessary to obtain the substance (e.g., visiting multiple doctors or driving long distances), use the substance (e.g., chain-smoking), or recover from its effects
(6) important social, occupational, or recreational activities are given up or reduced because of substance use
(7) the substance use is continued despite knowledge of having a persistent or recurrent physical or psychological problem that is likely to have been caused or exacerbated by the substance (e.g., current cocaine use despite recognition of cocaine-induced depression, or continued drinking despite recognition that an ulcer was made worse by alcohol consumption)

Specify if:
With Physiological Dependence: evidence of tolerance or withdrawal (i.e., either Item 1 or 2 is present)
Without Physiological Dependence: no evidence of tolerance or withdrawal (i.e., neither Item 1 nor 2 is present)

Course specifiers:
Early Full Remission
Early Partial Remission
Sustained Full Remission
Sustained Partial Remission
On Agonist Therapy
In a Controlled Environment

(Modified from American Psychiatric Association: *Diagnostic and statistical manual of mental disorders,* ed 4 [DSM-IV], Washington DC, 1994, American Psychiatric Press.)

Since it is usually a family member who brings the youth for an evaluation, a more complete picture can be obtained from an additional source. The formal DSM-IV diagnosis is relatively easy to generate once the psychosocial data are forthcoming. The criteria are straightforward and serve the physician well because of their checklist nature (Boxes 15-2 and 15-3).

Risk Factors

There are a number of risk factors that have been described as correlates to serious substance abuse in adolescents (Box 15-4). When the physician sees a teenager and family with these types of problems, alcohol and drugs need to be considered as part of the clinical picture. The most influential factor for a teenager having problems with alcohol and drugs is a relative, such as a parent, grandparent, aunt, or uncle, who has a history of alcohol or drug addiction. The physician should specifically ask whether a relative had problems with drugs and alcohol. Specific attitudes and a lack of achievement by the teenager also correlate with alcohol and substance abuse. Such attitudes include the teenager thinking poorly of herself, not liking school, not achieving or dropping out of school, and smoking cigarettes, as well as rebellious and delinquent behavior. The aggressive or impulsive teenager is at high risk for substance abuse. Additionally, if the teenager's friends have the same characteristics (that is, they are aggressive or delinquent) or if the teenager's friends use drugs or alcohol, the adolescent in question is at high risk for drug or alcohol use. In terms of family problems, disruption and dysfunction within the family correlate with alcohol and drug abuse in teenagers. Thus parental separation, divorce, lack of clear discipline, and especially the lack of positive relationships within the family all increase the likelihood that a teenager will use or abuse alcohol and drugs. Teenagers who have been sexually or physically abused, who have had a depressive episode, or who have had problems in school because of behavior, ADHD, or learning disabilities are at increased risk for alcohol and substance abuse.

Research indicates that teenagers become involved in alcohol and drugs through a pattern of progression, which begins with abstention and moves to the use of beer or wine and cigarettes, hard liquor, marijuana, and then other drugs (Box 15-5). Thus it is extremely unusual for a teenager who is using cocaine to never have tried marijuana. In contrast with adults, teenagers often do not give up the drug of the previous stage but continue to use it along with the new drugs. Therefore teenagers tend to be multiple drug users. For example, many abuse alcohol, marijuana, and LSD during the same period. Cigarette use is a method of learning to smoke and thereby is a gateway to the use of marijuana. An exception to this pattern of staged progression is that of inhalants, where eighth graders have the highest rate of use; inhalant use may precede any alcohol or drug use.

BOX 15-4

RISK FACTORS FOR SERIOUS SUBSTANCE ABUSE IN ADOLESCENTS

Parent or other relative with substance abuse or dependency problems
Low achievement, especially in school
Poor self-esteem
Aggressive or impulsive personality
Family instability
History of sexual or physical abuse
Psychiatric disorder, especially depression

BOX 15-5

GATEWAY DRUGS

Cigarettes
Beer and wine
Inhalants

Assessment

Because of the widespread use and possible severe detrimental consequences, the primary care physician should screen all adolescents for substance use or abuse. Early detection and treatment saves lives.

When talking to the teenager and his family about alcohol and drug use, the physician must be knowledgeable and comfortable approaching these issues. The teenager who is abusing alcohol and drugs will quickly notice if the physician knows little about the way drugs and alcohol are abused, their effects, and the problems associated with their use. However, if the physician has personal experience with drugs or alcohol, this fact should not be mentioned. Additionally, the physician should not become too chummy, since the teenager will then treat the physician as he would treat another teenager. An attitude of interest, concern, and seriousness mixed with a little humor in the context of the physician's usual style is often the best approach. Any change in feelings, mood, behavior, or cognitive functioning may be related to problems with alcohol and drugs.

Anglin describes a framework for interviewing teenagers about their alcohol and drug use. This commonly used framework includes a psychosocial assessment, whereby home and family relationships are explored in detail and functioning at school is covered. Peer relationships, leisure activities and employment, and self-perceptions are carefully reviewed. Of course, these issues must also be explored with the family. Teenagers tend to deny and hide their drug use. Therefore changes in feelings, actions, and thinking must be carefully explored in an open nonaccusatory way with the family. The physician must at all times act as an ally of the parents and as a knowledgeable and concerned professional who is there to help the teenager. To explore alcohol and substance use with a teenager, Anglin suggests an ordered discussion of the substances the teenager ingests. Thus questions move from dietary patterns to prescribed medications, over-the-counter medica tions, and the use of other substances. The discussion of actual substance abuse may move from tobacco to alcohol, marijuana, and other drugs. If a teenager is reluctant to discuss his own actions, asking what his peers do and do not do may give insight to what he does or does not do. It is often helpful to ask a questions such as, "How many times a month do you smoke pot?" rather than, "Do you smoke pot?" This may help the teenager to lower his defenses and prevent him from immediately answering, "No" to every question.

Halikas, in a study of adolescents and delinquency, developed specific key questions to examine patterns of use and abuse in teenagers. Questions related to alcohol are in the following list:

1. Do you drink on school grounds?
2. When you are truant, do you ever go drinking?
3. Do you miss school because of drinking or being hung over?

He found that a positive answer to one of these questions correlated highly with severe alcohol problems. Three key questions related to drug use are in the following list:

1. Do you mix alcohol and drugs?
2. Is your family concerned about your drug use?
3. When you are truant, do you get high on drugs?

A positive answer to one of these questions correlated highly with severe drug problems.

Teenagers should also be questioned about the following important issues:

- Taking risks, such as driving or being in a car when using alcohol or drugs
- Doing things that they would not otherwise have done
- Breaking the law
- Somatic effects, such as memory difficulties resulting from marijuana use
- Changes in school achievement

The physician should ask specific details of a teenager's activities and experiences, since these reveal the details of his life. For example, asking, "How's school?" yields little. Asking about the details of the day, what a teacher is like, the nature of the teenager's relationship to the teacher, and grades in a specific course often reveals much important data. Be aware that the parents often do not know the extent of their child's alcohol and drug abuse.

Confidentiality

Issues of confidentiality are difficult in their clinical application and vary with the style and judgment of the physician. Although promising the teenager absolute confidentiality may yield more information, this can be extremely problematic. Much of the information may be of a life-threatening nature (for example, the teenager may reveal that she drives while tripping on LSD), and this needs to be brought to the attention of the parents. If a teenager is clearly endangering herself or others, this is an indication for confidentiality to be broken. The risks of drugs and alcohol are often life-threatening but may not be immediate and clear. This calls for the consideration of relationships and the involvement of judgment in the decision-making process. One method of handling the situation is to interview the teenager alone and then conduct a second interview in the presence of the parents; thus the teenager reveals the specifics of the high-risk behavior directly to her parents.

Urine Drug Screening

Issues of judgment and risk taking also involve judgments about urine drug screening. The physician

PEARLS & PERILS

DRUG AND ALCOHOL ABUSE

- If there is a problem in the teenage years, alcohol and drugs may be involved.
- If there are any problems in feelings, actions or thinking, drugs and alcohol may be causing the problems.
- The greater the problem with alcohol and drugs, the more the teenager will lie about his drug and alcohol use. Therefore information from family, peers, and school is important.
- Teenagers tend to be multiple drug users.
- The Imaginary Urine Drug Screen is a useful tool.
- If a teenager is not asked about drugs and alcohol, he will not volunteer this information.

should be familiar with the local laboratory, the types of urine drug screening that can be done, and the cutoff points for positive tests. A urine drug screen is only valid if it is unadulterated and if it is actually the teenager's urine. Therefore, urine for drug screens needs to be obtained under observed conditions. The Imaginary Urine Drug Screen helps the physician recognize the relationship between the teenager's attitude toward giving the urine and the urine test results. Jaffe et al. have shown that in a treatment program for a drug-abusing population, resistance to giving a urine specimen for a drug screen correlated with whether the urine was positive or negative for marijuana. Thus the more resistant the teenager was, the higher the chance of being positive for marijuana. Teenagers who ask, "Don't you trust me?" should be answered with, "No. Show me you are not using." Adults should not be put off by the numerous ploys of shifting the issue from the teenager's possible drug use to issues concerning relationships or others. Urine drug screens should not be done on a routine basis but only when there is reasonable suspicion of drug use. Adolescent urine drug

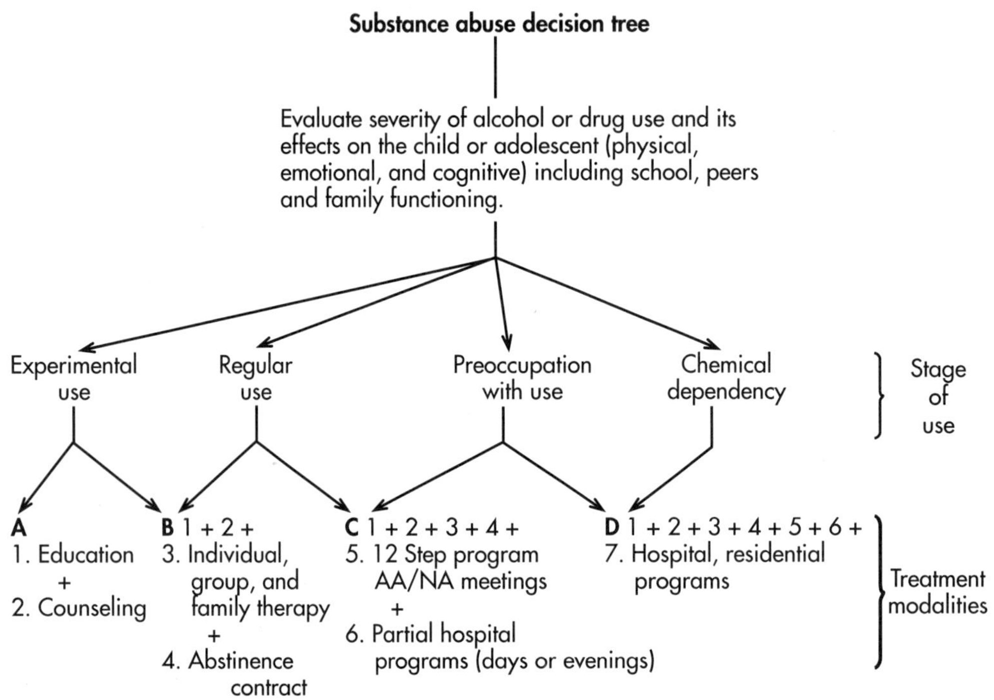

- Full psychiatric evaluation is needed because substance abuse often coexists with one or more psychiatric disorders (especially mood disorders, behavior disorders such as ADHD and CD, and anxiety disorders)
- Failure of treatment usually indicates that a more advanced stage of use was actually present. Treatment modalities of this more advanced stage are indicated.
- Detoxification is not usually needed for adolescents because of the following:
  —adolescents tend to be in better physical condition than adults
  —adolescents tend to use multiple drugs
  —marijuana, LSD, and cocaine, which are commonly used by adolescents, do not require detoxification
  —heavy alcohol abuse is often episodic without the development of physical addiction
- Although it is rare in adolescents, physical addiction to alcohol, sedatives, or other minor tranquilizers can have life-threatening withdrawal symptoms and necessitates detoxification.

FIGURE 15-1 Substance abuse decision tree.

screening mainly shows evidence of marijuana use, because cannaboids last for 3 to 4 weeks after they are smoked. Most other drugs are only present for 1 to 2 days.

Determining Stage of Involvement and Treatment Strategies

When determining how to deal with alcohol and drug abuse in teenagers, understanding the stage of involvement is often extremely helpful. For the teenager who is only involved in experimental or social use, education and counseling is needed. If the teenager has progressed to more regular use, then the addition of individual, group, and family therapy, as well as an abstinence contract, is needed. The abstinence contract involves the teenager who is using drugs more than occasionally but maintains that he will have no problem stopping. The teenager agrees to regular urine testing and counseling and promises not to use drugs or alcohol.

In this treatment strategy, the teenager's progress determines whether more intensive treatment modalities are needed. For example, a teenager who has been doing poorly in school and has had hostile confrontations with his family may agree to counseling and an abstinence contract. If this teenager stops smoking marijuana, his urine drug screens will be negative after the 2 or 3 weeks it takes for the tetrahydrocannabinol (THC) to be eliminated from the body, and his behavior relationships and school achievement will return to their predrug levels. More intensive treatment will not be needed. However, if the teenager is unable to abstain from drugs and alcohol, further rules will be broken, family relationships will be disrupted, failures will increase at school, at work, and elsewhere, and deteriorating behavior will help the physician determine that a more intensive treatment program is needed (Figure 15-1). Additional treatment methods include a partial hospital program, 12-step program, and residential treatment (Box 15-6). Box 15-7 shows the names and addresses of self-help and advocacy groups that may be helpful, resources for recovering teenagers and their families.

It is important to note that teenagers who are serious abusers of alcohol and drugs may have numerous coexisting disorders, especially ADHD, learning disabilities, depression, or histories of physical or sexual abuse. Full evaluation of coexisting psychiatric disorders is needed. Because of the extensive use, abuse, and high risk of drugs and alcohol in the teenage population, it is essential for all physicians working with teenagers to become knowledgeable and effective in dealing with this aspect of a teenager's life.

If the teenager tells a physician about alcohol and drug problems, it is imperative for the physician to explore these issues, educate the teenager and his family, determine the extent and stage of usage, and help the teenager obtain treatment.

BOX 15-6

TREATMENT METHODS FOR TEENAGERS WHO USE DRUGS AND ALCOHOL.

Experimental (recreational use)

Education—helps adolescent and parents learn about alcohol and drugs and their detrimental effects. Excellent information and pamphlets for distribution may be obtained at no charge from the National Clearinghouse for Alcohol and Drug Information Publications Catalog (1-800-729-6686).

Counseling—talking with the adolescent about his life and drug use.

Regular use

Individual, group and family therapy—done by a mental health professional.

Abstinence Contract—written agreement not to use drugs, to have regular urine drug screens, and to abide by home rules (privileges and consequences) as developed by the parents and the adolescent.

Preoccupation with use

12-Step Program—attending regular meetings of Alcoholics Anonymous or Narcotics Anonymous; establishing a sponsor and completing the steps.

Partial Hospital Program—attending a program during the day or evening that includes therapy groups, family programs, individual therapy, creative activities, and school.

Chemical dependency

Hospital Program—acute and intermediate level of care.

Residential Program—long-term intermediate level of 24-hour care and therapeutic program.

BOX 15-7

SELF-HELP AND ADVOCACY GROUPS

National Clearinghouse for Alcohol and Drug Information (NCADI); P.O. Box 2345; Rockville, MD 20852; (301)468-2600

National Federation of Parents for Drug-Free Youth (NFP); 8730 Georgia Avenue, #200; Silver Spring, MD 20910; (301)585-5437. Activities include Project Graduation and Safe Homes.

Parent Resources and Information for Drug Education (PRIDE); Robert Woodruff Building, Volunteer Service Center, Suite #1012; 100 Edgewood Avenue NE, Atlanta, GA 30303; (800)241-9746. Information and referral resource for parents and others.

Alcoholics Anonymous/Narcotics Anonymous; 16155 Wyandotte Street; Van Nuys, CA 91406; (818)780-3951. Narcotics Anonymous (NA) is a national network of more than 2000 regional groups. They are closely patterned after Alcoholics Anonymous (AA). NA groups are conducted by recovered drug addicts, who follow the AA program to aid in rehabilitation. NA publishes a variety of helpful materials for its members, including a directory of group meetings.

Mothers Against Drunk Driving (MADD); 669 Airport Freeway, Suite #310; Hurst, TX 76053; (817)268-MADD. Membership is open to all parents, including fathers; Promotion of public policy against drunk driving.

National Parent-Teachers' Association (PTA); 700 North Rush Street; Chicago, IL 60611; (312)787-0977. The nation's largest child advocacy association.

Families Anonymous (FA); P.O. Box 528; Van Nuys, CA 91408; (818)989-7841. Self-help group patterned after AA.

Adult Children of Alcoholics (ACOA); P.O. Box 880517; San Francisco, CA 94188; (415)931-2262. Addresses the trauma of growing up in an alcoholic family.

Safe Rides: Provides free and confidential safe rides for young people. Commonly associated with local Boy Scout troops.

Students Against Driving Drunk (SADD); P.O. Box 800; Marlboro, MA 01752; (617)481-3568. Chapters in high schools and colleges; weekend hot-line service to provide safe rides.

(Adapted from American Academy of Pediatrics: *Evaluation by interview.* In Schonberg, SK editor: *Substance Abuse: a guide for health professionals,* Elk Grove Village, Ill., 1988, author.)

CONSIDER CONSULTATION WHEN . . .

- There is life-threatening behavior
- The youth is unable to abide by an abstinence contract

Annotated Bibliography

Anglin TM: Interviewing guidelines for the clinical evaluation of adolescent substance abuse, *Pediatr Clin North Am* 34:381-398, 1987.
This article provides a wonderful detailed description of an interview method.

Halikas J: *Substance abuse in children and adolescents.* In Garfinkel BD, Carlson GA, Weller EB, editors: *Psychiatric disorders in children and adolescents,* Philadelphia, 1990, W.B. Saunders.
This is a good review chapter.

Jaffe SL et al: *Validity of the adolescent imaginary urine drug screen: association between attitude when giving urine and test results.* Presented at the annual meeting of the American Psychiatric Association Miami, Fl., May, 1995 (manuscript in preparation).
This is a discussion of a study in which adolescents' resistant attitudes to giving the urine specimen correlated with their urine being positive for marijuana.

Jaffe SL: *The step workbook for adolescent chemical dependency recovery,* Washington DC, 1990, American Psychiatric Press.
This is a workbook in which an adolescent writes answers to specific questions to examine the consequences of his alcohol or drug use. These answers are then discussed with a counselor. It is especially useful for groups and outpatient/inpatient programs.

Schwartz RH, Cohen PR, Bilair GO: Identifying and coping with a drug-using adolescent: some guidelines for pediatricians and parents, *Pediatr Rev* 7:133-139, 1985.
This article describes concrete strategies for treating resistant adolescents.

Stowell RJA: Dual diagnosis issues, *Psychiatr Ann* 21:98-104, 1991.
This article summarizes a study demonstrating multiple diagnoses in substance-abusing adolescents.

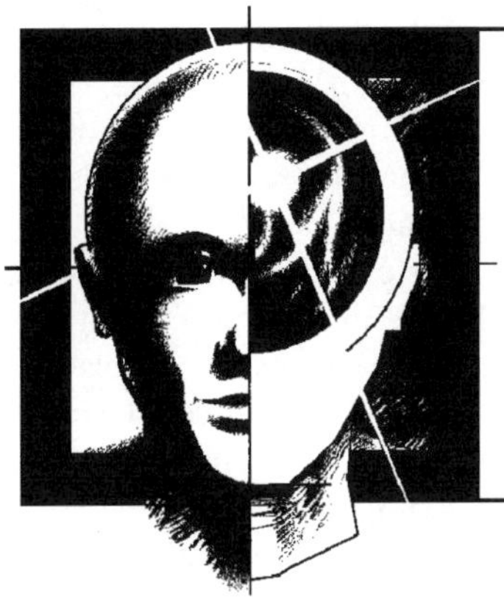

chapter 16

Children and Abuse

Cheryl Al-Mateen, MD and Stanley E. Hemsley, Jr., MD

Sequelae of Abuse
Neglect
Emotional Abuse
Physical Abuse
Sexual Abuse
Interventions and Treatment
Summary

Jason was born to a 27-year-old single woman after 27 weeks of pregnancy. He was successfully treated for premature lung disease and apnea. When he was 65 days old, he was discharged with a cranky disposition and resolving bronchopulmonary dysplasia that required oxygen therapy. At 4 months of age, he was brought to the emergency room by his grandmother after several hours of uncontrollable crying and 2 hours of being unarousable. A physical examination confirmed that the infant was unresponsive and had periodic apnea, a bulging anterior fontanel, dilated and fixed pupils, and multiple bruises, some old and some new. Resuscitation was unsuccessful. The skeletal survey and autopsy showed multiple healing fractures, including a new depressed skull fracture, cerebral edema, and a splenic hemorrhage.

Jason's case is an all-too-common event in the news. Fortunately, the death of an infant from maltreatment is the least common occurrence of child abuse. Whereas abused infants are most likely to die of their injuries, infancy is the time of least abuse. Because maltreatment occurs often before it is considered life-threatening from a public health perspective, there are opportunities for intervention.

In the United States more than 1.5 million children are maltreated each year, and between 2000 and 5000 children die of their injuries each year. Although the maltreatment of children is thought by some to be a new phenomenon in America, only the reporting of it is new. The maltreatment of children has been an undocumented, pervasive epidemic for at least several decades, if not since our society's origins.

The idea of child abuse is a societally determined phenomenon. What is deemed abusive to children continues to evolve in the United States based on medical, sociologic, and psychologic research. Society's ever-changing concept of child abuse has been reflected politically and legally through laws and legal systems. Whereas societies and institutions can foster the maltreatment of children, it is individuals that society holds legally responsible for the acts.

The first protective laws for children limited the use of children in the workplace and required the education of children to a certain age. These laws attempted to reduce physical and emotional abuse, as well as the exploitation of children for profit. In the last several decades, each state has passed laws and set up protective service agencies attempting to protect children from continuous neglect, physical abuse, and emotional harm. Although each state's laws are somewhat different, each recognizes the categories of neglect, physical abuse, sexual abuse, and exploitation. Each state also mandates that health care providers and other professionals who work with children report suspected maltreatment of a child. Mandated reporting has widened knowledge about the maltreatment of children and provides benchmarks for monitoring prevention programs.

Sequelae of Abuse

The disruption in development that occurs because of physical, sexual, or emotional abuse is widespread. Depending on the age at the time of occurrence and on the nature and severity of abuse, there may be symptoms in one or more spheres of intrapsychic, social, occupational, or academic functioning (Boxes 16-1 and 16-2). An abused child may not recollect the abuse or show any symptoms. A child who is the victim of one assault and who subsequently reports it, is believed, and is adequately supported may experience no psychologic symptoms.

The potential for long-term effects of abuse is great. Abused children may experience low self-esteem, major depression, dysthymia, and suicidality, and they may engage in self-injury. Dissociative symptoms may be seen. Self-injurious behavior includes self-cutting or burning, substance abuse, and other high-risk behavior. Aggressive and disruptive behavior may be seen. There may be eating disorders, somatic complaints, and major health problems such as chronic treatment-resistant pain, headaches, and pelvic pain.

There are more psychiatric symptoms in people with histories of physical and sexual abuse. Adult survivors of abuse may have poor interpersonal relationships, anxiety disorders, sleep disturbances, learning disabilities, dissociative disorders, and substance abuse disorders. The severity of the initial trauma is related to the severity of symptoms later in life. A significant number of adults with borderline personality disorder have experienced sexual or physical abuse or witnessed domestic violence. Sexual abuse has a clearer relationship to borderline personality disorder. The chronic dysphoria and derealization symptoms found in borderline personality disorder have been found to be predictive of a history of sexual abuse in childhood. It has also been noted that borderline personality traits may stem from an initial insult of attachment difficulties, which is the result of physical or emotional unavailability of the parent compounded by severe abuse. People with a history of abuse have significantly lower IQ scores than

BOX 16-1

SYMPTOMS OF ABUSE
preschool children

Anxiety
Withdrawal
Guilt
Somatic complaints
Appetite disturbance
Separation anxiety
Sleep difficulties
Nightmares
Hyperactivity
Lying
Impaired trust
Phobias
Regression in toilet training or other behaviors
Age-inappropriate sexual knowledge
Age-inappropriate sexual behavior
Aggression
No symptoms

BOX 16-2

SYMPTOMS OF ABUSE
school-age children and adolescents

Anxiety
Withdrawal
Guilt
Somatic complaints (vague abdominal pain)
Appetite disturbance
Sleep difficulties
Enuresis
Encopresis
Nightmares
Depression
Phobias
School difficulties (school phobia or truancy)
Panic attacks
Poor peer relationships
Running away
Suicide attempts
Tics
Hostility and oppositionality
Aggression
Passivity
Delinquency
Sexual acting out (sexually preoccupied talk)
Obsessions
Psychosis
Poor self-esteem
No symptoms

people with no such history. Sexual abuse was again more strongly related to this finding. Verbal IQ was the score most significantly affected. People with a history of physical abuse have an increased rate of nonlethal suicide attempts, whereas those who experienced sexual abuse do not attempt suicide as often. However, individuals who have been rejected or abused by their mothers also make suicide gestures.

EEG abnormalities have been found in survivors of physical abuse. These findings may possibly be related to head injuries during abuse, although EEG abnormalities have also been found in victims of sexual abuse. Neuropsychiatric studies of both genders have shown limbic system impairment, with people suffering both physical and sexual abuse having higher levels of dysfunction than those who experienced only one type of abuse. Symptoms of impairment affect the realms of memory, sensation, and behavior. Dysregulation of the hypothalamic-pituitary-adrenal axis has also been found.

Lenore Terr, who has conducted research on several types of childhood trauma, has found that besides the presence of other psychiatric disorders, adults with a history of childhood abuse have the following four types of symptoms:

- Visualized or repeatedly perceived memories of the trauma
- Repetitive behavior
- Trauma-specific fears
- Changed attitudes about people, life, and the future

Significant, long-term damage from childhood abuse affects the capacity of an individual to form and maintain close and sustaining interpersonal relationships. The abuse survivor often develops a pattern of seeking out abusive relationships and remaining in them. Additionally, if the survivor has children, they are at risk for a second generation of abusive behavior.

General Notes on Assessment

There are general signs that suggest that a child is being mistreated in some way. These signs are not pathognomonic. It is important to realize that sexual abuse, physical abuse, and emotional abuse do not necessarily occur in isolation but are likely to occur in combination. A change in the child's usual behavior or school performance is a marker for some significant change in relationships at home or with peers, and abuse is a possibility. Worrisome signs include particularly watchful behavior from the child, as if she were preparing for a negative event. The child may come to school early, stay late, or say that she does not want to go home. She may be seen as too responsible or as an overachiever. In short, the child who is being abused may have many, few, or no signs of a problem.

> PEARLS & PERILS
>
> **CHILD MALTREATMENT**
>
> - There are initial and long-term effects of abuse.
> - The various types of abuse are likely to occur in combination.
> - Some children may have no psychiatric symptoms or signs of abuse.

Neglect

Definition and Epidemiology

Physical neglect is the most reported form of maltreatment. Of the approximately 2.7 million reports of child abuse each year, more than one half are reports of physical neglect. Physical neglect is the failure of a caregiver to provide the basic physical needs of a child to the extent that these omissions could result in physical harm to the child. Most states limit basic needs to food, clothing, and sanitary living conditions. The second part of the definition, which implies that neglect could result in physical harm, is usually ill-defined. This ambiguity results in nonreporting or in inappropriate reporting, depending on the observer's interpretation. A parent or guardian cannot be held responsible for neglect if the factors that led to the neglect were beyond the caregiver's control.

Medical neglect is the failure of a parent to seek prompt medical attention or noncompliance with a prescribed medical regimen that is considered important for the child's health and well-being. Although society and the legal system agree with a person's right to make informed decisions about medical care based on moral or religious beliefs, a parent is not allowed to withhold medical care that is health- or lifesaving for the child.

Emotional neglect is the failure to provide needed emotional supports, such as love, protection, and supervision. Such lack of protection can result in accidents and poisonous ingestions. Educational neglect includes the failure to provide appropriate intellectual stimulation or schooling. Poor household sanitation, hygiene, or nutrition; unsafe living conditions; and abandonment may also fall into the realm of neglect.

Etiology

Poor attachment between a child and a caregiver leads to neglect. It occurs most commonly in the least educated part of the lower socioeconomic classes. Large family size and close spacing can place any child at risk for neglect. The mothers of neglected infants are less able to use available supports, appear to have fewer positive emotions, and are more likely to capriciously stop feedings.

The largest number of confirmed cases of abuse and neglect occurs in children born to adolescent mothers. Reasons for this include poverty and low educational levels, a high incidence of prematurity and low birth weight, and fussy temperaments of children. The younger the mother at the age of her first pregnancy, the more likely she is to have more closely spaced children during her teenage years. Because of their own age, these mothers are less likely to be prepared for the emotional rigors of parenting or to have learned the necessary parenting skills. Consequently they may rely on their own mothers to care for their children. This is likely to increase parent-child conflict in that sphere, resulting in depression, low self-esteem, and other symptoms that increase the likelihood of neglect.

Sequelae

There are few studies that have focused on the effects that neglect has on the long-term psychologic development of children. The effects of neglect are an interaction of what is omitted and what the child's needs are at the time. In infancy, a lack of nutrition or emotional bonding results in failure to thrive (see Chapter 12 and Box 16-3). A continuation of poor attachment behavior between the child and the caregiver leads to deficient social skill development, low self-esteem, poor coping skills, and a slower development of autonomy in relationships (Box 16-4). Furthermore, there may be high levels of anger, which are expressed in violent criminal activity.

Emotional Abuse

Definition

Emotional abuse is rarely reported and difficult to prove when it is suspected. It is the failure to provide psychologic nurturance to the child. Briere has noted that the following eight types of behavior characterize emotional abuse: (1) deliberate rejection; (2) degrading or devaluing; (3) terrorizing; (4) isolating; (5) corrupting; (6) exploiting; (7) denying essential emotional stimulation, responsiveness, or availability; and (8) unreliable and inconsistent parenting. Usually, there is a combination of these, as well as other forms of abuse.

Etiology

Emotional abuse can occur when a parent is not certain how to best discipline a child. More than parents who use other forms of abuse, the emotionally abusive parent abuses alcohol or other substances. As with the other forms of abuse, it is likely that an abusive parent had similar experiences during her own development.

Sequelae

The most pervasive emotional consequence of emotional abuse is low self-esteem. This leads to difficulties in academics, peer relations, and trusting relationships.

PEARLS & PERILS

NEGLECT

- Neglect is related to poor attachment between the caregiver and the child.
- Sequelae of neglect include failure to thrive, poor attachment, poor social skills, and anger.

PEARLS & PERILS

EMOTIONAL ABUSE

- Emotional abuse is strongly related to substance abuse.
- Sequelae of emotional abuse include low self-esteem, depression, and difficulties in relationships.

DSM-IV DIAGNOSTIC CRITERIA

BOX 16-3 FEEDING DISORDER OF INFANCY OR EARLY CHILDHOOD

A. Feeding disturbance as manifested by persistent failure to eat adequately with significant failure to gain weight or significant loss of weight over at least 1 month.

B. The disturbance is not due to an associated gastrointestinal or other general medical condition (e.g., esophageal reflux).

C. The disturbance is not better accounted for by another mental disorder (e.g., Rumination Disorder) or by lack of available food.

D. The onset is before age 6 years.

(From American Psychiatric Association: *Diagnostic and statistical manual of mental disorders,* ed 4 [DSM-IV], Washington DC, 1994, American Psychiatric Press.)

BOX 16-4 REACTIVE ATTACHMENT DISORDER OF INFANCY OR EARLY CHILDHOOD

DSM-IV DIAGNOSTIC CRITERIA

A. Markedly disturbed and developmentally inappropriate social relatedness in most contexts, beginning before age 5 years, as evidenced by either (1) or (2):

(1) persistent failure to initiate or respond in a developmentally appropriate fashion to most social interactions, as manifest by excessively inhibited, hypervigilant, or highly ambivalent and contradictory responses (e.g., the child may respond to caregivers with a mixture of approach, avoidance, and resistance to comforting, or may exhibit frozen watchfulness)

(2) diffuse attachments as manifest by indiscriminate sociability with marked inability to exhibit appropriate selective attachments (e.g., excessive familiarity with relative strangers or lack of selectivity in choice of attachment figures)

B. The disturbance in Criterion A is not accounted for solely by developmental delay (as in Mental Retardation) and does not meet criteria for a Pervasive Developmental Disorder.

C. Pathogenic care as evidenced by at least one of the following:

(1) persistent disregard of the child's basic emotional needs for comfort, stimulation, and affection

(2) persistent disregard of the child's basic physical needs

(3) repeated changes of primary caregiver that prevent formation of stable attachments (e.g., frequent changes in foster care)

D. There is a presumption that the care in Criterion C is responsible for the disturbed behavior in Criterion A (e.g., the disturbances in Criterion A began following the pathogenic care in Criterion C).

Specify type:

Inhibited Type: if Criterion A1 predominates in the clinical presentation

Disinhibited Type: if Criterion A2 predominates in the clinical presentation

(From American Psychiatric Association: *Diagnostic and statistical manual for mental disorders,* ed 4 [DSM-IV], Washington DC, 1994, American Psychiatric Press.)

A child often feels that he has done something bad for which he is being punished; such children often go on to misinterpret the comments and nonverbal expressions of others as critical. As they grow older, survivors of emotional abuse are likely to have symptoms of dysthymic disorder or major depressive disorder (MDD) (Boxes 16-5 and 16-6).

Physical Abuse

Definition and Epidemiology

Physical abuse is the second most reported form of child abuse. More than 1 million children are estimated to be physically abused each year. Physical abuse is the commission of a physical act to a child that could lead to permanent physical damage to that child. With the improved understanding of the mechanisms of physical injury, the identification of acute physical child abuse has become easier. These improvements have led to more valid reporting by health care professionals.

Eighty percent of physical abuse is at the hands of the parents. Roughly 10% of physical abuse is committed by other family members, with the remainder committed by outsiders such as babysitters or school and day care personnel. Age is the most consistent predictor of severe injury, with young children suffering greater abuse. Boys are more likely to suffer serious injury from birth through age 12, whereas girls are more likely to be seriously injured after age 13. Data from 1990 to 1992 suggest that 87% of children whose deaths resulted from physical abuse were younger than age 5, and 46% were under age 1. Black children are overrepresented in studies of known child abuse fatalities, but socioeconomic status may be a confounding factor.

Etiology

There is no one picture of a physically abusive family. Family patterns may reflect a multigenerational failure of being nurtured and being unable to nurture. This is called a *cycle of violence.* The parent may have been reared this way and not realize that he was abused.

The Interactive Model of Child Abuse proposes that physical abuse is the result of the interactions of characteristics of the child, the abuser, and the social environment. According to this model, the abused child is more demanding of the caregiver in some way. This "special child" may be mentally or physically disabled, chronically physically ill, or hard to console (for example, a baby with colic). The child may be hyperactive or exhibit defiant behavior. He may be premature or the re-

DSM-IV DIAGNOSTIC CRITERIA

BOX 16-5 DYSTHYMIC DISORDER

A. Depressed mood for most of the day, for more days than not, as indicated either by subjective account or observation by others, for at least 2 years. **Note:** In children and adolescents, mood can be irritable and duration must be at least 1 year.

B. Presence, while depressed, of two (or more) of the following:
(1) poor appetite or overeating
(2) insomnia or hypersomnia
(3) low energy or fatigue
(4) low self-esteem
(5) poor concentration or difficulty making decisions
(6) feelings of hopelessness

C. During the 2-year period (1 year for children or adolescents) of the disturbance, the person has never been without the symptoms in Criteria A and B for more than 2 months at a time.

D. No Major Depressive Episode has been present during the first 2 years of the disturbance (1 year for children and adolescents); i.e., the disturbance is not better accounted for by chronic Major Depressive Disorder, or Major Depressive Disorder, In Parital Remission.

Note: There may have been a previous Major Depressive Episode provided there was a full remission (no significant signs or symptoms for 2 months) before development of the Dysthymic Disorder. In addition, after the initial 2 years (1 year in children or adolescents) of Dysthymic Disorder, there may be superimposed episodes of Major Depressive Disorder, in which case both diagnoses may be given when the criteria are met for a Major Depressive Episode.

E. There has never been a Manic Episode, a Mixed Episode, or a Hypomanic Episode, and criteria have never been met for Cyclothymic Disorder.

F. The disturbance does not occur exclusively during the course of a chronic Psychotic Disorder, such as Schizophrenia or Delusional Disorder.

G. The symptoms are not due to the direct physiological effects of a substance (e.g., a drug of abuse, a medication) or a general medical condition (e.g., hypothyroidism).

H. The symptoms cause clinically significant distress or impairment in social, occupational, or other important areas of functioning.

Specify if
Early Onset: if onset is before age 21 years
Late Onset: if onset is age 21 years or older

Specify (for most recent 2 years of Dysthymic Disorder):**With Atypical Features**

(From American Psychiatric Association: *Diagnostic and statistical manual of mental disorders,* ed 4 [DSM-IV], Washington DC, 1994, American Psychiatric Press.)

sult of an unwanted pregnancy. In situations where physical abuse begins during adolescence, the youth is likely to be involved in the developmental tasks of individuation, which result in conflict with parents.

There are many risk factors for a parent to become abusive, including a lack of personal maturity and difficulty dealing with anger; a history of having been abused; poor understanding of child development and the role of the parent; and a psychiatric diagnosis, including substance abuse problems. Abusive parents have unrealistic and rigid expectations of their children, and they subjectively report themselves as unhappy in their interpersonal relationships. For adolescents who are abused, one or both of the parents may be experiencing a significant midlife developmental crisis. Environmental risk factors are unemployment, social isolation of the family, poverty, single parenthood, and lack of peer support.

Sequelae

The individual with a history of physical abuse may develop a wide range of emotional, behavioral, and in-

BOX 16-6 MAJOR DEPRESSIVE EPISODE

DSM-IV DIAGNOSTIC CRITERIA

A. Five (or more) of the following symptoms have been present during the same 2-week period and represent a change from previous functioning; at least one of the symptoms is either (1) depressed mood or (2) loss of interest or pleasure.

Note: Do not include symptoms that are clearly due to a general medical condition, or mood-incongruent delusions or hallucinations.

(1) depressed mood most of the day, nearly every day, as indicated by either subjective report (e.g., feels sad or empty) or observation made by others (e.g., appears tearful). **Note:** In children and adolescents, can be irritable mood.
(2) markedly diminished interest or pleasure in all, or almost all, activities most of the day, nearly every day (as indicated by either subjective account or observation made by others)
(3) significant weight loss when not dieting or weight gain (e.g., a change of more than 5% of body weight in a month), or decrease or increase in appetite nearly every day. **Note:** In children, consider failure to make expected weight gains.
(4) insomnia or hypersomnia nearly every day
(5) psychomotor agitation or retardation nearly every day (observable by others, not merely subjective feelings of restlessness or being slowed down)
(6) fatigue or loss of energy nearly every day
(7) feelings of worthlessness or excessive or inappropriate guilt (which may be delusional) nearly every day (not merely self-reproach or guilt about being sick)
(8) diminished ability to think or concentrate, or indecisiveness, nearly every day (either by subjective account or as observed by others)
(9) recurrent thought of death (not just fear of dying), recurrent suicidal ideation without a specific plan, or a suicide attempt or a specific plan for committing suicide

B. The symptoms do not meet criteria for a Mixed Episode.

C. The symptoms cause clinically significant distress or impairment in social, occupational, or other important areas of functioning.

D. The symptoms are not due to the direct physiological effects of a substance (e.g., a drug of abuse, a medication) or a general medical condition (e.g., hypothyroidism).

E. The symptoms are not better accounted for by Bereavement, i.e., after the loss of a loved one, the symptoms persist for longer than 2 months or are charactrized by marked functional impairment, morbid preoccupation with worthlessness, suicidal ideation, psychotic symptoms, or psychomotor retardation.

(From American Psychiatric Association, *Diagnostic and statistical manual of mental disorders,* ed 4 [DSM-IV], Washington DC, 1994, American Psychiatric Press.)

terpersonal problems that can be long-lasting and difficult to treat. Many people with bonafide psychiatric diagnoses have histories of having been physically abused. Certainly, any child or adolescent who develops a serious emotional disorder should be evaluated for past and current physical abuse. In particular, children who become violent have the highest likelihood of having been abused, and they are also at a greater risk for depression, suicidal behavior, and substance abuse. Conduct disorder (CD) is a likely sequelae of physical abuse (Box 16-7). If an abused child can maintain a positive relationship with a nonabusive parent, then there is a better chance that the cycle of violence will not be repeated when the child is a parent.

Special Notes on Assessment

General aspects of assessment apply in evaluating the child who may have been physically abused. The parent may have an unrealistic perception of the child or his injuries, which can be gleaned through history-gathering. Through proper interviewing and an abuse screening, many high-risk children can be identified. A Child's World Screen should be completed annually. Sample questions are shown in Box 16-8. This is an interview that assesses psychosocial risk factors and supports available to the family. Anticipatory guidance can be focused toward particular areas of concern. For children age 5 or older, questions about their world should be age-appropriately addressed to them with parental

DSM-IV DIAGNOSTIC CRITERIA

BOX 16-7 CONDUCT DISORDER

A. A repetitive and persistent pattern of behavior in which the basic rights of others or major age-appropriate societal norms or rules are violated, as manifested by the presence of three (or more) of the following criteria in the past 12 months, with at least one criterion present in the past 6 months:

Aggression to people and animals

(1) often bullies, threatens, or intimidates others
(2) often initiates physical fights
(3) has used a weapon that can cause serious physical harm to others (e.g., a bat, brick, broken bottle, knife, gun)
(4) has been physically cruel to people
(5) has been physically cruel to animals
(6) has stolen while confronting a victim (e.g., mugging, purse snatching, extortion, armed robbery)
(7) has forced someone into sexual activity

Destruction of property

(8) has deliberately engaged in fire setting with the intention of causing serious damage
(9) has deliberately destroyed others' property (other than by fire setting)

Deceitfulness or theft

(10) has broken into someone else's house, building, or car
(11) often lies to obtain goods or favors or to avoid obligations (i.e., "cons" others)
(12) has stolen items of nontrivial value without confronting a victim (e.g., shoplifting, but without breaking and entering; forgery)

Serious violations of rules

(13) often stays out at night despite parental prohibitions, beginning before age 13 years
(14) has runaway from home overnight at least twice while living in parental or parental surrogate home (or once without returning for a lengthy period)
(15) is often truant from school, beginning before age 13 years

B. The disturbance in behavior causes clinically significant impairment in social, academic, or occupational functioning.

C. If the individual is age 18 years or older, criteria are not met for Antisocial Personality Disorder.

Specify type based on age at onset:
Childhood-Onset Type: onset of at least one criterion characteristic of Conduct Disorder prior to age 10 years
Adolescent-Onset Type: absence of any criteria characteristic of Conduct Disorder prior to age 10 years

Specify severity:
Mild: few if any conduct problems in excess of those required to make the diagnosis **and** conduct problems cause only mild harm to others
Moderate: number of conduct problems and effect on others intermediate between "mild" and "severe"
Severe: many conduct problems in excess of those required to make the diagnosis **or** conduct problems cause considerable harm to others

(From American Psychiatric Association: *Diagnostic and statistical manual of mental disorders,* ed 4 [DSM-IV], Washington DC, 1994, American Psychiatric Press.)

support of information. Children this age are able to understand what is good or bad and what actions are taken against them if they are bad. The child may innocently say, "Daddy hits with a belt when I am bad," thus providing helpful information to the primary care physician. For the teen, the psychosocial screen is called HEADSS. Sample HEADSS questions are in Box 16-9.

The office-based medical professional may not see the acute symptoms of physical abuse; subacute findings are much more likely. Although many injuries can

BOX 16-8

CHILD'S WORLD QUESTIONS

Prenatal

How do you feel about the pregnancy?
What are your concerns about being a parent?
How do you feel about how you were raised?
What would you keep the same? What would you change?
How does the father feel about the pregnancy?
What are his concerns?
How does the father feel about how he was raised?
What would he keep the same? What would he change?
Who will help you after the baby is born?
How do you think having a baby is going to change your life?
How will it change the father's life?

Newborn

How was the delivery? Any problems?
All parents have difficulties with their babies. What difficulties have you had?
How does having this baby differ from what you expected?
What type of help with the baby do you have?
Which term would describe your baby? Sleepy? Cranky? Irritable? Pleasant?
How does this child compare to your other children when they were babies?

Toddlers

What do you and your child do for fun?
What do your child and the father do for fun?
What types of things does your child do that makes you happy?
What do you do when this happens?
What types of things does your child do that makes the father happy?
What does he do when this happens?
What types of things does your child do that upsets you?
What do you do when this happens?
What types of things does child do that upsets the father?
What does he do when this happens?
What type of help do you have with the children?

Childhood

Same as the toddler's questions plus the following:
Is your child in daycare?
How does your child interact with other children?
What difficulties has your child had with the teacher?
What difficulties has your child had with peers?

occur accidentally, lesions that occur on the face (excluding the forehead and chin), buttocks and hips, thorax, or pelvis; lesions in multiple sites; or lesions that have evidence of being sustained at different times are highly suggestive of abuse. During the physical examination, the physician needs to inquire how previously undocumented fractures, injuries, and skin manifestations of injury occurred (see the annotated bibliography at the end of this chapter for works dedicated to this subject).

PEARLS & PERILS

PHYSICAL ABUSE

- Physical abuse may be related to a "cycle of violence" and is a result of interactions of the characteristics of the child, the abuser, and the social environment.
- Sequelae of physical abuse include violent behavior, depression, substance abuse, and difficulties in relationships.

Sexual Abuse

Definition and Epidemiology

Sexual abuse is the use of a child by an adult or person of authority for sexual gratification. Sexual exploitation is the use of a child in sexual acts for the profit of an adult. Although research on sexual maltreatment of children is in its infancy, studies suggest that as many as half a million children are sexually maltreated each year. One half of all sexually abused children are between 9 and 12 years old. Nationally, 27% of adult women and 16% of adult men report being sexually abused before their eighteenth birthday.

Sexual abuse includes oral, anal, and genital intercourse, genital fondling, and exhibitionism. There is usually a progression of sexual contact, starting with genital fondling (the most common form of sexual abuse) and advancing to frottage (orgasm achieved by rubbing genitals against body parts), oral-genital contact, and then penetration with fingers or objects. Next there may be vulvar intercourse, in which the child feels penetrated but the hymen is intact, and then finally oral, vaginal, or anal intercourse.

Sexual abuse occurs at the same rate in every ethnic group, religious group, and socioeconomic class. Despite this fact, it should be noted that sexually abused children among whites and in the higher socioeconomic classes are the least likely to be reported to legal authorities or CPS.

BOX 16-9

SAMPLE HEADSS QUESTIONS

Home

Who lives at home with you?
How do you get along with your mother? father? siblings?
What happens when you and your parents disagree?
What happens with your parents when you do something right? wrong?
Have you ever felt like running away from home?

Education

What school do you attend?
What grade are you in now?
How are you doing in school? A's, B's, C's, D's, or F's?
How does that compare to your grades last year?
Do you think that you can do better? How?
How do you think you would like to do after finishing school?
Do you ever worry about your safety in school?

Activities

Would you say you have many friends, a best friend, or no friends?
Give me examples of what you and your friends do together.
What do you like to to do for fun?
When was the last time you were in a fight?

Drugs

Have any of your friends tried smoking?
Have you ever tried smoking?
How many of your friends have tried an alcoholic drink such as beer, wine, or a mixed drink?
How often do you drink alcoholic drinks? Do you ever drink to get drunk?
Have any of your friends experimented with drugs? What kind?
Have you ever tried any drugs? When? What type?

Sex

Have any of your friends had sex? Has your best friend had sex?
What is sexual intercourse? Have you ever had sexual intercourse? With boys, girls, or both?
How old were you when you first had sex? How many partners have you had in your life? How old have your partners been?
What do you enjoy about having sex? Has anyone ever forced you to have sex with them?
What do you use to protect yourself from sexually transmitted diseases? How often do you use this protection?
What do you or your partner use to protect against pregnancy? Have you ever been or gotten your partner pregnant?

Suicide

Would you describe yourself as happy, sad, or sometimes both?
What makes you happy? What makes you sad? Have you ever thought about hurting yourself?

Although the vast majority of abusers are men, there is no single "type" of abuser. Up to 90% of perpterators are known to the victim, and 65% are family members. Although brothers and uncles are the most common perpetrators, parental incest is most often reported.The majority of extrafamilial perpetrators are people known to the family. Only 10% of all abusers are unknown to the victim.

For many years, sexual abuse was felt to be a problem that affected primarily girls. However, studies suggest that boys are also commonly abused, with the ratio felt to be as high as two girls to one boy. For boys who are victims, up to 43% of perpetrators are women, although the research on how and by whom boys are sexually abused is limited compared with that on girls who are victims. Society's double standard for boys and girls confuses the definition of what is abusive to boys. This is most unclear in the cases of young teenage boys having sex with adult women. Some perceive this as "making a man out of the boy" and actively encourage it, whereas others see it as abusive. Surveys of adult males suggest that approximately 20% had sex with an adult woman when they were teenagers. These adult women were current or past babysitters, friends of the family, distant relatives, or mothers of the boys' friends. Boys are more commonly abused by individuals outside the home, such as distant relatives, religious leaders, school personnel, other group leaders, parents' friends, or their friends' parents. Most abusers are known to the victim and his family; however, in many instances the abuser is known only to the boy and not his family.

Etiology

The literature on the causes of sexual abuse is vast. Finkelhor and Krugman have stated that the following four conditions must be present for the sexual abuse of a child to occur:

- The perpetrator must experience sexual arousal when with children. Sexual abuse must fill some

need for the abuser, whether it is pure sexual arousal or some emotional need. In some instances, the perpetrator feels that all other means of sexual fulfillment are blocked.
- The perpetrator must overcome inhibitions. Inhibitions may be decreased through alcohol or drug abuse or because of emotional disturbance, social tolerance of sexual interest in children (which "justifies" the behavior), and weak criminal penalties against offenders (which prevents limitation of behavior by fear of consequences).
- There must be an external opportunity. Examples include absence of parental supervision, social isolation of the family, and unusual sleeping or rooming conditions that bypass normal external inhibitors.
- The child must be vulnerable. For example, the child may crave attention, and the abuser may take advantage of this need by first enticing and then using coercion when the child resists.

Understanding each of these conditions helps in the recognition, assessment, and treatment of sexual abuse. Lanning has described a situational type of child molester and a preferential type; the individual who is sexually aroused by children fits into one or the other of these categories. The situational child molester does not have a sole preference for sex with children but exploits others as well. This may be the situation in some incest cases. The preferential child molester, or pedophile, prefers sexual activity with children over adults and is likely to have a large number of victims. The abuser may use coercion, threat, or intimidation. Coercion includes seduction, bribery, manipulation, and deception, and the abuser may make statements such as, "I will kill your parents," or "You won't be able to come and visit me if you don't do this."

Compared with male sexual offenders, little has been written about the female sexual offender. Although it has generally been considered rare for a woman to sexually molest a child, it is likely that these episodes of victimization are underreported and that these offenders are underrecognized. There are three categories of female sexual offenders, and all are likely to have experienced abuse in childhood or adolescence. The teacher-lover molester initiates the abuse and sees the child or adolescent as her equal; she does not appreciate the abusive nature of the relationship. She feels that the experience was a positive one for the child. The predisposed or intergenerational offender also initiates the abuse and is more likely to have deviant sexual fantasies that she considers shameful. She is likely to engage in self-injurious or suicidal behaviors. The male-coerced offender fits the "classic" description of the female sexual offender. She is extremely dependent on males, has low self-esteem, and feels powerless in relationships. As part of a relationship, she may agree to engage in abusive behaviors. To continue the relationship, she may later initiate these behaviors herself.

A child may be vulnerable simply because she is the gender and age preferred by the abuser. The child may show some early curiosity about sexual matters, thereby "justifying" the molester's intentions. Children who become victims of sexual abuse often have low self-esteem that results in a high need for love and approval. They may not feel emotionally close to the mother, or they may feel isolated and be unable to make friends easily. Factors that contribute to the external opportunity to abuse are described in the following section.

Profiles of Abuse

Intrafamilial Sexual Abuse

Father-Daughter

These families are usually socially and perhaps physically isolated. There is a great deal of resentment and anger caused by excessive dependence and the inability to meet one another's needs. In these families, the daughter who is sexually abused may develop anger and resentment toward her mother. The mother may be perceived as inadequate because she has been unable to protect the daughter from her father. There is more risk with a stepfather, because he has had less parental contact, which decreases the inherent sexual nature of many parent-child interactions. There may be role confusion in a blended family. The daughter may be the eldest or only girl, and she may have early sexual maturation. The mother may have delegated certain duties to her. The daughter has typically had inadequate socialization with peers, and may be kept from her peers by her father. In the dependent-domineering pattern, the father is dependent and the mother is domineering. As the mother becomes increasingly weary of her husband's dependency, she withdraws from him and he turns to the daughter for fulfillment of his needs. He may also be under the influence of alcohol or some other substance. In the possessive-passive family, the father is extremely controlling and views his wife and children as possessions. Because the daughter is a possession, the father feels that he may use her sexually. He may rationalize this by stating that he is "breaking her in" and showing her that he treats her better than others. In the incestrogenic or dependent-dependent family, one or both parents may have a history of sexual abuse by a family member. They are unable to meet each other's emotional needs and look to their children for emotional sustenance.

The child's initial response to father-daughter incest may not be negative. She is often convinced that she has a special, close relationship with her father. She may feel that she has power over her siblings, and she may have privileges that they do not have. She may crave the attention that she is getting from this man whom she has every reason to trust. She may receive special gifts, and she enjoys feeling like an adult. However, this is a difficult position to maintain, since the abuse interferes with the establishment of normal peer and child-adult relationships.

The father may not want his daughter to interact with peers for fear that she will reveal the secret. As the abuse becomes more and more sexually intrusive, she becomes more frightened. More coercion and threatening become necessary. She may feel as if she is responsible because she did not (or felt she could not) tell her mother or someone else immediately. She is prone to feel guilty because of any physical or emotional pleasure she may have experienced as a result of the incest. If the daughter is able to tell the mother and the mother believes her, then a healing process can start. If the mother disbelieves her, the child will feel abandoned, unprotected, and at the mercy of the father's sexual desires. The following factors contribute to the abusive situation: (1) secrecy, which is necessary for the abuse to continue; (2) helplessness, which describes the child's feelings about stopping the abuse; (3) entrapment, or the feeling that she cannot tell when the abuse has occurred more than once; and (4) accommodation, the means by which the daughter emotionally tolerates the abuse. The results of a delayed disclosure may result in the retraction of the accusation. Each of these factors is ultimately a focus of treatment.

Siblings

Sibling incest is not uncommon, although it is not commonly reported. Roughly 13% of the population has been involved with sibling incest. The abusive sibling is likely to have been sexually abused himself. Because of the closeness in age, the impact of the abuse may be minimized by family members. However, force and coercion are involved in most cases. A lack of parental physical or emotional presence contributes to the sexual abuse of a child by a sibling; this can include abandonment, focus on career, substance abuse, mental illness, or repetitive pregnancies. Additionally, parents may stimulate a sexual climate in the home by engaging in intercourse within their children's view or by sexually abusing or being overly seductive with one or more of the children, thereby creating an environment with poor relationship boundaries.

Grandparent-Child

In abuse by grandparents, grandfathers are generally the perpetrators, and granddaughters are the victims. Step-grandfathers are often responsible for more severe forms of abuse. Grandfathers more commonly limit their abuse to fondling without penetration, but they do make explicit threats and overtly assault their grandchildren. The vast majority of abusive grandfathers have abused their daughters as well as their granddaughters.

Extrafamilial Sexual Abuse

Knowledge about the prevalence of extrafamilial sexual abuse is not as extensive as that surrounding intrafamilial abuse, because mandatory reporting laws are often not applicable. Certain states require that only caregivers must be reported to CPS. Therefore, these situations may not be reported or examined. There are sociologic factors that contribute to a child's vulnerability to extrafamilial sexual abuse. Divorce affects two out of three marriages in the United States and brings children into ongoing close contact with new adults: stepparents, parents' new boyfriends or girlfriends, and new child care providers. Children and parents may be emotionally devastated after a divorce, leaving the children simultaneously more emotionally needy and less protected. Children often leave the family to go to day care, school, and organized recreational activities, and they spend more time away from their families. As a result, they are more vulnerable. Poor parental supervision of a child's activities and whereabouts can increase the risk of abuse. A substitute caregiver is more likely to sexually abuse a child than the mother. Boys are more likely than girls to be sexually abused outside of the home.

The extrafamilial sexual abuser is likely to be a preferential child molester who finds a job that provides access to children and then initiates an abusive relationship. However, the abuser may be a situational molester who does not recognize the attraction to children. Day care situations, schools, and youth group gatherings are common situations for either type of abuser.

Child prostitution and sex rings are additional situations in which children are abused by adults. There are three types of sex rings: the solo ring, the transition ring, and the syndicated ring. In the solo ring, there is one offender and several victims. The perpetrator usually has legitimate access to the victims. In the transition ring, there are several perpetrators. The victims are usually adolescents. In the syndicated ring, there is a highly organized system that may extend across geographic areas. In these situations, children are usually abused in a group, or are at least aware of the other children involved. The children may be manipulated to become competitive for the adults' favor and special attention by receiving special favors for various behaviors. As the child grows older, she may be used to obtain other children for the ring. The children develop strong bonds with one another and their abusers; as such, they are unlikely to disclose their abuse to anyone. Children and adolescents in these situations may be prostituted or may participate in group or dyadic sex with adults and peers; pornography may be developed from their activities.

Sequelae

Sexual abuse may result in a range of disturbed and disturbing behaviors and emotional symptoms. In preschoolers, there may be a regression in attained skills or vague complaints. Inappropriate sexual behavior may be seen (see Boxes 16-1 and 16-2). The sexually abused adolescent or older child may have vague abdominal pain, school phobias, advanced sexual talk, secondary enuresis, secondary encopresis, defiance, panic attacks, and passive behavior.

It is important to recognize that some children may not show any signs of distress or dysfunction in reaction to sexual abuse. It is very possible that symptoms may not manifest until puberty, adolescence, or even adulthood. A history of abuse may be discovered only when an adult is unable to have stable, satisfying romantic relationships.

Sexual abuse disrupts normal psychosexual development. This traumatic sexualization results in a child's sexuality being inappropriately and dysfunctionally shaped. The sexual relationship and stimulation that is experienced becomes a matter that may obsess the child and prevent psychologic development in other areas. School-age children who have been sexualized in this manner do not have the ability to repress or sublimate interest in sexual activity as do others their age, who are able to spend this energy learning and developing appropriate social relationships.

Long-term effects of sexual abuse include a range of symptoms and characterologic abnormalities. Both male and female victims of sexual abuse can develop psychiatric disorders related to the abuse. Borderline personality disorder is strongly correlated with survivors of sexual abuse (Box 16-10). The full clinical picture is often seen only in late adolescence or adulthood. Similarly, dissociative identity disorder may occur in an abused child (Box 16-11). Self-injurious behaviors are common. Sexual difficulties that a victim may experience include difficulty with arousal, vaginismus, flashbacks to abusive events, sexual guilt and anxiety, and low sexual self-esteem. Furthermore, these individuals are at a higher risk for sexual victimization in adolescence and adulthood.

Finkelhor and Browne's model of traumagenic dynamics elucidates personality characteristics seen in those with a history of sexual abuse. Four dynamic factors, traumatic sexualization, betrayal, powerlessness, and stigmatization, are experienced by victims of childhood sexual abuse. These symptoms may also be seen in victims of other types of trauma, but the particular combination of these factors in a child who has been sexually abused results in their unique nature. The researchers conclude that these dynamics affect the child's cognition and emotions regarding the abuser, herself, and the world in general.

As a result of traumatic sexualization, the child receives an emotional or tangible reward for behavior that is not developmentally appropriate. She may associate terrifying memories with sexual activity for the remainder of her life, or she may think that sexual behaviors are appropriate for children.

BOX 16-10 BORDERLINE PERSONALITY DISORDER

DSM-IV DIAGNOSTIC CRITERIA

A pervasive pattern of instability of interpersonal relationships, self-image, and affects, and marked impulsivity beginning by early adulthood and present in a variety of contexts, as indicated by five (or more) of the following:

(1) frantic efforts to avoid real or imagined abandonment. **Note:** Do not include suicidal or self-mutilating behavior covered in Criterion 5.
(2) a pattern of unstable and intense interpersonal relationships characterized by alternating between extremes of idealization and devaluation
(3) identity disturbance: markedly and persistently unstable self-image or sense of self
(4) impulsivity in at least two areas that are potentially self-damaging (e.g., spending, sex, substance abuse, reckless driving, binge eating). **Note:** Do not include suicidal or self-mutilating behavior covered in Criterion 5.
(5) recurret suicidal behavior, gestures, or threats, or self-mutililating behavior
(6) affective instability due to a marked reactivity of mood (e.g. intense episodic dysphoria, irritability, or anxiety usually lasting a few hours and only rarely more than a few days)
(7) chronic feelings of emptiness
(8) inappropriate, intense anger or difficulty controlling anger (e.g., frequent displays of temper, constant anger, recurrent physical fights)
(9) transient, stress-related paranoid ideation or severe dissociative symptoms

(From American Psychiatric Association: *Diagnostic and Statistical Manual of Mental Disorders,* ed 4 [DSM-IV], Washington DC, 1994, American Psychiatric Press.)

BOX 16-11 DISSOCIATIVE IDENTITY DISORDER — DSM-IV DIAGNOSTIC CRITERIA

A. The presence of two or more distinct identities or personality states (each with its own relatively enduring pattern of perceiving, relating to, and thinking about the environment and self).

B. At least two of these identities or personality states recurrently take control of the person's behavior.

C. Inability to recall important personal information that is too extensive to be explained by ordinary forgetfulness.

D. The disturbance is not due to the direct physiological effects of a substance (e.g., blackouts or chaotic behavior during Alcohol Intoxication) or a general medical condition (e.g., complex partial seizures). **Note:** In children, the symptoms are not attributable to imaginary playmates or other fantasy play.

(From American Psychiatric Association: *Diagnostic and statistical manual of mental disorders,* ed 4 [DSM-IV], Washington DC, 1994, American Psychiatric Press.)

In betrayal, the child comes to understand that someone whom she trusted and depended on manipulated and hurt her deliberately. Furthermore, another trusted person disbelieved, was unable, or even worse, was unwilling to protect her from harm. Symptoms resulting from betrayal include extreme dependency or clingi ness in relationships because of the need to establish a trusting relationship. Similarly, the victim may show poor judgment about the trustworthiness of others because she had no model of an appropriately trusting relationship. As an adolescent and adult, the survivor of sexual abuse is particularly vulnerable to later victimization and may become involved in relationships that involve the physical, emotional, or sexual abuse of herself or her children. She may also have absolute distrust of all male-female relationships, which leads to poor heterosexual relationships.

In powerlessness, the child's will and sense of ability to master any threatening situation are continually undermined. She ultimately sees herself as someone who cannot be effective in any venue. Some sense of empowerment may be regained if the child is eventually able to stop the abuse. Symptoms related to this dynamic are nightmares and phobias, as well as clinginess and hypervigilance. The impaired sense of efficacy and coping skills can lead to learning problems, suicide gestures and attempts, and running away.

Stigmatization refers to the shame and guilt that are part of the ongoing abuse and that become part of the child's self-concept. These negative emotions come from secrecy, demeaning statements made by the abuser, and the disapproving reactions of others to the abuse or to other victims of trauma. Resulting symptoms include low self-esteem, a persistent sense of guilt and shame, and the victim's belief that she is alone in having survived such an experience.

Special Notes on Assessment

Disclosure of sexual abuse has been found not to be an event, but a process. Young children are most likely to accidentally disclose sexual abuse; for example, when she is having a bath a child might tell her mother what Uncle Fred would do if he were giving the bath. In contrast, adolescents most often purposefully inform someone about what has been happening to them, and they often tell out of anger. Either type of disclosure often happens shortly before or after the child spends time with the perpetrator.

SEXUAL ABUSE — PEARLS & PERILS

- Sexual abuse is a result of interactions of characteristics of the child, the abuser, and the social environment.
- Sequelae include self injurious behaviors, borderline personality disorder, dissociative disorders, depression, low self-esteem, sexual problems, and difficulties in relationships.

A youngster might make an inappropriate statement that promotes suspicion in the parent. In another situation, a young girl might share a secret with a friend, who then may tell her parent or a teacher. Purposeful disclosure may result from a school program that teaches children about inappropriate touching; a child may learn from such a program that activities in which she has been engaged are not sanctioned. She may be encouraged by peers to disclose. A child may simply feel that it is the right time to tell what has been happening.

Approximately 75% of all children deny any abuse after their initial disclosure and the first stages of a formal investigation. Of these children, only a few immediately continue the disclosure and describe the events again. The remainder go through a stage of tentative disclosure, in which they make discounting statements such as, "I forgot," or, "I was only teasing." They may distance themselves from the abuse by saying, "It happened a long time ago," or, "It happened to Ricky, not me."

Minimizing or self-empowering statements, such as, "It only happened once," or, "He wanted to hurt me, but I karate-chopped him," may be made. Another type of tentative disclosure statement involves a description of dissociation; for example, a child may say, "When that happens, I go to a special place." The majority of children progress to active disclosure from tentative disclosure.

After active disclosure, the child or adolescent is faced with the consequences of having revealed her traumatization. As a result, from 12% to 33% of children then recant their allegations. This is often found in situations where the child is faced with the possibility of loss, specifically of love or of family. In incest cases, the impending loss of a parent through someone moving out of the home or the remaining parent having to choose between spouse and child may compel the victim to recant. The fear of meeting with the police and representatives from social services or of appearing in court may similarly result in such recantation. However, 92% of those who recant go on to reaffirm that they were sexually abused.

A full evaluation of suspected sexual abuse includes the developmental history, the medical and psychiatric histories, an assessment of cognitive functioning, any history of previous abuse or trauma, and any parental history of abuse. In instances where intrafamilial abuse is alleged, an understanding of any allegiance to one parent over the other is paramount. Ultimately, the evaluation serves to determine whether abuse has occurred, whether the child is in need of protection, and whether treatment is indicated. In some settings, a multidisciplinary team is used for evaluation and treatment of the family. Cooperation between agencies is paramount. It is recommended that the child be seen by the fewest number of professionals as possible to minimize stress. Multiple interviewers may foster confabulation, because the child may think that additional information is sought by the agencies and clinicians.

When conducting an interview with a suspected victim of sexual abuse, the physician should ask open-ended questions, such as, "What brings you here?" and not, "Who hurt you?" It is imperative to put the child as much at ease as possible. Toys, games, and other age-appropriate activities such as coloring or drawing are helpful. Genitalia on human drawings can suggest the possibility of sexual abuse. However, the absence of genitalia does not rule out the possibility of sexual abuse. It is imperative that the developmental level of the child be considered when assessing drawings; there is a normal age range in which children may produce anatomically correct drawings (see Chapter 19). The use of anatomically correct dolls is controversial and may or may not be helpful.

Adolescents should be questioned privately about HEADSS issues. Special attention should be given to drug and alcohol activity (see Chapter 15). Chronic use of drugs or alcohol many be the only way an adolescent can live with the abuse. Adolescents who run away or who have attempted suicide have a high risk of having been and of being abused, both physically and sexually. Refer to the annotated bibliography at the end of this chapter for further readings about the assessment of child abuse.

False Allegations of Sexual Abuse

The physician should consider the possibility of false allegations in all instances of reported abuse where there is potential secondary gain, particularly in situations of divorce or if the report is coming from an adult and not the child. The child's disclosure should be the primary source of information. Pathognomonic signs of abuse are trauma to genitalia of a preverbal child and sexually transmitted disease in a child. Again, it is most important not to ask leading questions, since they may lead to problems in court later. No pressure should be put on the child to disclose (such as, "You can't eat until you tell me") because children respond to pressure and perhaps confabulate a response.

Faller has found four reasons for a mother to make allegations of sexual abuse in the context of divorce:

- The mother discovers the abuse and decides to divorce her husband
- Revelation of abuse during the breakup
- Abuse precipitated by the break-up
- Altogether false allegations

Faller reports that about one half of women who discover abuse divorce their husbands. In the second instance, she notes that a child may finally feel safe enough to reveal the abuse. The mother who may have been in denial about certain behaviors in the household may now be able to recognize the true significance of them. Faller also reports that it is possible that the mother may have been aware of the abuse but fearful of reporting it during the marriage. In the third category, the father's sexual predilection for children may have been controlled by the existence and structure of the marriage itself. The emotional losses inherent in the separation and divorce may disinhibit the abusive parent. In general, false allegations stem from a parent, not the child. However, as more is taught about such matters (for example, in the useful Good Touch/Bad Touch

PEARLS & PERILS

FALSE ALLEGATIONS OF SEXUAL ABUSE

- False allegations are often seen in the context of divorce.

programs in schools), the angry child or adolescent may make such allegations for purposes of revenge regarding another matter. An adolescent may deliberately lie about sexual abuse out of vengeance against an adult or to cover up her own sexual activity. The emotional trauma of the divorce may result in misperception of the child's behaviors, which results in allegations. Similarly, a child with a history of abuse may misinterpret an adult's behaviors. The parent may recognize acutal signs of abuse but assume it is by the former spouse and not the actual perpetrator. Although rare, the remaining possibility is that the parent consciously lies to incriminate the ex-spouse.

When a child is prompted by a parent to deliberately lie, the history of sexual abuse is much more likely to be garnered easily during the first session. The child may often check with the mother during this first disclosure. The child is much more likely to confront the father either alone or in the mother's presence. In contrast, in a genuine case of sexual abuse, the child is reluctant to disclose events of the abuse, either with her mother or the therapist. She is also unlikely to confront her father with his actions because of fear or guilt. She may appear frightened or uncomfortable in his presence (however, this may not be the case if the molestation is more seductive and nonthreatening).

Interventions and Treatments

The act of reporting is the first intervention. Reporting serves to protect the child, and it ensures that the physician is fulfilling a legal obligation and acting in the best interests of the child. In the case of abuse suspected by a parent or guardian the primary care physician may need to keep the child in the office or admit the child to the hospital until CPS can assume care of the child. Practitioners are protected under law for reporting and arranging a safe environment if such actions are done in good faith and without malice.

At the time of reporting, the physician should make the family aware of any concerns about child abuse and of the legal obligation to report the concerns to CPS. Protecting the child from further harm is the first priority; then the physician should try to forge and maintain a professional relationship with the suspected abusive parent and with others in the family. The goal of CPS, after ensuring the immediate safety of the child, is to work with the family (and often the abusive parent) so they can move on to provide a safe and healthful environment for the child.

When the alleged abuse has been perpetrated by someone outside of the family, the criminal justice system proceeds to prosecution, hoping to protect the child in question as well as other children.

There is an array of psychotherapeutic services that can be used to help an abused child, the family, and the abusive parent who wishes to become a better parent. Depending on the age and developmental needs of the child, individual and group therapies, as well as special educational support services have been found beneficial. Young children use play therapy to integrate the traumatic experiences and develop coping skills for age-appropriate functioning in the family, school, and peer group. Adolescents use group therapy to validate their feelings of anger and despair and to get support to stay in school, to stay off drugs, and to set realistic, prosocial goals for their lives. Various family therapy approaches have been found useful for pulling families back together, assisting parents with parenting skills, and helping the children to feel a part of a family that is working together to heal.

Considerable skill, patience, and understanding of the dynamics of abusive families is required for therapists who choose to work with cases of abuse. For instance, in individual therapy, the abused child may test the therapist's capacity to control his own anger by behaving provocatively. The child must sense that there is unconditional acceptance, but must also realize that the physician has the ability to set firm limits on destructive or manipulative behaviors. The family therapist must likewise be able to remain neutral but catalytically involved when issues about continuing a marriage between an abusing and a nonabusing parent arise. There is no single prescribed therapy with proven effectiveness for all cases; rather, children and families have achieved stabilization after abuse through a combination of psychotherapeutic approaches and community resources.

The Role of the Primary Care Physician

The role of the primary care physician is limited to the time that it takes to participate in an evaluation of suspected abuse and that can be made to work with the family (including the abusing family member) to support change and reintegration. A critical endeavor is to help the child and the family obtain good psychotherapy; as noted in the previous section, working with abuse cases is difficult, special training is needed, and the personality of the therapist is important. The well-established primary care physician should know which child psychiatrists, psychologists, or social workers are best suited for abuse cases in the community.

Summary

Because of long-term involvement with individual children and families in a community, the physician has a unique role in the prevention of child abuse. Specifically, the physician can have an impact on prevention as a community educator, a child care advocate, a researcher, and a teacher of patients and families.

As a community educator, the physician can provide volunteers, community organizations, and public officials with a greater awareness of potential child abuse situations, as well as methods to develop appropriate antiabuse programs. As a child care advocate, the physician can speak out for increasing comprehensive health and financial support for children in poverty and family situations that include teenage mothers and drug or alcohol abuse. We know what factors contribute to child abuse, and unfortunately, many political endeavors restrict intervention programs for situations of abuse.

As a researcher, the physician should learn what intervention programs and techniques really make a difference. Locally, the physician can determine which day care settings are best, how CPS evaluates and intervenes, and which therapists in the community do good work. Finally, the physician who is familiar with normal child development, risk factors for abuse, symptoms of abused children, and the evaluation of children and families for both their health and psychosocial problems will be able to prevent child abuse.

CONSIDER CONSULTATION WHEN . . .

- Behaviors prevent normal, age-appropriate interactions with others
- There are aggressive or self-injurious behaviors

Annotated Bibliography

Fleisher G, Ludwig S: *Textbook of pediatric emergency medicine,* ed 2, Baltimore, 1983, Williams and Wilkens.

This is an excellent resource for the primary care physician on emergency room diagnosis of acute physical abuse.

Kaplan SJ, Pelcovitz D, editors: Child abuse, *Child Adolesc Psychiatr Clin North Am* 3:645-893.

This is a current update including sections on new developments, psychopathology, therapy, and legal issues regarding all forms of abuse and neglect.

Krugman RD: Recognition of sexual abuse in children, *Pediatr Rev* 8:25-30, 1986.

This is an excellent review of the signs and symptoms of sexual abuse.

Schetky DH, Benedek E: *Clinical handbook of child psychiatry and the law,* Baltimore, 1992, Williams & Wilkins.

This is an overview of legal issues surrounding abuse and other areas of child and adolescent psychiatry.

Schetky DH, Green AH: *Child sexual abuse: a handbook for health care and legal professionals,* New York, 1988, Brunner Mazel.

This is a classic volume that is an excellent overview of issues for all health care providers.

The national directory of children, youth, and family services, ed 9, Longmont, Colo., 1993-1994, Marion Peterson Publishing.

This is a resource guide to find contact persons and telephone numbers in your locality.

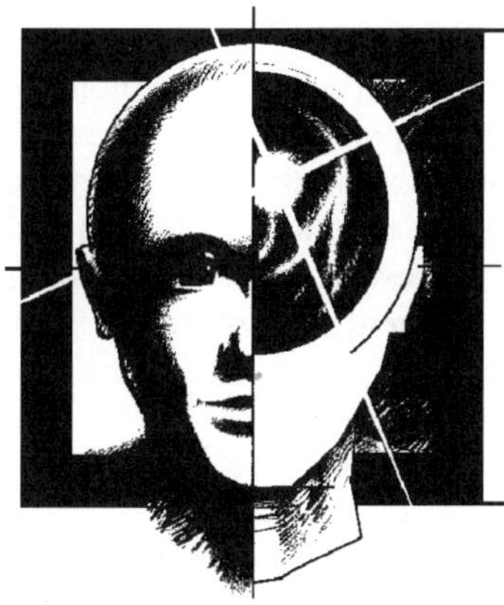

chapter 17

Problem Behaviors in Children with Developmental Disabilities

Cynthia R. Ellis, MD, Nirbhay N. Singh, PhD, and E. Vennecia Jackson, MD

Prevalence
Etiology
Assessment
Treatment
Specific Behavior Disorders
Summary

There are predictable phases in the normal development of a child, during which behavior problems typically occur (for example, temper tantrums in the "terrible twos"). Most problems are easily solved by the parents. However, biologic and environmental influences make some children more vulnerable to these problems and predispose them to greater difficulties during these phases. For example, a developmental disability influences the behavior and development of some children. Children with developmental disabilities may have a variety of handicapping conditions, including mental retardation, cerebral palsy, pervasive developmental disorders (PDDs), and specific learning disorders. Generally, behavior problems occur more often in children with developmental disabilities than in the general population. For example, some children with cerebral palsy may have high rates of emotional lability, irritability, impulsivity, hyperactivity, and attention deficits. Children with a PDD exhibit self-injury, stereotypy, and aggression, and children with learning disabilities have psychosocial and behavioral difficulties. Although high rates of behavior problems occur in children with developmental disabilities in general, the best data we have on the prevalence of behavior problems come from studies of children with mental retardation.

Prevalence

The prevalence of behavior problems and psychopathologic conditions is higher in children with mental retardation than it is in the general population. For example, Rutter, Tizard, and Whitmore examined an entire cohort of children from the Isle of Wight, ages 9 to 11, for the presence of emotional and behavioral problems. Based on parent and teacher interviews, they found that the prevalence of emotional and behavioral disorders for the entire cohort was 7%. However, the prevalence rates were much higher for children with mental retardation, ranging from 30% (parent reports) to 42% (teacher reports). Generally, the prevalence of mental illness in children with mental retardation is between 20% and 35%. In addition to having a higher overall prevalence of behavior problems, some behavior problems (for example, aggression and noncompliance) occur more often in children with developmental disabilities than in children from the general population. Furthermore there are behavior problems (such as self-injury, stereotypy, pica, and rumination disorder) that are more specific to children with developmental disabilities and are only rarely seen in children from the general population.

Etiology

The occurrence of some behavior problems is to be expected in most children during specific developmental periods. However, some children show a delay or deviance in their development because they have a developmental disability. This alteration in the normal developmental process can influence the course of developmentally appropriate behavior problems. For example, the course of temper tantrums seen in a typical 2-year-old child may be quite different in a child with mental retardation. In light of the discrepancy between the mental and chronologic age of the child with mental retardation, the onset of temper tantrums may occur at an older chronologic age. Additionally, because the child with mental retardation develops at a slower rate than his nonhandicapped peers, the duration of the phase when temper tantrums occur may be prolonged. However, all behavior problems seen in children with developmental disabilities cannot be attributed solely to the presence of a disability. Indeed, the increased overall prevalence of behavior problems in this population suggests that other factors may be involved.

Psychiatric, Medical, and Biologic Etiologies

The cause of some behavior problems in children with developmental disabilities may be related to psychiatric disorders and organic or medical conditions. In many cases, a behavior problem may have multiple origins and more than one causal factor may be involved.

Psychiatric Disorders

Children with developmental disabilities exhibit the entire spectrum of childhood psychiatric disorders. Although it is often difficult to differentiate between the behavioral manifestations of a psychiatric disorder and those behaviors that are the result of faulty learning or are controlled by the environment, the distinction is important because they lead to differential treatments. For example, aggression and self-injury are behavioral symptoms often associated with obsessive-compulsive disorder (OCD), bipolar disorder, and anxiety disorders in children with developmental disorders, and the treatment is directed at the underlying psychiatric disorder. However, the same behaviors can also be learning-based and, in this case, are better dealt with directly through behavioral management procedures.

Medical Conditions

Unrecognized medical conditions, including dental problems, occult infections, and musculoskeletal problems, are also associated with some behavior problems in children with developmental disabilities. These children are at risk for these types of problems because of their greater health care needs, their increased difficulties in expressing and communicating their symptoms, or a lack of effective health care services. For example, up to 20% of behaviorally disordered children with mental retardation have an occult medical condition, the most common of which is undiagnosed or suboptimally treated epilepsy. A large number of other medical conditions, including hypothyroidism, anemia, cardiac and gastrointestinal disorders, unrecognized pain, and sleep disorders may all manifest as behavioral symptoms.

Side Effects of Medication

Side effects of medication are another common medical factor related to behavior problems in children with developmental disabilities. Psychotropic medications are often used in this population, and many of them, even at therapeutic doses, have adverse behavioral side effects. For example, antipsychotic medication may cause mental confusion, sedation, impaired psychomotor activity, and paradoxic aggravation of psychotic symptoms. Anxiolytic medication may result in sedation, decreased cognitive performance, and behavioral disinhibition, including overexcitement, hyperactivity, increased aggressivity, and irritability. Additionally, other nonpsychotropic medications (for example, theophylline, antihypertensives, and corticosteroids) may also have behavioral side effects.

Other Biologic Etiologies

There are a number of syndromes or disorders that have been associated with the occurrence of specific behavioral problems. For example, self-injury is commonly associated with Lesch-Nyhan Syndrome and de Lange's syndrome, and stereotypic hand-wringing is characteristically seen in children with Rett's disorder. Neurobiologic abnormalities have also been associated with some behavior problems, such as self-injury, in children with developmental disabilities. For example, several neurochemical hypotheses have implicated the endogenous endorphin system or specific neurotransmitter dysfunctions, such as serotonin dysfunction, in the genesis and maintenance of self-injurious behavior (Box 17-1).

BOX 17-1

EXAMPLES OF BIOLOGIC ETIOLOGIES

OCD
Bipolar disorder
Anxiety
Occult infections
Musculoskeletal problems
Hypothyroidism
Anemia
Cardiac problems
Gastrointestinal problems
Unrecognized pain (dental problem)
Sleep disorders
Side effects of medication
Lesch-Nyhan syndrome
de Lange's syndrome
Rett's disorder

Behavioral Etiologies

From a behavioral perspective, problem behaviors are viewed as constellations of behavioral excesses and skills deficits that serve a functional purpose for the child. Indeed, most of the research on the causes of behavior problems in this population has focused on behavioral causes (Box 17-2). The four major behavioral hypotheses associated with problem behaviors include positive reinforcement, negative reinforcement, self-stimulation, and communication.

BOX 17-2

EXAMPLES OF BEHAVIORAL ETIOLOGIES

The child learns that problem behaviors result in increased attention.
The child learns that problem behavior stops an aversive event.
The behavior increases stimulation.
The behavior decreases stimulation.
The child uses the behavior to communicate.

Positive and Negative Reinforcement

According to the positive reinforcement hypothesis, a problem behavior is learned when the child is reinforced for its occurrence, typically with attention. For example, a child with mental retardation may accidently learn that she receives increased attention from parents and teachers when she is aggressive. Thus the child may then use aggression to elicit this form of social interaction from parents and teachers. According to the negative reinforcement hypothesis, a problem behavior is maintained by the termination of an aversive event. For example, if the child is able to avoid or terminate an undesirable activity (such as picking up toys) by engaging in a specific problem behavior (such as a temper tantrum), she will learn to use that behavior to escape or avoid the activity. In other words, if a child knows that her parents stop asking her to pick up toys after play if she engages in a temper tantrum, it is likely that she will engage in temper tantrums everytime her parents ask her to pick up toys.

Self-Stimulation

There are two related hypotheses that implicate self-stimulation in the occurrence of specific behaviors: hypoarousal and hyperarousal. According to the hypoarousal hypothesis, if a child is receiving less than optimal levels of stimulation, he may engage in a repetitive behavior (such as stereotypy or self-injury) to provide increased vestibular, tactile, kinesthetic, or other sensory stimulation. According to the hyperarousal hypothesis, if a child is in an overstimulating environment, he will engage in a behavior that reduces sensory stimulation. Thus a child may engage in self-stimulation if he is participating in group activities that are overly stimulating for him.

Communication

In some cases, a child with no language ability or delayed language development may use a maladaptive behavior to communicate needs to others. For example, a child with limited expressive language abilities may engage in head banging to alert his parents to physical pain, which may be caused by an ear infection. In such cases, we assume that the problem behavior has a communicative intent and that direct treatment of the problem behavior will not solve the problem. The child must be taught a more socially acceptable method of communicating, such as using signs or a communication board.

Assessment

A comprehensive approach is required to assess behavior problems in a child with developmental disabilities. In addition to a detailed analysis of the behavior itself, the assessment commonly involves an evaluation of the child's medical and psychiatric status, as well as speech, language, and other skills. This type of assessment identifies not only the problems and needs of the child but also the resources that are required for treatment and their availability. The role of the family in the assessment process cannot be overstated. Parents know their child best and are usually a good source of accurate information. Furthermore an understanding of the family's daily routine, their treatment goals, and their anticipated outcome is important when designing a comprehensive treatment plan.

Before beginning a formal assessment of a problem behavior, it is important to determine when the behavior constitutes enough of a problem to warrant an active treatment. There are a number of subjective elements that contribute to this decision, including the degree of physical danger the behavior presents to the child and others, interference with the child's learning caused by the behavior, the risk that the behavior will become more serious if left untreated, the degree to which the behavior is out of the normative range of behaviors for that child's peer group, and any decrement the behavior causes in the quality of life for the child and his family. When it is clear that the behavior requires treatment, a structured assessment should be undertaken. This assessment may consist of a number of components, including parental (and child, when appropriate) interviews, the use of checklists and rating scales, direct observation, a functional analysis of the problem behavior, and a medical and psychiatric evaluation. Depending on the severity of the problem behavior, the assessment may be best accomplished by a multidisciplinary team, integrating the skills and knowledge of a number of disciplines (for example, psychology, behavioral pediatrics, psychiatry, social work, and nursing). The objective of the assessment process is to clearly identify the problem behavior in terms of its nature and observable characteristics and to set realistic treatment goals. The model of assessment and diagnosis of mental illness in individuals with mental retardation developed by Singh et al. incorporates both psychiatric and behavioral methods and is appropriate for use in the assessment of behavior problems in children with developmental disabilities.

Interviews

The first step in the assessment process is an interview with the child's parents and other caregivers who interact regularly with the child and know him well. It is important to seek information from as many sources as possible (for example home, school, and day care). A primary focus of the interviews is to obtain a detailed description of the problem behavior. A common format for the acquisition of this type of information is to inquire about the ABCs of the behavior (the *a*ntecedents, the *b*ehavior itself, and the *c*onsequences of the behavior). To determine the antecedents of a behavior, it is necessary to identify the conditions under which the problem behavior occurs, such as the time of day, activities the child is engaged in just before its occurrence, and the nature of the environment (for example, the level of stimulation, the presence of specific persons, and requests being made of the child at the time). Similarly, it is important to identify the conditions under which the problem behavior does not occur. Information about the characteristics of the problem behavior (such as the frequency, intensity, duration, and severity) should also be obtained. Finally, the physician should inquire about the consequences of the behavior; that is, the way parents and teachers respond to the child's problem behavior. At this point, it is often instructive to ask the parents if they have any particular insights into why the behavior is occurring and what treatments might be successful. Furthermore, it is useful to discuss with them their previous attempts to control the problem behavior and the outcome of such attempts.

In addition to details about the problem behavior, other information should also be solicited during the parent interview. If the child is not already well known to the physician, a detailed medical history should be obtained. Parents should be asked about any family history of medical, developmental, or psychiatric problems, because certain familial factors may have a negative effect on the psychologic and educational outcomes for the child. Parental psychopathologic conditions may be particularly relevant, because they significantly influence the parents' coping abilities and perceptions of their child's problems. Additionally, a detailed social history should be obtained, and the extent and quality of social support networks should be determined, because social support is related to the quality of parent-child interaction and the perceived quality of life for the family. The physician should ask about sources of emotional, informational, and material supports (resources) available and accessed by the family. Factors such as parental rejection or overprotectiveness may also be pertinent in some cases.

In many cases, the child can be directly interviewed about the problem behavior. However, the nature and extent of the child's disability may be a limiting factor. For example, the level of mental retardation and receptive and expressive language capabilities are important considerations in the usefulness of interviews with children.

Checklists and Rating Scales

There are a number of behavioral checklists and rating scales that can be used in the assessment of problem behavior in children (see Chapter 2). Some of these are global in scope and are useful for screening purposes, whereas others provide specific information on selected behaviors or disorders. The majority of these instruments have been devised for use with children in the general population and not for children with developmental disabilities. However, there are a few instruments that have been developed specifically for use with some groups of children with developmental disabilities, particularly for children with mental retardation. Examples include the Aberrant Behavior Checklist (ABC), the Reiss Screen for Maladaptive Behavior, the Psychopathology Instrument for Mentally Retarded Adults, and the Diagnostic Assessment for the Severely Handicapped scale. Although a majority of these instruments are not diagnostic in nature, they can be used to screen for a number of disorders or problems. They often yield information that directs the physician to areas that warrant further investigation. Whereas the information obtained through rating scales and checklists is subjective and limited to the scope of the instrument, these instruments require little or no training to use and can help the physician gather preliminary information from a variety of sources (such as teachers, parents, and day care providers).

Behavioral Observations

Behavioral observations can be performed by the physician or by a trained observer. However, useful information can also be obtained from parental observations, as well as from individuals who regularly interact with and know the child well. Behavioral observations can be performed in the child's natural environment, such as home or school, or in a clinical or laboratory setting. They may be general in nature and record a narrative of the range of behaviors that occur, or they can be more structured and consist of observing the child for occurrences of well-defined behaviors. Data can also be collected on elements in the child's environment that may be related to the behavior (for example, settings, activities, or the presence of certain individuals). Behavioral observations can provide useful information on the frequency, severity, intensity, and duration of the problem behavior, as well as its environmental antecedents and consequences.

Functional Analysis

In addition to direct behavioral observations, a functional analysis is often helpful in determining the motivating factors for a specific behavior. In a functional analysis, hypotheses about the cause of the problem behavior are tested experimentally to determine which variable is most responsible for its occurrence. Although a functional analysis is usually conducted by a trained behavioral psychologist in a laboratory setting, parents and teachers can also be taught to use this procedure. Such an analysis may help physicians differentiate those behaviors that are learned from those that are of organic or medical origin. If the behavior is of learned origin, it may serve several functions, including self-stimulation, communication, escape or avoidance from a demand or request, and attention-seeking. A differential assessment of these functions helps the physician devise a learning-based intervention to teach the child a socially acceptable replacement behavior that may serve the same function as the problem behavior.

Medical and Psychiatric Evaluation

A comprehensive medical and psychiatric assessment, including a complete physical and neurologic examination, is an important component in the evaluation of a problem behavior. The need for laboratory or diagnostic testing should be determined on a case-by-case basis. The physician should also thoroughly review all medications prescribed for the child, as well as their potential side effects. The psychiatric evaluation should include a mental status examination before a psychiatric diagnosis is established. This is often difficult to do in a child with a developmental disability because of the nonspecificity of the behavioral symptoms the child may have.

Treatment

The primary goals of a treatment plan are the reduction of one or more problem behaviors and an increase in the patient's quality of life. Thus a comprehensive assessment and analysis is a prerequisite to matching the most appropriate treatment to a specific behavior problem. Approaches to the treatment of behavior problems in children with developmental disabilities are similar to those for children without disabilities. In many cases, variations of the same treatment modalities, including behavior therapy, pharmacotherapy, psychotherapy, and socioenvironmental therapy, can be used. It is not uncommon for the treatment of a behavior problem to consist of some components of different treatments. However, all therapeutic interventions must be specifically tailored to the child and must take into account the child's chronologic age, developmental level, type of disability, family and cultural contexts, and the problem behavior to be addressed.

The choice of a particular treatment is usually based on a number of factors, including the risk the behavior poses to the child and the urgency with which reduction of the problem behavior is needed; the underlying motivation or function of the behavior; the availability of practical and effective treatments for the behavior; the technical sophistication of the parents, caregivers, or clinicians to implement the intervention; and parental preferences. In light of the general concern over the aversive nature of many treatments, physicians should use the least restrictive but most effective alternative available.

In many cases, the child's primary care physician alone can be instrumental in providing the necessary treatment for a specific problem. Primary care physicians typically focus on parent and teacher education, as well as working directly with the child. However, with some training, parents and other caregivers can also meaningfully participate in the assessment, design, and implementation of a treatment program. In other cases, treatment decisions are made by a multidisciplinary team consisting of the child's parents and professionals from a variety of disciplines who work with the child and family. Although some of the more common problem behaviors can be treated easily, more difficult cases should be referred to a specialist such as a behavioral psychologist, behavioral pediatrician, or child psychiatrist.

To be successful, a treatment must result in an improvement of the problem behavior across various settings in the child's natural environment, such as home and school. Another important measure of success is the degree to which the behavior reduction is maintained after discontinuation of active treatment. Additionally, merely controlling a problem behavior is often not enough if it does not make a significant life-style change for the child. Treatment modalities that can be used to control problem behaviors and achieve life-style changes are described in the following sections.

Behavior Modification

Behavior management techniques can be used to increase a desired behavior, decrease an undesirable behavior, or teach a new behavior. These techniques have been the mainstay in the management of behavior problems in children with developmental disabilities. Although behavior reduction procedures can be used alone, they are typically used in conjunction with other treatments, such as skills training, educational interventions, and pharmacologic management. The selection of an appropriate behavioral treatment is based on an understanding of the cause or function of the problem behavior for the child. In some cases, the factors that initially caused the behavior to occur may no longer be present, but the behavior may persist because of the environmental response it elicits. For example, head banging in reaction to an ear infection may persist once the ear infection has been treated because the head banging still occasions parental attention. The use of some behavioral interventions can be relatively labor intensive and may require implementation and ongoing monitoring by trained personnel. In other cases, the procedures can be simplified and implemented by parents or teachers with minimal training. However, all treatments require a system based on ongoing data collection and an evaluation of the outcomes as treatment proceeds so necessary changes in the treatment protocol can be made.

Behavioral interventions are based on the relationship between a behavior and its antecedents and consequences (Box 17-3). The goal of behavior therapy is to change (that is, strengthen or weaken) the relationship between a behavior and its maintaining contingencies. If the contingent relationships between the behav-

BOX 17-3

BEHAVIORAL THERAPY

Use least restrictive, but most effective means of treatment available.

Behavior modification can increase, decrease, or teach a new behavior.

Antecedent interventions identify conditions that immediately precede and influence a behavior.

Positive reinforcement uses a reinforcer to increase the likelihood of a behavior recurring.

Negative reinforcement increases the frequency of a behavior that is followed by the removal of a negative reinforcer.

Punishment decreases the likelihood of a behavior recurring through an action taken immediately after the behavior.

PEARLS & PERILS

MANAGEMENT OF BEHAVIOR IN CHILDREN WITH DEVELOPMENTAL DISABILITIES

- Mental retardation is primarily a problem of learning—drugs don't teach these children; parents and teachers do.
- Behavior problems occur with greater frequency in children who have developmental disabilities than in children in the general population.
- Unrecognized medical conditions and side effects of medications will not be appreciated unless a thorough medical evaluation is included in the evaluation of problem behaviors.
- Parents are usually the people who know the child best, and they must be included in the multidisciplinary team.
- To be successful, a treatment strategy that reduces a problem behavior must replace that behavior with another, more appropriate behavior.
- The success of a treatment can best be judged on the basis of the improvement in the quality of life it produces for the child and family.

ior and its antecedents and consequences can be identified, then they can be manipulated in a consistent manner to change the frequency of the behavior. Antecedent strategies involve the modification of conditions that result in a behavior, and response contingent strategies involve the modification of the consequences of the behavior.

Antecedent Treatment Strategies

Antecedent interventions involve the identification and systematic manipulation of the environmental conditions that occur immediately before and influence the occurrence of the problem behavior. There are a large number of potential antecedent conditions that can precede and facilitate the occurrence of a behavior. For example, if a child engages in an undesirable behavior for self-stimulation because of an uninteresting environment, enriching the environment or providing alternate sensory activities may decrease the frequency of the problem behavior. Training in alternative forms of communication when a problem behavior is used as a form of communication may also result in a reduction in the undesired behavior. The selection of an antecedent strategy should be based on the assessment and analysis of the conditions that maintain the behavior. Antecedent strategies are usually used as a first-line intervention because they are safe, nonaversive, and socially acceptable. Furthermore, antecedent strategies do not require the labor-intensive manipulation of the problem behavior.

Positive Reinforcement Interventions

Positive reinforcement procedures use reinforcers to increase the likelihood of a behavior recurring in the future. A reinforcer is an item or activity that the child desires and will work to obtain. It must immediately follow the occurrence of a specific behavior. Although positive reinforcement procedures are typically used to increase the frequency of a behavior, they can also be used to decrease a behavior by making reinforcement differentially contingent on the nonoccurrence of that behavior. There are a number of differential reinforcement procedures that can be used with children who have developmental disabilities. Differential reinforcement of other behavior (DRO) involves the reinforcement of the absence of the target behavior and the occurrence of any other behavior. In differential reinforcement of alternative behavior (DRA) and differential reinforcement of incompatible behavior (DRI), reinforcement is contingent on the replacement of the problem behavior with an appropriate alternative response or a behavior that is physically incompatible with the problem behavior.

Differential reinforcement procedures clearly indicate to a child which behaviors are appropriate and which are not. However, to be successful the reinforcer must be one that the child wants. The procedures must be consistently implemented by all caregivers in all settings where the child exhibits the problem behavior. These procedures require a period of learning by the child and may not be appropriate for life-threatening problems (such as some forms of self-injury) that require rapid reduction.

Negative Reinforcement Interventions

Negative reinforcement procedures increase the frequency of a response that is followed by the termination or removal of a negative reinforcer. For example, a parent may ask the child to do something that the child dislikes doing (such as pick up the toys after play). To avoid or escape from doing this task, the child may engage in a temper tantrum when the parent makes a such a demand. If the parent stops asking or does not make the child complete the task because of the temper tantrum, the parental task demand is the negative reinforcer for the child. There are three possible outcomes. First, if the parent stops asking because of the anticipated temper tantrums, the child has effectively avoided doing the task. Second, should the parent keep asking the child without making him complete the task at each request, the frequency of temper tantrums will increase. Third, should the parent prevent the child from avoiding the task by making the child complete it despite the temper tantrums, it is very likely that the temper tantrums will decrease and disappear. This happens because the child quickly learns that throwing temper tantrums does not allow him to avoid a task or escape from completing it. There is much evidence in the research literature to show that many behavior problems of children, both with and without developmental disabilities, are maintained by negative reinforcement.

Punishment

Punishment consists of an action taken immediately after the occurrence of a behavior. The punishment decreases the likelihood that the behavior will recur under similar conditions in the future. There are three general ways of delivering punishment for a problem behavior. Punishment can consist of the presentation of an aversive (undesirable) stimulus contingent on the occurrence of the problem behavior. Examples include the use of verbal reprimands or other procedures that cause discomfort or restrict movement, such as water mist-sprays, noxious tastes and odors, facial screening, or brief physical restraint. Punishment can also consist of the withdrawal of something the child likes after the occurrence of a problem behavior. For example, time out involves removing the child from a reinforcing situation after the occurrence of a specific behavior. Response cost also involves the loss of a reinforcer or the imposition of a penalty, such as the removal of a token, privilege, or other reward that the child has previously earned, on the occurrence of a problem behavior. Finally, punishment may require the child to engage in an undesirable, aversive behavior immediately after exhibiting a problem behavior. For example, the child may be required to engage in a forced-arm exercise after an aggressive act.

To be effective, punishment procedures must be implemented consistently and immediately after the problem behavior. They must be combined with positive reinforcement procedures, and they must be a part of an overall program designed to teach functional and appropriate skills. Punishment techniques can effectively decrease and eliminate severe or dangerous problem behaviors. Some behavioral experts suggest that punishment procedures should be considered after reasonable attempts with positive reinforcement procedures have failed, when the behavior poses a threat to the child's physical well-being, or when the behavior interferes with the child's ability to reach her maximum potential and integration in the community. The advantages of punishment techniques are that they are rapid and generally effective at bringing about behavioral change. However, they may also result in the emergence of avoidance behaviors or aggression, they do not teach appropriate replacement behaviors, and there is a potential for physical harm to the child.

There is some controversy over the use of aversive or punishment procedures as a result of ethical concerns over inflicting pain or discomfort on children in need of therapy. Additionally, some professionals and parents have argued that punishment procedures are not necessary because other, nonaversive, alternative treatments are available. Decisions about using aversive or punishment procedures should involve parents and guardians, as well as human rights and peer review committees to review treatment plans and determine if they are humane and warranted.

Psychopharmacotherapy

The use of psychotropic medication is commonly incorporated into treatment plans for severe problem behaviors in children with developmental disabilities. Individuals with developmental disabilities, particularly those with mental retardation, are the most medicated group in our society. In addition to the use of medication to treat psychiatric disorders in people who have developmental disabilities, aggressive behavior, self-injury, agitation, property destruction, and stereotypy also commonly lead to medication in this population. Furthermore, the use of medication increases as the number and severity of a child's problem behaviors increase. Historically, medication was used primarily for its sedative effects and behavioral control; however, concern over the impact of these medications on learning, as well as recent legislation and litigation, has resulted in a more judicious use of psychotropic medication in this population. At present, about one in five individuals with developmental disabilities is likely to be on psychotropic medication for behavior problems or psychiatric illness.

In general, medication is a single component in a broad treatment model, with the selection of a particular drug based on a comprehensive assessment and diagnosis of the problem behaviors. There are few methodologically sound studies that examine the efficacy of medication in treating behavior problems in individuals with developmental disabilities (particularly in children), and medication prescription is often based more on clinical judgment than on robust scientific findings. However, there are good theoretic rationales available for using psychopharmacologic treatments for some behaviors, such as self-injury. In general, it is useful to remember that medication should be used to improve the child's general functioning and quality of life rather than strictly for reducing an undesirable behavior.

Before instituting treatment with medication, it is important to discuss with the parents and child, if appropriate, the risks and benefits of using a particular medication. Evaluation of the drug response with repeated assessment measures, such as rating scales and behavioral observations, and monitoring of side effects is necessary to determine the effects of the treatment. Standard medication management principles should be followed, including appropriate dosage titration and monitoring. Finally, periodic reassessment of the need for continued medication should be undertaken at least once every 30 to 90 days to avoid unnecessarily prolonged treatment. In the rare case that a child is on medication for more than a year, it is critical that a drug holiday is instituted every year to determine the continued need for the medication.

It is standard practice to combine psychopharmacologic treatment with behavioral and other interventions, particularly skills training. Medication is typically considered in the treatment of a problem behavior when behavioral interventions have been unsuccessful or when there is no apparent motivation for the behavior and it is presumed to be of organic origin. Before prescribing psychotropic medication, the physician must be convinced that the behavior is not the result of medical conditions (for example, otitis media or migraine headaches) or environmental and psychosocial factors (living conditions, peer taunting, or abuse). Furthermore, it is the physician's responsibility to monitor the effects of medication and determine that the child does indeed have a better quality of life as a result of medication.

Antipsychotics

Antipsychotics, particularly chlorpromazine (Thorazine), thioridazine (Mellaril), and haloperidol (Haldol), are the most commonly prescribed medications for the management of hallucinations and delusions, as well as for behavior problems in patients with developmental disabilities. These drugs are often used in children who are aggressive, explosive, violent, destructive, and self-injurious. Although early studies with chlorpromazine indicated that it was beneficial in treating a number of problem behaviors, more recent and better controlled studies have shown that it may have a suppressive and detrimental effect on appropriate behaviors in some individuals. Unless valid and reliable data are available to show otherwise, physicians should refrain from using this drug. Thioridazine, the most prescribed of the antipsychotics, is probably the most effective of the three in controlling hyperactivity, aggression, and stereotypy in individuals with developmental disabilities. Haloperidol is also used to treat problem behaviors such as hyperactivity, aggression, and impulsivity because of its lower sedative effect, but it is more likely to cause extrapyramidal syndromes.

Other antipsychotics, such as fluphenazine (Prolixin), mesoridazine (Serentil), trifluoperazine (Stelazine), thiothixene (Navane), and loxapine (Loxitane), are used in institutional settings to control problem behaviors in individuals with mental retardation, but primary care physicians should be aware of the fact that there is little scientific data attesting to their efficacy. Additionally, most of these drugs have not been approved by the FDA for use in this population. Furthermore the same caution applies to the newer antipsychotics such as clozapine (Clozaril) and risperidone (Risperdal).

The antipsychotics have well-known side effects, including dystonia, akathisia, pseudo-parkinsonism, tardive dyskinesia, drowsiness and sedation, hypotension, and anticholinergic side effects (dry mouth, dry eyes, constipation, urinary retention, blurred vision, and tachycardia). Although all of these side effects are important and must be monitored, when prescribing antipsychotics for children with developmental disabilities, primary care physicians should be particularly sensitive to the following conditions: (1) akathisia because it is often mistaken for behavioral problems such as agitation and aggression; (2) tardive dyskinesia because children with mental retardation are often prescribed antipsychotics for long periods without the benefit of occasional drug holidays; and (3) those side effects that are not easily observed, because many children with mental retardation cannot verbally tell their parents or teachers about these side effects.

Although knowledge of this area is relatively incomplete because of the paucity of well-controlled studies, it is generally understood that cognitive and academic impairment may be serious side effects of antipsychotics in children, especially those with mental retardation. Thus primary care physicians should require parents and teachers to monitor the child's adaptive, social, and academic behaviors during dosage adjustment, as well as while on maintenance medication to see if any of these behaviors are adversely affected. At all times, the physician's goal should be to use the lowest dosage to treat the problem behavior without affecting the learning potential of the child. After all, the ultimate objective is not to control the behavior but to teach the child alternative ways of behaving so there will be no need for the medication.

Given that the half-lives of orally administered antipsychotics range from 10 to 20 hours, physicians tend to use either a large bedtime dose to avoid daytime drowsiness or two or three divided doses, with the largest dose given at bedtime. Although doses may vary with individual cases, children under age 12 typically receive an average daily dose of 75 to 200 mg/day of chlorpromazine and thioridazine and between 2 to 5 mg/day of haloperidol. Furthermore, it is advisable to prescribe an anticholinergic drug if the physician anticipates that therapeutic doses of chlorpromazine, thioridazine, and haloperidol will produce extrapyramidal side effects. A number of anticholinergics can be used for this purpose, including benztropine (Cogentin), biperiden (Akineton), ethopropazine (Parsidol), trihexyphenidyl (Artane), and procyclidine (Kemadrin). However, it must be remembered that in addition to controlling some extrapyramidal side effects, the anticholinergics also produce adverse reactions that may need to be monitored.

Finally, it is critical that primary care physicians monitor the effects of prescribed medication on the problem behavior of children with developmental disabilities. Although no single assessment instrument can be used for all disorders and with all children, the Aberrant Behavior Checklist (ABC) is the only instrument designed specifically for evaluating the effects of psychotropic drugs in children and in adults with mental retardation. This rating scale covers the primary problem behaviors for which antipsychotics and other drugs are usually prescribed, as well as a range of other behaviors that may show medication-related changes. Furthermore, the primary care physician is well advised to monitor the possible emergence of tardive dyskinesia caused by exposure to neuroleptic medication. At present, the best instrument to use for this purpose is the Dyskinesia Identification System-Coldwater, a scale devised specifically for measuring tardive dyskinesia in individuals with developmental disabilities. When tardive dyskinesia is suspected, a referral to a neurologist is in order.

Antidepressants

Antidepressants have been relatively infrequently used in this population compared with the antipsychotics. However, they are increasingly used to manage problem behaviors in individuals with developmental disabilities even though there is little hard data to support such practice. In at least one well-controlled study, imipramine resulted in a significant behavioral deterioration in irritability, social withdrawal, and acting-out behaviors. There is some evidence that second-generation antidepressants (for example, fluoxetine) may be beneficial in the treatment of self-injury in some individuals with mental retardation. However, primary care physicians should be cautious in their use of antidepressants for treating behavior problems in this population, because there is a paucity of research evidence attesting to their efficacy.

Antiepileptics

Up to 20% of individuals with mental retardation and 50% of those with mental retardation and cerebral palsy have a seizure disorder. Typically, antiepileptics are used to control the seizures of these individuals. However, a few antiepileptics are used for their psychotropic effects in the treatment of behavior disturbances.

The primary psychiatric use of antiepileptics in children and adolescents with developmental disabilities is for affective disorders such as mania, bipolar disorder, or schizoaffective disorder, especially if a disturbance has been resistant to traditional treatment. Carbamazepine (Tegretol), valproic acid (Depakene) and, to a much lesser extent, clonazepam (Klonopin) are currently being used for this purpose. In the absence of hard data, most of the enthusiasm for the use of these drugs to control behavior disturbances in children with developmental disabilities is based on clinical experience and uncontrolled case studies. However, the use of other antiepileptics, such as phenytoin (Dilantin) and phenobarbital (Luminal), is not recommended with this population. These drugs have serious side effects (for example, aggression, lower frustration tolerance, hyperactivity, self-injury, screaming, and irritability) that parents and teachers may assume to be additional behavior or psychiatric problems. The use of recently approved antiepileptic drugs by the FDA, such as felbamate (Felbatol) and gabapentin (Neurontin), is not recommended, because there is absolutely no information about them with regard to their efficacy in treating behavior disturbances in individuals with developmental disabilities.

There are good reasons why primary care physicians should be careful about using antiepileptics for behavior control in children with developmental disabilities. First, there is almost no scientific data supporting their use for this purpose in this population. Additionally, the antiepileptics are potentially sedating and produce cognitive loss, thus impeding new learning in the child. If such drugs are to be used, the physician must evaluate the child at least monthly for signs of cognitive loss and obtain periodic laboratory studies, including a complete blood count and hepatic and renal function tests. Furthermore, the following side effects must be monitored regularly: sedation, nystagmus, ataxia, dysarthria, drowsiness, decline in memory and learning ability, psychomotor restlessness, headache, and behavioral side effects (such as hyperactivity, irritability, and agitation). Finally, as with other psychotropic medications, the physician must initiate a drug holiday at least annually to determine the continued need for the medication.

Anxiolytics

These drugs are used primarily for treating anxiety. However, antianxiety agents are also used for their purported psychotropic effects in controlling such behaviors as hyperactivity, agitation, aggression, and disruption. However, there is scant scientific literature on the use of anxiolytics in individuals with developmental disabilities, and the few well-controlled studies that are available suggest that problem behaviors do not improve and may even worsen as a result of taking these drugs. Buspirone (BuSpar), a relatively new serotoninergic anxiolytic, has been used in the management of behavior problems in children and adults with developmental disabilities, and the available case studies suggest that it may be effective with only some individuals. Clearly, we need more data on the efficacy of the anxiolytics with this population, but in the meantime a cautious approach to their use is advised.

Stimulants

Stimulant medications, particularly methylphenidate (Ritalin) and dextroamphetamine (Dexedrine), are commonly used in the treatment of attention-deficit/hyperactivity disorder (ADHD) and hyperactivity in children. The efficacy of stimulant treatment in children with ADHD and mild to moderate mental retardation is close to that of children in the general population, although those with mental retardation have a higher rate of adverse effects from the medication (such as tics and social withdrawal). However, stimulant medication does not have a beneficial effect on the behavior of children with severe and profound mental retardation.

In one of the few studies reporting the use of stimulants on a behavior other than those associated with ADHD in children with developmental disabilities, the frequency of pica decreased in three adolescents with profound mental retardation who were taking methylphenidate. The change is possibly the result of the diminished dopaminergic neurotransmission associated with the drug.

At present, we know little about the effects of stimulants on cognition, learning, and skills training in children with developmental disabilities. However, stimulants are used fairly widely in this population, and primary care physicians will invariably be asked to prescribe them for behavior problems. Our current understanding of the research suggests that stimulants may be of benefit to young children with only mild or moderate levels of mental retardation and for problem behaviors such as hyperactivity, inattention, and distractibility. If stimulants are to be used, physicians must encourage parents and teachers to closely monitor their effects not only on the problem behaviors but also on the child's cognition, learning, and rehabilitation.

Antimanics

Lithium is the drug of choice for treating bipolar or recurrent unipolar depression in individuals with developmental disabilities. It appears to be useful in treating those individuals who have nonspecific behavior disorders with a strong family history of bipolar disorder, severe behavior disorders that are cyclic in nature, and uncontrolled, explosive, aggressive behavior. As with most drugs used to control problem behavior in individuals with developmental disabilities, there is a paucity of well-controlled research on the effects of lithium. However, given the potential toxicity of lithium, primary care physicians should restrict its use to only those cases that have proven intractable to standard behavioral and psychopharmacologic treatments.

Opioid Antagonists

The opioid antagonists, naloxone and naltrexone, have been used in the treatment of behavior problems in some individuals with developmental disabilities, specifically self-injury in individuals with mental retardation. The theory that a dysfunction of the endogenous opioid system may be the causal factor in some cases of self-injury provides a good rationale for the use of these medications. Although it is limited, research does suggest that opioid antagonists may be effective in controlling the self-injury of some individuals with developmental disabilities.

The use of naloxone is not advised because of its short action. Physicians wishing to use naltrexone should note that although this drug has shown some reduction of self-injury in some cases, the changes have been small and not quite as dramatic as might be expected from the theoretic rationale. We suspect that the reduction in self-injury may in fact be a result of the sedative side effect of the drug and may have little to do with a dysfunction of the endogenous opioid system in these children.

Psychotherapy

Traditional forms of psychotherapy, including individual and group therapy, are often included in the comprehensive treatment of a problem behavior, especially if the child only has mild or moderate mental retardation. The clinician providing the therapy should be a skilled child psychotherapist, have knowledge of and experience with children who have developmental disabilities, and be able to adapt the therapy to the child's abilities. Individual therapy can be supportive, cognitive, behavioral, or multimodal in nature and can address such issues as self-esteem, coping strategies, and social skills training. Group therapy typically consists of peer, family, or heterogeneous groups. Peer groups may be beneficial if they focus on issues common to children with similar or different abilities. Additionally, a peer group provides a natural setting for the teaching and practice of appropriate skills and behaviors. Regardless of the nature and degree of a child's disability, inclusion of the family in the therapeutic process is recommended. Issues related to overall family stress and support can be addressed, as can specific issues relative to their child, including expectations and relationship satisfaction.

Socioenvironmental Therapy

Socioenvironmental therapy consists of a number of possible services designed to support the child and family. These range from psychoeducational programs and family support services to psychiatric day care, inpatient hospitalization on a specialized treatment unit, and foster care. Other sources of socioenvironmental therapy include recreational and camping programs specific to children with developmental disabilities, court and corrections services, and private residential schools.

Specific Behavioral Disorders

The full range of behavioral and psychiatric problems that are seen in children in the general population are also seen in children with developmental disabilities. In addition to having a higher overall prevalence of problem behaviors, there are certain behaviors, such as aggression and noncompliance, that are more commonly reported in children with developmental disabilities. For example, although the prevalence of conduct disorder (CD) is about 3% to 4% in children in the general population, estimates among those with mental retardation range from 12% to 45%.

Aggression

In this population, the increased occurrence of aggressive behavior may be caused by a child's inability to verbalize feelings and by poor impulse control, in contrast to the premeditated, predatory aggression and violence common in children with CD. A child's mental age and developmental level must be considered when evaluating aggression, because the behavior may represent a normal developmental stage or serve a communicative function. Additionally, there are many psychiatric disorders, including psychotic disorders, ADHD, and bipolar disorder, in which aggression may be a symptom. The treatment of choice for learning-based aggression in this population is typically behavioral intervention. Psychopharmacologic treatment can also be used alone or combined with behavioral therapies, but its efficacy is not well established.

Pica

Pica is the persistent eating of nonnutritive substances for at least 1 month. It must be inappropriate for a child's developmental level and not part of a culturally sanctioned practice. It may be nonspecific, such as when nonfood items are consumed indiscriminately, or it may be specific for certain substances, such as dirt (geophagia) or feces (coprophagia). Pica is more common in children with developmental disabilities than in the general population, and it is the most common eating disorder in individuals with mental retardation. In addition to the psychologic and social sequelae of pica, there are a number of potentially severe medical complications, including constipation, gastric obstruction, toxic ingestions, and even death. A number of etiologic theories for pica have been proposed, including nutritional deficiencies (for example, deficiencies of zinc, iron, and specific vitamins), the inability to discriminate between food and nonfood items, and biochemical dysfunctions (such as diminished dopaminergic neurotransmission). However, it is generally accepted that most cases of pica in this population are learned.

Although nutritional and pharmacologic treatments have been used, the majority of cases have been treated with behavioral intervention. Virtually all behavior reduction procedures have been used to control pica, some more successfully than others. Antecedent strategies that have been used include environmental enrichment, discrimination training, and the provision of alternate sensory activities. Response contingent strategies that have been used include differential reinforcement, visual screening, noxious tastes (such as lemon juice) and odors (aromatic ammonia), water mist, brief physical restraint, and overcorrection. An understanding of the causes and treatment of pica in this population is incomplete, but enough treatment regimens are available to control the problem in most cases.

Rumination Disorder

Rumination disorder is the repeated and deliberate regurgitation and rechewing of previously ingested food, not secondary to a gastrointestinal or other medical condition, for a period of at least 1 month following a period of normal functioning. It is typically observed in infants and individuals with mental retardation, with prevalence ranging from 6% to 10% for individuals with mental retardation in residential-care settings. Complications from this disorder may be mild (for example, tooth decay), or they may be potentially life-threatening and include extreme weight loss, anemia, and malnutrition. The evaluation of a child with rumination disorder includes a comprehensive history and physical examination to rule out medical conditions with similar symptoms, such as gastroesophageal reflux, pyloric stenosis, or food allergies. The medical assessment may include radiologic studies, endoscopy, gastrointestinal manometry, and biopsy. A complete psychiatric and behavioral assessment are also indicated.

Although a number of psychopharmacologic, surgical, and psychotherapeutic treatments have been used in the management of rumination disorder, their efficacy other than to correct an underlying medical condition has not been established. Behavioral treatments are generally regarded as the intervention of choice, and several techniques have been demonstrated to be successful. Antecedent strategies, such as special feeding techniques and food satiation, have been used. A number of response-contingent therapies, including differential reinforcement, electric shock, aversive gustatory stimulation, physical exercise, oral hygiene procedures, and overcorrection, have also been used successfully.

Self-Injury

Self-injury is usually defined as any nonfunctional behavior that results in physical injury to oneself without apparent willful intent for self-harm (that is, the definition excludes suicidal gestures and other behaviors with intent for self-harm). It represents a heterogeneous group of behaviors that include head rubbing, nail-picking, eye poking, biting, and head banging. In most cases, there is a repetitive and rhythmic quality to the behavior. In the DSM-IV diagnostic classification system, self-injury is categorized within stereotypic movement disorder (formerly stereotypy/habit disorder) along a continuum with other stereotypic behaviors that do not result in injury and are not better accounted for by a compulsion, a tic, a stereotypy that is part of a PDD, or hair pulling. Self-injury can be a manifestation of a co-morbid psychiatric disorder, such as OCD, depression or psychosis, or a medical condition such as an ear infection or seizure disorder. It can also be symptomatic of a neurobiologic disturbance, such as in Lesch-Nyhan syndrome and de Lange's syndrome. In most cases, self-injury is a learned behavior. For example, self-injurious behavior in a nonverbal child may serve a communicative function, either to get attention or to escape an undesirable task or situation. In other cases, self-injurious behavior may serve a self-stimulatory function, as in a child with a sensory deficit or an unstimulating environment.

Although some normal children younger than age 5 engage in self-injurious behavior, particularly head banging, it is rarely seen in the general pediatric population. Severe cases of self-injury generally occur in individuals with developmental disabilities, most notably in those with autistic disorder and mental retardation. Studies have shown an inverse relationship between the prevalence of self-injurious behavior and intellectual abilities; that is, the more severe the level of mental retardation a child has, the greater the prevalence of self-injurious behavior is.

Despite considerable research, no single therapy has emerged as the treatment of choice for self-injury, probably because there is no single cause. Pharmacologic approaches, behavioral interventions, and protective strategies have all been demonstrated to be effective in reducing the frequency and morbidity of self-injurious behavior in some cases. Pharmacologic treatments are generally recommended when an individual has not responded to behavioral interventions, particularly when the motivation cannot be identified and it is suspected to be of organic origin. Few drugs have been shown to be totally effective for this behavior. Recent research suggests that newer drugs, such as fluoxetine and buspirone, are promising in their effectiveness. However, the majority of cases of self-injury can be treated with behavioral procedures, probably because about 80% of cases are of learned origins, with the best results being obtained when the treatment is matched to the hypothesized function of the behavior. Protective equipment, such as a helmet and padded clothing, is sometimes necessary to protect the individual from physical harm in the initial stages of treatment. However, by themselves, protective equipment does not constitute effective treatment, because the child does not have an opportunity to learn an alternative, socially acceptable behavior.

Summary

Given the high prevalence and broad spectrum of problem behaviors and psychopathologic conditions seen in children with developmental disabilities, physicians working with these children and their families will, at some point, undoubtedly be faced with the task of managing problem behaviors. Although many of these problem behaviors can be attributed to a biologic or behavioral cause and successfully treated, some are complex in nature and require a comprehensive, multimodal approach to assessment and treatment to achieve a lasting result. The ultimate goal, of course, is to provide treatments that improve the quality of life of the child and the family.

CONSIDER CONSULTATION WHEN . . .

- There are persistent aggressive or self-injurious behaviors
- The family is overwhelmed by the child's behaviors

Annotated Bibliography

Aman MG: *Assessing psychopathology and behavior problems in persons with mental retardation: a review of available instruments,* Rockville, Md., 1991, U.S. Department of Health and Human Services.

This book provides a comprehensive description of assessment instruments and interview techniques for evaluating psychopathologic conditions and behavior disorders in people with mental retardation.

Aman MG, Singh NN: *Psychopharmacology of the developmental disabilities,* New York, 1988, Springer-Verlag.

This book covers a number of issues related to the use of psychotropic medications in individuals with developmental disabilities, including information on specific psychotropic drug groups, vitamin and dietary treatments for behavioral control, the assessment of drug effects in their natural contexts, and pertinent ethical and legal concerns.

Singh NN: *Prevention and treatment of severe behavior problems: models and methods in developmental disabilities,* Pacific Grove, Calif., 1995, Brooks/Cole.

This up-to-date reference written specifically for clinicians provides detailed descriptions of treatment strategies for specific behavior problems commonly exhibited by individuals with developmental disabilities.

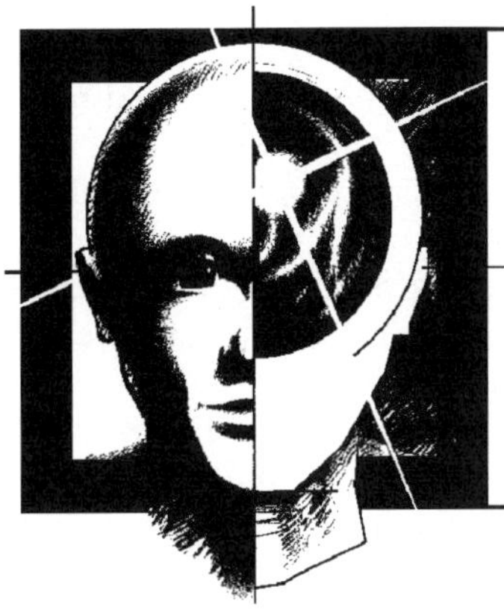

chapter 18

Chronic Illness in Children and Adolescents

Daniel N. Davidow, MD

Childhood Developmental Considerations
The Process of Acceptance
Dimensions of the Patient and Family
Illness-Specific Variables
Effective Utilization of Resources
Special Considerations
The Role of the Consultant

Perhaps William Shakespeare would have said that some are born ill, some acquire illness, and some have illness thrust upon them. When an illness becomes protracted, there are ramifications of constant stress, inherent psychosocial factors, and specific attributes of patients and family systems that these effects are separate from the physical impact of the disease process but which directly or indirectly influence the management of the medical condition. Consider the case of an 8-year-old boy whose parents have been recently divorced and who has been admitted to the hospital for investigation of the symptoms of diabetes mellitus. The security of his family unit has already been threatened, and now he faces an insult to his health and well being. He feels somehow responsible for the break-up of his family and believes that he deserves diabetes as a punishment. To whom will the child turn for guidance during the difficult process of assimilating this diagnosis into his self-concept? How successfully will the patient and family move through the process of grief over the boy's lost health status, from shock to acceptance? What tools will assist them in successfully managing this chronic illness? This chapter discusses those aspects of caring for the patient who has the type of illness that becomes a part of the patient's life and demands daily attention. The physician must effectively support the child and the family through their turmoil of emotion and confusion and help them reach a point of informed acceptance.

Specialized care provided by individual health providers may be necessary to address the various facets of a chronic condition; however, diversified care increases the risk that the treatment process will become disjointed. In most circumstances, a coordinated team of professionals is essential to achieve an optimal outcome. By developing a better awareness and understanding of the relevant concerns, the primary care physician can play a more effective role as coordinator of the management team. Other members of the team include the patient, the family, and other essential health care professionals, such as specialist consultants, a nutritionist, a nurse educator, a primary nurse, a social worker, a psychotherapist, a teacher, or a rehabilitation therapist.

Childhood Developmental Considerations

Just as there are differing medical considerations in the care of a 1-year-old child compared with the care of a 12-year-old child, there are also differing psychosocial considerations. Therefore an appreciation of a child's developmental process is of primary importance when creating a perspective from which to view the impact of chronic illness on a child. From infancy through adolescence, the successful completion of developmental tasks determines, in part, how well a patient can cope with adversity, internalize a positive ego-identity, and master social competence.

Chronic disease in infancy may disrupt parent-child bonding and interfere with the development of basic trust. A heightened degree of parental anxiety may be communicated to the child, thus creating insecurity. Repeated hospitalization or uncomfortable procedures can provoke intense separation fears in some children. Such children may seem irrationally immune to reassurance.

During the toddler stage, illness may impact a child's ability to explore the environment through mobility to gain mastery. This ability is critical to the child's ultimate accomplishment of separation and individuation from the family. The stage may be set for long-term enmeshment or dependency.

In early childhood, children are prone to "magical" thinking and often view illness as punishment earned through imaginary wrongdoing. Their worldview may be shaped by guilt or resentment, and they may accept illness as part of their identity. They may become passive or complacent. If the 8-year-old boy with diabetes responded to education about his illness by becoming particularly stoic or compliant, red flags of suspicion should be raised about his emotional adjustment.

In middle childhood, industriousness or productivity may be adversely affected by the disease process or by some secondary manifestation, such as school absence. A cycle of failure may be generated through self-fulfilling prophecy. Acceptance by same-sex peers becomes an important goal that is easily impeded by an illness, such as asthma or spina bifida, that impacts a child's appearance, ability, or stamina. Children ostracized by their peers may become introverted or depressed. The school-age child generally displays an acute appreciation of life's "fairness" principles. An insult to these principles, such as being saddled with a chronic illness, can provoke narcissistic outrage. Such anger may make an otherwise cooperative child resistant or oppositional. The child with spina bifida who refuses to perform self-catheterization may be making such a statement.

Adolescence encompasses further developmental sequences in the areas of physical, emotional, intellectual, and moral growth that are not necessarily temporally coordinated. Identity-acceptance and separation-individuation issues are intensified and may create power struggles that resemble oppositional behavior but are really designed to assert the emerging ego. These struggles are often amenable to face-saving compromise. For example, a teenager with cystic fibrosis may allow his uncle to perform chest PT for him but may refuse to allow his mother to do so. The adolescent's sense of omnipotence often presents more of a challenge than a power struggle. This feeling of indestructibility, combined with the lack of ability to project vision into the future or anticipate consequences, can result in noncompliance with medical treatments or even more self-endangering counterphobic behavior. If the adolescent with cystic fibrosis insists on smoking cigarettes, he may be attempting to master his fears of dying by facing high-risk situations, or he may be trying to prove that he is not different from his peers. Family conflict is often generated when parental attempts to offer guidance or to protect the child are viewed as attempts to control by teenagers who are already ambivalent over the amount of parenting they need.

The emergence of sexuality during the teenage years often creates further family tension. Teens with chronic illness are acutely aware of stigma related to their conditions that impact their body image or sexual attractiveness. Except for sexual function, upper body strength seems to be the attribute of most importance to the adolescent boy's sexual identity. A young woman's sexual identity, by contrast, more directly depends on the normal shape and proportion of her lower body and legs. Therefore an adolescent boy might be expected to have a more difficult adjustment to limb-girdle dystrophy, and a girl would have a hard time adjusting to polyarticular rheumatoid arthritis.

The final task of adolescence is to settle on a career goal and develop a means of becoming self-reliant. Illness may create genuine or imagined impediments to the accomplishment of this task, including, but not limited to, financial stresses and physical limitations. A seizure disorder may not only preclude certain career options; it may also prevent the attainment of a driver's license, which is considered to be the icon of independence.

The expectation for each patient's involvement in the care of an illness must be appropriately geared to the child's ability according to the stage of development. It is reasonable for a child to take part in self-management and to become educated about the illness, as long as the parent provides adequate protective structure and monitoring. It is probably better to err on the side of not giving the child enough responsibility than to over-burden a young child and set him up for failure. For example, the child with diabetes may be ready for the responsibility of learning to inject his own insulin sometime between the ages of 9 and 12, but he will likely still need parental supervision of the injection technique and assistance with diabetic problem-solving well into adolescence.

Feeling confused or overwhelmed can easily result in incompetence or nonadherence. A child must have an adequate understanding of the medical procedures involved to properly carry them out, and she may prefer to be considered lazy rather than admit she does not understand. If the rationale for a procedure is also given, compliance may be enhanced. Certain conditions that affect cognition, such as spina bifida, AIDS, and seizure disorders, can directly impede learning, concentration, or initiative. The secondary effects of medications, chemotherapy, or CNS radiation can have similar detrimental consequences on cognitive processing. They can even produce organic behavior disturbances. The sequencing and memory deficits associated with spina bifida, for instance, directly interfere with accomplishment of necessary but complex procedures, such as self-catheterization, wheelchair transfers, or skin self-inspection. A patient with spina bifida who needs to be prompted by extrinsic visual or auditory cues throughout the day should not consider herself a failure. For certain patients with mental disability, interdependence is a more realistic goal than independence.

The child's or teenager's attitude may fluctuate between wanting complete responsibility and wanting none at all. Parents and health care providers must be willing to search for possible reasons for this fluctuation, but also to be flexible enough to adapt the level of supervision and assistance to the evident need, as the young person proves more capable. Some of the many reasons that help explain patient nonadherence and some suggestions for intervention are summarized in Table 18-1.

The Process of Acceptance

Progress made toward curing transient illness and toward finding successful treatments for those conditions that cannot be cured is shifting the emphasis of health care toward the population of patients with chronic illness who require efforts to improve their quality of life and health maintenance. However, these same medical advances increase the public's expectation that all

TABLE 18-1

FACTORS INFLUENCING NONADHERENCE TO MEDICAL REGIMEN

Reason for nonadherence	May be related to:	Treatment considerations
Lack of acceptance	Poor adjustment to condition Denial or fantasy as defense Premorbid characteristics Modeling negative behavior Family dynamics Cultural or religious beliefs	Counseling Psychotherapy Family therapy Psychotropic medication
Complexity	Confusion Feeling overwhelmed or incompetent Lack of motivation or energy	Simplify treatment Educate and reeducate
Developmental stage issue	Separation or individuation struggle Ego identity or sexual identity concern Lack of ability to project consequences into the future	Protective structure Counseling Wait it out
Impact on life-style	Inconvenience or restriction Stigma Financial stress	Social services consult Simplify treatment
Discomfort	Pain Side effects of treatment	Attempt to relieve or minimize
Need to be ill	Need to escape conflict Dependency Need for attention or nurturance Treatment or symptoms are pleasurable	High index of suspicion for abuse Psychotherapy Family therapy Protective confinement
No reason to be well	Lack of direction or career goals Terminal condition	Career planning Help patient discover the meaning in life

medical problems are temporary and can be cured by a competent physician. With prolonged illness, an eventual accommodation must be made to the realities and to the long-term stressors by all those who are affected. Such accommodation involves coming to terms with the losses of health, comfort, appearance, security, or functional ability, that are associated with the condition.

Dr. Kübler-Ross has described stages of the grief process that people adjusting to situations such as chronic illness experience. The stages are shock, denial, anger, depression, bargaining, and acceptance or resignation (Figure 18-1). Each family member progresses through these stages at a different rate relative to the patient and to other family members. The specific response that is manifest at each stage may be either adaptive or maladaptive.

Desirable coping techniques are patterns of behavior that allow for effective functioning, regardless of whether they promote movement through the stages of grief. For example, shock and denial may serve a protective function by temporarily buffering the emotional response to trauma. Intellectualization occurs when information that a patient or family member obtains is used to defend against feelings of shock, anger, or depression. Intellectualization can be helpful if the expertise developed is ultimately used to allow for more direct involvement as a member of the health management team. An example of intellectualization as a defense mechanism is seen in the mother of a child born with congenital renal disease who goes back to school to obtain her nursing degree. Rationalization of the reason for a condition may be required by some people to enable them to accept evident realities and should not necessarily be challenged. Repression of severely distressing information may be critical for the patient's psychologic well being; for example, a terminally ill patient may pursue productive activities even in the face of relentless deterioration. Attempts at compensation (or more commonly, overcompensation), often seen among teenagers who feel stigmatized by their illness, are not always of concern and may in fact be useful. For example it may be acceptable for a teenager with spina bifida to deny his limitations on the playing field to his peers. However, it may not be acceptable for him to deny the risk that his new athletic shoes may cause pressure sores.

However, some defense mechanisms can be maladaptive by interfering with a person's ability to cooperate with the health care team or by having a negative impact on his state of well-being and social or emotional adjustment. Shock or depression may result in complete incapacitation or regression to a state of dependency. Such dependence on others can ultimately generate resentment, especially in adolescents who yearn to be independent. Anger may be acted out, in the form of noncompliance or even conduct disturbances, instead of expressed directly. A patient with diabetes may completely refuse to accept any responsibility for her medical care. Bargaining may be manifest as an internal spiritual or psychologic struggle, or it may take the form of attempting to justify trading off one stressor for another. For example, the patient with diabetes may decide to take her insulin but to skip checking her blood sugars. Bargaining or noncompliance can include the projection of blame, with or without anger. This is usually a destructive process that can result in guilt reactions, such as self-punishment or self-deprecation, or in creating a negative self-concept. Isolation, retreat into fantasy, or actual dissociation are all attempts to escape from emotional distress and may create varying degrees of social disability. A child with Tourette's disorder may develop symptoms of school phobia and request home schooling rather than face embarrassment in the classroom. Alternatively, the patient might react with false bravado, in an effort to deny his fears to himself or others. Such denial may even take the form of self-destructive activities, provoking the need for adults to make protective boundaries more clear or more rigid.

Adequate assessment of the patients or family member's level or mechanism of adaptation is not merely an academic exercise; rather it is crucial to the determination of the need, type, and level of intervention required. The role of the physician is to facilitate movement through this process by using modalities such as education, counseling, psychotherapy, or exposure to a support group. However, the natural course of the pro-

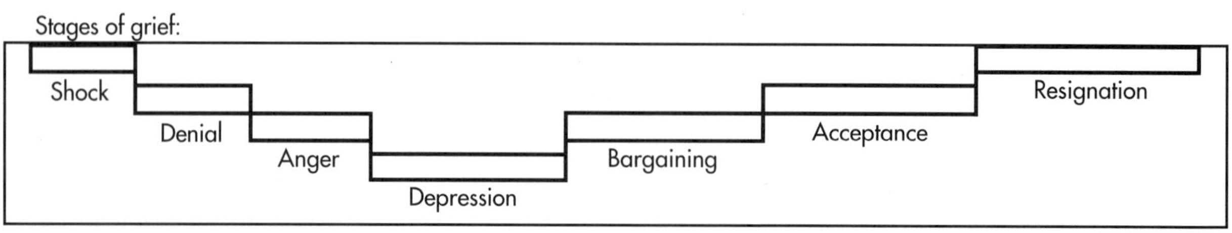

FIGURE 18-1 Stages of the grief process described by Dr. Kübler-Ross.

cess must also be appreciated as should the function served by coping mechanisms that are already evident. Any intervention should be specifically suited to the situation.

Dimensions of the Patient and Family

Unique characteristics of each patient and specific dynamics of each family must be separately appreciated for the bearing they have on adjustment to chronic illness. Families display specific temperament levels, character traits, personality styles, and pathologic states, as do the individuals that comprise a family. Additionally, the cultural heritage or religious belief system of the family often plays a strong role in determining the level of cohesiveness and the manner in which the members respond to stressful situations. These factors influence how capably the parents will supervise the child's care, follow through on recommended treatments, accommodate to alterations in life-style, help the patient adapt, and interface with the health care team. Interview is the simplest method of assessing family functioning, although some standardized instruments with questionnaires are available. The physician who fails to take family attributes into account may find therapeutic efforts frustrated by lack of cooperation or resistance. Response styles vary from hyperreactive and enmeshed to passive and disengaged, with a broad spectrum between these extremes. Some families are easily overwhelmed by loss, financial burdens, and complex information, whereas others are resilient. Some are chaotic, and others are highly organized with a specific hierarchy. Some families revolve around the child with chronic illness or value a dependent child, but in other families, a sick child may be resented, scapegoated, or even abused. Certain religious beliefs, such as an opposition to traditional medical treatments, can challenge the physician's ethical tenets or moral views. Every effort must be made to understand the perspective from which the family system operates in such situations, to relate effectively, and to negotiate a compromise solution. Therapeutic intervention for the family may be crucial if the concerns of the child are jeopardized. The social services network may be an invaluable support system and can work in coordination with other members of the health care team.

An individual patient may either conform to family patterns, rebel against them, or cooperatively differentiate from them. The child is likely to have been indoctrinated with the family belief system and will not begin to question it or to develop personal values until middle or late adolescence. Modeling of learned behavior or patterned responses that children display can be either valuable or detrimental. For example, a child may model parental virtues such as tolerance or inquisitiveness, or she may model unhealthy habits or noncompliant behaviors if she has been exposed to them. The child's temperament may also have a bearing on such factors as the degrees of acceptance vs. resignation or assertiveness vs. submissiveness that will be displayed. Specific character traits also impact adaptation to chronic illness. Ego strength, phobias, or anxious tendencies are aspects of a person's character that influence the manner in which she responds to external or internal stressors. Personality traits make some patients inherently more vulnerable to feeling hopeless or helpless, whereas they help others display innate strength in the face of adversity.

Just as the patient's behavior can complicate the management of an illness, the converse is also true. An illness such as Lupus, or the prednisone used to manage it, can be associated with behavioral consequences ranging from irritability to paranoia. To adequately assess a situational concern in a chronically ill patient, the physician must consider all of the relevant dimensions, including the patient's personality characteristics, the family dynamics, and specific variables relating to the illness or its treatment, in an effort to identify the root cause. A targeted intervention may involve the use of modalities such as individual, group, or family psychotherapy, CBT, or psychotropic medication, or it may simply involve education or adjustment of the treatment regimen.

Illness-Specific Variables

There are aspects relative to each specific condition that directly influence the ease of accommodation that can be anticipated. These factors include the level of intensity or severity of the illness, its degree of visibility to others, the degree of discomfort created by it, the predictability of its course, and the expected prognosis.

The intensity implies the impact on the patient or family's life-style and may range from inconvenience to restriction. However, the level of intensity must be personally interpreted, since an inconvenience to some (for example, having to eat meals at a certain time of day) may be considered by others to be an extreme constraint. Therefore intensity describes how often the condition is brought to mind each day. The degree of financial stress imposed by an illness is usually directly related to the intensity but also relates to the cost of medication and supplies. There is variable expression of almost every chronic condition. The level of involvement expressed by a particular condition is relative to the severity of symptoms. In many illnesses, such as cystic fibrosis or diabetes, the level of compliance with recommended treatments directly influences severity, whereas in others, such as sickle cell anemia, there is little direct correlation.

One might imagine that a more visible illness is more stigmatizing and therefore more difficult to accept. However, it appears that if all other factors are equal, acceptance generally comes more easily to patients whose conditions are obvious. It may be that people with evident challenges receive more validation of their efforts from the community than those whose hardships are not apparant to others.

Predictability is another variable aspect of chronic illness. Flare-ups or crisis-level complications that occur erratically and are unrelated to adherence to a prescribed regimen can be difficult to tolerate emotionally, because they involve an element of anxiety generated by hopelessness and loss of control. Such incidents might occur in patients with asthma, seizure disorders, or diabetes, and they are often wrongly attributed to patient noncompliance, compounding the detrimental effect. An attempt should be made to explore possible contributing factors with patients in a nonaccusatory manner and to help them understand the variables that are under their control. The temptation to question a patient's level of cooperation with treatment should be restrained unless a specific pattern of problematic management is evident.

Conditions that cause intermittent or chronic pain, such as sickle cell anemia or arthritis, or those that have painful treatments, such as thalassemia or renal failure, warrant special consideration. The tendency to avoid painful experiences can lead to noncompliance or narcotic-seeking behaviors that can complicate medical management. Cognitive ability, social functioning, and motivation can also be adversely affected by pain. Physicians should be sympathetically aware of the level of discomfort created by the imposed treatments, so efforts can be made to keep these to a minimum. It is also reasonable to explore alternative methods of pain control, such as relaxation techniques, hypnotherapy, biofeedback, transdermal electrical stimulation, or acupuncture to help patients become maximally functional and reduce the risk of narcotic addiction.

The issue of prognosis is sometimes sidestepped if the physician is uncomfortable confronting it directly. The course of a chronic condition may be stable for long periods; in contrast, it may be characterized by improvement, deterioration, unpredictable exacerbations, and remissions; or it may be relentlessly fatal. The physician is often challenged by ethical dilemmas regarding how much to inform children about their conditions. These are usually generated by paternalistic concerns. The object of informing patients is not to destroy their hope or break down defense mechanisms. Offering the hope of future medical advances that may improve their outcome, when this is realistic, is not incompatible with a straightforward discussion of future potential risks. The more predictable the outcome, the better chance the patient and family have of accommodating and responding constructively to the inevitable situations that arise. However, families can also work toward preparing for anticipated crises if an illness has a "predictably unpredictable" course. Therefore in most circumstances, information that has a bearing on prognosis is better shared than withheld if it is presented in the least threatening manner and at the child's level of comprehension.

Effective Utilization of Resources

An awareness that resources of time, money, and emotional and physical energy are limited demands that the health care team examine and remain acutely aware of the use of these resources and that the team create a strategy for the most efficient functioning (Table 18-2). Expenditures early in the course of illness that set the stage for optimal support and responsiveness can significantly reduce long-term costs.

Education of the patient and family is a critical process that can be facilitated by such members of the team as the nutritionist, the nurse educator, and the primary nurse. The need for periodic reeducation should not be overlooked, because reeducation can help the physician dispel misconceptions, evaluate current practices, and provide updates on prevailing medical theories. Financial planning for the family by a social service worker or career planning for the patient by a vocational counselor are other types of educational efforts that should not be overlooked.

Psychologic prophylaxis can also pay future dividends. A social worker, school counselor, or psychotherapist can help facilitate the development of certain characteristics that are found in families who function more effectively when challenged by circumstances beyond their control. The parents in such families are competent and in charge, set clear boundaries, and provide protective structure for their children. They offer positive reinforcement for desired behavior without being overly rigid, controlling, or demanding. Open communication and a flexible problem-solving approach are used. The support of extended family, the community, and the peer group is encouraged. Often, there are specific support groups within the community that can be used, providing a valuable resource at minimal cost. Families should be assisted and encouraged to access such services (Box 18-1).

Follow-up care must be often and sensitive enough to detect early signs of decompensation of the social system, as well as of the clinical condition. Indicators of concern include disruption of the family routine, social isolation, family conflict, financial stress, school or job performance or attendance problems, and lack of adherence to the prescribed treatment regimen. The

TABLE 18-2

RESOURCES FOR FAMILIES AND PHYSICIANS

	Human resources	Agencies and organizations	Protective structures
Medical	Primary care physician Nurse educator Nutritionist Rehabilitation therapists School nurse Specialist physician	Specialty agency or foundation (i.e., Easter Seals Society, American Diabetes Association, National Center for Youth with Disabilities)	Acute hospital Rehabilitation hospital Subacute hospital Nursing home
Emotional	Therapist School counselor Psychiatric consultant Developmental specialist Religious leader	Support group Group therapy Religious organization	Therapeutic day treatment Group home Residential treatment
Social	Extended family Family friends Social worker Case manager	Social services CPS Big Brothers and Sisters	Emergency shelter Placement with relative or friend Foster care
Educational and vocational	Teacher School official Vocational consultant	School Dept. of vocational rehabilitation services career counseling center	Job corps Boarding school Military school
Recreational	Coach Recreational therapist	Clubs Organized sports Fitness centers Boy/Girl Scouts	Experiential (wilderness) program
Legal	Advocate Probation officer Lawyer	Legal aid society Dept. for Rights of People with Disabilities Juvenile justice system	Children in Need of Supervision (CHINS) petition Probation House arrest Detention facility

BOX 18-1

COMMUNITY RESOURCES

Roberts N: *Living your own life: a handbook for teenagers by young people and adults with chronic illness and disabilities,* Minneapolis, 1993, PACER.
$8 From PACER Center; 4826 Chicago Ave. South, Minneapolis, MN 55417

Mackenzie L: *The complete directory for people with chronic illness, 1994,* Lakeville, CT, 1994, Grey House Publishing.

National Center for Youth with Disabilities (NCYD); Nancy A. Okinow, Executive Director; Telephone: 800-333-6293, FAX: 612-626-2134; University of Minnesota; Box 721-UMHC, Minneapolis, MN 55455
CYDLINE Reviews (annotated bibliography and resource list). Examples include:

- Youth with disabilities and chronic illnesses: an introductory guide for youth and parents
- Adolescents with chronic illness: issues for school personnel
- Developing social skills: issues for adolescents with chronic illnesses and disabilities
- Issues in sexuality for adolescents with chronic illnesses and disabilities
- Legal issues for adolescents with chronic illnesses and disabilities and their families
- Promoting decision making skills by youth with disabilities: health, education, and vocational choices
- Race and ethnicity: issues for adolescents with chronic illnesses and disabilities
- Self-esteem: issues for adolescents with chronic illnesses and disabilities
- Substance use by youth with disabilities and chronic illnesses
- Transition from pediatric to adult health care for youth with disabilities and chronic illnesses
- Vulnerability and resiliency: focus on children, youth and families with disabilities

health management team members should confer when necessary to ensure dissemination of information and coordination of care. It is important to remember that the patient and family are members of this team.

Rehabilitative therapists providing physical, occupational, or speech therapy services to the patient are also integral members of the health care team, as are specialist physicians who provide consultation to the primary care physician. Meetings may be carried out by conference call if face-to-face sessions are impractical. The broad goals of the team to maximize function and prevent deterioration should be kept foremost in mind and not overshadowed by the confusing cascade of day-to-day details. Ideally, the same management team would be available if the patient were to require hospitalization to provide for continuity of care.

Special Considerations

Changing standards in the health care arena are clouding the horizon and will invariably alter the concept and practice of medicine in the future. As resources become more tightly managed, the inevitable result will be rationing of services or treatments to those who cannot purchase them independently of a third party payer. The coordinating physician is often requested to serve as the patient's advocate or arbitrator. This role is not inappropriate as long as there is no conflict of interest. Most physicians will feel compelled to reexamine their abilities and limitations to more clearly delineate the range within which they feel competent to operate within this arena. Trained advocates for patients, such as case managers or legal representatives of a state's Department for the Rights of Citizens with Disabilities, might be available as alternative resources to patients with chronic conditions. The patient's community services board may also be required to provide special school programming or to explore funding options to meet the expenses of specialized care. Such issues concerning the utilization of resources can create difficult ethical dilemmas.

Other ethical concerns unique to the management of chronically ill patients are being raised. For example, the age at which a minor can consent to or refuse life-saving procedures was debated in the case of a young man who declined a liver transplant and chose to die. It is ironic that the same dramatic advances of medical science and technology that offer such hope to those afflicted by chronic disease are creating new dimensions to complicate the provision of care by physicians who take up the challenge.

The Role of the Consultant

The psychiatric consultant serves the health care team by providing an external perspective and special expertise. When initial efforts have failed to bring about a resolution of the conflict that threatens to put the patient's health at risk, or when team members feel that psychologic factors are preventing stabilization or recovery, more intensive intervention strategies may be necessary. The psychiatrist may help in a decision about the use of psychotropic medication or give advice regarding the need for admission to a day treatment program, hospital program, or residential treatment program. Except in critical situations, the criteria for admission into such a program should include failure of less restrictive alternatives. Family involvement in treatment is crucial to achieve a successful result. Only in rare circumstances when the family dynamics are destructive and inflexible is family exclusion or out-of-home placement considered. It may be difficult to visualize a parent's failure to supervise or control their child as neglect, but the consequences of such conditions can be life-threatening. The child's welfare must be the foremost consideration. Strong suspicions of abuse should be raised if a child with chronic illness is often readmitted to the hospital, because this may be a veiled attempt to escape from an intolerable situation. Even in this event, the possibility of placing the child with a close relative or friend is preferable to a foster family or group home.

If psychiatric intervention is indicated, it must be provided concurrently with the medical management and the efforts of other team members to be productive. Psychotropic medication may result in interactions between drugs or other unacceptable side effects that are first detected by the primary physician or other observer.

PEARLS & PERILS

CHRONIC ILLNESS

- The treatment of chronic illness requires a team effort. The patient and family are part of the team.
- The physician should consider the impact of the condition on the patient, as well as potential side effects of treatments or medications.
- When noncompliance is observed, the cause must be elucidated.
- Defense mechanisms may be adaptive or maladaptive.
- The patient's level of adaptation and coping styles may differ from those of family members.
- Cultural and religious beliefs may strongly influence behavior.
- When recurrent hospitalizations are necessary, the physician should keep a high index of suspicion for abuse or neglect in the home.
- Homebound education is rarely helpful or necessary.

The interrelated aspects of caring for chronically ill patients are challenging to coordinate, but the rewards of meeting this challenge can be surprising. An investment in helping patients find successful problem solving strategies and create advantages to overcome their barriers pays dividends in the form of encouragement and inspiration to the physician.

CONSIDER CONSULTATION WHEN . . .

- Persistent noncompliance with the medical regimen becomes life-threatening
- The youth consistently cannot or will not accept appropriate self-care responsibilities
- The family is overwhelmed by the youth's condition

Annotated Bibliography

Hymovitch D, Hagopian G: *Chronic illness in children and adults: a psychosocial approach,* Philadelphia, 1992, W.B. Saunders.

This book has many practical suggestions and is written from a nursing perspective.

Taner Leff P, Walizer EH: *Building the healing partnership: parents, professionals, and children with chronic illnesses and disabilities,* Cambridge, Mass., 1992, Brookline Books.

This is a readable book with many case vignettes. It may also be used as a resource for families.

Eisner C: *Growing up with a chronic disease: the impact on children and their families,* Philadelphia, 1993, J. Kingsley.

This book provides a good overview, and it is readable. The emphasis is on the developmental process.

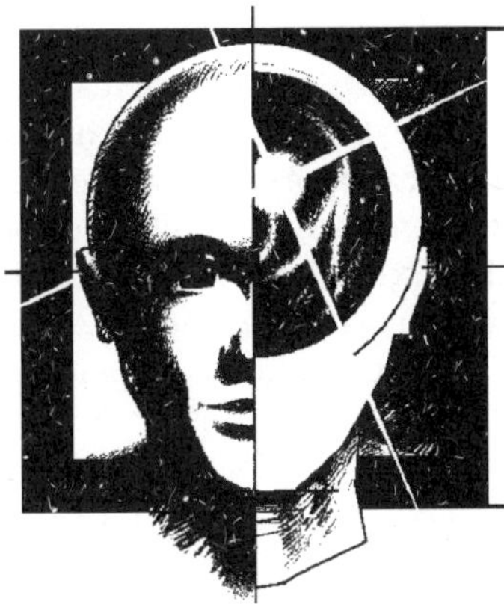

chapter 19

Sexuality

Debbie R. Carter, MD, Cheryl Al-Mateen, MD, and Richard R. Brookman, MD

Theories of Sexual Development in Childhood and Adolescence
Normal Sexual Development
Assessment
Special Topics in Child and Adolescent Sexuality
Prevention
Summary

Sexuality is recognized as an essential aspect of human development that is expressed throughout the lifespan. In the United States, child and adolescent sexuality is expressed in the context of cultural, environmental, family, and religious influences. In a cross-cultural analysis of sexual permissiveness, the United States ranked as having one of the most sexually restrictive cultures. A child in this society is faced with the task of developing a significant component of identity amidst ambiguous messages about sexuality. Children and adolescents who are also members of an ethnic cultural or ethnic minority group must incorporate into their sexual identities the values, behavior, expressions, and accepted sexual activities of the dominant group as well as those of the ethnic or minority culture.

The definitions of sexuality help define the confluence of components that comprise normal sexual development (Box 19-1). Biologic sex is incorporated by the child into a self-perception of being male or female that is referred to as core gender identity. An initial sense of core gender identity can be observed in children at an average age of 18 months. A stable core gender identity is established by 30 months. At this age, children can acknowledge that girls become women and boys become men.

Gender role behavior, or sex role behavior, is the term used to describe the behaviors and actions that a culture or society views as typically masculine and feminine. These are nonsexual attributes that are di-

BOX 19-1

DEFINITIONS OF SEXUALITY

Core gender identity—self-perception of being male or female

Gender role behavior—behaviors described as typically masculine or feminine

Gender role identity—self-image of exhibiting maleness or femaleness

Sexual orientation—self-identification as gay or lesbian, heterosexual, or bisexual

Sexual identity—recognition of sexual orientation and the disclosure of that to others

chotomous for men and women. Gender role behaviors include characteristics such as speech patterns, mannerisms, display of emotions, physical grooming, and appearance.

Gender role identity is the child's psychologically constructed self-image of an individual who exhibits femaleness or maleness. This identity is dynamic and is altered by the child's psychologic growth and development. The environments of the child (initially the family and then peers and cultural institutions) enhance or challenge the individual's expression of this gender identity by accepting or rejecting roles the child performs. For example, some sports activities and careers in the United States are viewed primarily male pursuits; women are not allowed to participate or are recipients of minimal economic rewards for performing in the sport or career. Similarly, there are careers that have historically been deemed inappropriate for men.

Sexual orientation refers to the individual's self-identification as essentially heterosexual, gay, or lesbian. The expression of sexual orientation is influenced by biologic and environmental factors and includes cognitions, affects, and fantasies. It is the compilation of erotic and romantic fantasies, as well as activities directed to the preferred sex over the other sex for the development of intimate attachments. In this chapter the term *homosexual* is used to refer to sexual behavior. The terms *gay* and *lesbian* are used in reference to an individual's concept of identity. Research on bisexuality in adolescents is still preliminary and is not discussed in this chapter.

Sexual identity involves the recognition of one's sexual orientation and the disclosure of that information to others. This term relates to the results of the "coming out" process in gay or lesbian individuals. There are three components to sexual identity. An individual may think of himself as homosexual in relation to romantic and sexual settings; this is the self-identity. The perceived identity involves how the individual feels she is seen by others. The announcement of oneself in a particular situation as gay or lesbian is the presented identity. The identity is most fully realized when all three aspects agree.

Theories of Sexual Development in Childhood and Adolescence

Gender identity, gender role behaviors, and sexual orientation all comprise a person's sexual identity. Sexuality is a person's expression of sexual identity. There are a number of theories of sexual development that attempt to understand how a child incorporates each component into sexual identity.

Psychoanalytic Theories

Freud created the first systematic psychosexual development theory, a psychoanalytic theory. Freud noted that the sexual drive is an essential primary urge or instinct. The personality structure of the id, ego, and superego is influenced by the sexual drive. The oral stage of psychosexual development occurs in infancy. During the first year of life the infant is the object and recipient of its own sexual instinct. The infant derives great pleasure from oral exploration of its body and the world. Infants who breastfeed obtain erotic pleasure from the mother's nipple and the intimacy of feeding. The anal stage of psychosexual development occurs between the ages of 2 and 3. The child develops control of the anal sphincter and experiences increased autonomy. The child's sexual desire is evidenced by the child's retention and expelling of stool, and eroticism is attached to the act of defecation. The child also must cope with ambivalence about separation from the primary caregiver. The phallic stage occurs between the ages of 4 and 6. The child develops a primary interest in the genitals. The primary source of sexual pleasure for the child occurs through the manipulation and exhibition of the genitalia. The child engages in consensual sex play and is curious about male and female genital differences. The child engages in increasing sexual self-stimulation of the genitals and may use a number of inanimate masturbatory objects. The oedipal period is an important component of the phallic stage. The child is faced with the task of understanding and incorporating her genital difference from that of the opposite sex and developing an identification with the same sex parent. The conflict for the child in the oedipal period is over managing hostile feelings toward the same sex parent and competing for the affection of the opposite sex parent. In boys this conflict is exhibited by fears of loss of the penis or by castration anxiety. In girls the oedipal conflict results in anxiety of not having a penis. During the oedipal period, children who develop a primarily heterosexual orientation work through hostile emotions toward the same sex parent after realizing that they are unable to compete for the opposite sex parent. These children develop an identification with the same sex parent. Early psychoanalytic theory proposes that only a heterosexual resolution is normal.

Some homosexual boys enter the oedipal phase with the perception of being different. For example, a boy desires the attention of his father. The child's eroticized encounter attempts with the father lead to a conflicted father-son relationship. The father responds by distancing himself from the child's erotic inclinations. In lesbians the primacy of the initial dyadic mother-daughter relationship remains eroticized, and the child's sexual desire is directed toward feminine objects.

The latency stage occurs between the age of 6 and the onset of puberty. The child in this stage experiences a repression of sexual interests as a result of maturation of the ego and superego.

The final stage of psychosexual development occurs in adolescence. In the genital stage, the adolescent reworks the oedipal conflict and sexual desire begins to be expressed, channeled, or inhibited in a more adult fashion. The adolescent may experience turmoil as attempts are made to incorporate sexual identity into a consistent self-identity (Box 19-2).

Several psychoanalytic revisions of child and adolescent psychosexual development exist that have not been included in this discussion. A number of clinical observations of children and adolescents can be compared or contrasted with the psychosexual developmental theories. Genital arousal and masturbation in infancy is well-documented, which suggests that sexual desire is expressed through genital manipulation in infancy. Children remain interested in sex-based genital play during toilet training. Parental influence during toilet training has a great impact on the child's eroticism of the anus. The oedipal conflict is not universal in all cultures. In latency, children engage in masturbation and sex play. Many adolescents incorporate sexual identity without turmoil.

Erikson's psychosocial psychoanalytic theory of development emphasizes the process of a child's socialization over sexual instinct as a propelling force in development. In his model the sexual drive influences the child's ability to form intimate relationships. In the first stage of trust vs. mistrust, the infant's sexual drive is closely tied to eroticized body parts. The infant is afforded comfort and constancy by the primary caregivers. This relationship allows the infant to develop a basic sexual identification and basic trust. In the second stage, autonomy vs. self-doubt, the toddler age 18 months to 4 years struggles to gain control of elimination. The child becomes less impulsive, and the sexual drive is expressed in manipulation of inanimate objects. The toddler's sexual activities conform to acceptable societal standards. The third stage, initiative vs. guilt, occurs between the ages of 4 and 6. The child is aware of genital differences and sex role differences. The child responds to societal norms by identifying with the same sex parent or caregiver. Industry vs. inferiority is the fourth stage of development and occurs during elementary school years. The child continues to have sexual strivings, which are often translated into a desire to work, create, and engage in nonsexual play. The adolescent enters the fifth stage of identity vs. identity diffusion. The adolescent reexperiences dormant sexual desires and attempts to sustain a core sense of self. The adolescent completes the tasks in this stage after successfully integrating all identifications gained from previous relationships (Box 19-3).

BOX 19-2

FREUD'S ANALYTIC DEVELOPMENT STAGES

Oral—mouth and feeding is focus of pleasure
Anal—control of anal sphincter is learned
Phallic—primary interest is genital organs
Oedipal—understanding of difference from parent of opposite sex is incorporated
Latency—sexual interests are repressed
Genital—oedipal conflict is reworked

BOX 19-3

ERIKSON'S STAGES

Trust vs. mistrust—appreciates constancy, develops basic trust
Autonomy vs. self-doubt—gains control of self (toilet training) to conform to social standards
Initiative vs. guilt—is aware of gender/sex role differences, identifies with same sex parent
Industry vs. inferiority—translates sexual strivings into desire to work and play
Identity vs. identity diffusion—reexperiences sexual desires while establishing a core sense of self

Social Learning Theories

The social learning theories of development postulate the importance of sexuality as a component of a child's development. Central to the development of the child's identity is the pleasure derived from the socialized behaviors that maximize and promote relationships with the social environment.

The infant experiences sexuality in the complex communications that occur in the dyadic relationship with the primary caregiver. The caregivers in the child's life model sex-role differences, and by age 3 or 4 the child responds to the male and female role divisions in the culture by choosing models of sex-role stereotypes consistent with the same sex parent. This is accomplished by the child approximating the same sex parent's modeling of sex differences through identification. In adolescence these roles are resorted in conjunction with identifications, sexual fantasies, and sexual behavior options as the adolescent completes identity formation.

Cognitive Theories

The cognitive developmental theories of child development stress the role of intellectual competence in developing personality structures. The child interacts with the environment, and objects are perceived as having certain attributes and are categorized. Sexuality is one component of identity that evolves based on the intellectual growth of the child. In infancy the child perceives the environment as being organized by the body. By age 5, the child is aware of the sexual schema of male and female roles and uses anatomic differences to assist in perceiving socially acceptable male and female gender roles. The child identifies with the same sex parent. In adolescence the ability to perform formal operations allows the adolescent flexibility in using a number of intellectual perceptions, integrating sexuality into a self-identity. The adolescent is successful in integrating sexuality through achieving a heterosexual self-concept.

Sociologic analysis, which combines social learning and cognitive-based concepts, provides a construct to understand homosexual identity formation. Troiden's theory on the formation of homosexual identities is one of several models. From infancy to puberty the child is in the sensitization stage. The child assumes that she is heterosexual but experiences feelings of being different from same sex peers. The child may feel odd because of a preference for less rigid gender roles. In the second stage the adolescent reflects on feeling and behaviors that are potentially homosexual. This stage of identity confusion is characterized by the adolescent not being able to assume an automatic sexual identification as heterosexual. Stigma and lack of information about homosexuality add to the inner turmoil of the adolescent. The adolescent may deny homosexual components of her feelings, fantasies, or activities. The adolescent may attempt to extinguish these feelings by seeking professional treatment in an attempt to repair the earlier assumption and perception of being heterosexual. The adolescent may withdraw from activities perceived to be associated with homosexuality. The adolescent may attempt to avoid opposite sex peers to prevent others from discovering disinterest in heterosexual desire. The adolescent may avoid exposure to information about homosexuality or redefine homosexual feelings and activities as one-time events. Some adolescents employ self-destructive avoidance strategies, such as assuming homophobic intellectual stances, promiscuous heterosexual encounters to disprove homosexual feelings, or abusing alcohol and illicit substances. Typically, in late adolescence the third stage of identity assumption occurs. The adolescent incorporates a self-identity that includes the perception of being gay or lesbian (Box 19-4). This is accomplished after the strategies adopted in the previous stage fail to promote identity cohesion. In the stage of identity assumption the adolescent may decide to come out and present this aspect of personality to the world. In ethnic cultures and ethnic minority cultures, coming out may not occur since the individual may prefer to present only the minority group affiliation to greater society. Furthermore, these cultures may be particularly unaccepting of the gay or lesbian adolescent, forcing the teen to choose between the two groups. If the person chooses to identify with the minority culture, she may not be accepted by this group because of her homosexuality. If she chooses to identify with the dominant gay and lesbian culture she may lose contact with her minority culture.

BOX 19-4

TROIDEN'S STAGES

Sensitization—assumes heterosexuality, but feels different
Identity confusion—recognizes potential homosexuality
Identity assumption—incorporates self-identity that includes being gay or lesbian

Normal Sexual Development

Several investigators have studied the role of genetic, physiologic, and biologic determinants in the development of sexuality. Biologic and environmental factors, as well as the incorporation of feelings arising from intimate relationships, are intertwined in the development of sexual identity. Sexual orientation is believed to be a complex interaction of each child's sex of rearing, the positive and negative reactions of adults to expressions of sexuality throughout childhood, and the hormonal milieu of fetal life.

Intrinsic-Biologic Factors

Prenatal exposure to testosterone is required for the embryo to differentiate with male reproductive structures. Prenatal androgen exposure leads to nonsexual behavior differences, such as the difference in intensity of aggression in boys compared with that in girls. Studies of male pseudohermaphrodites with 5α-reductase deficiency tracked 18 infants who had prenatal exposure to testosterone but were assigned a gender identity of being female. In puberty the children underwent masculinization, and 16 of them changed their gender

PEARLS & PERILS

NORMAL SEXUAL DEVELOPMENT

- Sexual identity and sexual orientation are both the result of complex interactions of biologic and environmental factors.

identity to masculine. Girls with congenital adrenal hyperplasia (CAH) who are treated in infancy tend to exhibit higher energy levels than same-aged controls, and they also engage in more rough and tumble play. Overall, sexual development in children is remarkably similar.

Secretion of pituitary gonadotropins and growth hormone release heralds the onset of puberty. In girls, body fat increases. Ovary growth occurs approximately 1 year earlier than breast budding in response to the effect of follicle stimulating hormone. Ovarian estrogen stimulates breast development. This estrogen also promotes thickening of the vaginal mucosa, as well as vascularization and pigmentation of the labia majora. Uterine and clitoral enlargement occurs. Pubic and axillary hair growth approximates adult distribution as a result of the influence of adrenal androgens. In boys, pituitary gonadotropins and growth hormones lead to greater muscularity. Adrenal androgens promote pubic and axillary hair growth. Testicular enlargement occurs. Testosterone secretion in boys leads to enlargement of the epididymis, seminal vesicles, and prostate gland. The penis enlarges.

The adolescent must also cope emotionally and psychologically with physical changes that are occurring. Early puberty in girls and delayed puberty in boys can be associated with psychologic and social difficulties. These states may result in the adolescent feeling as if she is receiving undue attention (or lack thereof) from potential romantic objects, thus setting the teen apart from her peers.

Twin studies have shown that same sex orientation occurs more often in identical twins than in fraternal twins or in nontwin brothers. Similarly, heritability has also been shown in female homosexuality. Other studies have explored the effects of prenatal exposure to sex hormones, enzyme deficiencies in steroid synthesis pathways, or neuroanatomic differences. No conclusion has been reached as to the origin of homosexual orientation.

Extrinsic Factors

Clinicians have explored consistencies in sex differences perceived by society to be masculine or feminine. In a cross-cultural investigation, responses displayed over time from boys and girls that were indicative of sex-stereotyped behavior were highly shaped by the environment. Girls exhibited more social awareness of interpersonal responsibility and tended to seek comfort from the environment.

The child's family and ethnocultural heritage also significantly impact sexual development. Two examples may be useful in illustrating the effect of family and cultural norms on sexuality. For many children reared in African-American families, sexuality is viewed as a positive and natural part of life. Damaging myths about African-American sexuality may, however, promote antagonistic relationships. These myths include the essential unattractiveness of Africanized features, hair, and skin color. Black men are often portrayed as animalistic and oversexed. Black women are portrayed in conflicting stereotypes; sometimes they appear loose and exotic and at other times they are shown to be domineering or nurturing but sexless. Children and adolescents exposed to such negative models often struggle to establish a self-identity in which sexuality is a positive aspect of the personality. African-American caregivers provide intellectual categories of options concerning gender role behavior and sexual expression based on concepts such as mutual respect, cooperation, and social role fluidity that promotes group survival. In contrast, majority culture middle class and upper class members tend to repress a child's sexual interests and try to distract them from sexual interests or maintain their ignorance. A child's early misconceptions about sex are rarely acknowledged. Children are more likely to learn about sex from peers or from the media.

Gay and lesbian adolescents who are in the process of developing their sexual identities must also contend with ethnocultural heritage. Those who grow up in orthodox religious homes, in homes where the children are expected to live with the family until marriage, in homes where everyone is expected to marry and have children, or in homes with polarized gender role expectations will be the most in conflict with their families. Members of certain ethnic groups feel that it is impossible for other members of their group to be homosexual. Belonging to a specific ethnic culture and being homosexual may be perceived as mutually exclusive. This myth will remain unchallenged as long as homosexual members of that group remain closeted. Parents may blame the dominant culture for their child's sexual orientation. For example, a 20-year-old Pakistani-Canadian man explains that his parents are hurt because they believe homosexuality is against the Muslim faith. For his parents, homosexuality is an aspect of the dominant culture; their son learned to be gay from his white friends. To them, homosexuality is the result of a decadent, Western, urban society.

One reason that adolescent sexual activity occurs at such a high rate in our culture is that sex has been enshrined in our media-driven culture. Media images are synthesized with the mores of the family, community, and society at large. The adolescent's decision to be sexual or not is processed by a series of filters, each representing the influences of media, family, and society. These filters can be referred to as youth culture screens. In the first screen, the adolescent assesses the meaning of sexuality in a particular situation and determines whether to be active or inactive. The second screen is the process the adolescent and partner go through to negotiate which sexual activities will occur. The third screen is the perception of danger of the sexual acts. This screen can be shaded by the adolescent's sense of invulnerability.

Normal Sexual Behavior

Studies of normal sexual interactions in children highlight aspects of sexual development. Infants and children exhibit pleasure when engaged in autoerotic activities such as thumb sucking and masturbation. During diaper changes, children enjoy being cleaned and often explore their genitals and anus. Children exhibit genital pride in play activities such as "doctor." When children enter elementary school, same sex peer groups tend to enforce gender role behavior boundaries by using verbal slurs. Sex play often occurs in organized group games such as "truth or dare" or "strip poker."

Many gay and lesbian adults report persistent involvement in cross-gender behavior during childhood. The actual percentage of homosexual adults who exhibited such behavior as children is unclear, but the relationship is consistent in empirical studies.

Normal sexual activity in youngsters is consensual, between peers of the same age with ongoing friendly relationships. The range of normal behaviors is wide, and may include touching, peeking, kissing, hugging, and even pretend intercourse. Up to 3% of children under age 12 engage in intercourse. It is not uncommon for boys between the ages of 8 and 13 to engage in genital exhibition, group masturbation, or mutual masturbation. Although the children may be embarrassed when they are discovered by an adult, shame and guilt are not seen; the emotions attached to the experiences are generally lighthearted and playful. Furthermore, when they are directed by the adult to stop the behavior children do stop (at least in the presence of the adult). Children involved in these normal exploratory activities have interests in other undertakings as well and do not seem overly preoccupied with sexual issues. Box 19-5 shows an overview of normal sexual behaviors of children.

Adolescents are preoccupied with the normality of their sexual thoughts, feelings, impulses, and behaviors. As a developmental group, they do not consider the potential harmful consequences of their behaviors. A child reaches early adolescence when she is just entering pu-

BOX 19-5

NORMAL SEXUAL BEHAVIORS OF CHILDREN

Preschool children

- Touch own genitals when diapers changed, anxious, or sleepy
- Touch genitals and breasts of familiar people

Preschool or young school-age children

- Look for differences between boys and girls; men and women
- Ask about genitals, intercourse, and babies and where they come from
- Enjoy own nudity, may offer to show others genitalia
- Are interested in watching people use the bathroom
- Are interested in own feces
- May use "dirty" words for toileting or sexual functions
- Play doctor
- Out of curiosity, insert objects in genitals or rectum of self or other
- Play house, acting as mommy or daddy
- Have erections (boys)

Young school-age children

- Think other gender children are "gross," but chase them
- Talk about sex or play games related to sex with friends
- Want privacy in bathroom or when changing clothes
- Like "dirty" jokes
- Look at nude pictures of adults or nude adults
- Put genitalia on human figure drawings
- Compare genitals with same age friends; want to touch same age friends and be touched
- Kiss familiar adults and children
- Are interested in animals breeding

(Adapted from Johnson: Assessment of sexual behavior problems in preschool-aged and latency-aged children, *Child Adolesc Psychiatry Clin North Am* 2:431-449, 1993).

berty. Young adolescents are intensely aware of the physical changes of their body, observing and comparing with peers for any evidence of abnormality. They tend to exaggerate and fret over physical symptoms, yet they see themselves as invulnerable. As puberty progresses, masturbation may be (re)discovered. Close relationships with same sex peers may result in sexual experimentation out of curiosity. The intensity of relationships with members of the opposite sex is diminished by the distance of the telephone or interaction in mixed sex groups. There are crushes on important adult figures in the adolescent's life. Some of these crushes may be on adults of the same gender. Conversation involves a lot of sexual innuendo. The majority of young adolescents are not involved in sexual intercourse; only 16% of 13-year-old children have had intercourse.

In middle adolescence (ages 14 to 18), puberty is generally complete. Although the adolescent is already physically mature and able to reproduce, psychosocial development progresses. There is frustration because the teenager does not have social permission to express sexuality in an adult manner. The middle adolescent wants to show off his new adult body to simultaneously impress peers and perhaps shock adults. Peer approval is constantly sought. The adolescent continues to feel invulnerable and experiments in risk-taking behaviors such as driving, substance use, (nicotine, alcohol, and drugs) and sexual activity. There is a range of sexual behaviors, and in some, sexuality may be used as rebellion. Most middle adolescents masturbate with varying frequency. Fifty-six percent of girls and 73% of boys have intercourse before the age of 18. For boys, sexual intercourse or active anal intercourse is viewed as an enhancement of the masculine image. Girls tend to view sexual activity as an expression of greater intimacy in a romantic relationship. Adolescents may be unaware of the range of normal human sexual responses or of the common occurrence among adults of less-than-satisfactory sexual encounters. They tend not to discuss these concerns because of embarrassment about revealing a personal failure.

Late adolescence begins at age 17 or 18 and lasts through the early twenties. Generally, there is a well-established sexual identity and an ability to form and maintain mutually satisfying intimate relationships.

Assessment

The assessment of a young person's sexual behavior first involves the usual history gathering. Routine visits should include questions about sexual development and sexuality concerns. Particularly with adolescents, it is important to ensure accurate and appropriate levels of confidentiality. It is reasonable to promise that private information will not be shared with parents. However, confidentiality cannot be promised in situations where CPS must be notified. Knowledge and understanding about puberty and human reproduction should be assessed, and misinformation should be corrected. A child or adolescent should be asked if she has been touched in an uncomfortable manner or if anyone has ever attempted to force her to do anything sexual against her will (see Chapter 16).

"Am I normal?" is a question that is common to most adolescents, even if it is not readily verbalized to parents or health professionals. Reassurance is often greatly appreciated. Adolescents should be allowed to express any concerns about physical developmental changes, masturbation, dating behavior, sexual feelings, and pressures related to intimacy. Usual sources of sexuality information, the extent of communication about sexuality within the family, and opportunities for formal sexual education should be determined.

Questions about sexuality should be asked in an orientation-neutral manner, and they should be repeated if the patient is seen on an ongoing basis. Questions such as, "Have you ever dated anyone?", "Have you had sex with another person?", and "Are you are involved with males, females, or both?" indicate a willingness to discuss homosexual as well as heterosexual activity. Furthermore, the recognition that heterosexuality is not assumed can decrease the fear many gay and

PEARLS & PERILS

COMING OUT IN GAY AND LESBIAN YOUTH

- Coming out is a high risk process for gay and lesbian youth.
- They will likely be initially rejected by family and perhaps friends.
- Physical and verbal abuse are likely after disclosure.
- Teenagers may also be afraid to come out to a physician.
- Because of rejection, there is a high risk for substance abuse, running away, suicide, and homelessness.

PEARLS & PERILS

ASSESSMENT

- Appropriate levels of confidentiality should be ensured.
- Sexuality questions should be asked in an orientation-neutral manner.
- Both boys and girls should be asked about contraception and safer sex procedures.
- Collateral information should be obtained when assessing inappropriate sexual behavior.

lesbian adolescents feel about revealing their sexual orientation to a physician. Gay and lesbian adolescents are at a higher risk for poor developmental adjustment as they go through the process of coming out. Almost all gay and lesbian adolescents are at least initially spurned by their families when they disclose their sexual orientation. Many also lose friends and are the victims of verbal or physical abuse at the hands of their peers. There may be a decline in school performance. If these teenagers feel unsupported, they are ultimately at serious risk for substance abuse, running away, and suicide. Gay and lesbian youth are statistically overrepresented in the homeless population. It is suspected that up to 30% of teenagers who commit suicide are gay or lesbian.

Adolescents should be asked if they have ever had sexual intercourse. Those who have should be asked how often they have engaged in sexual activity. They should also be asked about the kinds of intimate sexual behaviors they have been involved in, possible exposures to infection, their knowledge and use of any preventive measures (both boys and girls), and a history of any health consequences such as infection, preg-

TABLE 19-1

ABNORMAL SEXUAL BEHAVIORS OF CHILDREN

Age	Concern necessary when children...	Mental health evaluation necessary when children...
Preschool or young school-age children	• Touch genitals in public after being told many times not to	• Touch self in public or private instead of other activities
	• Ask about genital differences or babies after all questions answered	• Play mommy or daddy with sadness, anger, or aggression; hate one sex
	• Touch genitals or breasts of (or ask to be touched by) unfamiliar adults	• Sneakily touch others or demand that others touch them
	• Stare at nude people after seeing many nude people	• Ask others to take off their clothes; try to undress others
	• Have continuous erections	• Have painful erections
	• Keep watching people in bathroom	• Won't give others privacy in bathroom
	• Want to be naked in public after parents say no	• Will not wear clothes; show self to others after being reprimanded
	• Use "dirty" words after parents say no	• Use dirty words after being reprimanded
	• Smear feces more than once on wall, floor, furniture	• Often play in or smear feces after being reprimanded
	• Play doctor after being told to stop	• Force others to play doctor
	• Put objects in rectum or genitals of self or others after being told no	• Cajole or force others to insert objects in rectum
	• Simulate sex with other children while clothed	• Simulate sex (without clothes) or engage in real intercourse; oral sex
Young school-age children	• Are fearful or anxious about sexual topics	• Ask constant questions about sex; know too much for age
	• Pretend to be having a baby for weeks or months (boys)	• Are fearful or angry about babies or intercourse
	• Play with feces or deliberately urinate outside of bowl	• Constantly play with feces or urinate on furniture
	• Get caught telling dirty jokes, making sexual sounds	• Tell dirty jokes when peers disapprove
	• Get in trouble for sex talk or think all relationships are romantic	• Talk about sex a lot; in constant trouble about sexual behavior
	• Get very upset if seen changing clothes	• Aggressively or tearfully demand privacy
	• Show fascination with nude pictures	• Masturbate to nude pictures or display them
	• Want to play sexual games with much younger or older children	• Force others to play sexual games
	• Draw genitalia only on one gender or out of proportion to body size	• Make genitalia most prominent features of artwork; draw intercourse or group sex
	• Want to be opposite sex	• Hate being own sex or hate own genitalia
	• French kiss, talk in sexual manner, are afraid of hugs or kisses from adults	• Are too familiar with strangers; sexual with unknown adults; anxious if in contact with adult stranger
	• Touch genitalia of animals	• Engage in sexual behavior with animals

(Adapted from Johnson, Assessment of sexual behavior problems in preschool-aged and latency aged children, *Child Adolesc Psychiatric Clin North Am* 2:431-449, 1993.)

nancy, genital injury, or abuse. Those who have had any health consequences should be asked about treatment, outcome, and their own as well as their parents' response to the problem. It is helpful to ensure that interviewing about sexuality be done privately, after some degree of rapport has been established. The adolescent and the interviewer should also understand each other's terminology, including street language and ethnocultural variations of definitions.

When there is concern about inappropriate sexual behavior with others, it is important to gather as much collateral information as possible. Information from the following list should be included:

- Number and types of sexual behaviors (past and current) (alone and others)
- History of sexual behavior problems
- Motivation for sexual behavior
- Other child's description, response to, and feelings about the activity
- Use of trickery, bribery, coercion, force
- Affect of the child regarding sexuality
- Full developmental history (history of abuse, placements outside the home, protective services involvement)
- All legal involvement, with records from court, probation officers, and other institutions or authorities
- Behavior in school or day care
- Psychiatric, legal, abuse, and substance abuse history of all family members
- Emotional and sexual climate in home

Normal behaviors in preschool and young school-age (under age 10) children were reviewed in Box 19-5. Table 19-1 reviews behaviors that may be grounds for concern or are definite indicators to seek the assistance of a mental health specialist.

An understanding of the household in which the child was raised helps provide insight into factors that contribute to a child's sexual behavior. The household emotional and sexual climate fits into a continuum of descriptors. In the *natural and healthy home,* the child is free to ask about sexuality. Parents and children touch each other in an appropriate and loving manner, with respect for physical and emotional space. In the *sexually neutral home,* there is no particular inclination or disinclination to discuss sexual topics. There is minimal physical expression of emotion. The *open or communal-living home* has a liberal attitude toward sex with free conversation; nudity may be common, and parents are open about their sexuality. In the *sexually repressed home,* sex is a forbidden subject and parents neither discuss it nor appear to engage in it. In *sex-is-dirty homes,* the mentioning of sex results in hostility; sex is for procreation, and any pleasure from it is bad. In the *home with overt values and covert norms,* sex is positive and used to revere God. However, there are covert extramarital affairs and abusive relationships that are never discussed. In the *home that is sexually overwhelming,* the parents are overtly sexual and share sexually explicit material with the children, whereas in *sexually and emotionally needy homes,* the needy adult may use the child as a substitute partner until another adult is available. Aggressive interactions may be common in this type of home. The next point on the continuum is the *home where sex is an exchange commodity,* in which sex is used to obtain money, drugs, or other items. Children may observe or be involved in these events. Physical agression is likely to occur in the home. The *sexually abusive home* has incest by one or both parents, and there may be aggression and substance abuse. Finally, the *multigenerational sexually abusive home* has sexual activity between many generations of the family. Power is abused routinely in these homes (Box 19-6).

BOX 19-6

HOME SEXUAL AND EMOTIONAL CLIMATE CONTINUUM

Natural and healthy
Sexually neutral
Open or communal
Sexually repressed
Sex is dirty
Overt values and covert norms
Sexually overwhelming
Sexually and emotionally needy
Sex is an exchange commodity
Sexually abusive
Multigenerational sexually abusive

Special Topics in Child and Adolescent Sexuality

Masturbation

Many older children and adolescents masturbate. Cultural and religious opposition to masturbation, coupled with remnants of the myths that masturbation may cause a variety of physical and mental disorders, may create significant feelings of guilt and fear. This safe, developmentally normal form of sexual expression

PEARLS & PERILS

MASTURBATION

- Masturbation is a safe, developmentally normal, and educational sexual activity.

may be rejected in favor of sexual intercourse, especially when surrounding adults are ambivalent of or intolerant about masturbation. Masturbation may help an adolescent learn about his own sexual responses and relieve sexual urges while postponing sexual intercourse.

An uncommon variant of masturbation is the sexual asphyxiation syndrome. This involves self-strangulation during autoerotic activity. The practice consists of arranging a belt or rope to compress the neck, viewing sexually explicit materials, and masturbating with the neck compressed to enhance orgasm. It often includes binding the extremities and wearing women's clothing. This practice can be fatal. The most common victims are adolescent males, possibly because of their ignorance or denial of the lethal potential. Those who survive usually describe themselves as heterosexual and deny depression or suicidal thinking. The behavior is private and is often repeated by those who avoid death. In time, it may involve a partner of the same sex and a shift to homosexual orientation.

Abnormal Sexual Behaviors

There are four groups of sexual behaviors in children and adolescents (Table 19-2). Group I children are involved in natural and healthy sexual exploration. Those in Group II are involved in sexually reactive behaviors, and Group III children are engaged in the full gamut of adult sexual behaviors. Group IV children are involved in sexually aggressive behaviors. Group I behaviors are described in the section on normal sexuality. Children may not be part of only a single group but move back and forth between groups in their behaviors.

Group II behaviors are generally seen in children who have a history of exposure to pornography, live in households with excessive sexual stimulation (including watching parents, older siblings, or too many soap operas), or are victims of sexual abuse. These children focus on sexuality to a degree that is out of proportion to the attention their peers give to the subject. They seem to have a compulsion to be engaged in sexual behaviors, either alone or with same age peers. They may not stop behaviors in the presence of an adult when asked. They do not force or coerce. These children may feel shame, guilt, or extreme anxiety about sex.

Group III children use sexual behavior to relate to their peers. Their behavior is more extensive than that of children in Group II. Preoccupied with sex, these children generally engage in sexual behaviors with same age peers and purposefully keep their activities secret from nearby adults. They may entice or persuade their peers to become involved in sexual behaviors. Their affect is matter of fact and without shame, guilt, or aggression. These children feel an inability to relate to adults, most likely because of a history of severe physical, emotional, and sexual abuse.

Group IV children and adolescents are sexual offenders. They are preoccupied with sex and coerce or aggressively force others of any age into sexual activity. Sexual behaviors may be impulsive and compulsive, increasing in severity over time. Additionally these children usually have numerous other behavior problems. It is rare that these individuals feel empathy for their victims. They often experience rage, loneliness, and fear; because of their life experiences, these emotions are associated with sex and aggression. Roughly 25% of these children and adolescents are girls. They will not stop their behaviors without specialized, intensive treatment, which is beyond the scope of this text. Without treatment, they are at great risk for continuing to develop as sexual perpetrators. The literature indicates that up to 80% of adult sexual offenders committed assaults during adolescence.

Of children who engage in abnormal sexual behaviors, Group II children come from sexually repressed

TABLE 19-2

TYPES OF ABNORMAL SEXUAL BEHAVIOR

Group	Behavior
Group I	
Natural and healthy sexual exploration	Consensual, between same age peers with lighthearted affect
Group II	
Sexually reactive behaviors	Compulsive behaviors accompanied by shame, guilt, or anxiety; may entice peer
Group III	
Mutual engagement in adult behaviors	May entice or persuade peer into activities; matter-of-fact affect
Group IV	
Sexually aggressive behaviors	Entice, coerce or force others of any age into activity; angry affect

PEARLS & PERILS

SEXUALLY AGGRESSIVE BEHAVIORS

- The majority of sex offenders committed assaults during adolescence.

homes or from homes further in the continuum. Some of these children may have been in open or communal living homes. Children in Group III are most likely from homes at or above the level of overt values and covert norms, whereas Group IV children come from homes at or above the sexually and emotionally needy level.

Gender Identity Disorder

In gender identity disorder (GID), the child has persistent discomfort and senses that the assigned sex is inappropriate. This is communicated through engagement in markedly cross-gender behaviors. Usually the behavior begins between the ages of 18 and 36 months, during the time in which the gender identity is solidified. Significant areas in assessing gender-appropriate behavior include the choice of toys, fantasy roles (Ken vs. Barbie), roles assumed in dress-up play, and gender of playmates. A high activity level and involvement in rough and tumble play are factors particularly associated with boys. A decrease in these behaviors is seen in boys with GID, and an increase is seen in girls with GID. In most instances, the child verbalizes or demonstrates a wish to be a member of the opposite gender; in a few cases, the child mistakenly believes that he is a member of the opposite sex (Box 19-7). A boy wishes for a disappearance of the penis, and a girl asserts that one will grow.

Boys are referred for treatment for GID more often than girls. This may be because more extreme cross-gender behavior is tolerated in girls before assistance

BOX 19-7 GENDER IDENTITY DISORDER

DSM-IV DIAGNOSTIC CRITERIA

A. A strong and persistent cross-gender identification (not merely a desire for any perceived cultural advantages of being the other sex).

In children, the disturbance is manifested by four (or more) of the following:

(1) repeatedly stated desire to be, or insistence that he or she is, the other sex
(2) in boys, preference for cross-dressing or simulating female attire; in girls, insistence on wearing only stereotypical masculine clothing
(3) strong and persistent preferences for cross-sex roles in make-believe play or persistent fantasies of being the other sex
(4) intense desire to participate in the stereotypical games and pastimes of the other sex
(5) strong preference for playmates of the other sex

In adolescents and adults, the disturbance is manifested by symptoms such as a stated desire to be the other sex, frequent passing as the other sex, desire to live or be treated as the other sex, or the conviction that he or she has the typical feelings and reactions of the other sex.

B. Persistent discomfort with his or her sex or sense of inappropriateness in the gender role of that sex.

In children, the disturbance is manifested by any of the following:in boys, assertion that his penis or testes are disgusting or will disappear or assertion that it would be better not to have a penis, or aversion toward rough-and-tumble play and rejection of male stereotypical toys, games, and activities; in girls, rejection of urinating in a sitting position, assertion that she has or will grow a penis, or assertion that she does not want to grow breasts or menstruate, or marked aversion toward normative feminine clothing.

In adolescents and adults, the disturbance is manifested by symptoms such as preoccupation with getting rid of primary and secondary sex characteristics (e.g., request for hormones, surgery, or other procedures to physically alter sexual characteristics to simulate the other sex) or belief that he or she was born the wrong sex.

C. The disturbance is not concurrent with a physical intersex condition.

D. The disturbance causes clinically significant distress or impairment in social, occupational, or other important areas of functioning.

Code based on current age:
Gender Identity Disorder in Children
Gender Identity Disorder in Adolescents and Adults
Specify if (for sexually mature individuals)
Sexually Attracted to Males
Sexually Attracted to Females
Sexually Attracted to Both
Sexually Attracted to Neither

(From American Psychiatric Association: *Diagnostic and statistical manual of mental disorders,* ed 4 [DSM-IV], Washington DC, 1994, American Psychiatric Press.)

is sought. More information is available about boys with GID. All children with GID do not verbalize a desire to change gender; older children and adolescents, because of their recognition of the stigma involved, are less likely to do so. These adolescents may express their dysphoria by idealizing the other gender or devaluing their own in conversation. Children with GID also have an increased incidence of other psychopathologic conditions; boys are generally found to have more internalizing problems on the Child Behavior Checklist (CBCL) (see Chapter 2).

The majority of adults with GID (formerly called adult transsexualism) recall cross-gender behaviors in childhood. However, adults who have this disorder are rare; therefore there is difficulty with accurate statistical interpretation of available information.

The cause of GID is unclear. Biologic and psychodynamic factors have been explored. There is some research in the area of prenatal effects of hormones; congenital adrenal hyperplasia is being studied in girls, and androgen-insensitivity is under investigation in boys. It has also been noted that some extremely feminine boys are quite attractive in a feminine manner and are often described as having the potential to "make a beautiful girl" by strangers. Parents may also subtly change the child's appearance to be consistent with the other gender, although studies find that parents do not do this because of an explicit wish for a child of a specific gender. There is likely to be a disturbed parent-child relationship in children with GID. The mothers and sons may be enmeshed, resulting in more expressed femininity in the son. With this model, the impairment in a mother-daughter relationship results in a disidentification, devaluation of femininity, and a commensurate overvaluation of masculinity. Alternately, if the mother is distant from the son, he may experience some separation anxiety and develop more feminine characteristics to engage the mother.

Treatment of GID in childhood and adolescence has several goals: the elimination of ostracism by peers, the treatment of any associated psychopathologic condition (depression, separation anxiety, difficulty with extreme emotions, and poor relationships with others), and the prevention of continued GID (transsexualism) in adulthood. There are also some physicians who treat GID in hopes of preventing homosexuality in adulthood. Gender identity conflict is most effectively addressed in childhood, and there is a poor prognosis after puberty. Behavioral therapists focus on correcting gender-specific behaviors, whereas psychodynamic therapists focus on psychopathologic states in the family as well as the child. Psychopathologic disruption in the family includes the ambivalence of the parents regarding their child's disorder and any covert support of the gender dysphoria. A combination of modalities is likely to be appropriate, although no empiric therapy outcome studies have been completed. Play therapy groups and individual therapy may help the child cope with trauma surrounding separation anxiety issues.

Paraphilias

A person who has a paraphilia is compulsively responsive to and obligatorily dependent on an unusual and personally or socially unacceptable stimulus. The stimulus may be perceived or it may be in the ideation and imagery of fantasy, but it is necessary for optimal initiation and maintenance of sexual arousal and for the facilitation or attainment of orgasm. Paraphilic imagery may occur in fantasy during masturbation or during intercourse with a partner. Although they are usually thought of as occurring in adulthood, the paraphilias have forerunners in childhood (as a protoparaphilia) and adolescence. Paraphilias are reported more often in males. Paraphilias generally become a focus for treatment when there are legal consequences for the behavior. There are over 40 paraphilias, but only a few come under the province of the judicial system. Studies of adults with paraphilias have shown that traumatic events with erotic implications occurred in the lives of these adults when they were about 8 years old.

The paraphilias include exhibitionism, fetishism, frotteurism, pedophilia, transvestic fetishism, voyeurism, sexual sadism, and sexual masochism. In exhibitionism, there is exposure of one's genitals to an unsuspecting stranger for sexual arousal (Box 19-8). Fetishism occurs when an animate or an inanimate object is required for sexual arousal (Box 19-9). Frotteurism involves touching or rubbing a nonconsenting person (Box 19-10), and pedophilia occurs when there is sexual arousal involving children (Box 19-11). In transvestic fettishism, a child has recurrent fantasies or persistently cross-dresses in order to achieve sexual excitation (Box 19-12). In voyeurism, an unsuspecting individual is observed while disrobing, naked, or engaging in sexual activity (Box 19-13). In sexual sadism and masochism, acts of causing or experiencing humiliation are found sexually stimulating (Boxes 19-14 and 19-15). The paraphilias are treated through the use of medroxyprogesterone acetate (Depo-Provera), which lowers circulating androgens. However, other psychotropic medications, including lithium, the antidepressants, and certain

PARAPHILIAS

- The paraphilias generally begin in adolescence, although precursors may be seen in childhood.

PEARLS & PERILS

BOX 19-8 EXHIBITIONISM

DSM-IV DIAGNOSTIC CRITERIA

A. Over a period of at least 6 months, recurrent, intense sexually arousing fantasies, sexual urges, or behaviors involving the exposure of one's genitals to an unsuspecting stranger.

B. The fantasies, sexual urges, or behaviors cause clinically significant distress or impairment in social, occupational, or other important areas of functioning.

(From American Psychiatric Association: *Diagnostic and statistical manual of mental disorders,* ed 4 [DSM-IV], Washington DC, 1994, American Psychiatric Press.)

BOX 19-9 FETISHISM

DSM-IV DIAGNOSTIC CRITERIA

A. Over a period of at least 6 months, recurrent, intense sexually arousing fantasies, sexual urges, or behaviors involving the use of nonliving objects (e.g., female undergarments)

B. The fantasies, sexual urges, or behaviors cause clinically significant distress or impairment in social, occupational, or other important areas of functioning.

C. The fetish objects are not limited to articles of female clothing used in cross-dressing (as in Transvestic Fetishism) or devices designed for the purpose of tactile genital stimulation (e.g., a vibrator).

(From American Psychiatric Association: *Diagnostic and statistical manual of mental disorders,* ed 4 [DSM-IV], Washington DC, 1994, American Psychiatric Press.)

BOX 19-10 FROTTEURISM

DSM-IV DIAGNOSTIC CRITERIA

A. Over a period of at least 6 months, recurrent, intense sexually arousing fantasies, sexual urges, or behaviors involving touching and rubbing against a nonconsenting person.

B. The fantasies, sexual urges, or behaviors cause clinically significant distress or impairment in social, occupational, or other important areas of functioning.

(From American Psychiatric Association: *Diagnostic and statistical manual of mental disorders,* ed 4 [DSM-IV], Washington DC, American Psychiatric Press.)

antipsychotics (clozapine and thioridazine) have been found helpful. All medications are used in conjunction with psychotherapy, including CBT.

Chronic Illness

Chronic illness can affect sexual development in several ways. The child's caregivers may inhibit the child's attempt at separation and individuation. Sexual development can be hampered by delays in psychosocial development. Societal responses to an adolescent with physical disabilities may mark the child as asexual. The adolescent who is restricted by chronic illness, disability, or hospitalization may use sexually provocative language or behavior to reassure herself and others that she is a normal teenager. The child may be excluded from peer interactions concerning sexuality. Children and concerned family members may be overly concerned about the child's fragility caused by medical or mental illnesses. The physician can assist children and their families by addressing this developmental issue along with concerns about management of the illness.

PEARLS & PERILS

CHRONIC ILLNESS

- Society may view the chronically ill child or adolescent as asexual.
- The adolescent may combat society's response to chronic illness with provocative sexual behavior.

BOX 19-11 PEDOPHILIA

DSM-IV DIAGNOSTIC CRITERIA

A. Over a period of at least 6 months, recurrent, intense sexually arousing fantasies, sexual urges, or behaviors involving sexual activity with a prepubescent child or children (generally age 13 years or younger).

B. The fantasies, sexual urges, or behaviors cause clinically significant distress or impairment in social, occupational, or other important areas of functioning.

C. The person is at least age 16 years and at least 5 years older than the child or children in Criterion A.

Note: Do not include an individual in late adolescence involved in an ongoing sexual relationship with a 12-or 13-year old.

Specify if:
Sexually Attracted to Males
Sexually Attracted to Females
Sexually Attracted to Both

Specify if:
Limited to Incest
Specify type:
Exclusive Type (attracted only to children)
Nonexclusive Type

(From American Psychiatric Association: *Diagnostic and statistical manual of mental disorders,* ed 4 [DSM-IV], Washington DC, 1994, American Psychiatric Press.)

BOX 19-12 TRANSVESTIC FETISHISM

DSM-IV DIAGNOSTIC CRITERIA

A. Over a period of at least 6 months, in a heterosexual male, recurrent, intense sexually arousing fantasies, sexual urges, or behaviors involving cross dressing.

B. The fantasies, sexual urges, or behaviors cause clinically significant distress or impairment in social, occupational, or other important areas of functioning.

Specify if:
With Gender Dysphoria; if the person has persistent discomfort with gender role or identity.

(From American Psychiatric Association: *Diagnostic and statistical manual of mental disorders,* ed 4 [DSM-IV], Washington DC, 1994, American Psychiatric Press.)

BOX 19-13 VOYEURISM

DSM-IV DIAGNOSTIC CRITERIA

A. Over a period of at least 6 months, recurrent, intense sexually arousing fantasies, sexual urges, or behaviors involving the act of observing an unsuspecting person who is naked, in the process of disrobing, or engaging in sexual activity.

B. The fantasies, sexual urges, or behaviors cause clinically significant distress or impairment in social, occupational, or other important areas of functioning.

(From American Psychiatric Association: *Diagnostic and statistical manual of mental disorders,* ed 4 [DSM-IV], Washington DC, 1994, American Psychiatric Press.)

BOX 19-14 SEXUAL SADISM

DSM-IV DIAGNOSTIC CRITERIA

A. Over a period of at least 6 months, recurrent, intense sexually arousing fantasies, sexual urges, or behaviors involving acts (real, not simulated) in which the psychological or physical suffering (including humiliation) of the victim is sexually exciting to the person.

B. The fantasies, sexual urges, or behaviors cause clinically significant distress or impairment in social, occupational, or other important areas of functioning.

(From American Psychiatric Association: *Diagnostic and statistical manual of mental disorders,* ed 4 [DSM-IV], Washington DC, 1994, American Psychiatric Press.)

BOX 19-15 SEXUAL MASOCHISM

DSM-IV DIAGNOSTIC CRITERIA

A. Over a period of at least 6 months, recurrent, intense sexually arousing fantasies, sexual urges, or behaviors involving the act (real, not simulated) of being humiliated, beaten, bound, or otherwise made to suffer.

B. The fantasies, sexual urges, or behaviors cause clinically significant distress or impairment in social, occupational, or other important areas of functioning.

(From American Psychiatric Association: *Diagnostic and statistical manual of mental disorders,* ed 4 [DSM-IV], Washington DC, 1994, American Psychiatric Press.)

Sexually Transmitted Diseases

Each year, 25% of sexually active teenagers contract a sexually transmitted disease. However, such diseases are underreported and underdiagnosed. Untreated gonorrhea or *Chlamydia* may lead to pelvic inflammatory disease, which is related to infertility or ectopic pregnancy. After one episode of unprotected sex with an infected partner, there is a 1% chance of acquiring HIV and a 30% or 50% chance of contracting genital herpes or gonorrhea. Adolescents who perceive themselves as invulnerable are less likely to use preventive methods when engaging in sexual behaviors. They are more likely to be frightened and deny symptoms of infection, delaying the receipt of effective treatment. Similarly, teenagers are likely to be embarrassed when they realize they have contracted an infection and may not follow through effectively on recommended treatment. Most adolescents benefit from repeated verbal education during follow-up visits. Subsequent visits should include observation of adverse effects on self-esteem, emotional adjustment, and interpersonal relationships with peers and family.

According to the results of the National Youth Risk Behavior Survey, high-risk sexual behaviors reported by high school students coincide with reports of alcohol, marijuana, cocaine, and other illicit drug use. Adolescents who do not engage in substance use are least likely to report having sexual intercourse. Other studies link a risk for sexually transmitted disease to substance abuse and use. D'Angelo studied HIV prevalence rates in adolescents across several populations. The HIV rate is highest in adolescents from cities in which AIDS is endemic who engage in high-risk sex and abuse illicit substances or alcohol. Education about abstinence, incorporation of safe sex practices, and education about sexually transmitted diseases must be included in adolescent assessments for medical or mental health visits.

SEXUALLY TRANSMITTED DISEASES AND PREGNANCY

PEARLS & PERILS

- The adolescent who feels invulnerable is less likely to take appropriate precautions.
- Those involved in substance use are more likely to engage in intercourse and contract sexually transmitted diseases or get pregnant.
- Education of the adolescent is key.

Adolescents who have HIV are permanently required to counter the developmental norm to prevent spreading the disease. Furthermore, the usually invulnerable teenager must confront impending mortality.

Pregnancy

The same sense of invulnerability that results in sexually transmitted diseases results in pregnancy, which is a significant public health issue for adolescents. Adolescents fail to use birth control for a number of reasons. Girls forgo birth control to add to the heightened sense of sexual intercourse as a spontaneous expression of romantic love. Boys tend to view birth control as a female concern. Some adolescents are ignorant about reproduction. Many teenage girls do not seriously consider the possibility of becoming pregnant until they experience a "scare" or actually become pregnant. Subconsciously, many teenagers think that pregnancy can't happen to them, at least not when they first become sexually active.

Pregnancy prevention is an appropriate preventive medical task. The consequences of early childbearing should be stressed. If the patient knows a friend who has had a baby, the physician may ask how the friend spends her time since giving birth, whether she still goes to school, if she still has time for extracurricular activities, and whether she still has time to socialize with her friends. Such questions may help the patient appreciate the potential impact of pregnancy on her life. Asking the patient about her plans for the next 5 years and how they might be affected if she has a baby may also help her plan more effectively.

For some adolescents, pregnancy provides access to instant adulthood. Pregnant teens have reported that pregnancy gives them someone to love. A girl is at particular risk for pregnancy if she does not have much academical or social success; she may see a pregnancy as a potential bright spot in an otherwise difficult life. Other risk factors include the following:

- A family history of early, unwed pregnancy
- The experience of early losses through divorce or death and a subsequent search for replacement of broken relationships
- Feelings of being unloved
- Abuse of drugs or alcohol, which decreases the likelihood of using contraception
- A life of poverty in an unstable family

The younger the patient, the more emotional her reaction to the pregnancy is likely to be. She needs a chance to express her feelings. She can be expected to progress though a cycle of reactions, including shock, denial, and anger, before arriving at acceptance. Immediate attention to the pregnancy must be encouraged, since adolescents typically receive less prenatal care and place their infants at risk for prematurity. The vast majority of teenagers who decide to have their babies keep them rather than surrender them to adoption or foster care. The physician can help the patient think realistically about how she will accomplish this goal. The patient should be encouraged to consider how she will continue her education, both before and after the baby is born. Some larger communities have special school programs for pregnant teenagers and their partners that offer health care, nutrition programs, job preparation, parenting education, daycare after the baby arrives, and follow-up information about contraception. It is recommended that physicians who work with adolescents develop a network of resources, including clinics, educational programs, and early parenting programs.

PEARLS & PERILS

RISK FACTORS FOR TEENAGE PREGNANCY

- The girl does not appreciate any "bright spots" in her life.
- There is a family history of early, unwed pregnancy.
- The girl has experienced early losses through divorce or death.
- The girl feels unloved.
- The girl abuses drugs or alcohol.
- The girl lives a life of poverty in an unstable family.

Prevention

Reproductive health care for adolescents is best served by the prevention of biopsychosocial consequences. Many adults believe that adolescents should refrain from sexual intercourse until marriage or until they have a mature committed relationship in which both partners are able and willing to take responsibility for any consequences. Many professionals believe that sexual intercourse should be postponed at least until the reproductive system is fully mature (late teens) and until there is sufficient psychosocial maturity for responsible behavior. It may be unrealistic to expect adolescents to abstain from all physical expressions of sexuality, especially if marriage is unlikely until the mid-to late-twenties.

Adolescents must be well informed about the risks of all forms of sexual intimacy, and they must be provided with the knowledge and methods for prevention of infection and pregnancy. They should be instructed about "safer sex," which may require a description or at least mention of practices that increase the risk of serious infections or injuries (such as anal intercourse). Sexually active teenagers, even those who consistently use barrier methods of contraception and have a single partner, should be screened yearly for infections. More frequent screening should be considered for high-risk adolescents such as gay and lesbian youth, runaways, drug abusers, and delinquents.

Sex education or family-life education does not guarantee prevention of consequences, will not ensure abstinence, and has not been shown to increase sexual experimentation. Family-life education of children and adolescents is a responsibility shared by parents, schools, health professionals, and other adults who provide services to youth. All contribute positively or negatively to each young person's understanding about and attitude toward human sexuality. Parents and other family members begin this process at childbirth and provide the primary influence in the development of personal values and beliefs. Society's unresolved debate about the content and timing of sexuality education and parental reluctance to discuss sexuality topics often leave youth uninformed or misinformed. Incomplete or inaccurate sexual information tends to be derived from friends, the media, and available written materials that range from dictionaries to sex-oriented adult magazines.

As children reach adolescence, the normal distancing from parents may interfere with open communication and effective education, even in the most enlightened and comfortable families. Health professionals can be important allies of parents and schools in providing scientific information and the latest technical advances, in supporting developmentally appropriate communication within families, and in helping the community accept the importance of lifelong comprehensive family-life education for all families. Professionals can assist individual parents in educating their children and themselves, and they can help and promote family-life education curricula and opportunities in schools, churches, and other community settings.

Summary

Children and adolescents are sexual beings. Providing good comprehensive health care requires that this aspect of child development is incorporated into any assessment of child and family health. Sensitivity to cultural and ethnic minority variances of development is essential. Competence in providing health care to children and adolescents includes having an understanding of normal development in heterosexual and homosexual children. Sexuality is an important aspect of human development, and additional research in the area of normative development is needed to assist children, families, and society in gaining an appreciation of comprehensive health.

CONSIDER CONSULTATION WHEN . . .

- There are sexually aggressive behaviors or behaviors that violate the rights of others
- A sexual behavior prevents normal, age-appropriate interactions with others
- You feel uncomfortable with the clinical presentation
- There are self-injurious behaviors

Annotated Bibliography

Stein TS, editor: *Changing perspectives of homosexuality.* In Odham J, Riba M, editors: *American psychiatric association annual review of psychiatry,* Washington DC, 1993, American Psychiatric Press.

The five chapters in this section provide a complete review of the current literature on gays and lesbians, including biologic theories of etiology, identity development, and the coming-out process.

Troiden RR: The formation of homosexual identities, *J Homosex* 17:43-73, 1989.

This classic article gives a solid understanding of the developmental processes a gay or lesbian adolescent undergoes in the task of identity synthesis.

Yates, Alayne, editor: *Child and adolescent psychiatric clinics of north america, issue on sexual and gender identity disorders,* July 1993.

This is a comprehensive review of normal and pathological topics in the sexualtiy of children and adolescents.

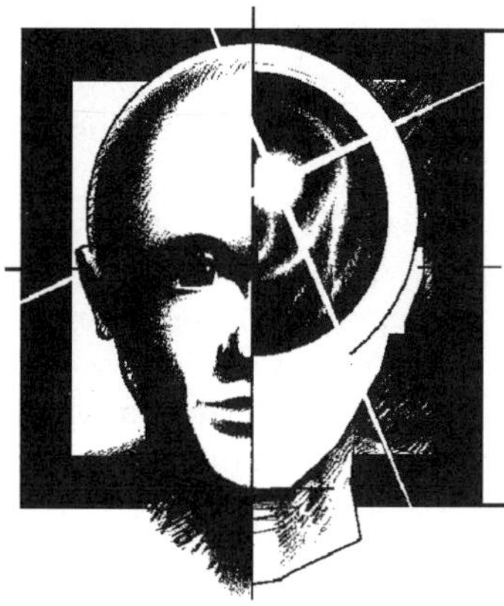

chapter 20

Common Behavioral Problems and Reactions to Stress

Katherine Grimes, MD

Stress
Elimination Disorders
Habits
Separation and Grief
Nightmares, Imaginary Friends, and Magic
Witness to Trauma
Summary

Although many of the problems described in this text could be treated by a child psychiatrist, that is not always possible. Psychiatry is often a scarce resource in rural areas, and a child psychiatrist may be even harder to find. Additionally cultural, linguistic, and financial barriers often exist even if child psychiatry is geographically available. Furthermore, parents commonly view the presence of psychiatric problems with shame and embarrassment. This makes disclosing them difficult. However, in a relationship where the parent is already comfortable, such as with the child's primary care physician or with the parent's own therapist, she is more likely to share her concerns.

Unfortunately, if a physician does not respond to the parent's attempts to obtain guidance about a child with sensitivity, the parent may not try again or delay seeking help, to the child's detriment. Therefore physicians should be prepared to address common questions about child development (including social and emotional development, intellectual growth, motor milestones, and self-care) that may lead to case identification and referral.

Some deviations from expected behavior are transient and therefore not clinically significant, such as a toddler's avoidance of balloons after one bursts in his face. Others, such as temper tantrums, are already managed routinely in primary care settings. Parents are often only seeking a sympathetic ear and some reassurance. However, it is prudent not to be too dismissive of the parent's complaint, remembering that it may be only a piece of a larger problem. It is also helpful to offer a follow-up consultation after a reasonable period.

Not only does this convey the physician's willingness to listen, but it also gives a standard against which to measure the significance of the behavior. Generally if the symptoms persist, they warrant further evaluation.

Nonspecialists commonly express apprehension about managing children's mental health issues. They are appropriately cognizant of the fact that children are different (if they are physicians for adults) or that emotional problems can be less straightforward than physical ones (if they are pediatric physicians). However, there are compelling reasons to take at least some initial steps when presented with direct evidence of, or queries regarding, children under stress. The first reason is that the physician's involvement may be the child's only chance. An abused 2-year-old boy who just happens to be brought along to his mother's emergency room visit for pneumonia may not have another opportunity for a responsible adult to intervene on his behalf. Those who know children who have died from neglect or abuse often report assuming that someone else must also have known of the situation and would do something about it. Such physicians do not think they are the right people or the best people to confront the parent or to contact social services. They fail to realize that they may be the only obstacles between the child and further harm.

A physician's intervention is of relevance even in a non–life-threatening situation. The mother who consults a physician for fatigue, which she attributes to the sleep disturbance her 4-year-old daughter is experiencing (or who brings the girl to the family practitioner for advice about bedtime rules), may mention that the girl is often up late with her father. However, unless there is a follow-up inquiry, she will not reveal that the father is taking his daughter with him to bars at night. If the physician does not explore the explanations for the woman's fatigue and the daughter's sleep disturbance, the mother may conclude that the father's behavior is acceptable. She may even say, "I told the doctor and she didn't seem concerned."

One reason for alertness on the part of the physician who is not a child psychiatrist is that some serious situations cannot be deferred until greater expertise is available. Another reason for vigilance is that insufficient response to a concern may be misheard as approval of the behavior and result in delayed treatment and greater morbidity. Still another reason for primary care physicians to participate in case-identification discussions with parents is that even if appropriate referrals are made and subspecialists are available, some families do not agree to go. Therefore the only person in a position to help is the physician who is already trusted. In this situation, it may take weeks or months of contending with major symptoms for the provider to persuade the family to participate in mental health treatment for the child. During this time, the primary care physician or the adult psychiatrist should consult often with the child mental health expert to get help with treatment suggestions and guidelines about levels of care. The eventual goal in these cases, if the problems persist or worsen, is to support the family's ability to accept the referral to an expert. A strategy that can be useful in such instances is to invite the consultant to join the physician in a scheduled visit, thus emphasizing the collaboration and lending the safety of the first relationship, by extension, to the new relationship.

If the referring physician truly recognizes and effectively communicates the value of the consultation, compliance will be greater. Patients often feel rejected when a physician sends them to a children's mental health expert. The family who is informed that a pediatric gastroenterology referral is necessary feels the primary care physician's concern and involvement; it is clear that the consultant will be communicating back to the family physician, to whom the case obviously belongs. The primary care physician knows what the consultation will offer and expects to continue with the case. Families rarely refuse this type of referral. However, when a primary care physician refers a family to a children's mental health specialist, it can sound like the physician is giving up, terminating the relationship, and transferring the case. Furthermore, physicians are sometimes poorly able to communicate the reason for the referral or what the patient can expect. It is no wonder that these referrals are met with less compliance. Therefore it is important (in areas where subspecialty expertise is available) that a good working relationship exist between different types of clinicians to demystify the clinical content and allow for easy communication about cases.

Finally there are settings where specialty referral is not possible. Physicians who feel they are being asked to manage clinical areas that lie beyond their training should first recognize that any effort to modulate the intensity of parent-child distress is probably beneficial and increases the chance for greater objectivity from the involved parties. The physician should also be sure to seek peer supervision if there is no specialist available. Strategic errors can often be picked up early by listeners outside of the direct encounter. Finally, a wealth of information is now available even in the most unpopulated areas through books, journals, and E-mail.

Stress

Opportunities and adverse events of daily life occur for children within the context of development. A visit to the zoo or a parent's weekend away on business has a quite different significance for a 3-month-old child, compared with that for a 3-year-old child, and still a different significance for a 10-year-old child. Additionally, a child's temperament and the capacity of the family (that is, physical and emotional health combined with intellectual, financial, and social resources) are important variables in the type of response the child has. Therefore the assessment of the historical or prospective impact of a stressor on a child must include the objective dimensions of the stressor, the child's developmental level, and the intrinsic and environmental supports available to the child.

It is worth noting that the repertoire of available mechanisms to respond to stress is also determined by developmental level. (An infant being bathed and an infant being abused may both cry.) It is important not to underrespond or make assumptions about the cause of a child's behavioral symptom, since there are limited ways for children to let adults know something is wrong. Careful history-taking from the parents (and child, when age permits) is critical to evaluate all the possible sources of stress contributing to a child's behavior. Parents often confuse what is stressful for them with what is stressful for the child. This may be the case, or it may be that the child is most burdened by something the parents are unaware of or would have thought insignificant.

Elimination Disorders

Enuresis

One of the most common behavioral complaints of parents to pediatricians is bed wetting (Box 20-1). The first question that must be asked is the age of the child; inexperienced or unrealistic parents may be expecting too much from a 2½-year-old or 4-year-old child. Nighttime enuresis is quite common until age 6 or 7, particularly for boys. Nocturnal enuresis can be normal and continue, with decreasing frequency, into adolescence, especially where there is a positive family history. Daytime accidents in new settings or during times of great excitement are also not uncommon in young children. Most children learn they can defer the need to go to the bathroom and then have at least some occasion

PEARLS & PERILS

STRESSOR SCALE

- Mild stressors are disruptive but not disabling (for example, a change of school or the birth of a sibling).
- Moderate stressors are somewhat disabling (for example, a parental divorce or a chronic illness).
- Severe stressors are significantly disabling (for example, sexual abuse, or the death of parent).

PEARLS & PERILS

ENURESIS

- Bed-wetting up to age 14 as a transient response to a major life event (new baby, move) can be normal.
- Day-time wetting is likely to be either organic or related to more serious emotional conditions.
- Enuresis may be the only symptom of sexual abuse.

DSM-IV DIAGNOSTIC CRITERIA

BOX 20-1 **ENURESIS**

A. Repeated voiding of urine into bed or clothes whether involuntary or intentional).

B. The behavior is clinically significant as manifested by either a frequency of twice a week for at least 3 consecutive months or the presence of clinically significant distress or impairment in social, academic (occupational), or other important areas of functioning.

C. Chronological age is at least 5 years (or equivalent developmental level).

D. The behavior is not due exclusively to the direct physiological effect of a substance (e.g., a diuretic) or a general medical condition (e.g., diabetes, spina bifida, a seizure disorder).

Specify type:
Nocturnal Only
Diurnal Only
Nocturnal and Diurnal

(From American Psychiatric Association: *Diagnostic and statistical manual of mental disorders,* ed 4 [DSM-IV], Washington DC, 1994, American Psychiatric Press.)

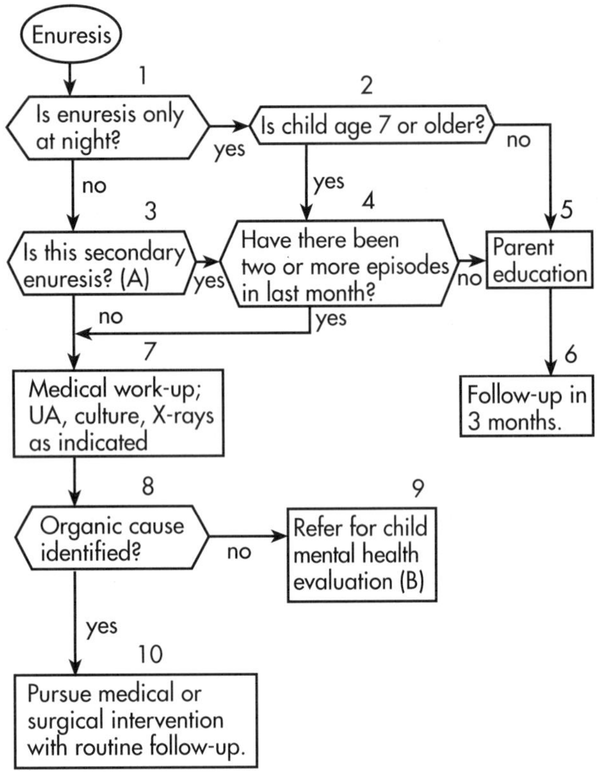

FIGURE 20-1 Decision points in the treatment of enuresis. *A* and *B* correspond to notes in Box 20-2.

> **BOX 20-2**
>
> **ENURESIS**
>
> **notes to figure 20-1**
>
> (A) Secondary enuresis is when loss of bladder control occurs after the child has been successfully toilet trained for more than three months.
>
> (B) Child psychiatric evaluation should include assessment for recent or past trauma, including sexual abuse.

when they defer too long. Therefore the response to the problem in the preschool years should be parent education. The algorithm in Figure 20-1 and the notes in Box 20-2 outline key decision points to consider in the treatment of enuresis.

Encopresis

Encopresis is culturally more offensive than enuresis and is usually of greater concern to parents and teachers. It may be associated with serious psychiatric conditions. Unfortunately, because of embarrassment some patients and families "forget" to report this symptom and clinicians rarely ask about it.

Important elements for the treatment of encopresis are highlighted in the algorithm shown in Figure 20-2 and Box 20-3. It is most common to encounter true encopresis in children between the ages of 7 and 12, and it occurs in boys more often than girls (Box 20-4). As with enuresis, it is important to clarify parental understanding at the beginning. Staining of underwear, even in grade-school children, that results from haste and poor hygiene is not encopresis and usually responds to instruction and support. True encopresis is significant both as a marker for emotional disturbance and for potential medical complications.

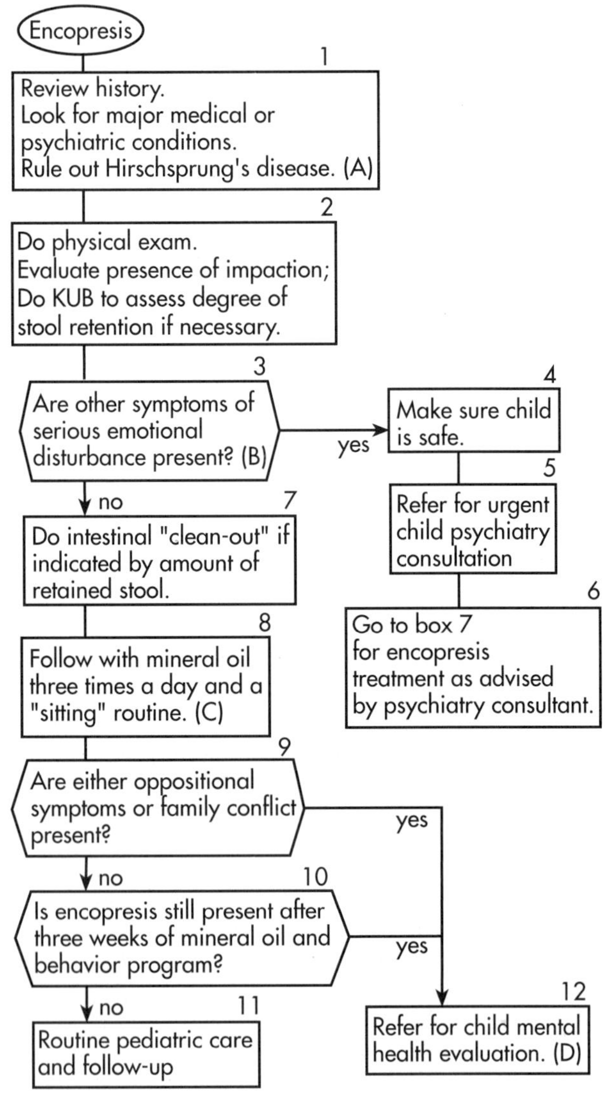

FIGURE 20-2 Decision points in the treatment of encopresis. *A, B, C,* and *D* correspond to notes in Box 20-4.

BOX 20-3

ENCOPRESIS

notes to figure 20-2

(A) Refer to Fleischer DR: Diagnosis and treatment of disorders of defecation in children, *Pediatric Gastroenterology: Pediatric Annals* Nov. 1976.

(B) It is important to look for violent conduct disorder (CD) suicidal or homicidal ideation, abuse, fire setting, and psychosis.

(C) "Sitting" is a common successful corrective intervention to teach the child to notice and respond to the urge to defecate. It will not be successful if the bowel is still distended by stool. After clean-out, a structured 5 to 10 minutes on the toilet after each meal usually begins to produce results within 10 days. The child is to be commended for complying with the sitting and not only if stool is passed.

(D) The physician should review the way family handles expressions of anger or aggression at home. Issues of control (and sometimes abuse) are often present and respond best to family therapy. Encopresis may be the only symptom of sexual abuse, particularly in cases of anal penetration.

PEARLS & PERILS

ENCOPRESIS

- It is important to always look for issues of control between parent and child.
- Encopresis suggests over- or undermodulation of aggression in the family.
- Sexual abuse and suicidal or homicidal ideation should be ruled out.

Habits

Thumbsucking, rocking, nailbiting, blinking, and stuttering are some of the common tension release mechanisms of the young latency-age child. Although thumbsucking or rocking may taper off earlier, 7- and 8-year-old children are particularly prone to what might otherwise be viewed as tic disorders (Boxes 20-5, 20-6, 20-7, and 20-8). Healthy, normal children in ordinary situations may demonstrate these habits as they struggle internally with large new issues such as power within a peer group or autonomy from parents. Mostly, these symptoms resolve themselves quickly if they are given little or no notice by others. Factors to consider when evaluating the need for a child to have a mental health evaluation include the degree to which the symptom pervades or dominates the child's life (preventing normal interactions with others), the extremity of the onset (from nothing to intense thumbsucking after a visit with a parent living outside the home), and the persistence of the symptom over time. A subsequent neurologic evaluation might be requested by the child psychiatrist if the habits are truly more like tics or are linked with other symptoms suggestive of a seizure disorder or a pervasive developmental disorder (PDD). The parent's role is to avoid criticizing or correcting the child (which usually worsens the problem), to protect the child from teasing by siblings, to make sure the child gets enough rest and is not overstimulated, and to be available to talk over any issues that might be bothering the child.

PEARLS & PERILS

HABITS

- The pervasiveness (intrusiveness) of a habit is a clue to a child's overall level of adjustment.
- The persistence of a habit may indicate an unaddressed problem (such as excess anxiety).
- Suddenness of onset may be caused by trauma.

DSM-IV DIAGNOSTIC CRITERIA

BOX 20-4 **ENCOPRESIS**

A. Repeated passage of feces into inappropriate places (e.g., clothing or floor) whether involuntary or intentional.

B. At least one such event a month for at least 3 months.

C. Chronological age is at least 4 years (or equivalent developmental level).

D. The behavior is not due exclusively to the direct physiological effects of a substance (e.g., laxatives) or a general medical condition except through a mechanism involving constipation.

Code as follows:
With Constipation and Overflow Incontinence
Without Constipation and Overflow Incontinence

(From American Psychiatric Association: *Diagnostic and statistical manual of mental disorders,* ed 4 [DSM-IV], Washington DC, 1994, American Psychiatric Press.)

BOX 20-5 TOURETTE'S DISORDER

A. Both multiple motor and one or more vocal tics have been present at some time during the illness, although not necessarily concurrently. (A *tic* is a sudden, rapid, recurrent, nonrhythmic, stereotyped motor movement or vocalization.)

B. The tics occur many times a day (usually in bouts) nearly every day or intermittently throughout a period of more than 1 year, and during this period there was never a tic-free period of more than 3 consecutive months.

C. The disturbance causes marked distress or significant impairment in social, occupational, or other important areas of functioning.

D. The onset is before age 18 years.

E. The disturbance is not due to the direct physiological effects of a substance (e.g., stimulants) or a general medical condition (e.g., Huntington's disease or post-viral encephalitis).

DSM-IV DIAGNOSTIC CRITERIA

(From American Psychiatric Association: *Diagnostic and statistical manual of mental disorders,* ed 4 [DSM-IV], Washington DC, 1994, American Psychiatric Press.)

BOX 20-6 CHRONIC MOTOR OR VOCAL TIC DISORDER

A. Single or multiple motor or vocal tics (i.e., sudden, rapid, recurrent, nonrhythmic, stereotyped motor movements or vocalizations), but not both, have been present at some time during the illness.

B. The tics occur many times a day nearly every day or intermittently throughout a period of more than 1 year, and during this period there was never a tic-free period of more than 3 consecutive months.

C. The disturbance causes marked distress or significant impairment in social, occupational, or other important areas of functioning.

D. The onset is before age 18 years.

E. The disturbance is not due to the direct physiological effects of a substance (e.g., stimulants) or a general medical condition (e.g., Huntington's disease or postviral encephalitis).

F. Criteria have never been met for Tourette's Disorder.

DSM-IV DIAGNOSTIC CRITERIA

(From American Psychiatric Association: *Diagnostic and statistical manual of mental disorders,* ed 4 [DSM-IV], Washington DC, 1994, American Psychiatric Press.)

BOX 20-7 TRANSIENT TIC DISORDER

A. Single or multiple motor and/or vocal tics (i.e., sudden, rapid, recurrent, nonrhythmic, stereotyped motor movements or vocalizations).

B. The tics occur many times a day, nearly every day for at least 4 weeks, but for no longer than 12 consecutive months.

C. The disturbance causes marked distress or significant impairment in social, occupational, or other important areas of functioning.

D. The onset is before age 18 years.

E. The disturbance is not due to the direct physiological effects of a substance (e.g., stimulants) or a general medical condition (e.g., Huntington's disease or postviral encephalitis).

F. Criteria have never been met for Tourette's Disorder or Chronic Motor or Vocal Tic Disorder.

Specify if:
Single Episode or **Recurrent**

DSM-IV DIAGNOSTIC CRITERIA

(From American Psychiatric Association: *Diagnostic and statistical manual of mental disorders,* ed 4 [DSM-IV], Washington DC, 1994, American Psychiatric Press.)

BOX 20-8

TIC DISORDER NOT OTHERWISE SPECIFIED

This category is for disorders characterized by tics that do not meet criteria for a specific Tic Disorder. Examples include tics lasting less than 4 weeks or tics with an onset after age 18 years.

(From American Psychiatric Association: *Diagnostic and statistical manual of mental disorders,* ed 4 [DSM-IV], Washington DC, 1994, American Psychiatric Press.)

Separation and Grief

Children's experiences of separation and loss may be as mild as a friend moving away or as extreme as the death of a parent. In fact, for children under age 7, the most salient aspect of mortality is separation. Despite sincere efforts by adults to explain death and dying, the bright 5-year-old child may still ask, "Why doesn't Mommy need her pocketbook?" months after her mother has died.

Parents often seek advice after the death of a pet, when a grandparent is dying, or as they face the prospect of divorce. It is helpful to remember that the most important feature for a child experiencing a loss is the reaction of the significant adults around her. If the child's loss is also a loss for the parents, this can be difficult. Physicians must first offer support and reassurance to the adult; the adult will then be able to give more support to the child. If the child feels that the parent is not able to endure the loss, the child's sense of loss is exponential (the original loss is multiplied by the withdrawal of the protective, nurturing function of the parent). The best intervention for the child may be psychiatric referral of the parents for help handling their own grief or depression.

Loss is also cumulative; if the cat and the grand-

BOX 20-9 **SEPARATION ANXIETY DISORDER**

DSM-IV DIAGNOSTIC CRITERIA

A. Developmentally inappropriate and excessive anxiety concerning separation from home or from those to whom the individual is attached, as evidenced by three (or more) of the following:

(1) recurrent excessive distress when separation from home or major attachment figures occurs or is anticipated
(2) persistent and excessive worry about losing, or about possible harm befalling, major attachment figures
(3) persistent and excessive worry that an untoward event will lead to separation from a major attachment figures (e.g., getting lost or being kidnapped)
(4) persistent reluctance or refusal to go to school or elsewhere because of fear of separation
(5) persistently and excessively fearful or reluctant to be alone or without major attachment figures at home or without significant adults in other settings
(6) persistent reluctance or refusal to go to sleep without being near a major attachment figure or to sleep away from home
(7) repeated nightmares involving the theme of separation
(8) repeated complaints of physical symptoms (such as headaches, stomachaches, nausea, or vomiting) when separation from major attachment figures occurs or is anticipated

B. The duration of the disturbance is at least 4 weeks.

C. The onset is before age 18 years.

D. The disturbance causes clinically significant distress or impairment in social, academic (occupational), or other important areas of functioning.

E. The disturbance does not occur exclusively during the course of a Pervasive Developmental Disorder, Schizophrenia, or other Psychotic Disorder and, in adolescents and adults, is not better accounted for by Panic Disorder With Agoraphobia.

Specify if:
Early Onset: if onset occurs before age 6 years

(From American Psychiatric Association: *Diagnostic and statistical manual of mental disorders,* ed 4 [DSM-IV], Washington DC, 1994, American Psychiatric Press.)

mother die within a brief span of time, the child's response to the illness of a teacher will be amplified. Parents should not be surprised at the child's increased need for care, trouble sleeping, or regression from previously acquired skills (Box 20-9).

Parallel to the child's need to know from her parent that grief caused by separation can be supported and falls within the boundaries of normal existence is the parents' need for reassurance from the physician that their child's response is normal. A parent who is experiencing grief (over the end of a marriage, a move to a new community, or the death of a family member) often feels helpless and guilty. It is easy for these feelings to fuel parental anxiety over whether his child has also been damaged (a double loss for the parent).

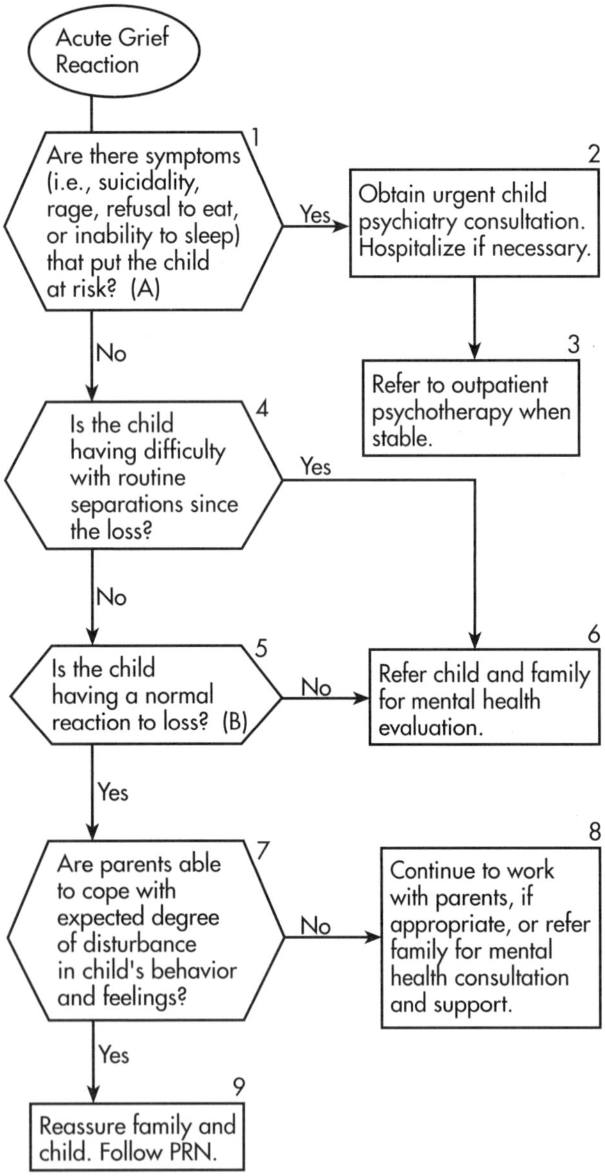

FIGURE 20-3 Decision points in the treatment of symptoms caused by separation. *A* and *B* correspond to notes in Box 20-10.

BOX 20-10

ACUTE GRIEF REACTION
notes to figure 20-3

(A) Extreme reactions of guilt, self-punishment, or rage can occur as extensions of acute bereavement. Loss of an adolescent's boyfriend or girlfriend is a common precipitant of suicide attempts in teenagers.

(B) A normal response to loss includes a degree of proportionality between the loss and the reaction. It is rare for a child to underrespond to the death of his father (and it is indicative of serious disturbance if it occurs); however, it is common for an overresponse to a less profound loss, such as the death of a neighbor, to be a marker for unaddressed fears or childhood depression. Another indication of a normal response is whether the child knows how to express his feelings and seeks support appropriately. A child whose sorrow is proportionate but entirely private also may benefit from intervention.

Additionally, a parent who has not been able to prevent the death of a spouse or of a child's sibling may seek consultation about the child's grief reaction because of a magnified sense of the child's vulnerability and a wish to bring the family life more under control. Parents in such situations are often less distressed by what the child is currently doing than they are by the fear that they will not be prepared for future threats to the child's well-being.

Death and Dying

The child or family that sustains a loss of one of its immediate family members (a parent or child) is likely to benefit from supportive psychotherapy at the time of the loss. Such therapy should be aimed at identifying and making understandable common aspects of bereavement (Figure 20-3 and Box 20-10). Other symptoms, such as separation anxiety disorder (SAD) or depression may appear later in both children and parents. In that event, a new course of treatment with the current developmental issues taken into consideration should be initiated.

A common question from parents after a death has occurred is whether their child should attend the funeral or other memorial event. A usual rule of thumb is that children 6 years old or younger are more likely to disrupt the adult's opportunity to participate and to be frightened by the spectacle of a group of distraught adults than they are to benefit from the exposure. Children age 7 or older should be asked if they would like to attend, and their wishes should be respected. A plan should be made in advance for any child who chooses to attend, so they can be taken out by a caring adult to wait for the occasion to be over if the need arises.

Helping the child talk about what they valued in the person who has died and what they miss gives them both permission to express their feelings and a model for the way memories assuage the pain of loss. Parents are sometimes concerned that the child's memories are so moving for the adult to hear that they may find themselves weeping. There is nothing injurious to the child in this as long as the adult neither appears frightened of his own grief nor seems incapable of responding to the child. It may be helpful to involve an array of adults (such as relatives and baby-sitters) in the child's care to provide the child with some variation in the emotional intensity and to allow the adults some time alone. Children may seem only mildly affected by the loss but then display an extreme reaction to some other, more minor disruption. They may need to be protected from the well-meaning but often intrusive queries of other adults (such as extended family or teachers). The first weeks and months are the hardest, since new routines are getting established. Everyone in the family needs extra time, attention, and patience at these times, whether or not they openly appear sad.

PEARLS & PERILS

ACUTE GRIEF

- Overreaction may signify underlying vulnerability to anxiety or depression and is a common childhood problem.
- Underreaction is rare and may be present in a young child, a child who feels she should protect others from her grief, or possibly a child with cognitive or emotional disturbance.
- Survivors of a death from suicide may experience extreme guilt, rage, and abandonment, which puts them at risk.

PEARLS & PERILS

DIVORCE

- It is critical for parents to avoid blaming the child for the problems in the marriage.
- Parents should avoid criticizing each other when the child can hear.
- Each parent should support contact with the other parent, or the child will hold the parent who is present responsible for the other's absence.

Divorce

Next to a death, divorce is the most powerful loss a child may experience. In many ways a child's reaction to divorce mirrors acute bereavement; however, there may be less visible support or acknowledgment from others. Whereas a death is usually a fairly public event in a family, separation and divorce are often managed, if not in secret, at least in private. This limits the number of outside resources the child (or parent) has access to. Additionally, the people that children do have access to may be the least able to listen neutrally or offer support regarding the child's concerns. When a 4-year-old boy cries at night after his father dies, his mother is the most likely person to echo his grief and offer him comfort. The 4-year-old who cries, "I miss Daddy," after a divorce often encounters a more complicated, less validating response, even in the most enlightened home. Furthermore, the child may be encouraged not to share the news of his or her loss with friends, creating an additional burden of shame and isolation. Younger children will and should say what they need to when they want to (for example, in the grocery store or at the playground) and may need much repetitive discussion on the topics they find most distressing. Even though her mother has explained it many times, a 6-year-old girl may still ask, "But how can Daddy still be my daddy if you get divorced?" It is important for parents to attempt to differentiate their issues from their children's issues and to maintain clarity about the distinction. Children of any age should be spared diatribes about the many faults of the other parent. Conflicted loyalty and loss of self-esteem (after all, they are the product of both parents) are the result of this behavior. Additionally, children complain that parents often seem more interested in fighting with each other than in attending to them. They quickly recognize that the struggles over custody and visitation that parents pursue "on behalf" of their children have other motives. "I feel like they're the bread and I'm the cheese," complained one little boy.

Another risk to children in the divorce process is a feeling of too much responsibility—either for the parental conflict itself or for the well-being of their parents. Children may engage in covert or overt bargaining with their helpfulness, cooperativeness, or other good behavior that should please parents enough to make the family stress go down so the parents can get back together. Conversely, children may succeed in creating an emergency by running away, lighting a fire, or doing poorly in school, which they imagine will draw the parents back together to save the child. These are not manipulations but are true expressions of the extreme situation in which the child finds himself. Along with efforts to repair the marriage, children may feel the burden of the adult sorrow or rage and an expectation to fill the gap that is now present in the adult's life. Distressed parents may yield to the temptation to share too much of their experience with their child and unconsciously recruit the nurture that they are missing. Details of parental anxiety about money or romance are not appropriate for children to worry over and amplify the child's fear of being unprotected.

Older children often seem to feel that the capacity for adult executive functioning has been lost with the divorce and that they must now make the decisions. This gets compounded when inquiries about the child's preferences regarding custody and visitation get heard as "you decide." It is important to clarify that even divorced parents are still parents and retain the major decision-making authority. Where this is not possible, a guardian ad litem or a judge (not the child) need to fill in.

A common inquiry from parents is what, if anything, should be said to the teacher regarding separation or divorce. It is usually a good idea to alert a teacher whenever a major event is befalling a student. However, it should be done with caution. It is disconcerting and often quite distressing to the older student, who has been successfully escaping the stress of family conflict at school, to know that a teacher is now privy to all the child has been avoiding. Parents should encourage the teacher to be aware that the child may not be at her best but to let any discussion be initiated by the child. The young child may be comforted to know that the teacher has been told; it can be a way for parents to communicate their permission for the child to confide in the teacher. The school guidance counselor may also be an appropriate contact. Some schools offer peer group discussions regarding separation and divorce that can be helpful.

Transitions are not only losses; they should also be presented as opportunities by parents whenever possible. It is appropriate to miss one's old school, but it is also possible to be excited about a new school. Change supports growth, and parents may need to be reassured that upcoming transitions may have beneficial elements for the child.

Nightmares, Imaginary Friends, and Magic

Nightmares

Even before a child can talk, parents may be aware of the presence of nightmares. A toddler may wake up with true *pavor nocturnus* (characterized by desperate crying, terror, and inconsolability), which can also be a frightening experience for parents and prompt them to seek advice. A child of any age may have routine nightmares that cause them to wake up. These nightmares can usually be described immediately on awakening. It is estimated that 20% to 30% of children have bedtime or night-awakening difficulties throughout their first 4 years. Nightmares are common, and parents who are either anxious or inexperienced may need reassurance about this. Nightmares can accompany medical illness (for example, a fever or a stomachache), frightening external events (a car accident or parental conflict), or frightening internal events (angry feelings or loss). Even positive accomplishments (such as graduating from diapers or learning to skate) can contribute to nightmares. Parents should listen for what might be making the child feel unprotected. It is of great importance, no matter how inconvenient, to convey parental availability to the child through the night. Parents commonly raise the question of whether this will encourage the child to have more nightmares. The answer is *no*. The underlying precipitant to all nightmares is some type of lack of modulation; there is physical discomfort that cannot be overridden by the usual mechanisms, or there is emotional discomfort. The child needs to know that when his supplies are insufficient, an adult is available to help modulate the overwhelming rage or fear he feels. It is that feeling of being overpowered that drives the nightmare. One reason that children ages 3 to 7 seem to be at greater risk for nightmares is that their competencies are expanding exponentially during this time. Another reason is that they have little sense of proportion at that age. Therefore a 3-year-old boy with complex ideas but limited language to explain them may be infuriated by his inarticulateness during the day, with consequent affective overflow into nightmares. A capable 7-year-old girl given a new chore may fear she has to take on more responsibility than she can manage and become overwhelmingly anxious, causing her nightmares.

A common family-system factor is when young children, often boys, feel there is no one in the house who is strong enough to tolerate their powerful feelings of anger, jealousy, and attachment. This is especially common in fatherless households, but it is also evident in homes where parents are not comfortable with their own anger and do not know how to help the child feel contained in the daytime.

PEARLS & PERILS

NIGHTMARES

- Nightmares may occur with physical illness (such as an earache or a fever).
- Nightmares may be caused by overwhelming external events (such as a car accident, fire, or domestic violence).
- Nightmares may be caused by overwhelming internal events (such as rage, guilt, or anxiety).
- Improved access to modulation of affect for both parents and child is usually helpful.

When behavioral problems and nightmares are combined, it is useful to review the way anger is handled in the family and to assess for the presence of loss of control or abuse.

Children who can obtain the support of a parent for their fears in the day or nighttime are not likely to have difficulty. If the parent feels the nightmares are increasing or has no idea what might be precipitating them, having someone else talk to the child is advisable.

Small requests, such as leaving the night light on or the door open should be honored and are in no way detrimental to the child's maturation. Bedtime routines, such as favorite songs and stuffed animals, often help the child go to sleep feeling safe, with the day's dramas no longer a threat. However, requests by the child to sleep with the parents should be redirected by the parent so that the child obtains the needed support but can distinguish the adult's bed, life, and body from his own. Sleeping in the same bed sounds like a straightforward solution for the child who is scared and for the adult who does not want to lose sleep. Unfortunately, if the parent agrees, the child inevitably concludes that the adult needs the child's company at night (and the child is often correct). As a result, the opposite of the desired message is sent. Instead of, "Don't worry; no matter how big your feeling or problem is, I can handle it," the child hears, "You're right; nighttime is cold and lonely, and we need to stick together." This only exacerbates the child's fear. Additionally, if a parent tries to set limits but yields when the child reacts to the limit (by arguing or crying), the child gets confirmation that his reaction is too big for the parent to manage. Since it is already too big for the child to manage, it leaves him feeling worse. Consistent, available limits set during the day by adults who mostly avoid either losing control or being overcontrolled is the best prevention for nightmares.

Imaginary Friends

Imaginary friends have an established place in child development, but physicians may still be perplexed about how to respond to parents' questions on this topic. Much depends on the child's age and state of mind. Children from around age 3 to age 7 have a rapidly increasing capacity for imagination, along with increased awareness of their own and others' feelings. Compelling topics (such as new siblings, power in relationship to others, major transitions) are commonly dealt with through displacement. That is, play allows the child to express feelings or ideas through a safe intermediary, such as a toy or storybook character. Traditional theory contends that imaginary friends or enemies carry those attributes that reside within the child about which she has strong feelings. The loyal little girl who wants her mother to think she is tidy but who also relishes seeing her own power when the enormous pile of books she has arranged tips over and lands on the living room floor may announce indignantly, "I didn't do it!" As she makes this statement, she is sincere. It is not that her memory fails her but that the "I" of whom she speaks would not have done such an openly aggressive thing. It is that other "I" who did it, the bad, morally backward one. Some children take this distinction a step further by naming the other "I." This entity, now called Lucy, was the one who knocked the books down. Parents can support the child's development better by avoiding direct confrontation on this point. Instead of saying, "You did it! I know you did!" or worse, "Stop lying," which is frightening and confusing to the child who is trying to indicate that she knows it was a wrong thing to do, it is preferable to say, "I see; well, Lucy needs to understand that the books can get torn this way and it is better to make towers out of blocks. Why don't you come help me pick them up?" This way the good "I," who didn't (expect to) do it, can redeem herself and be stronger against temptation next time. Alter egos are not injurious as "fall-guys" responsible for misdeeds; however, real children should be given opportunities to undo the harm they may have caused and thus to realign themselves with the parentally approved identity. It may be that the widespread access to TV and video characters has lessened the identification of homegrown, imaginary associates (since the need can be met by a known character). However, it is still a normal phase for a young child to go through and usually has the adaptive significance of helping the child work something out.

Two variations of the imaginary friend warrant more concern; the first is when the parent appears to be overinvolved in the existence of the child's imaginary friend. This signifies both an unhealthy intrusiveness on the part of the parent and an overly narcissistic need to direct the child's inner life. The parent should be warned to avoid inquiries about the imaginary friend and to only respond to what is offered by the child. Otherwise, the child's efforts to address issues of power and control cannot be effective.

Another potential problem is when the child's imaginative play becomes too real, is rigidified, or persists into later latency. In these situations either the child, or more often, the parent, has become worried. The child worries when the companion she has created apparently becomes a source of powerful feelings instead of a way to practice managing powerful feelings. This is one risk of parents pretending too much that they believe in the imaginary friend. The child finds the process outside of her control and becomes frightened.

Other times, serious psychologic stress can alter the child's perception of reality and she can no longer be sure she knows what is real. For children under age 5, this is less of a concern since they have a more fluid sense of reality as a baseline. They may just need reassurance (there are no such things as ghosts). However, older children may actually become psychotic and require urgent evaluation by a child psychiatrist for possible medication. Overly rigid, ritualized games, especially those that seem to replace usual family interactions or peer relations, are an appropriate cause for concern.

Magic

Much of what was said about imaginary companions can also be said about the role of magic in general. Magic is invoked either as the explanation for things too complex to be comprehended or as the resource to contend with forces too powerful to be contained. Children delight in magic because it gives them a fighting chance; a child may feel smaller than his enemies, but with magic he can even the odds. So much of what happens to children is marvelous (such as telephone calls from an invisible grandmother, videos that start with the push of a button, or snow falling) or terrifying (gentle Mommy changing into a furious giant, bowel movements disappearing down the toilet, or lightning flashing) that magic seems necessary to fill in their understanding. Somebody must be in charge of all these unseen forces.

If older children, including those over age 8 and approaching adolescence, continue to need magic, they may still be feeling bewildered and overwhelmed by their circumstances. It is a sign of emotional distress, and these children should be offered some private opportunity to share their worries. Again, it is preferable to avoid directly challenging the system the child has created but instead to gain access to what other subjects are on the child's mind and to look for sources of stress that can be removed. If the child's beliefs are delusional, then the child is at high risk and needs psychiatric assessment on an emergency basis.

Witness to Trauma

Domestic Violence

The awareness (and probably the prevalence) of domestic violence has mushroomed, and we know that many children have experienced significant amounts of fear and anxiety. The effects of violence are so serious that they can drive a 5-year-old girl to take up a kitchen knife against her father, trying desperately to protect her mother from assault. This same child may become suicidal in the face of her father's recurrent violence toward her mother and her mother's recurrent provocation of her father. Such despair is both common and dangerous. Recent studies indicate that witnessing violence is at least as harmful (and maybe more so) than directly experiencing it. Adults relate the helplessness they felt as children at not being able to protect their siblings or their parent. The anguish over the beloved victim's observed pain was far worse than their own direct experience of pain. Despite the public fascination with predatory strangers, the data collected on abuse consistently confirm that most violence takes place in the context of a relationship and most commonly within the home. Although supermarkets offer booklets titled *Don't Talk to Strangers* and gradeschool classrooms dwell on the hazards of Halloween, there is little support or direction offered to the child (or parent) who is living with the constant stress of family violence. Even in the absence of physical violence, the negative impact of chronic, bitter parental conflict or verbal abuse can also be enduring. Sexual abuse, whether it occurs to the child directly or is happening to another family member, is particularly damaging.

Most children who have experienced significant abuse and many who live in homes where there is violence have serious enough sequelae to be diagnosed as having Posttraumatic Stress Disorder (PTSD) (Box 20-11).

PTSD is discussed in depth in Chapter 7. Some children who witness domestic violence do not meet full criteria for PTSD, but they may exhibit some symptoms from a fairly broad continuum, including those in the following list:

- Obsessive fears, phobias
- Sleep disturbance
- Hypervigilance
- Tearfulness
- Lack of enthusiasm
- Impulsivity
- Hyperaggressiveness
- Peer conflict
- Psychosomatic complaints
- Frequent illness or accidents

If a parent or teacher is concerned about a child who has these symptoms, it is best to keep the possibility of domestic violence in mind and give the child some private chances to discuss it. It is also important for the physician to discuss with a parent (again, privately) that the assessment of the child is consistent with the possibility that he may have been traumatized. Parents should be asked whether they are aware of any major conflict or family stress at home. Parents and children should each be asked if they or anyone in the family has been hurt or threatened in the last month. A follow-up question that specifies the last year can sometimes be helpful. The child can also be asked about how the family handles anger. A nonthreatening way to begin is to ask who has the biggest temper at home and

DSM-IV DIAGNOSTIC CRITERIA

BOX 20-11 POSTTRAUMATIC STRESS DISORDER

A. The person has been exposed to a traumatic event in which both of the following were present:

(1) the person experienced, witnessed, or was confronted with an event or events that involved actual or threatened death or serious injury, or a threat to the physical integrity of self or others
(2) the person's response involved intense fear, helplessness, or horror. **Note:** In children, this may be expressed instead by disorganized or agitated behavior.

B. The traumatic event is persistently reexperienced in one (or more) of the following ways:

(1) recurrent and intrusive distressing recollections of the event, including images, thoughts, or perceptions. **Note:** In young children, repetitive play may occur in which themes or aspects of the trauma are expressed.
(2) recurrent distressing dreams of the event. **Note:** In children, there may be frightening dreams without recognizable content.
(3) acting or feeling as if the traumatic event were recurring (includes a sense of reliving the experience, illusions, hallucinations, and dissociative flashback episodes, including those that occur on awakening or when intoxicated). **Note:** In young children, trauma-specific reenactment may occur.
(4) intense psychological distress at exposure to internal or external cues that symbolize or resemble an aspect of the traumatic event
(5) physiological reactivity on exposure to internal or external cues that symbolize or resemble an aspect of the traumatic event

C. Persistent avoidance of stimuli associated with the trauma and numbing of general responsiveness (not present before the trauma), as indicated by three (or more) of the following:

(1) efforts to avoid thoughts, feelings, or conversations associated with the trauma
(2) efforts to avoid activities, places, or people that arouse recollections of the trauma
(3) inability to recall an important aspect of the trauma
(4) markedly diminished interest or participation in significant activities
(5) feeling of detachment or estrangement from others
(6) restricted range of affect (e.g., unable to have loving feelings)
(7) sense of a foreshortened future (e.g., does not expect to have a career, marriage, children, or a normal life span)

D. Persistent symptoms of increased arousal (not present before the trauma), as indicated by two (or more) of the following:

(1) difficulty falling or staying asleep
(2) irritability or outbursts of anger
(3) difficulty concentrating
(4) hypervigilance
(5) exaggerated startle response

E. Duration of the disturbance (symptoms in Criteria B, C, and D) is more than 1 month.

F. The disturbance causes clinically significant distress or impairment in social, occupational, or other important areas or functioning.

Specify if:
Acute: if duration of symptoms is less than 3 months
Chronic: if duration of symptoms is 3 months or more

Specify if:
With Delayed Onset: if onset of symptoms is at least 6 months after the stressor

(From American Psychiatric Association: *Diagnostic and statistical manual of mental disorders,* ed 4 [DSM-IV], Washington DC, 1994, American Psychiatric Press.)

what they get mad about. It does not matter if the child says he has the biggest temper; the story that goes with that statement will illustrate the family's style of conflict resolution.

Additionally, children should be interviewed about the presence of substance abuse in the home, both because it often functions as an amplifier for violence in relationships and because even where there is no violence, fear and concern for parents who are using substances can produce symptoms in children that are indistinguishable from trauma-related symptoms.

Although child abuse has been discussed in depth in Chapter 16, it is worth noting that both clinical experience and epidemiologic surveys demonstrate the high correlation between the presence of abuse or trauma and any symptoms related to a child's mental health. Depression and conduct disorder (CD) are commonly found in cases where there is either child abuse or family violence. Any child who is symptomatic should have a family assessment about violence as part of their review of systems.

If ongoing violence is found, the first step is to create a safety plan with the people at risk. It is appropriate to include a clinical team review (if one is available) to help with both the logistic and the emotional burdens of this type of work on the physician. Any time anyone in the family is being abused, all family members are suffering and in need of protection. An important therapeutic step for the witness of trauma is to emphasize the ways in which he was not helpless or did not behave helplessly. These can be minor acts of symbolic defiance, such as when an older brother yells for a watching child to shut the door as he rapes their sister, and the child goes away but refuses to close the door. They may be significant interventions, such as when a child tells his teacher that his father broke his mother's arm and the family is consequently referred to social services. Reporting an incident long after the fact is to be congratulated and validated as an active step in protecting others or aiding recovery. Children in a witness role often worry about the safety of everyone in the family, even the perpetrators. It is important to demonstrate compassion and concern for all parties to help the child to hand over this responsibility. Only when the child feels secure that someone else is guarding the whole family can he begin to attend to his own needs.

Community Violence

Community violence and family violence are, of course, not mutually exclusive, and when both are present it compounds the distress a child may experience. However, community violence alone interferes with a child's optimal development. The intrapsychic work a child needs to do is predicated on certain requirements from her external environment. These requirements include food, shelter, affection, and the illusion of safety. We know that infants who are malnourished or seriously ill do not progress with milestone acquisition. They conserve resources to stay alive. Harlow and Bowlby demonstrated that affection and attachment are as essential to life as food and shelter. Clinical experience indicates that the capacity to grow emotionally, intellectually, and physically is highly influenced by the psychologic environment. Failure to thrive, even in the presence of sufficient calories, is a well-established syndrome with an origin in interactional inadequacies between the child and his caregivers.

> **PEARLS & PERILS**
>
> **TRAUMA WITNESS**
>
> - Immediate safety is the most important concern; all other interventions should be secondary.
> - If one person is being abused, the whole family is suffering
> - The physician should emphasize ways the witness showed he was not helpless.

Unfortunately, even families who manage to provide appropriate and loving care are affected by traumatic events that may occur in their neighborhood or nearby. The more children can be buffered from hearing about or witnessing cruelty, murder, or rape, the more firmly the illusion of safety can be established. The assumption that evil is far away and that powerful adults will protect them provides children with a psychologic work-space where they can attend to their developmental tasks. On the other hand, if evil is in their midst and no one can protect them, the children's psychic energy must be redirected towards vigilance and there is room for little else.

One of the effects of television news, magazines, and other media is that even wars occurring across the globe do not seem far away to children. A man cutting up and eating other men in one city or a woman drowning her children in another are described with an immediacy that brings the danger into the child's own living room and are often traumatic to children. Thus in a sense, all violence becomes community violence, and children experience a cumulative toll when they are unprotected from this material.

However, the child who encounters a body in the stairwell of her apartment building as she goes out to catch the school bus or the child whose best friend was killed in a drive-by shooting is at a much greater risk of psychologic damage. Children can still defend themselves somewhat with the idea that the people involved in television or newspaper violence are "others" or "unlike" the child and her close circle of acquaintances. However, if those involved (as perpetrators or victims) come from the child's immediate environment, the possibility of psychologic defense against terror becomes remote.

Symptoms commonly encountered in children or adolescents in communities with high crime rates include those shown in the following list:

- Depression
- Sleep disturbance
- Anxiety
- School failure
- CD
- Substance abuse
- Pregnancy

There can be high degrees of fatalism, hopelessness, and helplessness that develop in the face of the awareness that risk is pervasive and that survival is somewhat randomly determined.

Cared for by adults, who may be similarly overwhelmed and unable to devote as much attention to the child as they might otherwise, children and adolescents in violent communities describe feeling that life is meaningless and brief, and that they have little significance or power. These feelings appear to contribute to the presence of risk-taking behaviors such as sexual activity and substance abuse, which offer sensual gratification, transient freedom from anxiety, and an enhanced sense of personal importance or identity. Similarly, the anger and depression that develop from the chronic experience of abandonment or lack of protection affect the child's investment in achievement or long-term goals and can contribute to an increased risk of suicide and homicide.

Any community can suffer from violence, and children appear to have endogenously different sensitivity to trauma that directly affects their resilience. An additional strategy that parents and providers can use to support resilience in young children is to try to shield the children from hearing or seeing more than they have the maturity or resources to assimilate. Some exposures to violence are unanticipated or unavoidable; some occur through lack of recognition by an adult that certain conversations or activities should not take place when children are present. The physician may need to guide parents in protecting their child from more than he can process. Part of feeling safe is feeling that the resources to contend with danger are available. Small children have neither the intellectual nor the emotional capacity to respond to stories of murder, arson, and rape. They should not be taken to watch buildings burn down or to hear courtroom testimony about a homicide. If a child is quiet as a result of the overpowering effect of an event or very active, overstimulated by its content, parents may mistakenly conclude that the child is unaware of the violence to which she has been exposed. The physician needs to assure them this is not the case.

Beyond avoidance of the traumatic material, validation and responsiveness to the events at the time, (or later if the event is being described) help the child restore the fabric of the protective illusion of safety. Recognition and articulation of the fact that it is not acceptable for an older child to assault a younger child or for a gang shooting to take place on the playground help the child maintain his sense of what should be. Appropriate emotional responses from the physician clarify for the child that what occurred was an aberration; advocacy from the physician restores the child's sense of hope. Interest and concern from a significant figure is commonly reported retrospectively by adults as a contributing factor to their survival under otherwise traumatizing circumstances.

Finally, it is important that either with schoolmates, family, or both, children be given the opportunity to jointly process the community violence they have witnessed (perhaps with professional guidance) to achieve some integration of the event and to begin to surround it with what will become the protective myth the group or family creates.

Summary

Children's development is like the melody line, with harmonics provided by the resources (endogenous and exogenous) available to them and variations introduced by the events that befall them. Mostly, the result is harmonious. However, the role of the professional with responsibility for evaluating a child's current status or overall progress is to be alert for "wrong notes." The earlier in a child's development that disproportionate stressors or insufficient resources can be identified, the more likely it is that intervention can be limited and the child's growth optimally supported. Recognition of common behavioral indicators of distress, and likely sources, enables physicians to better serve the children in their care.

CONSIDER CONSULTATION WHEN . . .

- The clinical presentation persists or worsens despite your intervention
- The symptom prevents normal, age-appropriate interactions with others

Annotated Bibliography

Ames LB: *Your three year old: friend or enemy,* New York, 1976, Dell.
This is one of a series of useful books written for parents. Anyone who has or works with children will enjoy them. Each volume deals with a designated age range and is filled with examples of predictable conflicts, explanations of developmental issues that might drive the behavior, and practical strategies for coping with them. The opportunity to expand one's data base from a particular child to a developmental cohort is commonly experienced by parents as a great relief.

Fraiberg SH: *The magic years,* New York, 1959, Scribners.
In recent years this author fell out of favor for a book that appeared to suggest that children should only be cared for by their mothers. It would be unfortunate if anyone involved with children avoided reading this classic because of a failure to appreciate the valuable contribution the author made to the field of child psychiatry. This work is best known for making sense out of nonsense; in other words, it helps us understand things from a child's point of view.

Gardner RA: *Boys and girls book about divorce,* New York, 1970, J. Aronson.
Now out of print, this book is worth locating in the library because of its gentle but straightforward handling of a familiar but painful topic. Common worries are reviewed with suggested strategies for discussing them. This book has been so popular with parents and children that it is often referred to in fictional books for children about divorce.

Koocher GP, Gudas LJ: *Grief and loss in childhood.* In Walker CE, Roberts MC, editors: *Handbook of clinical child psychology,* ed 2, New York, 1992, Wiley and Sons.
Consistent with Koocher's previous writings on grief in children, this chapter arms the physician with a clear understanding of the interplay between naturally occurring developmental events and unanticipated loss. The difference between adult and child perspectives is described and specific interventions that might prove of value to the child are explained.

Richters JE, Martinex P: The NIMH community violence project. I. Children as victims of and witnesses to violence, *Psychiatry* 56:262-264, February 1993.
This commonly quoted study was one of the first to definitively document that children could be, and were, traumatized by violence even if they were not physically touched. This article, among others, led to a shift in the thinking of physicians and protective service workers, some of whom had previously reported no risk to the children in a home where there was known spouse abuse. It also addressed the larger public health issue of how many children were suffering or being damaged in communities where violence was prevalent.

Bibliography

Chapter 1

American Psychiatric Association: *Diagnostic and statistical manual of mental disorders,* ed 4, DSM-IV, Washington, DC, 1994, American Psychiatric Association.

Diamond CB: *General issues in the clinical assessment of children and adolescents.* In Kestenbaum CJ, Williams DT, editors: *Handbook of clinical assessment of children and adolescents,* vol 1, New York, 1988, New York University Press.

Kaplan HI, Sadock BJ, Grebb JA, editors: *Synopsis of psychiatry,* ed 7, Baltimore, 1994, Williams & Wilkins.

Robson KS, editor: *Manual of clinical child and adolescent psychiatry,* rev ed, Washington, DC, 1994, American Psychiatric Press.

Rutter M, Tuma AH, Lann IS, editors: *Assessment and diagnosis in child psychopathology,* New York, 1988, The Guilford Press.

Simmons JE: *Psychiatric examination of children,* ed 4, Philadelphia, 1987, Lea & Febiger.

Chapter 2

Achenbach TM, Edelbrock CS: *Child behavior checklist and youth self-report,* Burlington, Vt., 1986a, Author.

Achenbach TM, Edelbrock CS: *Teacher's report form,* Burlington, Vt., 1986b, Author.

Aman MG, Singh NN: *Aberrant Behavior Checklist manual,* East Aurora, N.Y., 1986, Slosson Educational Publications.

Ammerman RT: *Physical abuse and neglect.* In Ollendick TH, Hersen M, editors: *Handbook of child and adolescent assessment,* Boston, 1993, Allyn & Bacon.

Barkley RA: *Child behavior rating scales and checklists.* In Rutter M, Tuma A, Lann IS, editors: *Assessment and diagnosis in child psychopathology,* New York, 1987, Guilford Press.

Bech P, Maier W, Ballus C: *Compendium of rating scales corresponding with DSM-III, DSM-III-R and ICD-10 syndromes,* Berlin, 1991, Springer.

Beck A et al: An inventory for measuring depression, *Arch Gen Psychiatry* 4:53-63, 1961.

Capra F: Bootstrap and Buddhism, *Am J Physics* 42:15-19, 1974.

Conners CK: *The Conners Rating Scales: instruments for the assessment of childhood psychopathology,* Unpublished manuscript, 1985.

Cooper Z, Fairburn CG: The Eating Disorder Examination: a semi-structured interview for the assessment of the specific psychopathology of eating disorders, *Int J Eat Disord* 6:1-8, 1987.

Costello AJ et al: *Report on the NIMH Diagnostic Interview Schedule for Children (DISC),* Washington, DC, 1984, National Institute for Mental Health.

Deluty RH: Children's Action Tendency Scale: a self-report measure of aggressiveness, assertiveness, and submissiveness in children, *J Consult Clin Psychol* 47:1061-1071, 1979.

Elliot DS, Ageton SS: Reconciling race and class differences in self-reported and official estimates of delinquency, *American Sociological Review* 45:95-110, 1980.

Eyberg SM, Robinson EA: Conduct problem behavior: standardization of a behavioral rating scale with adolescents, *J Clin Child Psychol* 12:347-354, 1983.

Freeman BJ et al: A scale for rating symptoms of patients with the syndrome of autism in real life settings, *J Am Acad Child Psychiatry* 25:130-136, 1986.

Funderburk BW, Eyberg SM: Psychometric characteristics of the Sutter-Eyberg Student Behavior Inventory: a school behavior rating scale for use with preschool children, *Behav Assess* 11:297-313, 1989.

Garner DM: *The Eating Disorder Inventory manual,* Odessa, Fla., 1991, Psychological Assessment Resources.

Garner DM, Garfinkel PE: The Eating Attitudes Test: an index of the symptoms of anorexia nervosa, *Psychol Med* 10:647-656, 1979.

Garner DM, Olmsted MP, Polivy J: *The Eating Disorder Inventory: a measure of cognitive-behavioral dimensions of anorexia nervosa and bulimia.* In Darby PL et al, editors: *Anorexia nervosa: recent developments in research,* New York, 1983, Alan R. Liss.

Hasher L, Zachs RT: Automatic and effortful processing in memory, *J Exp Psychol* 108:356-388, 1979.

Helzer JE et al: Renard Diagnostic Interview: its reliability and procedural validity with physicians and lay interviewers, *Arch Gen Psych* 38:393-398, 1981.

Hodges K et al: The development of a child assessment schedule for research and clinical use, *J Abnorm Child Psychol* 10:173-189, 1982.

Hodges K et al: Diagnostic concordance between the Child Assessment Scale (CAS) and the Schedule for Affective Disorders and Schizophrenia for School-Age Children (K-SADS) in an outpatient sample using lay interviewers, *J Am Acad Child Adolesc Psychiatry* 26:654-661, 1987.

Hoehn-Saric E, Maisami M, Wiegand D: Measurement of anxiety in children and adolescents using semistructured interviews, *J Am Acad Child Adolesc Psychiatry* 26:541-545, 1987.

Jastak S, Wilkinson GS: *Wide range achievement test-revised,* Wilmington, Del., 1981, Jastak Associates.

Jay SM, Elliott CH: Behavioral observation scale for measuring children's distress: the effects of increased methodological rigor, *J Consult Clin Psychol* 52:1106-1107, 1984.

Jensen P et al: Test-retest reliability of the Diagnostic Interview Schedule for Children (DISC 2.1), *Arch Gen Psychiatry* 52:61-71, 1995.

Kagan J et al: Information processing in the child: significance of analytic and reflective attitudes, *Psychol Monogr* 78:1, 1964.

Kaplan SL, Hong GK, Weinhold C: Epidemiology of depressive symptomatology in adolescents, *J Am Acad Child Adolesc Psychiatry* 23:91-98, 1984.

Katz ER, Kellerman J, Siegel SE: Behavior distress in children with cancer undergoing medical procedures: developmental considerations, *J Consult Clin Psychol* 48:356-365, 1980.

Kaufman AS, Kaufman NL: *Kaufman test of educational achievement,* Circle Pines, Minn., 1985, American Guidance Service.

Kazdin AE, Esveldt-Dawson K: The Interview for Antisocial Behavior: psychometric characteristics and concurrent validity with child psychiatric inpatients, *J Psychopathol Behav Assess* 8:289-303, 1986.

Kazdin AE et al: Hopelessness, depression, and suicidal intent among psychiatrically disturbed inpatient children, *J Consult Clin Psychol* 51:504-510, 1983.

Kovacs M: Rating scales to assess depression in school-aged children, *Acta Paedopsychiatr* 46:305-315, 1980.

Kovacs M: *The Interview Schedule for Children (ISC): ISC interrater and parent-child agreement,* Unpublished manuscript, 1983.

Kovacs M: The interview schedule for children (ISC), *Psychopharmacol Bull* 21:991-994, 1985a.

Kovacs M: The children's depression inventory (CDI), *Psychopharmacol Bull* 21:995-998, 1985b.

LeBaron L, Zeltzer L: Assessment of acute pain and anxiety in children and adolescents by self-reports, observer reports, and a behavioral checklist. *J Consult Clin Psychol* 52:729-738, 1984.

Loney J, Milich R: Hyperactivity, inattention and aggression in child practice, *Adv Dev Behav Pediatr* 3:113-147, 1982.

Luckasson R et al: *Mental retardation: definition, classification, and systems of supports,* Washington, DC, 1992, American Association on Mental Retardation.

Markwardt FC Jr: *Peabody individual achievement test-revised (PIAT-R),* Circle Pines, Minn., 1989, American Guidance Service.

Matson JL: *Manual for the PIMRA,* Orland Park, Ill., 1988, International Diagnostic Systems.

Matson JL et al: A scale for evaluating emotional disorders in severely and profoundly retarded persons: development of the Diagnostic Assessment for the Severely Handicapped (DASH) scale, *Br J Psychiatry* 159:404-409, 1991.

McGrath PA *The CHEOPS: a behavioral scale to measure postoperative pain in children.* In Fields HL, Dubner R, Cervero F, editors: *Advances in pain research and therapy,* New York, 1985, Raven Press.

Moos RH, Moos BS: *Family environment scale,* ed 2, Palo Alto, Calif., 1986, Consulting Psychologists Press.

Nihira K et al: *AAMD Adaptive Behavior Scale manual,* rev ed, Washington, DC, 1975, American Association on Mental Deficiency.

Palmer R et al: The Clinical Eating Disorder Rating Instrument (CEDRI): a preliminary description, *Int J Eat Disord* 6:9-16, 1987.

Pelham WE et al: Normative data on the IOWA-Conners Teacher Rating Scale, *J Clin Child Psychol* 18:259-262, 1989.

Pelham WE et al: Methylphenidate and attributions in boys with Attention-Deficit Hyperactivity Disorder, *J Consult Clin Psychol* 60:282-292, 1992.

Pfeffer CR: *The suicidal child,* New York, 1986, Guilford Press.

Piacentini J et al: The Diagnostic Interview Schedule for Children—Revised Version (DISC-R). III. Concurrent criterion validity, *J Am Acad Child Adolesc Psychiatry* 32:658-665, 1993.

Poznanski EO et al: Preliminary studies of the reliability and validity of the Children's Depression Rating Scale, *J Am Acad Child Adolesc Psychiatry* 23:191-197, 1984.

Prout HT, Strohmer DC: *Prout-Strohmer Personality Inventory manual,* Schenectady, N.Y., 1989, Genium Publishing Corporation.

Puig-Antich J, Chambers W: *The schedule for affective disorders and schizophrenia for school-age children (Kiddie-SADS),* New York, 1978, New York State Psychiatric Institute.

Quay HC, Peterson DR: *Manual for the Revised Behavior Problem Checklist,* Coral Gables, Fla., 1987, Author.

Reich W, Welner Z: *Diagnostic interview for children and adolescents,* Unpublished manuscript, 1988.

Reiss S: *Test manual for the Reiss Screen for Maladaptive Behavior,* Orland Park, Ill., 1988, International Diagnostic Systems.

Reynolds CR, Richmond BO: Factor structure and construct validity of "What I think and feel": The Revised Children's Manifest Anxiety Scale (RCMAS), *J Pers Assess* 43:281-283, 1978.

Reynolds WM: *Suicidal ideation questionnaire,* Odessa, Fla., 1987, Psychological Assessment Resources.

Rosvold HE et al: A continuous performance test of brain damage, *J Clin Consult Psychol* 20:343-350, 1956.

Ruttenburg BA et al: *Behavior rating instrument for autistic and other atypical children* rev ed, Philadelphia, 1977, Developmental Center for Autistic Children.

Schopler E, Reichler RJ, Renner BR: *The childhood autism rating scale,* Los Angeles, 1986, Western Psychological Services.

Schwab-Stone M et al: The Diagnostic Interview Schedule for Children—Revised Version (DISC-R). II. Test-retest reliability, *J Am Acad Child Adolesc Psychiatry* 32:651-657, 1993.

Shaffer D et al: *Results of a field trial and proposals for a new instrument (DISC-R),* Washington, DC, 1988, National Institute for Mental Health.

Shaffer D et al: *Diagnostic interview schedule for children (DISC-C): child version,* Unpublished manuscript, 1989.

Shaffer D et al: The Diagnostic Interview Schedule for Children—Revised Version (DISC-R). I. Preparation, field testing, interrater reliability, and acceptability, *J Am Acad Child Adolesc Psychiatry* 32:643-650, 1993.

Shaw EG, Routh DK: Effect of mother presence on the children's reaction to aversive procedures, *J Pediatr Psychol* 7:33-42, 1982.

Silverman WK, Nelles WB: The anxiety disorders interview schedule for children, *J Am Acad Child Adolesc Psychiatry* 27:772-778, 1988.

Singh NN: In search of unity: some thoughts on family-professional relationships in service delivery systems, *J Child Fam Stud* 4:1-16, 1995.

Sparrow SS, Balla DA, Cicchetti DV: *Vineland adaptive behavior scales,* Circle Pines, Minn., 1984, American Guidance Service.

Spielberger CD: *Preliminary manual for the State-Trait Anxiety Inventory for Children,* Palo Alto, Calif., 1973, Consulting Psychologists Press.

Strohmer DC, Prout HT: *Strohmer-Prout Behavior Rating Scale manual,* Schenectady, N.Y., 1989, Genium Publishing Corporation.

Ullmann RK, Sleator EK, Sprague RL: *Manual for the ADD-H Comprehensive Teacher's Rating Scale: ACTeRS,* Champaign, Ill., 1988, Meritrech.

Varni JW, Thompson KL, Hanson V: The Varni/Thompson Pediatric Pain Questionnaire: chronic musculosketetal pain in juvenile rheumatoid arthritis, *Pain* 28:27-38, 1987.

Walker HM, Rankin R: *The Walker-Rankin rating scale of adaptive and maladaptive child behavior in school,* Eugene, Ore., 1983, University of Oregon.

Woodcock RW: *Woodcock-Johnson Psychoeducational Battery: technical report,* Allen, Tex., 1977, DLM Teaching Resources.

Yesseldyke JE, Christenson SL: *The instructional environment scale,* Austin, Tex., 1987, Pro-Ed.

Chapter 3

Andreasen NC et al: Ventricular abnormalities in affective disorder: clinical and demographic correlates, *Am J Psychiatry* 147:893-900, 1990.

Arin DM, Bauman ML, Kemper TL: The distribution of Purkinje cell loss in the cerebellum in autism, *Neurology* 41(Suppl 1):307, 1991.

Barta PE et al: Auditory hallucinations and smaller superior temporal gyrus volume in schizophrenia, *Am J Psychiatry* 147:1457-1462, 1990.

Bauman ML: Microscopic neuroanatomic abnormalities in autism, *Pediatrics* 87(Suppl):791-796, 1991.

Belliveau JW et al: Functional mapping of the human visual cortex by magnetic resonance imaging, *Science* 254:716-719, 1991.

Botteron KN et al: Magnetic resonance imaging in childhood and adolescent bipolar affective disorder: a pilot investigation, *J Am Acad Child Adolesc Psychiatry* 31:258-261, 1992.

Cassanova MF, Naidu S, Goldberg TE: Quantitative magnetic resonance imaging in Rett syndrome, *J Neuropsychiatry Clin Neurosci* 3:66-72, 1991.

Castellanos FX et al: Quantitative morphology of the caudate nucleus in attention deficit hyperactivity disorder, *Am J Psychiatry* 151:1791-1796, 1994.

Chelune GJ et al: Frontal lobe disinhibition in attention deficit disorder, *Child Psychiatry Hum Dev* 16:221-234, 1986.

Chiron C et al: Changes in regional cerebral blood flow during brain maturation in children and adolescents, *J Nucl Med* 33:696-703, 1992.

Chugani HT, Phelps ME: Maturational changes in cerebral function in infants by 18FDG positron emission tomography, *Science* 231:840-843, 1986.

Chugani HT, Phelps ME, Mazziotta JC: Positron emission tomography study of human brain functional development, *Ann Neurol* 22:487-497, 1987.

Coffey CE et al: Quantitative cerebral anatomy in depression, *Arch Gen Psychiatry* 50:7-16, 1993.

Courchesne E, Press GA, Yeung-Courchesne R: Parietal lobe abnormalities detected with MR in patients with infantile autism, *AJR Am J Roentgenol* 160:387-393, 1992.

Courchesne E, Townsend J, Saitoh O: The brain in infantile autism, *Neurology* 44:214-223, 1994.

Courchesne E et al: Hypoplasia of cerebellar lobules VI and VII in infantile autism, *N Engl J Med* 318:1349-1354, 1988.

Dauphinais ID et al: Reduction in temporal lobe size in siblings with schizophrenia: a magnetic resonance imaging study, *Psychiatry Res: Neuroimaging* 35:137-147, 1990.

Demaerel P, Kingsley DPE, Kendall BE: Isolated neurodevelopmental delay in childhood: clinicoradiological correlation in 170 patients, *Pediatr Radiol* 23:29-33, 1993.

Duara R, Kushch A, Gross-Glenn K: Neuroanatomic differences between dyslexic and normal readers on magnetic resonance imaging scans, *Arch Neurol* 48:410-416, 1991.

Gaffney GR, Tsai LY: Magnetic resonance imaging of high level autism, *J Autism Dev Disord* 17:433-438, 1987.

Galaburda AM et al: Developmental dyslexia: four consecutive cases with cortical anomalies, *Ann Neurol* 18:222-223, 1985.

Garber HJ et al: A magnetic resonance imaging study of autism: normal fourth ventricle size and absence of pathology, *Am J Psychiatry* 146:532-534, 1989.

Geidd JN et al: *Quantitative magnetic resonance imaging (MRI) of human brain development: ages 4-18,* Poster session, American College of Neuropsychopharmacology, Dec 13-17, 1993.

Ghjaziuddin M et al: Utility of the head computerized tomography scan in child and adolescent psychiatry, *J Am Acad Child Adolesc Psychiatry* 32:123-126, 1993.

Grodzinsky GM, Diamond R: Frontal lobe functioning in boys with attention-deficit hyperactivity disorder, *Dev Neuropsych* 8:427-445, 1992.

Gur RC, Erwin RJ, Gur Raquel RE: Neurobehavioral probes for physiologic neuroimaging studies. *Arch Gen Psychiatry* 49:409-414, 1992.

Guze BH: Magnetic resonance spectroscopy, *Arch Gen Psychiatry* 48:572-574, 1991.

Hashimoto T et al: Brainstem involvement in high functioning autistic children, *Acta Neurol Scand* 88:123-128, 1993.

Hendren RL et al: *Neuropsychophysiologic study of children at risk for schizophrenia: a preliminary report,* Poster presentation, American Academy of Child and Adolescent Psychiatry Annual Meeting, New York, Oct. 1994.

Holttum JR et al: Magnetic resonance imaging of the posterior fossa in autism, *Biol Psychiatry* 32:1091-1101, 1992.

Hsu M et al: Absence of magnetic resonance imaging evidence of pontine abnormality in infantile autism, *Arch Neurol* 48:1160-1163, 1991.

Hynd GW, Semrud-Clikeman M: Dyslexia and brain morphology, *Psychol Bull* 106:447-487, 1989.

Hynd GW et al: Brain morphology in developmental dyslexia and attention deficit disorder/hyperactivity, *Arch Neurol* 47:919-926, 1990.

Hynd GW et al: Corpus callosum morphology in attention deficit-hyperactivity disorder: morphometric analysis of MRI, *Journal of Learning Disabilities* 24:141-146, 1991.

Jack CR et al: Magnetic resonance image-based hippocampal volumetry: correlation with outcome after temporal lobectomy, *Ann Neurol* 31:138-146, 1992.

Jernigan TL et al: Cerebral structure on magnetic resonance imaging in language and learning-impaired children, *Arch Neurol* 48:539-545, 1991a.

Jernigan TL et al: Maturation of human cerebrum observed in vivo during adolescence, *Brain* 114:2037-2049, 1991b.

Keshavan MS, Kapur S, Pettegrew JW: Magnetic resonance spectroscopy in psychiatry: potential, pitfalls and promise, *Am J Psychiatry* 148:976-984, 1991.

Kim S et al: Functional magnetic resonance imaging of motor cortex: hemispheric asymmetry and handedness. *Science* 261:615-617, 1993.

Kleiman MD, Neff S, Rosman NP: The brain in infantile autism: are posterior fossa structures abnormal? *Neurology* 42:753-760, 1992.

Kuperman S et al: Neuroimaging in child and adolescent psychiatry, *J Am Acad Child Adolesc Psychiatry* 29:159-172, 1990.

Kushch A et al: Temporal lobe surface area measurements on MRI in normal and dyslexic readers, *Neuropsychologia* 31:811-821, 1993.

Kwong KK et al: Dynamic magnetic resonance imaging of human brain activity during primary sensory stimulation, *Proc Natl Acad Sci USA* 89:5675-5679, 1992.

Larsen JP et al: MRI evaluation of the size and symmetry of the planum temporale in adolescents with developmental dyslexia, *Brain Lang* 39:289-301, 1990.

Lassonde M: *The facilitatory influence of the corpus callosum on interhemispheric processing.* In Lepore F, Ptito, and Jasper H, editors: *Two hemispheres-one brain,* New York, 1986, Alan R. Liss.

Leonard CM et al: Anomalous cerebral structure in dyslexia revealed with magnetic resonance imaging, *Arch Neurol* 50:461-469, 1993.

Lou HC, Henriksen L, Bruhn P: Focal cerebral dysfunction in developmental learning disabilities, *Lancet* 335:8-11, 1990.

Lou HC et al: Focal cerebral hypoperfusion in children with dysphasia and/or attention deficit disorder, *Arch Neurol* 41:825-829, 1984.

Lou HC et al: Striatal dysfunction in attention deficit and hyperkinetic disorder, *Arch Neurol* 46:48-52, 1989.

McKenna K, Gordon CT, Rapoport JL: Childhood-onset schizophrenia: timely neurobiological research, *J Am Acad Child Adolesc Psychiatry* 33:771-781, 1994.

Minshew NJ et al: A preliminary 31P MRS study of autism: evidence for undersynthesis and increased degradation of brain membranes, *Biol Psychiatry* 33:762-773, 1993.

Murakami JW et al: Reduced cerebellar hemisphere size and its relationship to vermal hypoplasia in autism, *Arch Neurol* 46:689-694, 1989.

Nasrallah HA et al: Cortical atrophy in young adults with a history of hyperactivity in childhood, *Psychiatry Res* 17:241-246, 1986.

Newhouse JH, Wiener JI: *Understanding MRI,* Boston, 1991, Little, Brown & Co.

Peterson B et al: Reduced basal ganglia volumes in Tourette's syndrome using three-dimensional reconstruction techniques from magnetic resonance images, *Neurology* 43:941-949, 1993.

Piven J et al: Magnetic resonance imaging evidence for a defect of cerebral cortical development in autism, *Am J Psychiatry* 147:734-739, 1990.

Plante E, Swisher L, Vance R: MRI findings in boys with specific language impairment, *Brain Lang* 41:52-66, 1991.

Raichle ME, Grubb RL, Jr Gado MH: Correlation between regional cerebral blood flow and oxidative metabolism: in vivo studies in man, *Arch Neurol* 33:523, 1976.

Reiss AL, Lee J, Freund L: Neuroanatomy of fragile X syndrome: the temporal lobe, *Neurology* 44:1317-1324, 1994.

Reiss AL et al: Neuroanatomy of fragile X females: the posterior fossa, *Am J Hum Genet* 49:279-288, 1991a.

Reiss AL et al: Neuromorphology of fragile X syndrome: the posterior fossa, *Neurology* 29:26-32, 1991b.

Reiss AL et al: Neuroanatomy of Rett syndrome: a volumetric imaging study, *Ann Neurol* 34:227-234, 1993.

Ritvo ER, Freeman BJ, Scheibel AB: Lower Purkinje cell counts in the cerebellas of four autistic subjects: initial findings of the UCLA-NSAC Autopsy Research Report, *Am J Psychiatry* 143:862-866, 1986.

Ritvo E, Garber JH: Cerebellar hypoplasia and autism, *N Engl J Med* 319:1152, 1988.

Rumsey JM et al: Hemispheric asymmetries, fourth ventricular size, and cerebellar morphology in autism, *J Autism Dev Disord* 18:127-137, 1988.

Schaefer GB, Bodensteiner JB: Evaluation of the child with idiopathic mental retardation, *Pediatr Neurol* 39:929-943, 1992.

Schaefer GB et al: Age-related changes in the relative growth of the posterior fossa, *J Child Neurol* 6:15-19, 1991.

Schultz RT et al: Brain morphology in normal and dyslexic children: the influence of sex and age, *Ann Neurol* 35:732-742, 1994.

Semrud-Clikeman M et al: Attention-deficit hyperactivity disorder: magnetic resonance imaging morphometric analysis of the corpus callosum, *J Am Acad Child Adolesc Psychiatry* 33:875-881, 1994.

Shaywitz BA et al: Attention deficit disorder: quantitative analysis of CT, *Neurology* 33:1500-1503, 1983.

Shenton ME et al: Abnormalities of the left temporal lobe and thought disorder in schizophrenia, *N Engl J Med* 327:604-612, 1992.

Shue KL, Douglas VI: Attention deficit hyperactivity disorder and the frontal lobe syndrome, *Brain Cogn* 20:104-124, 1992.

Singer HS et al: Volumetric MRI changes in basal ganglia of children with Tourette's syndrome, *Neurology* 43:950-956, 1993.

Sokoloff L: Relationships among local functional activity, energy metabolism, and blood flow in the central nervous system, *Fed Proc* 40:2311, 1981.

Steinmetz H et al: Anatomical left-right asymmetry of language-related temporal cortex is different in left and right-handers, *Ann Neurol* 29:315-318, 1991.

Stytz MR, Frieder O: Three-dimensional medical imaging modalities: an overview, *Crit Rev Biomed Eng* 18:1-25, 1990.

Suddath RL et al: Temporal lobe pathology in schizophrenia: a quantitative magnetic resonance imaging study, *Am J Psychiatry* 146:464-472, 1989.

Tzika AA et al: Cerebral perfusion in children: detection with dynamic contrast-enhanced T2-weighted MR images, *Pediatr Radiol* 187:449-458, 1993.

Williams RS et al: Autism and mental retardation, *Arch Neurol* 37:749-753, 1980.

Yazgan MY et al: *Functional correlates of basal ganglia alterations in Tourette's syndrome: a preliminary report,* Young Investigator's Poster Session at the 146th Annual Meeting of the American Psychiatric Association, San Francisco, 1993.

Zametkin AJ et al: Brain metabolism in teenagers with attention-deficit hyperactivity disorder, *Arch Gen Psychiatry* 50:333-340, 1993.

Zilbovicius M et al: Regional cerebral blood flow in childhood autism: a SPECT study, *Am J Psychiatry* 149:924-930, 1992.

Chapter 4

Anderson GM et al: Whole blood serotonin in autistic and normal subjects, *J Child Psychol Psychiatry* 28:885-900, 1987.

Anderson LT et al: The effects of haloperidol on discrimination learning and behavioral symptoms in autistic children, *J Autism Dev Disorder* 19:227-239, 1989.

Asperger H: *"Autistic psychopathy" in childhood.* In Frith U, editor: *Autism and Asperger syndrome,* New York, 1944, Cambridge University Press.

Astington JW, Harris PL, Olson DR, editors: *Developing theories of mind,* New York, 1988, Cambridge University Press.

Baron-Cohen S, Leslie A, Frith U: Does the autistic child have a "theory of mind"? *Cognition* 21:37-46, 1985.

Bauman ML: Microscopic neuroanatomic abnormalities in autism, *Pediatrics* 87(Part 2 Suppl):791-796, 1991.

Burd L, Fisher W, Kerbeshian J: A prevalence study of pervasive developmental disorders in North Dakota, *J Am Acad Child Psychiatry* 26:700-703, 1987.

Campbell M et al: *Pharmacotherapy in infantile autism: efficacy and safety.* In Shagass C et al, editors: *Biological psychiatry,* New York, 1985, Elsevier.

Campbell M et al: Naltrexone in autistic children: an acute open dose range tolerance trial, *J Am Acad Child Adolesc Psychiatry* 28:200-206, 1989.

Campbell M et al: Stereotypies and tardive dyskinesia: abnormal movements in autistic children, *Psychopharmacol Bull* 26:260-266, 1990a.

Campbell M et al: Naltrexone in autistic children: a double-blind and placebo-controlled study, *Psychopharmacol Bull* 26:130-135, 1990b.

Campbell M et al: Naltrexone in autistic children: behavioral symptoms and attentional learning, *J Amer Acad Child Adoles Psychiatry* 32:1283-1291, 1993.

Cantwell DP, Baker L, Rutter M: A comparative study of infantile autism and specific developmental receptive language disorder. IV. Analysis of syntax and language function, *J Child Psych Psychiatry* 19:351-363, 1978.

Coleman M, Gillberg C: *The biology of the autistic syndromes,* New York, 1985, Praeger.

Comings DE: The genetics of Rett syndrome: the consequences of a disorder where every case is a mutation, *Amer J Med Genet* 24 (Suppl):383-388, 1986.

Cook E: Autism: review of neurochemical investigation, *Synapse* 6:292-308, 1990.

Courchesne E: Neuroanatomic imaging in autism, *Pediatrics* 87 (Part 2 Suppl):781-790, 1991.

DeMyer MK: *Parents and children in autism,* Washington, DC, 1979, V.H. Winston and Sons.

DeMyer MK, Hingtgen JN, Jackson RK: Infantile autism reviewed: a decade of research, *Schizophr Bull* 7:388-451, 1981.

DeMyer MK et al: Prognosis in autism: a follow-up study, *J Autism Childhood Schizophr* 3:199-245, 1973.

Diagnostic and Statistical Manual of Mental Disorders, ed 3, Washington DC, 1980, American Psychiatric Association, Committee on Nomenclature and Statistics.

Diagnostic and Statistical Manual of Mental Disorders, ed 3 revised, Washington DC, 1987, American Psychiatric Association, Committee on Nomenclature and Statistics.

Diagnostic and Statistical Manual of Mental Disorders, ed 4, Washington DC, 1994, American Psychiatric Association, Committee on Nomenclature and Statistics.

Evans-Jones LG, Rosenbloom L: Disintegrative psychosis in childhood, *Dev Med Child Neurol* 20:462-470, 1978.

Fankhauser MP et al: A double-blind placebo-controlled study of the efficacy of transdermal clonidine in autism, *J Clin Psychiatry* 53:77-82, 1992.

Folstein SE, Piven J: The etiology of autism: genetic influences, *Pediatrics* 87 (Part 2 Suppl):767-773, 1991.

Folstein SE, Rutter M: Infantile autism: a genetic study of 21 twin pairs, *J Psychol Psychiatry* 18:297-321, 1977.

Folstein SE, Rutter M: Autism: familial aggregation and genetic implications, *J Autism Dev Disord* 18:3-30, 1988.

Gadow KD: Pediatric psychopharmacotherapy: a review of recent research, *J Child Psychol Psychiatry* 33:153-195, 1992.

Ghaziuddin M, Tsai L, Ghaziuddin N: A reappraisal of clumsiness as a diagnostic feature of Asperger syndrome, *J Autism Dev Disord* 22:651-656, 1992.

Ghaziuddin M et al: Three siblings with Asperger syndrome: a family case study, *Eur Child Adolesc Psychiatry* 2:44-49, 1993.

Gillberg C: Autistic symptoms in Rett syndrome: the first two years according to mothers' reports, *Brain Dev* 9:499-501, 1987.

Gillberg C: Asperger syndrome in 23 Swedish children, *Dev Med Child Neurol* 31:520-531, 1989.

Gillberg C: *Clinical and neurobiologic aspects of Asperger syndrome in six family studies.* In Frith U, editor: *Autism and Asperger syndrome,* Cambridge, 1991, University Press Cambridge.

Gordon CT et al: A double-blind comparison of clomipramine, desipramine, and placebo in the treatment of autistic disorder, *Arch Gen Psychiatry* 50:441-447, 1993.

Hagberg B: Rett's syndrome: prevalence and impact on progressive severe mental retardation in girls, *Acta Paediatr* 74:405-408, 1985.

Happe F, Frith U: Is autism a pervasive developmental disorder? Debate and argument: how useful is the PDD label? *J Child Psychol Psychiatry* 7:1167-1172, 1991.

Heller T: Dementia infantilis, *Zeitschrift für die Erforschung und Behandlung des Jugendlichen Schwachsinns (Journal for Research and Treatment of Juvenile Feeblemindedness)* 2:141-165, 1908.

Hill AE, Rosenbloom L: Disintegrative psychosis of childhood: teenage follow-up, *Dev Med Child Neurol* 28:34-40, 1986.

Hobson P: *Beyond cognition: a theory of autism.* In Dawson G, editor: *Autism: nature diagnosis and treatment,* New York, 1989, Guilford.

Hobson RP: What is autism? *Psychiatr Clin North Am* 14:1-18, 1991.

Hoshino Y et al: Dexamethasone suppression test in autistic children, *Jpn J Clin Psychiatry* 26:100-102, 1984.

Howlin P, Rutter M: *Treatment of autistic children,* New York, 1987, John Wiley and Sons.

Jaselskis CA et al: Clonidine treatment of hyperactive and impulsive children with autistic disorder, *J Clin Pharmacol* 12:322-327, 1992.

Kanner L: Autistic disturbances of affective contact, *The Nervous Child* 2:217-250, 1943.

Kanner L: Follow-up study of eleven autistic children originally reported in 1943, *J Autism Childhood Schizophr* 1:119-145, 1971.

Kanner L: *Dementia infantilis.* In Kanner L, editor, *Childhood psychosis,* Washington DC, 1973, V. Winston.

Kanner L, Rodriguez A, Ashenden B: How far can autistic children go in matters of social adaptation? *J Autism Dev Disord* 2:9-33, 1972.

Kerbeshian J, Burd L: Asperger's syndrome and Tourette syndrome, *Br J Psychiatry* 48:731-735, 1986.

Kerr AM, Stephenson JBP: Rett's syndrome in the west of Scotland, *BMJ* 291:579-582, 1985.

Kurita H: The concept and nosology of Heller's syndrome: review of articles and report of two cases, *Jpn J Psychiatry Neurol* 42:785-793, 1988.

LeCouteur A, Bailey A, Rutter M: Epidemiologically based twin study of autism. Paper presented at the First World Congress on Psychiatric Genetics, Cambridge, England, 1989.

LeCouteur A et al: Autism Diagnostic Interview: a standardized investigator-based instrument, *J Autism Dev Disord* 19:363-387, 1989.

Leslie AM: Pretense and representation: the origins of "theory of mind," *Psychol Rev* 94:412-426, 1987.

Lockyer L, Rutter M: A five to fifteen year follow-up study of infantile psychosis. IV. Patterns of cognitive ability, *Br J Soc Clin Psychol* 9:152-163, 1970.

Lord C: Autism diagnostic observation schedule, *J Autism Dev Disord* 19:185-212, 1988.

Lord C, Schopler E, Revicki D: Sex differences in autism, *J Autism Dev Disord* 12:317-330, 1982.

Malone RP et al: Repeated episodes of neuroleptic-related dyskinesias in autistic children, *Psychopharmacol Bull* 27:113-117, 1991.

Miles SW, Capelle P: Asperger's syndrome and aminoaciduria: a case example. *Br J Psychiatry* 147:397-399, 1987.

Minshew N, Rattan AI: *The clinical syndrome of autism: developmental and acquired disorders of childhood.* In Rapin I, Segalowitz SJ, editors: *Handbook of neuropsychology, vol 6, child neuropsychology,* Amsterdam, 1992, Elsevier Science Publishers.

Nelson KB: Prenatal and perinatal factors in the etiology of autism, *Pediatrics* 87(Part 2 Suppl):761-766, 1991.

Olsson B, Rett A: Autism and Rett syndrome: behavioral investigations and differential diagnosis, *Dev Med Child Neurol* 29:429-441, 1987.

Ozonoff S, Pennington BF, Rogers SJ: Executive function deficits in high-functioning autistic individuals: relationship to theory of mind, *J Child Psychol Psychiatry* 32:1081-1105, 1991.

Ozonoff S, Rogers SJ, Pennington BF: Asperger's syndrome: evidence of an empirical distinction from high-functioning autism, *J Child Psychol Psychiatry* 132:1107-1122, 1991.

Percy A et al: Rett syndrome and the autistic disorders, *Neurol Clin* 8:659-676, 1990.

Piven J et al: Magnetic resonance imaging evidence for a defect of cerebral cortical development in autism, *Am J Psychiatry* 147:734-739, 1990.

Piven J et al: The prevalence of fragile X in a sample of autistic individuals diagnosed using a standardized interview, *J Amer Acad Child Adolesc Psychiatry* 30:825-830, 1991a.

Piven J et al: Psychiatric disorders in the parents of autistic individuals, *J Amer Acad Child Adolesc Psychiatry* 30:471-478, 1991b.

Piven J et al: Magnetic resonance imaging in autism: measurement of the cerebellum pons and fourth ventricle, *Biol Psychiatry* 31:491-504, 1992a.

Piven J et al: Psychiatric disorders in the parents of autistic individuals [see comments], *J Amer Acad Child Adolesc Psychiatry* 30:471-478, 1991, *J Amer Acad Child Adolesc Psychiatry* 31:370-371, 1992b.

Ratey JJ et al: Open trial effects of beta-blockers on speech and social behaviors in 8 autistic adults, *J Autism Dev Disord* 17:439-446, 1987.

Raymond G, Bauman M, Kemper T: The hippocampus in autism: Golgi analysis, *Ann Neurol* 26:483-484, 1989.

Realmuto GM, August GJ, Garfinkel BD: Clinical effect of buspirone in autistic children, *Psychopharmacology* 9:122-125, 1989.

Ritvo ER et al: Elevated daytime melatonin concentrations in autism: a pilot study, *Eur Child Adolesc Psychiatry* 2:75-78, 1993.

Rutter M: Autistic children: infancy to adulthood, *Semin Psychiatry* 2:435-450, 1970.

Rutter M: The treatment of autistic children, *J Child Psychol Psychiatry* 26:193-214, 1983.

Rutter M, Schopler E: Classification of pervasive developmental disorders: some concepts and considerations, *J Autism Dev Disord* 22:459-479, 1992.

Schopler E et al: Toward objective classification of childhood autism: Childhood Autism Rating Scale (CARS), *J Autism Dev Disord* 10:91-103, 1980.

Schopler E et al: *Helping autistic children through their parents: the TEACCH model.* In Schopler E, Mesibov GB, editors: *The effects of autism on the family,* New York, 1984, Plenum Press.

Schopler E, Reichler R, Renner BR: *The childhood autism rating scale CARS,* Los Angeles, 1988, Western Psychological.

Smalley S, Asarnow R, Spence M: Autism and genetics: a decade of research, *Arch Gen Psychiatry* 45:953-961, 1988.

Steffenburg S et al: A twin study of autism in Denmark, Finland, Iceland, Norway, and Sweden, *J Child Psychol Psychiatry* 30:405-416, 1989.

Stern DN: *The interpersonal world of the infant: a view from psychoanalysis and developmental psychology,* New York, 1985, Basic Books.

Szatmari P, Bartolucci G, Bremner R: Asperger's syndrome and autism: comparisons on early history and outcome, *Dev Med Child Neurol* 31:709-20, 1989.

Szatmari P et al: A vote for Asperger's syndrome, *J Autism Dev Disord* 16:515-517, 1986.

Tantam D, Evered C, Hersov L: Asperger's syndrome and ligamentous laxity, *J Am Acad Child Adolesc Psychiatry* 93:769-774, 1990.

The ICD-10 Classification of Mental and Behavioral Disorders: clinical descriptions and diagnostic guidelines, Geneva, 1992, World Health Organization.

The Rett Syndrome Diagnostic Criteria Work Group: Diagnostic criteria for Rett syndrome, *Ann Neurol* 23:425-428, 1988.

Trevarthen C: *Communication and cooperation in early infancy: a description of primary intersubjectivity.* In Bullowa M, editor: *Before speech: the beginnings of human communication,* Cambridge, 1979, Cambridge University Press.

Tsai LK: Is Rett syndrome a subtype of pervasive developmental disorders? *J Autism Dev Disord* 22:551-561, 1992.

Volkmar FR: Childhood disintegrative disorder: issues for DSM-IV, *J Autism Dev Disord* 22:625-642, 1992.

Volkmar FR, Cohen DJ: Disintegrative disorder or "late onset" autism? *J Child Psychol Psychiatry* 30:717-724, 1989.

Volkmar FR, Cohen DJ: Debate and argument: the utility of the term pervasive developmental disorder, *J Child Psychol Psychiatry* 32:1171-1172, 1991.

Volkmar FR, Stier DM, Cohen DC: Age of recognition of pervasive developmental disorder, *Am J Psychiatry* 142:1450-1452, 1985.

Whitehouse DW, Harris J: Hyperlexia in infantile autism, *J Autism Dev Disord* 11:31-44, 1984.

Wing L: Asperger's syndrome: a clinical account, *Psychol Med* 11:115-129, 1981.

Wing L: *A guide for parents and professionals,* New York, 1985, Brunner/Mazel.

Wing L: *The relationship between Asperger's syndrome and Kanner's autism.* In Frith U, editor: *Autism and Asperger syndrome,* Cambridge, 1991, Cambridge University Press.

Wing L: The definition and prevalence of autism: a review, *Eur J Child Adolesc Psychiatry* 2:61-74, 1993.

Wing L, Gould J: Severe impairments of social interaction and associated abnormalities in children: epidemiology and classification, *J Autism Dev Disord* 9:11-12, 1979.

Witt-Engerstrom I: Rett syndrome: a retrospective pilot study on potential early predictive symptomatology, *Brain Dev* 9:481-486, 1987.

Zoghbi HY et al: Patterns of X chromosome inactivation in the Rett syndrome, *Brain Dev* 12:131-135, 1990.

Chapter 5

Abramowitz AJ et al: ADHD children's responses to stimulant medication and two intensities of a behavioral intervention, *Behav Modif* 16:193-203, 1992.

Anastopoulos AD et al: Stimulant medication and parent training therapies for attention deficit-hyperactivity disorder, *Journal of Learning Disabilities* 24:210-218, 1991 (Review).

Anastopoulos AD et al: Parent training for attention-deficit hyperactivity disorder: its impact on parent functioning, *J Abnorm Child Psychol* 21:581-596, 1993.

Angier N: The debilitating malady called boyhood, *New York Times* Jan. 24, 1994.

Arnold LE et al: Does hair zinc predict amphetamine improvement of ADD/hyperactivity? [see comments], *Int J Neurosci* 50:103-107, 1990.

Balon R: Buspirone for attention deficit hyperactivity disorder? [letter], *J Clin Psychopharmacol* 10:77, 1990.

Barkley RA: A review of stimulant drug research with hyperactive children, *J Child Psychol Psychiatry* 18:137-165, 1977.

Barkley RA et al: The adolescent outcome of hyperactive children diagnosed by research criteria. I. An 8-year prospective follow-up study, *J Am Acad Child Adolesc Psychiatry* 29:546-557, 1990.

Barkley RA et al: Comprehensive evaluation of attention deficit disorder with and without hyperactivity as defined by research criteria, *J Consult Clin Psychol* 58:775-789, 1990.

Barkley RA et al: *Stimulants.* In Werry JS, Aman MG, editors: *Practitioner's Guide to Psychoactive Drugs for Children and Adolescents,* New York, 1993, Plenum Medical Book Co.

Barrickman L et al: Treatment of ADHD with fluoxetine: a preliminary trial, *J Am Acad Child Adolesc Psychiatry* 30:762-767, 1991.

Bauermeister JJ et al: Are attentional-hyperactivity deficits unidimensional or multidimensional syndromes? Empirical findings from a community survey, *J Am Acad Child Adolesc Psychiatry* 31:423-431, 1992.

Biederman J et al: A double-blind placebo controlled study of desipramine in the treatment of ADD. I. Efficacy, *J Am Acad Child Adolesc Psychiatry* 28:777-784, 1989.

Biederman J et al: Family-genetic and psychosocial risk factors in DSM-III attention deficit disorder, *J Am Acad Child Adolesc Psychiatry* 29:526-533, 1990.

Biederman J et al: Further evidence for family-genetic risk factors in attention deficit hyperactivity disorder: patterns of comorbidity in probands and relatives psychiatrically and pediatrically referred samples, *Arch Gen Psych* 49:728-738, 1992.

Birmaher B et al: Sustained release methylphenidate: pharmacokinetic studies in ADDH males, *J Am Acad Child Adolesc Psychiatry* 28:768-772, 1989.

Boris M, Mandel FS: Foods and additives are common causes of the attention deficit hyperactive disorder in children, *Ann Allergy* 72:462-468, 1994 (Review).

Bradley W: The behavior of children receiving benzedrine, *Am J Psychiatry* 94:577-585, 1937.

Brown RT, Sexson SB: Effects of methylphenidate on cardiovascular responses in attention deficit hyperactivity disordered adolescents, *J Adolesc Health Care* 10:179-183, 1989.

Brown RT et al: Methylphenidate and cognitive therapy: a comparison of treatment approaches with hyperactive boys, *J of Abnorm Child Psychol* 13:69-87, 1985.

Buchsbaum M, Wender PH: Average evoked response in normal and minimally brain dysfunctioned children treated with amphetamine: a preliminary report, *Arch Gen Psychiatry* 29:764-770, 1973.

Calderon-Gonzalez R: Attention deficit disorders spectrum, neurological and neuropsychological basis, *Int Pediatr* 8:189-198, 1993.

Cantwell DP, Baker L: Attention deficit disorder with and without hyperactivity: a review and comparison of matched groups, *J Am Acad Child Adolesc Psychiatry* 31:432-438, 1992 (Review).

Cantwell DP, Satterfield BT: Multimodality treatment: a one-year follow-up of 84 hyperactive boys, *Arch Gen Psychiatry* 36:965-974, 1979.

Carter CM et al: Effects of a few food diet in attention deficit disorder, *Arch Dis Child* 69:564-568, 1993.

Casat CD et al: Bupropion in children with attention deficit disorder, *Psychopharmacol Bull* 25:198-201, 1989.

Chan YP et al: Methylphenidate hydrochloride given with or before breakfast. II. Effects on plasma concentration of methylphenidate and ritalinic acid, *Pediatrics* 72:56-59, 1983.

Chess S, Thomas A: Infant bonding: mystique and reality, *Am J Orthopsychiatry* 52:213-221, 1982.

Clay TH et al: Clinical and neuropsychological effects of the novel antidepressant bupropion, *Psychopharmacol Bull* 24:143-148, 1988.

Conners CK: The effects of dexedrine on rapid discrimination and motor control of hyperkinetic children under mild stress, *J Nerv Ment Dis* 142:420-433, 1966.

Conners CK: A teacher rating scale for use in drug studies with children, *Am J Psychiatry* 126:884-888, 1969.

Conners CK: Personal communication, May 27, 1993.

Conners CK: *Attention deficit hyperactivity disorder: assessment and treatment for children and adolescents.* North Tonawanda, N.Y., 1994, Multi-Health Systems, Inc.

Conners CK, Blouin AG: Nutritional effects on behavior of children, *J Psychiatr Res* 17:193-201, 1982.

Conners CK et al: Multimodality therapies: methodologic issues in research and practice, *Child Adolesc Psychiatr Clin North Am* 3:361-377, 1994.

Diagnostic and Statistical Manual of Mental Disorders, Third Edition, Washington, DC, 1980, American Psychiatric Association.

Diagnostic and Statistical Manual of Mental Disorders, Fourth Edition, Washington, DC, 1994, American Psychiatric Association.

Diamond JM: TCA toxicity, *J Am Acad Child Adolesc Psychiatry* 32:1307-1308, 1993.

Diamond JM: *QEEG Evaluation of Children With ADHD.* Presented at the annual meeting of the American Psychiatric Electrophysiology Association, Philadelphia, 1994.

Diamond JM, Deane FP: Conners Teacher's Questionnaire: effects and implications of frequent administration, *J Clin Child Psychol* 19:202-204, 1990.

DuPaul GJ et al: Teacher ratings of academic skills: the development of the Academic Performance Rating Scale, *School Psychology Review* 20:284-300, 1991.

Egger J et al: Controlled trial of oligoantigenic treatment in the hyperkinetic syndrome, *Lancet* 1:540-545, 1985.

Eichelbaum M: Defective oxidation of drugs: pharmacokinetics and their implications, *Clinical Pharmacokinet* 7:1-22, 1982.

Elia J et al: Thyroid function and attention-deficit hyperactivity disorder, *J Am Acad Child Adolesc Psychiatry* 33:169-172, 1994.

Feinberg M, Carroll BJ: Effects of dopamine agonists and antagonists in Tourette's disease, *Arch Gen Psychiatry* 36:979-985, 1979.

Feingold BF: Hyperkinesis and learning disabilities linked to artificial food flavors and colors, *Am J Nurs* 75:797-803, 1975.

Fischer M et al: The adolescent outcome of hyperactive children: predictors of psychiatric, academic, social, and emotional adjustment [see comments], *J Am Acad Child Adolesc Psychiatry* 32:324-332, 1993.

Fox AM, Rieder MJ: Risks and benefits of drugs used in the management of the hyperactive child, *Drug Safety* 9:38-50, 1993 (Review).

Fuller PW: Computer estimated alpha attenuation during problem solving in children with learning disabilities, *Electroencephalogr Clin Neurophysiol* 42:149-156, 1977.

Gadow KD: Relative efficacy of pharmacological, behavioral, and combination treatments for enhancing academic performance, *Clin Psychol Rev* 5:513-533, 1985.

Gadow KD et al: Methylphenidate in hyperactive boys with comorbid tic disorder. II. Short-term behavioral effects in school settings, *J Am Acad Child Adolescent Psychiatry* 31:462-471, 1992.

Giedd JN et al: Quantitative morphology of the corpus callosum in attention deficit hyperactivity disorder, *Am J Psychiatry* 151:665-669, 1994.

Gittelman R, Eskenazi B: Lead and hyperactivity revisited: an investigation of nondisadvantaged children, *Arch Gen Psychiatry* 40:827-833, 1983.

Gittelman R et al: Hyperactive boys almost grown up. I. Psychiatric status, *Arch Gen Psychiatry* 42:937-947, 1985.

Goyette CH et al: Normative data on revised Conners parent and teacher ratings scales, *J Abnorm Child Psychol* 6:221-236, 1978.

Greenhill LL: Attention-deficit hyperactivity disorder: the stimulants, *Child Adolesc Psychiatr Clin North Am* 4:123-168, 1995.

Grünewald-Zuberbier E, Grünewald G: *Event-related EEG changes in children with different abilities to concentrate,* Amsterdam, 1982, Elsevier.

Grünewald-Zurberbier E et al: Hyperactive behavior and EEG arousal reactions in children, *Electroencephalogr Clin Neurophysiol* 38:149-159, 1975.

Hall RA et al: Evoked potential, stimulus intensity, and drug treatment in hyperkinesis, *Psychophysiology* 13:405-418, 1976.

Halperin JM et al: Serotonergic function in aggressive and nonaggressive boys with attention deficit hyperactivity disorder, *Am J Psychiatry* 151:243-248, 1994.

Hassler F: The hyperkinetic child: a historical review, *Acta Paedopsychiatr* 55:147-149, 1992.

Hauser P et al: Attention deficit-hyperactivity disorder in people with generalized resistance to thyroid hormone [see comments], *N Engl J Med* 328:997-1001, 1993.

Hinshaw SP: On the distinction between attentional deficits/hyperactivity and conduct problems/aggression in child psychopathology, *Psychol Bull* 101:443-463, 1987.

Hinshaw SP et al: Cognitive-behavioral and pharmacologic interventions for hyperactive boys: comparative and combined effects, *J Consult Clin Psychol* 52:739-749, 1984.

Hohman LB: Postencephalitic behavior disorder in children, *Johns Hopkins Hosp Bull* 380:372-375, 1922.

Homatidis S, Konstantareas MM: Assessment of hyperactivity: isolating measures of high discriminant ability, *J Consult Clin Psychol* 49:533-541, 1981.

Horn WF et al: Additive effects of dexedrine and self-control training: a multiple assessment, *Behav Modif* 7:383-402, 1983.

Hoza B et al: An examination of the "dosage" effects of both behavior therapy and methylphenidate on the classroom performance of two ADHD children, *Behav Modif* 16:164-192, 1992.

Hunt RD et al: Strategies for study of the neurochemistry of attention deficit disorder in children, *Schizophr Bull* 8:236-252, 1982.

Hunt RD et al: Possible change in noradrenergic receptor sensitivity following methylphenidate treatment: growth hormone and MHPG response to clonidine challenge in children with attention deficit disorder and hyperactivity, *Life Sci* 35:885-897, 1984.

Hunt RD et al: Clonidine benefits children with attention deficit disorder and hyperactivity: report of a double-blind placebo-crossover therapeutic trial, *J Am Acad Child Psychiatry* 24:617-629, 1985.

Hunt RD et al: Clonidine in child and adolescent psychiatry, *J Child Adolesc Psychopharmacol* 1:87-102, 1990.

Hunt RD et al: Trial of guanfacine in the treatment of attention-deficit hyperactivity disorder, *J Am Acad Child Adolesc Psychiatry* 34:50-54, 1995.

Hynd GW et al: Attention deficit-hyperactivity disorder and asymmetry of the caudate nucleus, *J Child Neurol* 8:339-347, 1993.

Ialongo NS et al: The effects of a multimodal intervention with attention-deficit hyperactivity disorder children: a 9-month follow-up, *J Am Acad Child Adolesc Psychiatry* 32:182-189, 1993.

Ialongo NS et al: Effects of psychostimulant medication on self-perceptions of competence, control, and mood in children with attention deficit hyperactivity disorder, *J Clin Child Psychol* 23:161-173, 1994.

John ER: The role of quantitative EEG topographic mapping or 'neurometrics' in the diagnosis of psychiatric and neurological disorders: the pros, *Electroencephalogr Clin Neurophysiol* 73:2-4, 1989.

Johnston C et al: Psychostimulant rebound in attention deficit disordered boys, *J Am Acad Child Adolesc Psychiatry* 27:806-810, 1988.

Kuehne C et al: Differences between children with attention deficit disorder, children with specific learning disabilities, and normal children, *J School Psychol* 25:161-166, 1987.

Li XR et al: Diagnosis of attention deficit disorder with hyperactivity in Chinese boys, *J Am Acad Child Adolesc Psychiatry* 28:497-500, 1989.

Lou HC et al: Focal cerebral hypoperfusion in children with dysphasia and/or attention deficit disorder, *Arch Neurol* 41:825-829, 1984.

Lou HC et al: Striatal dysfunction in attention deficit and hyperkinetic disorder, *Arch Neurol* 46:48-52, 1989.

Lubar JF: Discourse on the development of EEG diagnostics and biofeedback for attention-deficit/hyperactivity disorders, *Biofeedback Self Regul* 16:201-225, 1991 (Review).

Lubar JO, Lubar JF: Electroencephalographic biofeedback of SMR and beta for treatment of attention deficit disorders in a clinical setting, *Biofeedback Self Regul* 9:1-23, 1984.

Mann CA et al: Quantitative analysis of EEG in boys with attention-deficit-hyperactivity disorder: controlled study with clinical implications, *Pediatr Neurol* 8:30-36, 1992.

Mannuzza S et al: Adult outcome of hyperactive boys: educational achievement, occupational rank, and psychiatric status, *Arch Gen Psychiatry* 50:565-576, 1993.

Matochik JA et al: Cerebral glucose metabolism in adults with attention deficit hyperactivity disorder after chronic stimulant treatment, *Am J Psychiatry* 151:658-664, 1994.

Matsuura M et al: A cross-national EEG study of children with emotional and behavioral problems: a WHO collaborative study in the Western Pacific Region, *Biol Psychiatry* 34:59-65, 1993.

Mattes JA, Gittelman R: Effects of artificial food colorings in children with hyperactive symptoms: a critical review and results of a controlled study, *Arch Gen Psychiatry* 38:714-718, 1981.

Mattes JA, Gittelman R: Growth of hyperactive children on maintenance regimen of methylphenidate, *Arch Gen Psychiatry* 40:317-321, 1983.

McMillen BA: CNS stimulants: two distinct mechanisms of action for amphetamine-like drugs, *Trends Pharmacol Sci* 4:429-432, 1983.

Morrison J, Stewart M: A family study of hyperactive child syndrome, *Biol Psychiatry* 3:189-195, 1971.

Morrison J, Stewart M: The psychiatric status of the legal families of adopted hyperactive children, *Arch Gen Psychiatry* 28:888-891, 1973.

Offord DR: Child psychiatric disorders: prevalence and perspectives, *Psychiatr Clin North Am* 8:637-652, 1985.

Patterson GR: *Families,* rev ed, Champaign, Ill., 1975, Research Press.

Patterson GR: *Living With Children,* rev ed, Champaign, Ill., 1976, Research Press.

Patterson GR, Forgatch M: *Family living series. I. Five cassette tapes to be used with "living with children and families,"* Champaign, Ill., 1975, Research Press.

Petti TA, Law W: Abrupt cessation of high-dose imipramine in children, *JAMA* 246:768-769, 1981.

Physician's Desk Reference, Montvale, N.J., 1994, Medical Economics Co.

Pisterman S et al: The role of parent training in treatment of preschoolers with ADDH, *Am J Orthopsychiatry* 62:397-408, 1992.

Pliszka SR: Tricyclic antidepressants in the treatment of children with attention deficit disorder, *J Am Acad Child Adolesc Psychiatry* 26:127-132, 1987.

Pollard S et al: The effects of parent training and Ritalin on the parent-child interactions of hyperactive boys, *Child Fam Ther* 5:51-69, 1983.

Popper CW, Elliott GR: Sudden death and tricyclic antidepressants: clinical considerations for children, *J Child Adolesc Psychopharmacol* 1:125-131, 1990.

Quiason N et al: Buspirone for aggression, *Am Acad Child Adolesc Psychiatry* 30:1026, 1991 (Letter).

Rapport MD et al: Attention deficit hyperactivity disorder and methylphenidate: the relationship between gross body weight and drug response in children, *Psychopharmacol Bull* 25:285-290, 1989.

Riddle MA et al: Sudden death in children receiving Norpramin: a review of three reported cases and commentary, *J Am Acad Child Adolesc Psychiatry* 30:104-108, 1991.

Riddle MA et al: Another sudden death in a child treated with desipramine, *J Am Acad Child Adolesc Psychiatry* 32:792-797, 1993 (Review).

Rockstroh B et al: *Biofeedback: evaluation and therapy in children with attentional dysfunctions,* New York, 1990, Springer-Verlag.

Rogeness GA et al: Attention deficit disorder symptoms and urine catecholeamines, *Psychiatry Res* 27:241-251, 1989.

Rutter M: Syndromes attributed to "minimal brain dysfunction" in childhood, *Am J Psychiatry* 139:21-33, 1982.

Rutter M: *Behavioral studies: questions and findings on the concept of a distinctive syndrome.* In Rutter M, editor: *Developmental Neuropsychiatry,* New York, 1983, Guilford Press.

Ryan ND: Heterocyclic antidepressants in children and adolescents, *J Child Adolesc Psychopharmacol* 1:21-31, 1990.

Safer DJ: A familial factor in minimal brain dysfunction, *Behav Genet* 3:175-186, 1973.

Safer DJ, Krager JM: A survey of medication treatment for hyperactive/inattentive students, *JAMA* 260:2256-2258, 1988.

Satterfield BT, Cantwell DP: A two-year evaluation of 61 hyperactive boys, *Arch Gen Psychiatry* 37:915, 1980.

Satterfield BT, Cantwell DP: Three-year multimodality treatment study of 100 hyperactive boys, *J Pediatr* 98:650-655, 1981.

Satterfield JH: EEG issues in children with minimal brain dysfunction, *Semin Psychiatry* 5:35-46, 1973.

Satterfield JH et al: EEG aspects in the diagnosis and treatment of minimal brain dysfunction, *Ann N Y Acad Sci* 205:273, 1973.

Satterfield JH et al: Therapeutic interventions to prevent delinquency in hyperactive boys, *J Am Acad Child Adolesc Psychiatry* 26:56-64, 1987.

Satterfield JH et al: Ontogeny of selective attention effects on event-related potentials in attention-deficit hyperactivity disorder and normal boys, *Biol Psychiatry* 28:879-903, 1990.

Sergeant J, Steinhausen H: European perspectives on hyperkinetic disorder, *Eur J Child Adolesc Psychiatry* 1:34-41, 1992.

Shaywitz BA et al: Paradoxical response to amphetamine in developing rats treated with 6-hydroxydopamine, *Nature* 261:153-155, 1976a.

Shaywitz BA et al: Selective brain dopamine depletion in developing rats: an experimental model of minimal brain dysfunction, *Science* 191:305-308, 1976b.

Shaywitz SE et al: *Monoaminergic mechanisms in hyperactivity.* In Rutter M, editor: *Dev Neuropsych,* New York, 1983, The Guilford Press.

Shaywitz SE, Shaywitz BA: *Attention deficit disorder: diagnosis and role of Ritalin in management.* In Greenhill LL, Osman BB, editors: *Ritalin, Theory and Patient Management,* New York, 1991, Mary Ann Liebert.

Shetty T: Alpha rhythms in the hyperkinetic child, *Nature* 234:476, 1971.

Shetty T: Some neurologic electrophysiologic and biochemical correlates of the hyperkinetic syndrome, *Pediatr Ann* 29:29-38, 1973.

Silva PA et al: Blood lead, intelligence, reading attainment, and behaviour in eleven year old children in Dunedin, New Zealand, *J Child Psychol Psychiatry* 29:43-52, 1988.

Stevenson J: Evidence for a genetic etiology in hyperactivity in children, *Behav Genet* 22:337-344, 1992.

Sunder TR: Attention deficit-hyperactivity disorder reductio ad absurdum, *J Child Neurol* 7:454-458, 1992.

Sverd J et al: Behavior disorder and attention deficits in boys with Tourette syndrome, *J Am Acad Child Adolesc Psychiatry* 27:413-417, 1988.

Sverd J et al: Methylphenidate treatment of attention-deficit hyperactivity disorder in boys with Tourette's syndrome, *J Am Acad Child Adolesc Psychiatry* 28:574-579, 1989.

Swanson JM et al: Methylphenidate hydrochloride given with or before breakfast. I. Behavioral, cognitive, and electrophysiologic effects, *Pediatrics* 72:49-55, 1983.

Taylor EA: Childhood hyperactivity, *Br J Psychiatry* 149:562-573, 1986 (Review).

Taylor MJ et al: Changes in event-related potentials with stimulant medication in children with attention deficit hyperactivity disorder, *Biol Psychol* 36:139-156, 1993.

Thomson GO et al: Blood-lead levels and children's behaviour—results from the Edinburgh Lead Study, *J Child Psychol Psychiatry* 30:515-528, 1989.

Urion DK: Attention deficit hyperactivity disorder: pharmacological response predicted by neurological subtype, *Ann Neurol* 24:314, 1988.

U.S. Department of Education: *Memorandum from the United States Department of Education, Office of Special Education and Rehabilitative Services to Chief State School Officers,* Sept. 16, 1991.

Viesselman JO et al: *Antidysthymic drugs.* In Werry JS, Aman MG, editors: *Practitioner's guide to psychoactive drugs for children and adolescents,* New York, 1993, Plenum Medical Book Co.

Wechsler D: *Manual for the Wechsler Intelligence Scale for Children—Revised,* San Antonio, 1974, The Psychological Corporation.

Wechsler D: *Manual for the Wechsler Intelligence Scale for Children—Third Edition,* San Antonio, 1991, The Psychological Corporation.

Weintraub S, Mesulam M: Right cerebral dominance in spatial attention: further evidence based on ipsilateral neglect, *Arch Neurol* 44:621-625, 1987.

Weiss B: Food additives and environmental chemicals as sources of childhood behavior disorders, *J Am Acad Child Psychiatry* 21:144-152, 1982.

Weiss B et al: Behavioral response to artificial food colors, *Science* 207:1487-1489, 1980.

Weiss RE et al: Attention-deficit hyperactivity disorder and thyroid function, *J Pediatr* 123:539-545, 1993.

Weizman A et al: Imipramine binding to platelets of children with attention deficit disorder with hyperactivity, *Biol Psychiatry* 23:491-496, 1988.

Wender PH: Some speculations concerning a possible biochemical basis of minimal brain dysfunction, *Life Sciences* 14:1605-1621, 1971.

Whalen CK, Henker B: Therapies for hyperactive children: comparisons, combinations, and compromises. *J Consult Clin Psychol* 59:126-137, 1991.

Wilens TE et al: Electrocardiographic effects of desipramine and 2-hydroxydesipramine in children, adolescents, and adults treated with desipramine, *J Am Acad Child Adolesc Psychiatry* 32:798-804, 1993.

Zametkin AJ et al: Phenylethylamine excretion in attention deficit disorder, *J Am Acad Child Psychiatry* 23:310-314, 1984.

Zametkin AJ et al: Cerebral glucose metabolism in adults with hyperactivity of childhood onset [see comments], *N Engl J Med* 323:1361-1366, 1990.

Zametkin AJ et al: Brain metabolism in teenagers with attention-deficit hyperactivity disorder, *Arch Gen Psychiatry* 50:333-340, 1993.

Chapter 6

Campbell N, Gonzalez NM, Silva RR: The pharmacologic treatment of conduct disorders and rage outbursts, *Psychiatr Clin North Am* 15:69-85, 1992.

Diagnostic and statistical manual of mental disorders, ed 4, Washington, 1994, American Psychiatric Press.

Egan J: *Oppositional defiant disorder.* In Wiener JM, editor: *Textbook of child and adolescent psychiatry,* Washington, 1991, American Psychiatric Press.

Hendren RL: *Conduct disorder in childhood.* In Wiener JM, editor: *Textbook of child and adolescent psychiatry,* Washington, 1991, American Psychiatric Press.

Hinshaw SP, Lahey BB, Hart EL: Issues of taxonomy and comorbidity in the development of conduct disorder, *Dev psychopathol* 5:31-50, 1993.

Keller MB et al: The disruptive behavior disorder in children and adolescents: comorbidity and clinical course, *J Am Acad Child Adolesc Psychiatry* 31:204-209, 1992.

Lahey BB et al: Oppositional defiant and conduct disorders: issues to be resolved for *DSM-IV, J Am Acad Child Adolesc Psychiatry* 31:539-546, 1992.

Laite G, Galvin MR: Conduct disorder: a review, *Indiana Med* 172-179, Mar 1990.

Lavin MR, Rifkin A: Diagnosis and pharmacotherapy of conduct disorder, *Prog Neuropsychopharmacol Biol Psychiatry* 17:875-885, 1993.

Lewis DO: *Adolescent conduct and antisocial disorders.* In Wiener JM, editor: *Textbook of child and adolescent psychiatry,* Washington DC, 1991, American Psychiatric Press.

Lewis DO: *Conduct disorder.* In Lewis M, editor: *Child and adolescent psychiatry, a comprehensive textbook,* Baltimore, 1991, Williams & Wilkins.

Loeber R: Antisocial behavior: more enduring than changeable? *J Am Acad Child Adolesc Psychiatry* 30:393-397, 1991.

Loeber R: Oppositional defiant disorder and conduct disorder, *Hosp Commun Psychiatry* 42:1099-1102, 1991.

Loeber R et al: Developmental pathways in disruptive child behavior, *Dev Psychopathol* 5:103-134, 1993.

Rey JM: Oppositional defiant disorder, *Am J Psychiatry* 150:1769-1778, 1993.

Zahn TP, Kruesi MJP: Autonomic activity in boys with disruptive behavior disorders, *Psychophysiology* 30:605-614, 1993.

Wood IK, Singh N: The neurobiology of conduct disorder. (Submitted for publication).

Chapter 7

Amaya-Jackson L, March JS: *Post traumatic stress disorder in children and adolescents.* In March JS, editor: *Anxiety disorders in children and adolescents,* New York, 1995, Guilford Press.

American Psychiatric Association: *Diagnostic and statistical manual of mental disorders: third edition,* Washington DC, 1980, American Psychiatric Press.

American Psychiatric Association: *Diagnostic and statistical manual of mental disorders: fourth edition,* Washington DC, 1994, American Psychiatric Press.

Anderson JC et al: DSM-III disorders in preadolescent children, *Arch Gen Psychiatry* 44:69-76, 1987.

Bandura A: *Social foundations of thought and action: a social cognitive theory,* Englewood Cliffs, N.J., 1986, Prentice-Hall.

Barrios B, O'Dell S: *Fears and anxieties.* In Mash EJ, Barkley RA, editors: *Treatment of childhood disorders,* New York, 1989, Guilford Press.

Bell-Dolan D, Brazeal TJ: Separation anxiety disorder, overanxious disorder, and school refusal, *Child Adolesc Psychiatr Clin North Am* 2:563-580, 1993.

Beidel DC, Morris TL: *Social phobia.* In March JS, editor: *Anxiety disorders in children and adolescents,* New York, Guilford Press (in press).

Beidel DC, Turner SM, Morris TL: The social phobia and anxiety inventory for children: psychometric characteristics. Manuscript in preparation.

Berg CJ, Rapoport JL, Flament M: The Leyton obsessional inventory-child version, *Psychopharmacol Bull* 21:1057-1059, 1985.

Berg CJ, Rapoport J, Wolff R: *Behavioral treatment for obsessive-compulsive disorder in childhood.* In Rapoport J, editor: *Obsessive-compulsive disorder in children and adolescents,* Washington DC, 1989, American Psychiatric Press.

Biederman J et al: Behavioral inhibition as a temperamental risk factor for anxiety disorders, *Child Adolesc Psychiatr Clin North Am* 2:667-683, 1993.

Birmaher B et al: Fluoxetine for childhood anxiety disorders, *J Am Acad Child Adolesc Psychiatry* 33:993-999, 1994.

Black B: Neurobiology of anxiety disorders, *Child Adolesc Psychiatr Clin North Am* 2:749-763, 1993.

Black B: *Separation anxiety disorder and panic disorder.* In March JS, editor: *Anxiety disorders in children and adolescents,* New York, Guilford Press (in press).

Black B, Uhde TW: Elective mutism as a variant of social phobia, *J Am Acad Child Adolesc Psychiatry* 31:1090-1094, 1992.

Black B, Uhde TW: Treatment of elective mutism with fluoxetine: a double-blind, placebo-controlled study, *J Am Acad Child Adolesc Psychiatry* 33:1000-1006, 1994.

Broberg A, Lamb ME, Hwang P: Inhibition: its stability and correlates in sixteen- to forty-month-old children, *Child Dev* 61:1153-1163, 1990.

Brown E, Wilson V, Laybourne PC: Diagnosis and treatment of elective mutism in children, *J Am Acad Child Adolesc Psychiatry* 2:605-617, 1963.

Chambers WJ et al: The assessment of affective disorders in children and adolescents by semistructured interview: test-retest reliability of the Schedule for Affective Disorders and Schizophrenia in School-Age Children, Present Episode Version, *Arch Gen Psychiatry* 42:696-702, 1985.

Charney DS et al: Serotonin function in obsessive compulsive disorder: a comparison of the effects of tryptophan and m-chlorophenylpiperazine in patients and healthy subjects, *Arch Gen Psychiatry* 45:177-185, 1988.

Cheek JM, Buss AH: Shyness and sociability, *J Pers Soc Psych* 41:330-339, 1981.

Clark DB: *Assessment of social anxiety in adolescent alcohol abusers.* Presented at the Anxiety Disorders Association of America Annual Convention, Charleston, S.C., March 1993.

Coplan JD et al: Amelioration of mitralvalve prolapse after treatment of panic disorder, *Am J Psychiatry* 149:1587-1588, 1992.

Costello EJ: Developments in child psychiatry epidemiology, *J Am Acad Child Adolesc Psychiatry* 28:836-841, 1989.

Crumley FE: The masquerade of mutism, *J Am Acad Child Adolesc Psychiatry* 29:318-319, 1990.

Davidson J: *Childhood histories of adult social phobics.* Presented at the Anxiety Disorders Association of America Convention, Charleston, S.C., March 1993.

Dulcan MK, Popper CW: *A concise guide to child and adolescent psychiatry,* Washington DC, 1991, American Psychiatric Press.

Eth S, Pynoos R: *Posttraumatic stress disorders in children,* Washington DC, 1985, American Psychiatric Press.

Flament MF et al: Clomipramine treatment of childhood obsessive-compulsive disorder: a double-blind controlled study, *Arch Gen Psychiatry* 42:977-983, 1985.

Flament MF et al: Obsessive-compulsive disorder in adolescence: an epidemiological study, *J Am Acad Child Adolesc Psychiatry* 27:764-771, 1988.

Francis G, Beidel D: Cognitive behavioral psychotherapy. In March JS, editor: *Anxiety disorders in children and adolescents,* New York, Guilford Press (in press).

Freud S: *Analysis of phobia in a five year old boy*, standard ed, London, 1909, Hogarth Press.

Freud S: *Beyond the pleasure principle* (1920). In Strachey J, editor: *Complete psychological works,* London, 1959, Hogarth Press.

Freud S: *Inhibitions, symptoms and anxiety* (1926), New York, 1959, WW Norton and Co.

Goodman WK, Price LH, Rasmussen SA: efficacy of fluvoxamine in obsessive-compulsive disorder: a double-blind comparison with placebo, *Arch Gen Psychiatry* 46:36-44, 1989.

Golwyn DH, Weinstock RC: Phenelzine treatment of elective mutism: a case report, *J Clin Psychiatry* 51:384-385, 1990.

Grinker R, Spiegel J: *Men under stress,* Philadelphia, 1945, Blakiston.

Hayden TL: Classification of elective mutism, *J Am Acad Child Adolesc Psychiatry* 19:118-133, 1980.

Helzer JE, Robbins LN, McEvoy L: Post-traumatic stress disorder in the general population: findings of the epidemiologic catchment area survey, *N Engl J Med* 317:1630-1634, 1987.

Herjanic B, Reich W: Development of a structured psychiatric interview for children: agreement between child and parent on individual symptoms, *J Abnorm Child Psychol* 10:307-324, 1982.

Hodges K: *The child assessment schedule,* unpublished manuscript, Eastern Michigan University.

Insel TR et al: Obsessive-compulsive disorder and serotonin: is there a connection? *Biol Psychiatry* 20:1174-1188, 1985.

Kagan J, Reznick JS, Snidman N: The physiology and psychology of behavioral inhibition in young children, *Child Dev* 58:1459-1473, 1987.

Kagan J et al: Behavioral inhibition to the unfamiliar, *Child Dev* 55:2212-2225, 1984.

Kashani JH, Orvaschel H: A community study of anxiety in children and adolescents, *Am J Psychiatry* 147:313-318, 1990.

Kendall PC, Chansky TE: Considering cognition in anxiety disordered children, *J Anxiety Dis* 5:167-185, 1991.

Kendall PC et al: Treating anxiety disorders in children and adolescents. In Kendall PC, editor: *Child and adolescent therapy,* New York, 1991, Guilford Press.

Klein RG, Koplewicz HS, Kanner A: Imipramine treatment of children with separation anxiety disorder, *J Am Acad Child Adolesc Psychiatry* 31:21-28, 1992.

Kolvin I, Fundudis T: Elective mute children: psychological, development, and background factors, *J Child Psychol Psychiatry* 22:219-232, 1981.

Kratochwill TR: *Selective mutism: implications for research and treatment,* Hillsdale, N.J., 1981, Lawrence Erlbaum Association.

Kratochwill TR, Brody GH, Piersel WC: Elective mutism in children, *Adv Clin Child Psychol* 2:194-240, 1979.

Labbe EE, Williamson DA: Behavioral treatment of elective mutism: a review of the literature, *Clin Psychol Rev* 4:273-294, 1984.

Last CG et al: Comparison of DSM-III separation anxiety and overanxious disorders: demographic characteristics and patterns of comorbidity, *J Am Acad Child Adolesc Psychiatry* 26:527-521, 1987.

Last CG et al: Anxiety disorders in children and their families, *Arch Gen Psychiatry* 48:928-934, 1991.

Leitenberg H, Callahan E: Reinforced practice and reduction of different kinds of fears in adults and children, *Behav Res Ther* 11:19-30, 1973.

Leonard HL, Lenane MC, Swedo SE: Obsessive-compulsive disorder, In Leonard HL, editor, *Child Adolesc Psychiatr Clin North Am* 2:655-666, Philadelphia, P.A., 1993, W.B. Saunders Co.

Leonard HL, Rapoport JL: Separation anxiety, overanxious and avoidant disorders. In Weiner JM, editor: *Textbook of child and adolescent psychiatry,* Washington DC, 1991, American Psychiatric Press.

Livingston R: *Anxiety disorders.* In Lewis M, editor: *Child and adolescent psychiatry: a comprehensive textbook,* Baltimore, 1991, Williams and Wilkins.

Lyons JA: Post-traumatic stress disorder in children and adolescents: a review of the literature, *Dev Behav Pediatr* 8:349-356, 1987.

Mahler MS, Pine F, Bergman A: *The psychological birth of the human infant: symbiosis and individuation,* New York, 1975, Basic Books.

March JS, Mulle K, Herbel B: Behavioral psychotherapy for children and adolescents with obsessive-compulsive disorder: an open trial of a new protocol driven treatment package, *J Am Acad Child Adolesc Psychiatry* 33:333-341, 1994.

Marks IM: *Fears, phobias and rituals,* New York, 1987, Oxford University Press.

McDougle CJ et al: *Haloperidol addition in fluvoxamine refractory OCD.* Presented at the American Psychiatric Association, Washington DC, May 1992.

McGee R et al: DSM-III disorders in large samples of adolescents, *J Am Acad Child Adolesc Psychiatry* 29:611-619, 1990.

Moreau D, Follett C: Panic disorder in children and adolescents, *Child Adolesc Psychiatr Clin North Am* 2:581-602, 1993.

Ollendick TH: Fear reduction techniques with children. In Hersen M, Eisler RM, Miller PM, editors: *Progress in behavior modification,* vol 8, New York, 1979, Academic Press.

Ollendick TH, King NJ, Hamilton DI: Origins of childhood fears: an evaluation of Rachman's theory of fear acquisition, *Behav Res Ther* 29:117-123, 1991.

Ornitz E, Pynoos R: Startle modulation in children with post-traumatic stress disorder, *Am J Psychiatry* 146:866-870, 1989.

Ost LG: Age of onset in different phobias, *J Abnorm Psychol* 96:223-229, 1987.

Perrin S, Last CG: Do childhood anxiety measures measure anxiety? *J Abnorm Child Psychol* 20:567-578, 1993.

Pigott TA et al: *A controlled trial of clonazepam augmentation in OCD patients with clomipramine or fluoxetine.* Presented at the American Psychiatric Association, Washington DC, 1992.

Popper CW: Psychopharmacologic treatment of anxiety disorders in adolescents and children, *J Clin Psychiatry* 54(suppl):52-63, 1993.

Riddle MA et al: Double-blind, crossover trial of fluoxetine and placebo in children and adolescents with obsessive-compulsive disorder, *J Am Acad Child Adolesc Psychiatry* 31:1062-1069, 1992.

Rosenbaum JF et al: Behavioral inhibition in children of parents with panic disorder and agoraphobia: a controlled study, *Arch Gen Psychiatry* 45:463-470, 1988.

Rosenbaum JF et al: Further evidence of an association between behavioral inhibition and anxiety disorders: results from a family study of children from a non-clinical sample, *J Psychiatric Res* 25:49-65, 1991.

Rutter M, Tizard J, Whitmore K: *Education, health and behavior,* London, 1970, Longmans.

Shear MK et al: A psychodynamic model of panic disorder, *Am J Psychiatry* 150:859-866, 1993.

Silverman WK, Eisen AR: Age differences in the reliability of parent and child reports of child anxious symptomatology using a structured interview, *J Am Acad Child Adolesc Psychiatry* (in press).

Silverman WK, Rabian B: Simple phobias, *Child Adolesc Psychiatr Clin North Am* 2:603-623, 1993.

Simeon JG et al: Clinical, cognitive and neurophysiological effects of alprazolam in children and adolescents with overanxious and avoidant disorders, *J Am Acad Child Adolesc Psychiatry* 31:29, 1992.

Stallings P, March JS: Assessment of anxiety in children and adolescents. In March JS, editor: *Anxiety disorders in children and adolescents,* New York, Guilford Press (in press).

Strauss CC et al: Overanxious disorder: an examination of developmental differences, *J Abnorm Child Psychol* 16:433-443, 1988.

Swedo S: Rituals and releasers: an ethological model of obsessive-compulsive disorder. In Rapoport JL, editor: *Obsessive-compulsive disorder in children and adolescents,* Washington DC, 1989, American Psychiatric Press.

Swedo SE et al: Obsessive-compulsive disorder in children and adolescents: clinical phenomenology of 70 consecutive cases, *Arch Gen Psychiatry* 46:335-341, 1989.

Terr L: Childhood traumas: an outline and overview, *Am J Psychiatry* 148:10-19, 1991.

Thomas A, Chess S: *Temperament and development,* New York, 1977, Brunner/Mazel.

Tramer M: Elektiver Mutismus bei Kindern, *Kinderpsychiatrie,* 1934.

Turner SM, Townsley RM, Beidel DC: Potential etiological factors in social phobia, manuscript in preparation, 1993.

Turner SM et al: Psychopathology of social phobia and comparison to avoidant personality disorder, *J Abnorm Psychol* 95:389-394, 1986.

Valleni-Basile LA et al: Frequency of obsessive-compulsive disorder in a community sample of young adolescents, *J Am Acad Child Adolesc Psychiatry* 33:782-794, 1994.

Von Korff MR, Eaton WW, Keyl PM: The epidemiology of panic attack and panic disorder: results of three community surveys, *Am J Epidemiol* 122:970-981, 1985.

Walker HM et al: Differential effects of reinforcing topographic components of free play social interaction: analysis and systematic replication, *Behav Modif* 3:291-321, 1979.

Wergeland H: Elective mutism, *Acta Psychiatr Scand* 59:218-228, 1979.

Whitaker A et al: Uncommon troubles in young people: prevalence estimates of selected psychiatric disorders in a non-referred adolescent population, *Arch Gen Psychiatry* 47:4897-4896, 1990.

Wilkins R: A comparison of elective mutism and emotional disorders in children, *Br J Psychiatry* 146:198-203, 1985.

Wolpe J: *Psychotherapy by reciprocal inhibition,* Stanford, Calif., 1958, Stanford.

Wright HH: Early identification and intervention with children who refuse to speak, *J Am Acad Child Adolesc Psychiatry* 24:739-746, 1985.

Chapter 8

Akiskal HA et al: Affective disorders in referred children and younger siblings of manic-depressives, *Arch Gen Psychiatry* 42:996-1003, 1985.

Ambrosini PJ et al: Antidepressant treatments in children and adolescents. I. Affective Disorders, *J Am Acad Child Adolesc Psychiatry* 32:1:1-6, 1993.

American Psychiatric Association: *Diagnostic and statistical manual of mental disorders,* ed 4, Washington, DC, 1994a, American Psychiatric Press.

American Psychiatric Association: *Practice guidelines for the treatment of patients with bipolar disorder,* Washington, DC, 151:12, 1994b.

Asarnow JR et al: Childhood-onset depressive disorders: a follow-up study of rates of rehospitalization and out-of-home placement among child psychiatric inpatients, *J Affect Disord* 15:245-253, 1988.

Beck A, Beamesderfer A: Assessment of depression: the revised Beck Depression Inventory, *Psychol Measurements Psychopharmacol* 7:151-169, 1974.

Biederman J et al: Evidence of familial association between attention deficit disorder and major affective disorders, *Arch Gen Psychiatry* 48:633-642, 1991.

Bird HR et al: Estimates of the prevalence of childhood maladjustment in a community survey on Puerto Rico: the use of combined measures, *Arch Gen Psychiatry* 45:1078-1084, 1988.

Boulos C et al: An open naturalistic trial of fluoxetine in adolescents and young adults with treatment-resistant major depression, *J Child Adolesc Psychopharmacol* 2:103-111, 1991.

Bowring MA, Kovacs M: Difficulties in diagnosing manic disorders among children and adolescents, *J Am Acad Child Adolesc Psychiatry* 31:611-614, 1992.

Brumback RA, Dietz-Schmidt SG, Weinberg WA: Depression in children referred to an educational diagnostic center: diagnosis and treatment and analysis of criteria and literature review, *Disord Nerv Syst,* 38:529-535, 1977.

Brumback RA, Weinberg WA: Mania in childhood. II. Therapeutic trial of lithium carbonate and further description of manic-depressive illness in children, *Am J Dis Child* 131:1122-1126, 1977.

Butler L et al: The effect of two school-based intervention programs on depressive symptoms in preadolescents, *Am Educ Research J* 17:111, 1980.

Carlson GA, Kashani JH: Manic symptoms in a non-referred adolescent population, *J Affect Dis* 15:219-226, 1988.

Delong GR: Lithium carbonate treatment of select behavior disorders in children suggesting manic-depressive illness, *J Pediatr* 93:689-694, 1978.

Delong GR, Alderschof AL: Long-term experience with lithium treatment in childhood: correction with clinical diagnosis, *J Am Acad Child Adolesc Psychiatry* 26:389-394, 1987.

Depue RA et al: A behavioral paradigm for identifying persons at risk for bipolar depressive disorder: a conceptual framework and five validation studies, *J Abnorm Psychol* 90:381-437, 1981.

Eastgate J, Gilmour L: Long-term outcome of depressed children: a follow-up study, *Dev Med Child Neurol* 26:68-72, 1984.

Emslie GJ et al: Children with major depression show reduced rapid eye movement latencies, *Arch Gen Psychiatry* 47:119-124, 1990.

Fleming JE, Boyle MH, Offord DR: The outcome of adolescent depression in the Ontario child health study follow-up, *J Am Acad Child Adolesc Psychiatry* 32:28-33, 1993.

Fristad MA, Weller MA, Weller RA: Bipolar disorder in children and adolescents, *Child Adolesc Psychiatr Clin North Am: Mood Disorders* 1:13-29, 1992a.

Fristad MA, Weller EB, Weller RA: The mania rating scale: can it be used in children? A preliminary report, *J Am Acad Child Adolesc Psychiatry* 31:252-257, 1992b.

Garrison CZ et al: A longitudinal study of depressive symptomatology in young adolescents, *J Am Acad Adolesc Psychiatry* 29:580-585, 1990.

Geller B, Fox LW, Clark KA: Rate and prediction of prepubertal bipolarity during follow-up of 6- to 12-year-old depressed children, *J Am Acad Child Adolesc Psychiatry* 33:461-468, 1994.

Geller B et al: Double-blind placebo-controlled study of nortriptyline in depressed children using a "fixed plasma level" design, *Psychopharmacol Bull* 25:101-108, 1989.

Geller B et al: A double-blind placebo-controlled study of nortriptyline in depressed adolescents using a "fixed plasma level" design, *Psychopharmacol Bull* 26:85-90, 1990.

Harrington R et al: Adult outcomes of childhood and adolescent depression, *Arch Gen Psychiatry* 47:465-473, 1990.

Isaac G: Bipolar disorder in prepubertal children in a special educational setting: is it rare? *J Clin Psychiatry* 52:165-168, 1991.

Isaac G: Misdiagnosed bipolar disorder in adolescents in a special educational school and treatment program, *J Clin Psychiatry* 53:133-136, 1992.

Janicak et al: *Principles and practice of psychopharmacotherapy,* Baltimore, 1993, Williams & Wilkins.

Jensen PS, Ryan ND, Prien R: Psychopharmacology of child and adolescent major depression: present status and future directions, *J Child Adolesc Psychopharmacol* 2:31-45, 1992.

Kahn et al: Comparison of cognitive-behavioral, relaxation, and self-modeling interventions for depression among middle-school students, *School Psychol Rev* 19:196, 1990.

Kandel DB, Davies M: Adult sequela of adolescent depressive symptoms, *Arch Gen Psychiatry* 43:255-262, 1986.

Kashani JH et al: Current perspectives on childhood depression: an overview, *Am J Psychiatry* 138:143-153, 1981.

Kashani JH et al: Psychiatric disorders in a community sample of adolescents, *Am J Psychiatry* 144:584-589, 1987.

Kovacs M: Rating scales to assess depression in school-aged children, *Acta Paedopsychiatr* 46:305-315, 1981.

Kovacs M, Goldston D: Cognitive and social cognitive development of depressed children and adolescents, *J Am Acad Child Psychiatry* 30:388-392, 1991.

Kovacs M et al: Depressive disorders in childhood. I. A longitudinal prospective study of characteristics and recovery, *Arch Gen Psychiatry* 41:229-237, 1984a.

Kovacs M et al: Depressive disorders in childhood. II. A longitudinal study for the risk of subsequent major depression, *Arch Gen Psychiatry* 41:643-649, 1984b.

Kovacs M et al: Depressive disorders in childhood. III. A longitudinal study of comorbidity with and risk for conduct disorders, *J Affect Disord* 15:205-217, 1988.

Lewinsohn PM et al: Cognitive-behavioral treatment for depressed adolescent, *Behav Ther* 21:385-401, 1990.

McCauley E et al: Depression in young people: initial presentation and clinical course, *J Am Acad Child Adolesc Psychiatry* 32:714, 1993.

McCracken JT: The epidemiology of child and adolescent mood disorders, *Child Adolesc Psychiatr Clin North Am: Mood Disorders* 1:53-72, 1992.

McGlashen TH: Adolescent versus adult onset of mania, *Am J Psychiatry* 145:221-223, 1988.

Mokros HB, Poznanski EO, Merrick WA: Depression and learning disabilities in children: a test of an hypothesis, *J Learn Disabil* 22:230-233, 1989.

Myers JK et al: Six month prevalence of psychiatric disorders in three communities, 1980 to 1982, *Arch Gen Psychiatry* 41:959-967, 1984.

Papatheodorou G, Kutcher SP: Divalproex sodium treatment in late adolescent and young adult acute mania, *Psychopharmacol Bull* 29:213-219, 1993.

Petti TA: Depression in hospitalized child psychiatry patients: approaches to measuring depression, *J Am Acad Child Psychiatry* 17:49-59, 1978.

Post RM et al: Dysphoric mania: clinical and biologic correlates, *Arch Gen Psychiatry* 46:353-358, 1989.

Poznanski EO, Krahenbuhl V, Zrull JP: Childhood depression: a longitudinal perspective, *J Am Acad Child Psychiatry* 15:491-501, 1976.

Poznanski EO, Mokros HB, Grossman J et al: Diagnostic criteria in childhood depression, *Am J Psychiatry* 142:1168-1173, 1985.

Puig-Antich J et al: Psychosocial functioning in prepubertal major depressive disorders. I. Interpersonal relationships during the depressive episode, *Arch Gen Psychiatry* 42:500-507, 1985.

Puig-Antich J et al: Imipramine in prepubertal major depressive disorder, *Arch Gen Psychiatry* 44:81-89, 1987.

Puig-Antich J et al: A controlled family history study of pubertal major depressive disorder, *Arch Gen Psychiatry* 46:406-418, 1989.

Reynolds WM, Coats KI: A comparison of cognitive-behavioral therapy and relaxation training for the treatment of depression in adolescents, *J Consul Clin Psychol* 54:653, 1986.

Riddle M, Geller B, Ryan N: Another sudden death in a child treated with desipramine, *J Am Acad Child Adolesc Psychiatry* 32:792-797, 1993.

Ryan ND et al: Neuroendocrine response to L-5-hydroxytryptophan challenge in prepubertal major depression, *Arch Gen Psychiatry* 49:843-851, 1992a.

Ryan ND et al: A secular increase in child and adolescent onset affective disorder, *J Am Acad Child Adolesc Psychiatry* 31:600-605, 1992b.

Schaffer D, Fisher P: The epidemiology of suicide in children and adolescents, *J Am Acad Child Psychiatry* 20:545-565, 1981.

Stark KD, Reynolds WM, Kaslow N: A comparison of the relative efficacy of self-control therapy and a behavioral problem-solving therapy for depression in children, *J Abnorm Child Psychol* 15:91-113, 1987.

Strober M: The pharmacotherapy of depressive illness in adolescence. III. Diagnostic and conceptual issues in studies of tricyclic antidepressants, *J Child Adolesc Psychopharmacol* 2:23-29, 1992.

Strober M et al: A family study of bipolar disorder in adolescents: early onset of symptoms linked to increased familial loading and lithium resistance, *J Affect Disord* 15:255-268, 1988.

Strober M et al: Relapse following discontinuation of lithium maintenance therapy in adolescents with bipolar I illness: a naturalistic study, *Am J Psychiatry* 147:457-461, 1990.

Strober M et al: The course of major depressive disorder in adolescents. I. Recovery and risk of manic switching in a follow-up of psychotic and non-psychotic subtypes, *J Am Acad Child Adolesc Psychiatry* 32:34-42, 1993.

Varanka TM et al: Lithium treatment of manic episodes with psychotic features in prepubertal children, *Am J Psychiatry* 145:1557-1559.

Weinberg WA, Emslie GJ: Adolescents and school problems: depression, suicide, and learning disorders. In Feldman RA, Stiffman AR, editors: *Advances in adolescent mental health, vol 3: depression and suicide,* Greenwich, Conn., 1988, JAI Press.

Weinberg WA, Emslie GJ: Attention deficit hyperactivity disorder: the differential diagnosis, *J Child Neurol* 6(Suppl):521-534, 1991.

Weinberg WA, Rehmet A: Childhood affective disorder and school problems. In Cantwell DP, Carlson GA, editors: Affective disorders in childhood and adolescence: an update, Jamaica, N.Y., 1983, Spectrum.

Weinberg WA et al: Depression in children referred to an educational diagnostic center: diagnosis and treatment, *J Pediatr* 83:1065-1072, 1973.

Weller EB, Weller RA, Fristad MA: Lithium dosage guide for prepubertal children: a preliminary report, *J Am Acad Child Adolesc Psychiatry* 31:611-614, 1986.

West SA et al: Open trial of valporate in the treatment of adolescent mania, *J Child Adolesc Psychopharmacol* 4:263-267, 1994.

West SA et al: Attention deficit disorder in adolescent mania, *Am J Psychiatry* 152:271-273, 1995.

Wilkes TCR, Rush AJ: Adaptations of cognitive therapy for depressed adolescents, *J Am Acad Child Adolesc Psychiatry* 27:381-386, 1988.

Wilkes TCR et al: *Cognitive therapy for depression in adolescents,* New York, Guilford (in press).

Wilson H, Staton RD: Neuropsychological changes in children associated with tricyclic antidepressant therapy, *Int J Neurosci* 24:307-312, 1984.

Yaylayan S, Weller EB, Weller RA: Neurobiology of depression. In Shafi M, Shafi SL, editors: *Clinical Guide to Depression in Children and Adolescents,* 1992 American Psychiatric Press.

Chapter 9

Agras WS et al: Pharmacologic and cognitive-behavioral treatment for bulimia nervosa: a controlled comparison, *Am J Psychiatry* 149:82-87, 1992.

American Psychiatric Press: *Diagnostic and statistical manual of mental disorders,* ed 4, Washington DC, 1994, American Psychiatric Press.

Chatoor I: Eating and nutritional disorders of infancy and early childhood. In Wiener JM, editor: *Textbook of child and adolescent psychiatry,* Washington DC, 1991, American Psychiatric Press.

Erikson EH: *Childhood and society,* ed 2, New York, 1963, WW Norton.

Fairburn CG: Cognitive-behavioral treatment for bulimia. In Garner DM, Garfinkel PE, editors: *Handbook of psychotherapy for anorexia nervosa and bulimia,* New York, 1985, Guilford Press.

Fluoxetine Bulimia Nervosa Collaborative (FBNC) Study Group: Fluoxetine in the treatment of bulimia nervosa, *Arch Gen Psychiatry* 49:139-147, 1992.

Gryboski JD et al: Eleven adolescent girls with severe anorexia: intestinal disease or anorexia nervosa? *Clin Pediatr* 7:684-690, 1968.

Guedalia JSB et al: A reversible case of Klüver-Bucy syndrome in association with shigellosis, *J Child Neurol* 8:313-315, 1993.

Harel Z, Biro FM: Hyperthyroidism in an adolescent with bulimia nervosa, *J Adolesc Health* 15:342-344, 1994.

Hughes PL et al: Treating bulimia with desipramine, *Arch Gen Psychiatry* 43:182-186, 1986.

Kron L et al: Anorexia nervosa and gonadal dysgenesis: further evidence of a relationship, *Arch Gen Psychiatry* 34:332-335, 1977.

Lewin K, Mattingly D, Millis RR: Anorexia nervosa associated with hypothalamic tumor, *Br Med J* 2:629-630, 1972.

Mascari MJ et al: The frequency of uniparental disomy in Prader-Willi syndrome, *New Engl J Med* 326:1599-1607, 1992.

Mitchell JE, Raymond N, Specker S: A review of the controlled trials of pharmacotherapy and psychotherapy in the treatment of bulimia nervosa, *Int J Eat Disord* 14:229-247, 1993.

Pope HG et al: Bulimia treated with imipramine: a placebo-controlled, double-blind study, *Am J Psychiatry* 140:554-558, 1983.

Rodin GM et al: Eating disorders in female adolescents with insulin dependent diabetes mellitus, *Int J Psychiatry Med* 16:49-57, 1986-87.

Smith MS, Christie DL: An adolescent with vomiting and weight loss, *J Adolesc Health Care* 5:279-282, 1984.

Varadaraj R, Cooper AJ: Addison's disease presenting with psychiatric symptoms [letter], *Am J Psychiatry* 143:553-554, 1986.

Waller DA et al: Recognizing and managing the adolescent with Kleine-Levin syndrome, *J Adolesc Health* 5:139-141, 1984.

Walsh BT et al: Phenelzine vs. placebo in 50 patients with bulimia, *Arch Gen Psychiatry* 45:471-475, 1988.

Chapter 10

American Academy of Child and Adolescent Psychiatry: Schizophrenia in children, *Facts for families* 49, 1994, The Academy.

American Psychiatric Association: *Diagnostic and statistical manual for mental disorders,* ed 3, Washington DC, 1980, American Psychiatric Press.

American Psychiatric Association: *Diagnostic and statistical manual for mental disorders,* ed 3 (revised), Washington DC, 1987, American Psychiatric Press.

American Psychiatric Association: *Diagnostic and statistical manual for mental disorders,* ed 4, Washington DC, 1994, American Psychiatric Press.

Andreasen NC: Negative symptoms in schizophrenia, *Arch Gen Psychiatry* 39:784-788, 1982.

Andreasen NC: *Scale for the assessment of positive symptoms (SAPS),* Iowa City, Ia., 1984, University of Iowa.

Beitchman JH: Childhood schizophrenia: a review and comparison with adult-onset schizophrenia, *Psychiatr Clin North Am* 8:793-814, 1985.

Birmaher B et al: Clozapine for the treatment of adolescents with schizophrenia, *J Am Acad Child Adolesc Psychiatry* 31:160-164, 1992.

Blanz B, Schmidt MH: Clozapine for schizophrenia (letter), *J Am Acad Child Adolesc Psychiatry* 32:223-224, 1993.

Bleuler E: *Dementia praecox or the group of schizophrenias,* New York, 1950, International Universities Press (Translated by J Zimkin).

Brierre de Boismont M: On the insanity of early life, *J Psychol Med Ment Pathol* 10:622-638, 1857.

Burke P et al: Hallucinations in children, *J Am Acad Child Psychiatry* 24:71-75, 1985.

Campbell M et al: Neuroleptic-induced dyskinesias in children, *Clin Neuropsychopharmacol* 6:207-222, 1983.

Campbell M et al: Schizophrenic and psychotic disorders. In Weiner JM, editor: *Textbook of child and adolescent psychiatry,* Washington DC, 1991, American Psychiatric Press.

Cantor-Graae E et al: Are neurological abnormalities in well discordant monozygotic co-twins of schizophrenia the result of perinatal trauma? *Am J Psychiatry* 151:1194-1199, 1984.

Cantor-Graae E et al: Link between pregnancy complications and minor physical anomalies in monozygotic twins discordant for schizophrenia, *Am J Psychiatry* 151:1188-1193, 1994.

Caplan R, Guthrie D, Foy JG: Communication deficits and formal thought disorder in schizophrenic children, *J Am Acad Child Adolesc Psychiatry,* 31:151-159, 1992.

Caplan R et al: Middle childhood onset of interictal psychosis, *J Am Acad Child Adolesc Psychiatry* 30:893-896, 1991.

Chambers WJ: Psychotic symptoms in prepubertal major depressive disorder, *Arch Gen Psychiatry* 39:921-927, 1982.

Chouinard G, Arnott W: Clinical review of risperidone, *Can J Psychiatry,* 38 (suppl):S89-S95, 1993.

Cozza SJ, Edison DL: Risperidone in adolescents, *J Am Acad Child Adolesc Psychiatry* 33:1211, 1994.

De Sanctis S: On some varieties of dementia praecox. In Howells JG, editor: *Modern perspectives in international child psychiatry,* Edinburgh, 1969, Oliver and Boyd (translated by ML Osborn; originally published in *Revista sperimentale di freniatria* 32:141-165).

Eggers C: Course and prognosis of childhood schizophrenia, *J Autism Childhood Schizophr* 8:21-36, 1978.

Fish B et al: Infants at risk for schizophrenia: sequelae of a genetic neurointegrative defect, *Arch Gen Psychiatry* 49:221-235, 1992.

Goldstein MJ, Doane JA: Family factors in the onset, course and treatment of schizophrenic spectrum disorders, *J Nerv Ment Dis* 170:692-700, 1982.

Gottesman II, McGuffin P, Farmer AE: Clinical genetics as clues to the "real" genetics of schizophrenia: a decade of modest gains while playing for time, *Schizophr Bull,* 13:23-47, 1987.

Green WH et al: Schizophrenia with childhood onset: a phenomenological study of 38 cases, *J Am Acad Child Adolesc Psychiatry* 31:968-976, 1992.

Gualtieri CT et al: Tardive dyskinesia in young mentally retarded individuals, *Arch Gen Psychiatry* 43:335-340, 1986.

Hanson DR, Gottesman II: The genetics, if any, of infantile autism and childhood schizophrenia, *J Autism Childhood Schizophr* 6:209-234, 1976.

Jackson HJ, Smith N, McGorry P: Relationship between expressed emotion and family burden in psychotic disorders: an exploratory study, *Acta Psychiatr Scand* 82:243-249, 1990.

Jenkins JH, Karno M: The meaning of expressed emotion: theoretical issues raised by cross-cultural research, *Am J Psychiatry* 149:9-10, 1992.

Kallman FJ, Roth B: Genetic aspects of preadolescent schizophrenia, *Am J Psychiatry* 112:599-606, 1956.

Kennedy J et al: Evidence against linkage of schizophrenia to markers on chromosome 5 in a northern Swedish pedigree, *Nature* 336:167-169, 1988.

Kolvin I: Studies in childhood psychoses. I. Diagnostic criteria and classification, *Br J Psychiatry,* 118:381-384, 1971a.

Kolvin I et al: Studies in the childhood psychoses. III. The family and social background in childhood psychoses, *Br J Psychiatry* 118:396-402, 1971b.

Kraepelin E: *Dementia praecox and paraphrenia,* Huntington, N.Y., 1971, Robert E. Krieger Publishing (translated by RM Barclay, originally published 1919).

Kydd RR, Werry JS: Schizophrenia in children under 16 years, *J Autism Dev Disord* 12:343-357, 1982.

Levkovitch Y et al: Clozapine for Schizophrenia (letter), *J Am Acad Child Adolesc Psychiatry* 33:431, 1994.

Loebel AD et al: Duration of psychosis and outcome in first-episode schizophrenia, *Am J Psychiatry* 149:1183-1188, 1992.

Lombroso PJ, Pauls DL, Leckman JF: Genetic factors in the etiology of childhood psychiatric disorders. In Rothenberger A, editor: *Brain behavior in child psychiatry,* New York, 1990, Springer-Verlag.

Loranger AW: Sex difference in age at onset of schizophrenia, *Arch Gen Psychiatry* 41:157-161, 1984.

McAllister CG et al: Increased numbers of CD5+ B lymphocytes in schizophrenic patients, *Arch Gen Psychiatry* 46:890-894, 1989.

McClellan J, Werry J, Ham M: A follow-up study of early onset psychosis: comparison between outcome diagnoses of schizophrenia, mood disorders, and personality disorders, *J Autism Dev Disord* 23:243-262, 1993.

McKenna L et al: Looking for childhood-onset schizophrenia, *J Am Acad Child Adolesc Psychiatry* 33:616-635, 1994.

Mednick SA et al: Adult schizophrenia following prenatal exposure to an influenza epidemic, *Arch Gen Psychiatry* 45:189-192, 1988.

Menkes DB: Clozapine in the management of schizophrenia: risperidone is less toxic but equally effective (letter), *Br Med J* 307:200, 1993.

Orvaschell H, Tabrizi ML, Chambers W: *Schedule for affective disorders and schizophrenia for school-age children-epidemiologic version (Kiddie-SADS-E),* ed 3, New York, New York State Psychiatric Institute and Yale University School of Medicine.

Padilla RV: The National Alliance for the Mentally Ill-Children and Adolescents Network (NAMI-CAN): moving mountains in the mental health arena, *J Child Adolesc Psychopharmacol,* 2:145-147, 1992.

Pauls DL: Genetic influences on schild psychiatric conditions. In Lewis M, editor: *Child and adolescent psychiatry: a comprehensive textbook,* Baltimore, 1990, Wilkins & Wilkins.

Russell AT, Bott L, Sammons C: The phenomenology of schizophrenia occurring in childhood, *J Am Acad Child Adolesc Psychiatry* 28:399-407, 1989.

Rutter M: Psychotic disorders in early childhood. In Coppens A, Walk A, editors: *Recent developments in schizophrenia: British journal of psychiatry special publication No. 1,* Ashford, England, 1967, Royal Medico-psychological Association, Headley Bros.

Rutter M: Childhood schizophrenia reconsidered, *J Autism Child Schizophr* 2:315-338, 1972.

Rutter M et al: Genetic factors in child psychiatric disorders. I. A review of research strategies, *J Child Psychol Psychiatry* 31:3-37, 1990a.

Rutter M et al: Genetic factors in child psychiatric disorders. II. Empirical findings, *J Child Psychol Psychiatry* 31:39-93, 1990b.

Schneider, K: *Klinische Psychopathologie,* ed 9, Stuttgart, 1971, Thieme.

Sherrington R et al: Localization of a susceptibility locus for schizophrenia on chromosome 5, *Nature* 336:164-167, 1988.

Spencer EK et al: Haloperidol treatment of schizophrenic children, *Scientific proceedings of the 145th Annual Meeting of the American Psychiatric Association* Washington, DC, 1992, American Psychiatric Press.

Tamminga CA et al: Limbic system abnormalities identified in schizophrenia using positron emission tomography with fluorodeoxyglucose and neocortical alterations with deficit syndrome, *Arch Gen Psychiatry* 49:522-530, 1992.

Watkins JM, Asarnow RF, Tanguay PE: Symptom development in childhood onset schizophrenia, *J Child Psychol Psychiatry* 29:865-878, 1988.

Werry JS: *Schizophrenia in childhood* [Cassette Recording]. *Fifteenth annual review in child and adolescent psychiatry,* Chicago, 1990, American Academy of Child and Adolescent Psychiatry.

Werry JS: Child and adolescent (early onset) schizophrenia: a review in light of DSM-III-R, *J Autism Dev Disord* 22:601-625, 1992.

Chapter 11

Aaron P: *Dyslexia and hyperlexia: diagnosis and management of developmental reading disabilities,* Boston, 1989, Kluwer Academic Publishers.

Aaron P, Simurdak J: *Reading disorders: their nature and diagnosis.* In Obrzut J, Hynd G, editors: *Neuropsychological foundations of learning diabilities: a handbook of issues, methods and practice,* San Diego, 1991, Academic Press.

American Psychiatric Association: *Diagnostic and statistical manual of mental disorders,* ed 4, Washington DC, 1994, American Psychiatric Press.

Badian N: The prediction of good and poor reading before kindergarten entry: a four-year follow-up, *J Spec Educ* 16:309-318, 1982.

Badian N: Improving the prediction of reading for the individual child: a four-year follow-up, *J Learn Disab* 21:98-103, 1986.

Badian N: Prediction of good and poor reading before kindergarten entry: a nine-year follow-up, *J Learn Disab* 21:98-103, 1988.

Banks J: *Multiethnic education: theory and practice,* Boston, 1988, Allyn & Bacon.

Barkley R: *Attention-deficit hyperactivity disorder: a handbook for diagnosis and treatment,* New York, 1990, Guilford Press.

Bauer R: Memory processes in children with learning disabilities: evidence for deficient rehearsal, *J Exp Child Psychol* 24:415-430, 1979.

Bauer R, Emhert J: Information processing in reading-disabled and nondisabled children, *J Exp Child Psychol* 37:271-281, 1984.

Baum D, Duffelmey F, Geelan M: Resource teacher perceptions of the prevalence of social dysfunction among students with learning disabilities, *J Learn Disab* 21:380-381, 1988.

Bender W: *Learning disabilities: characteristics, identification and teaching strategies,* Boston, 1995, Allyn & Bacon.

Benson D: *Aphasia, alexia, and agraphia,* New York, 1979, Churchill Livingston.

Bereiter C, Scardamalia M: *From conversation to composition: the role of instruction in a developmental process.* In Glaser R, editor: *Advances in instructional psychology,* vol 2, Hillsdale, N.J., 1982, Lawrence Erlbaum.

Berk L: *Child development,* Boston, 1991, Allyn & Bacon.

Berninger V: Multiple orthographic codes: key to alternative instructional methodologies for developing the orthographic-phonological connections underlying word identification, *School Psychology Review,* 19:518-533, 1990.

Bigler E: Acquired cerebral trauma: epidemiology, neuropsychological assessment, and academic/educational deficits, *J Learn Disab* 20:516-517, 1987.

Bingol N et al: Terotegenicity of cocaine in humans, *J Pediatr* 10:93-96, 1987.

Birch H: *Nutritional factors in mental retardation.* Paper presented at Fifth Annual Neuropsychology Workshop, University of Victoria, Victoria, B.C., Canada, 1970.

Blachman B: Relationship of rapid naming in language analysis skills to kindergarten and first grade reading achievement, *J Educ Psychol* 76:610-622, 1984.

Blalock J: Persistent auditory language deficits in adults with learning disabilities, *J Learn Disab* 15:604-609, 1982.

Bos C, Filip D: Comprehension monitoring in learning disabled and average students, *J Learn Disab* 17:229-223, 1984.

Bos C, Vaughn S: *Strategies for teaching students with learning and behavior problems,* Boston, 1991, Allyn and Bacon.

Brackbill Y, McManus K, Woodward L: *Medication in maternity: infant exposure and maternal information.* Ann Arbor, Mi., 1985, University of Michigan Press.

Bradley L, Bryant P: *Rhyme and reason in reading and spelling,* Ann Arbor, Mi., 1985, University of Michigan Press.

Brady S, Shankweiler D, Mann V: Speech perception and memory coding in relation to reading ability, *J of Exp Child Psychol* 35:345-367, 1983.

Brandt I: Brain growth, fetal malnutrition, and clinical consequences, *J Perinat Med* 9:3-26, 1981.

Brandt J, Rosen J: Auditory phonemic perception in dyslexia: categorical identification and discrimination of stop consonants. *Brain Lang* 9:324-337, 1980.

Breitmeyer B, Ganz L: Implications of sustained and transient channels for theories of visual pattern masking, *Psychol Rev* 83:1-36, 1976.

Brown A, Palincsar A: Inducing strategic learning from texts by means of informed, self-controlled training, *Top Learn Learn Disab* 2:1-18, 1982.

Bruck M: The adult outcomes of children with learning disabilities, *Ann Dyslexia,* 37:252-263, 1987.

Bruck M: Word-recognition skills of adults with childhood diagnoses of dyslexia, *Dev Psychol* 26:439-454, 1990.

Burd L, Kauffman D, Kerbeshian J: Tourette syndrome and learning disabilities, *J Learn Disab* 25:598-604, 1992.

Cardon L et al: Quantitative trait locus for reading disability on chromosome 6, *Science,* 266:276-279, 1994.

Carlisle H: The use of morphological knowledge in spelling derived forms by learning-disabled and normal students, *Ann Dyslexia* 37:90-108, 1987.

Carnine D, Silbert J, Kameenui E: *Direct instruction reading,* Columbus, Ohio, 1990, Merrill.

Carpenter R: Mathematics instruction in resource rooms: instruction time and teacher competence, *Learn Disab Q* 8:95-100, 1985.

Catts H: *Phonological processing deficits and reading disabilities.* In Kamhi A, Catts H, editors: *Reading disabilities: a developmental language perspective,* Austin, Tex., 1989, PRO-ED.

Chee P et al: Effects of event rate and display time on sustained attention in hyperactive, normal, and control children, *J Abnorm Child Psychol* 17:371-391, 1989.

Chun R, Shapiro S: *Movement disorders.* In David R, editor: *Pediatric neurology for the clinician,* Norwalk, Conn., 1992, Appleton & Lange.

Colletti L: Relationship between pregnancy and birth complications and the later development of learning disabilities, *J Learn Disab* 12:659-663, 1979.

Coltheart M: *Reading, phonological recording and deep dyslexia.* In Coltheart M, Patterson K, Marshall J, editors: *Deep dyslexia,* London, 1987, Kegan Paul.

Conte R: *Attention disorders.* In Wong B, editor: *Learning about learning disabilities,* San Diego, 1991, Academic Press.

Cowen E et al: Long-term follow-up of early detected vulnerable children, *J Consult Clin Psychol* 41:438-446, 1973.

Cunningham C, Barkley R: The role of academic failure in hyperactive behavior, *J Learn Disab* 11:15-21, 1978.

Decker D, Vandenburg S: *Colorado twin study of reading disability.* In Gray D, Kavenagh J, editors: *Biobehavioral measures of dyslexia,* Baltimore, 1985, York Press.

DeFries J, Decker S: *Genetic aspects of reading disability: a family study.* In Malatesha R, Aaron P, editors: *Reading disorders: varieties and treatments,* New York, 1982, Academic Press.

DeFries J, Fulker D, LaBuda C: Evidence for a genetic aetiology in reading disability of twins, *Nature* 329:537-539, 1987.

DeFries J, Gillis J: *Etiology of reading deficits in learning disabilities: quantitative genetic analysis.* In Obrzut J, Hynd G, editors: *Neuropsychological foundations of learning disabilities,* San Diego, 1991, Academic Press.

Denckla M: *Childhood learning disabilities.* In Heilman K, Valenstein E, editors: *Clinical neuropsychology,* New York, 1979, Oxford University Press.

Denckla M, Rudel R: Rapid "automatized" naming (R.A.N.): dyslexia differentiated from other learning disabilities, *Neuropsychologia* 14:471-479, 1976.

Diamond G: The birthdate effect: a maturational effect? *J Learn Disab* 16:161-164, 1983.

Di Lollo V, Hanson D, McIntyre J: Initial stages of visual information processing in dyslexia, *J Exp Psychol: Human Perceptual Performance,* 9:923-935, 1983.

Donahue M: *Linguistic and communicative development in learning-disabled children.* In Ceci S, editor: *Handbook of cognitive, social, and neuropsychological aspects of learning disabilities,* Hillsdale, N.J., 1986, Lawrence Erlbaum.

Downey J et al: Cognitive ability and everyday functioning in women with Turner syndrome, *J Learn Disab* 24:32-39, 1991.

Drake W: Clinical and pathological findings in a child with a developmental learning disability, *J Learn Disab* 1:486-502, 1968.

Duane D: *Biological foundations of learning disabilities.* In Obrzut J, Hynd G, editors: *Neuropsychological foundations of learning disabilities,* San Diego, 1991, Academic Press.

Duffy F et al: Dyslexia: regional differences in brain electrical activity by topographic mapping, *Ann Neurol* 5:412-420, 1980.

Duffy F et al: *Neurophysiological studies in dyslexia.* In Plum F, editor: *Language, communication and the brain,* New York, 1988, Raven Press.

Ehri L, Wilce L: Movement into reading: is the first stage of printed word learning visual or phonetic? *Read Res Q* 20:163-179, 1987.

Elbert J: Short-term memory encoding and memory search in the word recognition of learning-disabled children, *J Learn Disab* 17:342-345, 1984.

Ellis A: *Spelling and writing (and reading and speaking).* In Ellis W, editor: *Normality and pathology in cognitive functions,* London, 1982, Academic Press.

Ellis E et al: An instructional model for teaching learning strategies, *Focus Except Child* 23:1-23, 1991.

Feinstein C, Aldershof A: *Developmental disorders of language and learning.* In Wiener J, editor: *Textbook in child and adolescent psychiatry,* Washington, DC, 1991, American Psychiatric Press.

Finucci J, Gottfredson L, Childs B: A follow-up study of dyslexic boys, *Ann Dyslexia* 35:117-136, 1985.

Fischer F, Shankweiler D, Liberman I: Spelling proficiency and sensitivity to word structure, *J Mem Lang* 24:423-441, 1985.

Fisher W, Burd L, Kerbeshian J: Markers for improvement in children with pervasive developmental disorders, *J Ment Defic Res* 32:357-369, 1988.

Flavell J: *Metacognitive aspects of problem solving.* In Resnick L, editor: *The nature of intelligence,* Hillsdale, N.J., 1976, Lawrence Erlbaum.

Fleischner J: *Diagnosis and assessment of mathematics learning disabilities.* In Lyon G, editor: *Frames of reference for the assessment of learning disabilities,* Baltimore, 1994, Brookes.

Fleischner J, Nuzum M, Marzola E: Devising an instructional program to teach arithmetic problem-solving skills to students with learning disabilities, *J Learn Disab* 20:214-217, 1987.

Fletcher J, Satz P: *Cluster analysis and the search for learning disability subtypes.* In Rourke B, editor: *Neuropsychology of learning disabilities: essentials of subtype analysis,* New York, 1985, Guilford Press.

Frankenberger W, Fronzaglio K: A review of states' criteria and procedures for identifying children with learning disabilities, *J Learn Disab* 24:495-500, 1991.

Frith U: *Beneath the surface of developmental dyslexia.* In Patterson K, Marshall J, Coltheart M, editors: *Surface dyslexia: neuropsychological and cognitive studies of phonological reading,* Hillsdale, N.J., 1985, Lawrence Erlbaum.

Gaddes W: *Learning disabilities and brain function: a neuropsychological approach,* New York, 1985, Springer-Verlag.

Gaddes W, Edgell E: *Learning disabilities and brain function: a neuropsychological approach,* New York, 1994, Springer-Verlag.

Galaburda A: Developmental dyslexia: current anatomical research, *Ann Dyslexia* 33:41-53, 1983.

Galaburda A, Kemper T: Cytoarchitechtonic abnormalities in developmental dyslexia: a case study, *Ann Neurol* 6:94-100, 1979.

Galaburda A, Rosen G, Sherman G: *The neural origin of developmental dyslexia: implications for medicine, neurology and cognition.* In Galaburda A, editor: *From reading to neurons,* Cambridge, Mass, 1989, MIT Press.

Galaburda A et al: Developmental dyslexia: four consecutive patients with cortical anomalies, *Annals of Neurol* 18:222-233, 1985.

Garner R: Monitoring of passage inconsistency among poor comprehenders: a preliminary test of the "piecemeal processing" explanation, *J Educ Res* 74:159-162, 1981.

Garner R, Alexander P, Chou-Hare V: *Reading comprehension failure in children.* In Wong B, editor: *Learning about learning disabilities,* San Diego, 1991, Academic Press.

Geschwind N: *Selected papers on language and the brain,* Boston, 1974, Reidel.

Geschwind N: *Anatomical foundations of language and dominance.* In *The neurological bases of language disorders in children: methods and directions for research, NINCDS Monograph* 22:145-157, 1979.

Goldstein D, Dundon W: *Affect and cognition in learning disabilities.* In Ceci S, editor: *Handbook of cognitive, social, and neuropsychological aspects of learning disabilities,* vol 2 Hillsdale, N.J., 1987, Lawrence Erlbaum.

Goldstein K: *Language and language disturbance,* New York, 1948. Grune & Stratton.

Gregg N: *Expressive writing.* In Hooper S, Hynd G, Mattison R, editors: *Developmental disorders: diagnostic criteria and clinical assessment,* Hillsdale: N.J., 1992, Lawrence Erlbaum.

Grunau R, Low M: Cognitive and task-related EEG correlates of arithmetic performance in adolescents, *J Clin Exp Neuropsychol* 9:563-574, 1987.

Hagerman R, Smith A: *The heterozygous female.* In Hagerman R, McBogg P, editors: *The fragile X syndrome: diagnosis, biochemistry, and intervention,* Dillon, Colo., 1983, Spectra Publishing.

Hagin R, Kugler J: *School problems associated with Tourette's syndrome.* In Cohen D, Brunn R, Leckman J, editors: *Tourette's syndrome and tic disorders: clinical understanding and treatment,* New York, 1988, Wiley.

Hallihan D, Reeve R, *Selective attention and distractibility.* In Keogh B, editor: *Advances in special education,* vol 1, Greenwich, Conn., 1980, JAI Press.

Halperin J et al: Reading disabled hyperactive children: a distinct subgroup of attention deficit disorder with hyperactivity? *J Abnorm Child Psychol* 12:1-14, 1984.

Hammill D et al: A new definition of learning disabilities, *J Learn Disab* 20:109-112, 1987.

Hanna P, Hodges R, Hanna J: *Spelling: structure and strategies,* Boston, 1971, Houghton-Mifflin.

Harris A, Sipay E: *How to increase reading ability: a guide to developmental and remedial methods,* New York, 1990, Longman.

Harris E: *The contribution of twin research to the study of etiology of reading disability.* In Smith S, editor: *Genetics and learning disabilities,* San Diego, 1986, College Hill Press.

Hartzell H, Compton C: Learning disability: a ten-year follow-up, *Pediatrics,* 74:1058-1064, 1984.

Haslam R et al: Cerebral asymmetry in developmental dyslexia, *Arch Neurol* 38:679-704, 1981.

Hayes J, Flower L: Writing research and the writer, *Am Psychol* 41:1106-1113, 1986.

Healy J, Aram D: Hyperlexia and dyslexia: a family study, *Ann Dyslexia* 36:237-252, 1986.

Hecaen H, Albert M: *Human neuropsychology,* New York, 1978, Wiley.

Heller K, Holtzman W, Messick S: *Placing children in special education: a strategy for equity,* Washington DC, 1982, National Academy Press.

Hetzel B, Hay I: Thyroid function, iodine nutrition and fetal brain development, *Clin Endocrinol* 11:445-460, 1979.

Hier D et al: Developmental dyslexia: evidence for a subgroup with a reversal of cerebral asymmetry, *Arch Neurol* 35:90-92, 1978.

Hooper S et al: *Measurement of written language expression.* In Lyon G, editor: *Frames of reference for the assessment of learning disabilities,* Baltimore, 1994, Brookes.

Houselander J et al: Infants born to narcotic addicted mothers, *Psychol Bull* 2:453-468, 1982.

Hulme C: The implausibility of low-level visual deficits as a cause of children's reading difficulties, *Cogn Neuropsychol* 5:369-374, 1988.

Hynd G: Neurological aspects of dyslexia: comments on the balance model, *J Learn Disab* 25:110-113, 1992.

Hynd G, Semrud-Clikeman M, Lyytinen H: *Brain imaging in learning disabilities.* In Obrzut J, Hynd G, editors: *Neuropsychological foundations of learning disabilities,* San Diego, 1991, Academic Press.

Hynd G et al: Brain morphology in developmental dyslexia and attention deficit disorder/hyperactivity, *Arch Neurol* 47:919-926, 1990.

Janesick V: *Our multicultural society.* In Meyen E, Skrtic T, editors: *Special education and student disability,* Denver, 1995, Love.

Johnson C: The learning disabled adolescent and young adult: an overview and critique of current practices, *J Learn Disab* 17:386-391, 1984.

Johnson D, Blalock J: *Young adults with learning disabilities,* New York, 1987, Grune & Stratton.

Johnson D, Myklebust H: *Learning disabilities: educational principles and practices,* New York, 1967, Grune & Stratton.

Jorm A: *The psychology of reading and spelling disabilities,* London, 1983, Routledge & Kegan Paul.

Kaluger G, Kolson C: *Reading and learning disabilities,* Columbus, Ohio, 1978, Merrill.

Kamhi A, Catts H, editors: *Reading disabilities: a developmental language perspective,* Austin, Tex., 1989, PRO-ED.

Kanner L: *Child psychiatry,* ed 1, Baltimore, 1935, Charles C. Thomas.

Kanner L: *Child psychiatry,* ed 3, Baltimore, 1957, Charles C. Thomas.

Kaplan E, Goodglass H: *Aphasia-related disorders.* In Sarno M, editor: *Acquired aphasia,* New York, 1981, Academic Press.

Kavale K: The reasoning abilities of normal and learning-disabled readers on measures of reading comprehension, *Learn Disab Q* 3:34-45, 1980.

Kavale K, Forness S: *The science of learning disabilities,* San Diego, 1985, College-Hill Press.

Kavanagh J, Truss T: *Learning disabilities: proceedings of the national conference,* Parkton, Md., 1988, York Press.

Kearney C, Drabman R: The right-say method for improving spelling accuracy in children with learning disabilities, *J Learn Disab* 26, 52-56.

Keller C, Sutton J: *Specific mathematics disorders.* In Obrzut J, Hynd G, editors: *Neuropsychological foundations of learning disabilities: a handbook of issues, methods, and practice,* San Diego, 1991, Academic Press.

Kemper M et al: Cognitive profiles and the spectrum of clinical manifestations in heterozygous fragile X females, *Am J Med Genet* 23:139-156, 1986.

Keogh B, Margolis J: Learn to labor and wait: attentional problems of children with learning disorders, *J Learn Disab* 9:276-286, 1976.

Keogh B, Sears S: *Learning disabilities from a developmental perspective: early identification and prediction.* In Wong B, editor: *Learning about learning disabilities,* San Diego, 1991, Academic Press.

Kinsbourne M, Caplan P: *Children's learning and attention problems,* Boston, 1979, Little, Brown.

Kochanek T, Kabacoff R, Lipsitt L: Early identification of developmentally disabled and at-risk preschool children, *Except Child* 56:528-538, 1990.

Kosc L, Developmental dyscalculia, *J Learn Disabil* 7:164-177, 1974.

Krupski A: *Attention processes: research, theory, and implications for special education.* In Keogh B, editor: *Advances in special education,* vol 1, Greenwich, Conn., 1980, JAI Press.

La Buda M, DeFries J: Cognitive abilities in children with learning disabilities and controls: a follow-up study, *J Learn Disab* 21:562-566, 1988.

Larsen J et al: MRI evaluation of the size and symmetry of the planum temporal in adolescents with developmental dyslexia, *Brain Lang* 39:289-301, 1990.

Leong C: *Children with specific reading disabilities,* Amsterdam, 1987, Swets and Zeitlinger.

Lerner J: *Learning disabilities: theories, diagnosis and teaching strategies,* Boston, 1993, Houghton Mifflin.

Liberman I: *Should so-called modality preferences determine the nature of instruction for children with reading disabilities?* In Duffy F, Geschwind N, editor: *Dyslexia: a neuroscientific approach to clinical evaluation,* Boston, 1985, Little, Brown, & Co.

Liberman I, Shankweiler D: Phonology and the problem of learning to read and write, *Remedial and Special Education,* 6:41-55, 1985.

Livingstone M, Hubel D: Psychophysical evidence for separate channels for the perception of form, color, movement, and depth, *J Neurosci* 7:3416-3468, 1987.

Lloyd J, Loper A: Measurement and evaluation of task-related learning behaviors: attention to task and metacognition, *School Psychol Rev* 15:336-345, 1986.

Lovegrove W, Martin F, Slaghuis W: A theoretical and experimental case for a visual deficit in specific reading disability, *Cogn Neuropsychol* 3:225-267, 1986.

Lyle J, Goyen J: The effect of speed of exposure and difficulty of discrimination on visual recognition of retarded readers, *J Abnorm Psychol* 84:673-676, 1975.

Lyon G, Moats L: *An examination of research in learning disabilities: past practices and future directions.* In Lyon G et al, editors: *Better understanding learning disabilities,* Baltimore, 1993, Brookes.

Lyon G et al: *Neuropsychology and learning disabilities.* In Wong B, editor: *Learning about learning disabilities* San Diego, 1991, Academic Press.

Lyytinen H, Lorys-Vernon A: Neurodevelopmental changes in ERP components associated with automatic attention (MMN), *J Clin Exp Neuropsychol* 11:28, 1988.

Madison L, George C, Moeschler J: Functioning in the fragile X syndrome: a study of intellectual memory and communication skills, *J Ment Defic* 3:129-148, 1986.

Mandler G: *Cognitive psychology,* Hillsdale, N.J., 1985, Lawrence Erlbaum.

Manis F: Acquisition of word identification skills in normal and disabled readers, *J Educ Psychol* 27:28-90, 1985.

Mann V: Longitudinal prediction and prevention of early reading difficulty, *Ann Dyslexia* 34:117-136, 1985.

Mann V: *Language problems: a key to early reading problems.* In Wong B, editor: *Learning about learning disabilities,* San Diego, 1991, Academic Press.

Mann V, Cowin E, Schoenheimer J: Phonological processing, language comprehension and reading ability, *J Learn Disab* 22:76-89, 1989.

Mann V, Liberman I: Phonological awareness in verbal short-term memory: can they presage early reading success? *J Learn Disab* 17:592-598, 1984.

Mann V, Liberman I, Shankweiler D: Children's memory for sentences and word strings in relation to reading ability, *Mem Cogn* 8:329-335, 1980.

Mann V, Shankweiler D, Smith S: The association between comprehension of spoken sentences and early reading ability: the role of phonetic representation, *J Child Lang* 11:627-643, 1985.

Mason W: Specific (developmental) dyslexia, *Dev Med Child Neurol* 9:183-190, 1976.

Mastropieri M, Scruggs T, Shiah S: Mathematics instruction for learning disabled students: a review of research, *Learn Disab Res Pract* 6:89-98, 1991.

Mattis S, French J, Rapin T: Dyslexia in children and young adults: three independent neuropsychological syndromes, *Dev Med Child Neurol* 17:50-163, 1975.

McCloskey M et al: *Cognitive representations and processes in number production: evidence from cases of acquired dyscalculia.* In Caramazza A, editor: *Cognitive neuropsychological and neurolinguistics: advances in models of cognitive function and impairment,* Hillsdale, N.J., 1990, Lawrence Erlbaum.

McCulloch C: *The Slingerland approach: is it effective in a specific language disability classroom?* Unpublished Master's thesis, Seattle Pacific University, Seattle, Washington, 1985.

McGee R, Share D: Attention deficit disorder-hyperactivity and academic failure: which comes first and what should be treated? *J Am Acad Child Adolesc Psychiatry* 27:318-325, 1988.

McKinney J, Feagans L: Adaptive classroom behavior of learning disabled students, *J Learn Disab* 16:360-367, 1983.

Mercer C: *Students with learning disabilities,* New York, 1992, Merrill.

Moats L: *Assessment of spelling in learning disabilities research.* In Lyon G, editor: *Frames of reference for the assessment of learning disabilities,* Baltimore, 1994a, Brookes.

Moats L: *Honing the concepts of listening and speaking: a prerequisite to the valid measurement of language behavior in children.* In Lyon G, editor: *Frames of reference for the assessment of learning disabilities,* Baltimore, 1994b, Brookes.

Monroe M: *Children who cannot read,* Chicago, 1932, University of Chicago Press.

Montague M, Bos C: The effect of cognitive strategy training on verbal math problem solving performance of learning disabled adolescents, *J Learn Disab* 19:26-33, 1986.

Moray N: *Attention: selective processes in vision and hearing,* London, 1969, Hutchinson.

Morrison G, Polloway E: *Mental retardation.* In Meyen E, Skrtic T, editors: *Special education and student disability: an introduction,* Denver, Colo., 1995, Love.

Myklebust H: *Development and disorders of written language, picture story language test,* vol 1, New York, 1965, Grune & Stratton.

Myklebust H: *Development and disorders of written language: studies of normal and exceptional children,* vol 2, New York, 1973, Grune & Stratton.

Naeye R, Peters E: Mental development of children whose mothers smoked during pregnancy, *Obstet Gynecol* 64:301, 1984.

Nieburg P et al: The fetal tobacco syndrome, *J Am Med Assoc* 253:2998-2999, 1985.

Novick B, Arnold M: *Fundamentals of clinical child neuropsychology,* Philadelphia, 1988, Grune & Stratton.

Ogle J: Aphasia and agraphia, *Report of the medical research counsel of Saint George's Hospital* 2:83-122, 1867.

O'Hare A, Brown J: Childhood dysgraphia. I. An illustrated clinical classification, *Child Care Health Dev* 15:79-104, 1989.

Olivarez A, Palmer D, Guillemard L: Predictive bias with referred and non-referred black, Hispanic, and white pupils, *Learn Disab Q* 15:175-186, 1992.

Orton S: "Word-blindness" in school children, *Arch Neurol Psychiatry* 14:581-615, 1925.

Owings R et al: Spontaneous monitoring and regulation of learning: a comparison of successful and less successful fifth graders, *J Educ Psychol* 72:250-256, 1980.

Ozols E, Rourke B: Characteristics of young learning-disabled children classified according to patterns of academic achievement: auditory-perceptual and visual-perceptual abilities, *J Clin Child Psychol* 17:44-52, 1988.

Palinscar A, Brown A: Reciprocal teaching of comprehension-fostering and monitoring activities, *Cogn Instr* 1:117-175, 1984.

Parker J, Asher S: Peer acceptance in later personal adjustment: are low-accepted children "at risk"? *Psychol Bull* 102:357-389, 1987.

Pasamanick B, Knoblock H: *The epidemiology of reproductive causality.* In Sapir S, Nitzburg A, editors: *Children with learning problems: reading in a developmental interaction approach,* New York, 1973, Brunner/Mazel.

Pearl R, Donahue M, Bryan T: *Social relationships of learning-disabled children.* In Torgesen J, Wong B, editors: *Psychological and educational perspectives on learning disabilities,* New York, Academic Press.

Pennington B: *Diagnosing learning disorders: a neuropsychological framework,* New York, 1991, Guilford Press.

Perfetti C: *Reading skill,* Hillsdale, N.J., 1985, Lawrence Erlbaum.

Peterson S, Mercer C, O'Shea L: Teaching learning disabled students place value using the concrete to abstract sequence, *Learn Disab Res* 4:52-56, 1988.

Plomen R: *Development, genetics, and psychology,* Hillsdale, N.J., 1986, Erlbaum.

Posner M: *Psychobiology of attention.* In Gazzaniga M, Blakemore C, editors: *Handbook of psychobiology,* New York, 1975, McGraw-Hill.

Raskin L et al: *Early brain damage and attentional deficit disorder: an animal model.* In Almli C, Finger S, editors: *Early brain damage: research orientations and clinical observations,* vol 1, New York, 1984, Academic Press.

Reid D, Hresko W: Mathematics [Editorial comment], *Topics in Learning and Learning Disabilities* 1:vii-ix, 1981.

Richards G et al: Sustained and selective attention in children with learning disabilities, *J Learn Disab* 23:129-136, 1990.

Roberts R et al: CT asymmetries in developmentally dyslexic adults, *Dev Neuropsychol* 43:231-237, 1988.

Roeltgen D: *Agraphia.* In Heilman K, Valenstein E, editors: *Clinical neuropsychology,* New York, 1985, Oxford University Press.

Rosenberger P, Hier D: Cerebral asymmetry and verbal intellectual deficits, *Ann Neurol* 8:300-304, 1980.

Rosenblith J, Sims-Knight J: *In the beginning: development in the first two years,* Monterey, 1985, Brooks-Cole.

Rourke B: Central processing deficiencies in children: toward a developmental neuropsychological model, *J Clin Neuropsychol* 4:1-18, 1982.

Rourke B: *Outstanding issues in research on learning disabilities.* In Rutter M, editor: *Developmental neuropsychiatry,* New York, 1983, Guilford Press.

Rourke B: *Nonverbal learning disabilities: the syndrome and the model,* New York, 1989, Guilford Press.

Rourke B, Finlayson M: Neuropsychological significance of variations in patterns of academic performance: verbal and visual-spatial abilities, *J Abnorm Child Psychol* 6:121-133, 1978.

Rovet J: The psychoeducational characteristics of children with Turner syndrome, *J Learn Disab* 26:333-341, 1993.

Rumsey J et al: Magnetic resonance imaging of brain anatomy in severe developmental dyslexia, *Arch Neurol* 43:1045-1046, 1986.

Rutter N: *Prevalence and types of dyslexia.* In Benton A, Pearl D, editors: *Dyslexia: an appraisal of current knowledge,* New York, 1978 Oxford Press.

Sandler A: Neurodevelopmental study of writing disorders in middle childhood, *Dev Behav Pediatr* 13:17-23, 1992.

Satterfield J et al: Topographic study of auditory event-related potentials in normal boys and boys with attention deficit disorder with hyperactivity, *Psychophysiology* 25:591-606, 1988.

Scarborough H: Very early language deficits in dyslexic children, *Child Dev* 61:1728-1743, 1990.

Scholevar G: *M.D. discusses assessment, treatment of depression, suicidal tendencies in children with learning disabilities,* Rosemont, Pa., 1987, Hilltop Preparatory School (ERIC document reproduction service no. Ed 309 602).

Segalowitz S, Brown D: Mild head injury as a source of developmental disabilities, *J Learn Disab* 24:551-559, 1991.

Sell E et al: Early identification of learning problems in neonatal intensive care graduates, *Am J Dis Child* 139:460-463, 1985.

Shafrir U, Siegel L: Preference for visual scanning strategies versus phonological rehearsal in university students with reading disabilities, *J Learn Disab* 27:583-588, 1994.

Shafrir U, Siegel L: Subtypes of learning disabilities in adolescents and adults, *J Learn Disab* 27:123-134, 1994.

Shankweiler D et al: The speech code and learning to read, *J Exp Psychol: Human Percep Performance* 5:531-545, 1979.

Shapiro T: *Diagnosis and diagnostic formulation.* In Wiener J, editor: *Textbook of child and adolescent psychiatry,* Washington, DC, 1991, American Psychiatric Press.

Shaywitz B: *Hyperactivity/attention-deficit disorder.* In *Learning disabilities: a report to U.S. Congress.* Washington DC, 1987, Interagency Committee on Learning Disabilities.

Shaywitz S, Cohen D, Shaywitz B: Behavior and learning difficulties in children of normal intelligence born to alcoholic mothers, *J Pediatr* 96:978-982, 1980.

Shaywitz S, Shaywitz B: *Attention deficit disorder: current perspectives.* In Kavanaugh J, Truss T, editors: *Learning disabilities: proceedings of the national conference,* Parkton, Md., 1988, York Press.

Shaywitz B, Shaywitz S, Fletcher J: *Learn Disab* 3:1-12, 1992.

Shaywitz S et al: Evidence that dyslexia may represent the lower tail of normal distribution of reading ability, *N Engl J Med* 326:145-150, 1992.

Siegel L, Heaven R: *Categorization of learning disabilities.* In Ceci S, editor: *Handbook of cognitive, social and neuropsychological aspects of learning disabilities,* vol 1, Hillsdale, N.J., 1986, Lawrence Erlbaum.

Silver A, Hagin R: Maturation of perceptual functions in children with specific reading disabilities, *Reading Teacher* 19:253-259, 1966.

Silver A, Hagin R: *Prevention of learning disorders.* In Shaffer D, Silverman M, Washington A, editors: *Prevention of mental disorders, alcohol and other drug use in children and adolescents,* Washington DC, 1989, Office of Substance Abuse Prevention (Monogr No. 2), U.S. Department of Health and Human Services.

Silver A, Hagin R: *Disorders of learning in childhood,* New York, 1990, Wiley.

Silver L: *The faces of MBD: psychiatric aspects.* Address to SUNY Upstate Medical Center and CIBA Conference, Understanding Minimal Brain Dysfunction, Syracuse, N.Y., November 1977.

Smith C: *Learning disabilities: the interaction of learner, task, and setting,* Boston, 1994, Allyn & Bacon.

Smith S, Mann V, Shankweiler D: Spoken sentence comprehension by good and poor readers: a study with the Token Test, *Cortex* 22:627-632, 1986.

Smith S et al: Familial dyslexia: use of genetic linkage data to define subtypes, *J Am Acad Child Adolesc Psychiatry* 29:204-213, 1990.

Speece D, McKinney J, Appelbaum M: Longitudinal development of conversation skills in learning disabled children, *J Learn Disab* 19:302-307, 1986.

Spreen O, Haaf R: Empirically derived learning disability subtypes: a replication attempt and longitudinal patterns over fifteen years, *J Learn Disab* 19:170-180, 1986.

Stanovich K: Matthew effects in reading: some consequences of individual differences in the acquisition of literacy, *Read Res Q* 21:360-406, 1986.

Stanovich K, Cunningham A, Cramer B: Assessing phonological awareness in kindergarten children: issues of task comparability, *J Exp Child Psychol* 38:175-190, 1984.

Stein, 1989. See Whyte, 1989.

Stevenson J et al: A twin study of genetic influences on reading and spelling ability and disability, *J Child Psychol Psychiatry* 28:229-247, 1987.

Swanson H: Relations among metamemory, rehearsal activity and word recall in learning disabled and nondisabled readers, *J Educ Psychol* 53:186-194, 1983.

Swanson H: Semantic and visual memory codes in learning disabled readers, *J Exp Child Psychol* 37:124-140, 1984.

Swanson H: Do semantic memory deficiencies underlie disabled readers encoding processes? *J Exp Psychol* 41:461-488, 1986.

Swanson H, Cochran K, Ewers C: Working memory and reading disabilities, *J Abnorm Child Psychol* 17:745-756, 1989.

Swanson H, Cooney J: *Learning disabilities and memory,* In Wong B, editor: *Learning about learning disabilities,* San Diego, 1991, Academic Press.

Swanson H, Rhine B: Strategy transformation in learning disabled children's math performance: clues to the development of expertise, *J Learn Disab* 18:596-603, 1985.

Swanson L: A study of nonstrategic linguistic coding on visual recall of learning disabled readers, *J Learn Disab* 16:209-216, 1983.

Tallal P: *Developmental language disorders.* In Kavanagh J, Truss T, editors: *Learning disabilities: proceedings of the national conference,* Parkton, Md., 1988, York Press.

Tarnowski K, Prinz R, Nay, S: Comparative analysis of attentional deficits in hyperactive and learning disabled children, *J Abnorm Psychol* 95:341-345, 1986.

Thorpe H, Borden K: The effect of multisensory instruction upon the on-task behavior and word reading accuracy of learning disabled children, *J Learn Disab* 18:279-286, 1985.

Tindal G, Parker R: Identifying measures for evaluating written expression, *Learn Disab Res Pract* 6:211-218, 1991.

Torgesen J: The role of nonspecific factors in the task performance of learning-disabled children: a theoretical assessment, *J Learn Disab* 10:27-34, 1977.

Torgesen J: Factors related to poor performance on rote memory tasks in reading-disabled children, *Learn Disab Q* 2:17-23, 1979.

Torgesen J: Studies of children with learning disabilities who perform poorly on memory span tasks, *J Learn Disab* 21:605-612, 1988.

Torgesen JK et al: Improving sight-word recognition skills in LD children: an evaluation of three computer program variations, *Learn Disab Q* 11:125-133, 1988.

Touwen B, Huisjes H: *Obstetrics, neonatal neurology, and later outcome.* In Almli C, Finger S, editors: *Early brain damage: research orientations and clinical observations,* vol 1, New York, 1984, Academic Press.

Ullman C: Teachers, peers, and tests as predictors of adjustment, *J Educ Psychol* 48:257-267, 1957.

Vaughn S, Hogan A: *Social competence and learning disabilities: a prospective study.* In Swanson H, Keogh B, editors: *Learning disabilities: theoretical and research issues,* Hillsdale, N.J., 1990, Erlbaum.

Vellutino F: *Dyslexia: theory and research,* Cambridge, Mass, 1979, MIT Press.

Vellutino F et al: Visual form perception in deficient and normal readers as a function of age and orthographic linguistic familiarity, *Cortex* 11:22-30, 1975.

Voeller K: *Techniques for measuring social competency in children.* In Lyon G, editor: *Frames of reference for the assessment of learning disabilities,* Baltimore, 1994, Brookes.

Vogel S: Levels and patterns of intellectual functioning among learning disabled students: clinical and educational implications, *J Learn Disab* 19:71-79, 1986.

Waldie K, Spreen O: The relationship between learning disabilities and persisting delinquency, *J Learn Disab* 26:417-423.

Whyte J: Progress in dyslexia research: an overview of dyslexia: current research issues, *Ir J Psychol* 10:465-478, 1989.

Wiener J: *Textbook of child and adolescent psychiatry,* Washington DC, 1991, American Psychiatric Press.

Wilen D, Sweeting C: Assessment of limited English proficient Hispanic students, *School Psychology Review,* 15:59-75, 1986.

Williams J, Richman L, Yarbrough D: Comparison of visual-spatial performance strategy training in children with Turner syndrome and learning disabilities, *J Learn Disab* 25:658-664, 1992.

Willows D: *Visual processes and learning disabilities.* In Wong B, editor: *Learning about learning disabilities,* San Diego, 1991, Academic Press.

Willows D, Corcos E, Kershner J: Disabled and normal readers' visual processing and visual memory of item and spatial-order information in unfamiliar symbol strings. Paper presented at the XXIV International Congress of Psychology, Sydney, Australia, August 1988.

Wolf M: Naming, reading and the dyslexias: a longitudinal overview, *Ann Dyslexia* 34:87-115, 1984.

Wong B: The effects of directive cues on the organization of memory and recall in good and poor readers, *J Educ Res* 72:32-38, 1978.

Wong B: Strategic behaviors in selecting retrieval cues in gifted, normal achieving and learning disabled children, *J Learn Disab* 15:33-37, 1982.

Wong B: *Learning about learning disabilities,* San Diego, 1991, Academic Press.

Wong B, editor: *Contemporary intervention research in learning disabilities: an international perspective,* New York, 1992, Springer-Verlag.

Wong B et al: The efficacy of a self-questioning summarization strategy for use by underachievers and learning-disabled adolescents, *Learn Disab Focus* 2:20-35, 1986.

Wright-Strawderman C, Watson B: The prevalence of depressive symptoms in children with learning disabilities, *J Learn Disab* 25:258-264.

Yopp H: The validity and reliability of phonemic awareness tests, *Read Res Q* 23:159-177, 1988.

Chapter 12

Achenbach TM, Edelbrock CS, Howell CT: Empirically based assessment of the behavioral/emotional problems of 2- and 3-year-old children, *J Abnorm Child Psychol* 15:629-650, 1987.

Adnopoz JA, Forsyth BWC, Nagler SF: Psychiatric aspects of HIV infection and AIDS on the family, *Child Adolesc Psychiatr Clin North America* 3:543-555, 1994.

American Psychiatric Association: *Diagnostic and statistical manual of mental disorders,* ed 4, Washington DC, 1994, American Psychiatric Press.

Blackman JA: *Developmental screening: infants, toddlers, and preschoolers.* In Levine et al, editors: *Developmental-behavioral pediatrics,* ed 2, 1992, Philadelphia, W.B. Saunders.

Bowlby J: *Attachment and loss,* New York, 1969, Basic Books.

Capute AJ et al: The clinical linguistic and auditory milestone scale (CLAMS), *Am J Dis Child* 140:694-698, 1986.

Costello EJ et al: How can epidemiology improve mental health services for children and adolescents? *J Am Acad Child Adolesc Psychiatry* 32:1106-1113, 1993.

Developmental stages prenatal, perinatal and infancy: a plan for prevention services, 30-52, 1988, Department of Mental Health, Mental Retardation and Substance Abuse Services of Virginia.

First LR, Palfrey JS: The infant or young child with developmental delay, *N Engl J Med* 330:478-483, 1994.

Gonzalez NM, Campbell M: Cocaine babies: does prenatal exposure to cocaine affect development? *J Am Acad Child Adolesc Psychiatry* 33:16-19, 1994.

Griffith DR et al: Three-year outcome of children exposed prenatally to drugs, *J Am Acad Child Adolesc Psychiatry* 33:20-27, 1994.

Hoon AH Jr et al: Clinical adaptive test/clinical linguistic auditory milestone scale in early cognitive assessment, *J Pediatr* 123:S1-S8, 1993.

March of Dimes Birth Defects Foundation: *March of dimes statbook statistics for healthier mothers and babies,* 1993.

Maurer HM: The growing neglect of American children, *Am J Dis Child* 145:540-541, 1991.

Oleske JM: The many needs of the HIV-infected child, *Hosp Pract* 63-69, Sept. 1994.

Osofsky JD: *Handbook of infant development,* ed 2, New York, 1987, John Wiley & Sons.

Price RH et al: Fourteen ounces of prevention: case book for practitioners, Washington, DC, 1988, American Psychological Association.

Richardson GA, Day NL: Detrimental effects of prenatal cocaine exposure: illusion or reality? *J Am Acad Child Adolesc Psychiatry* 33:28-34, 1994.

Verhulst F, Koot H: Child psychiatric epidemiology concepts, methods and findings, Newbury Park, Calif., 1992, Sage Publications.

Zero to Three/National Center for Clinical Infant Programs: *Diagnostic classification of mental health and developmental disorders of infancy and early childhood,* Arlington, Va., 1994, author.

Chapter 13

American Psychiatric Association: *Diagnostic and statistical manual of mental disorders,* ed 4, Washington, DC, 1994, American Psychiatric Press.

Aponte HJ, VanDuesen JM: *Structural family therapy.* In Gurman AS, Kniskern DP, editors: *Handbook of family therapy,* vol 1, New York, 1981, Brunner/Mazel.

Campbell M, Small AM, Green WH: Behavioral efficacy of haloperidol and lithium carbonate: a comparison in hospitalized aggressive children with conduct disorder, *Arch Gen Psychiatry* 41:650-656, 1984.

Carlson GA et al: Lithium in hospitalized children at 4 and 8 weeks: mood, behavior, and cognitive effects, *J Child Psychol: Psychiatry, and Allied Disciplines* 33:411-425, 1992.

Connor DF: Beta blockers for aggression: a review of the pediatric experience, *J Child Adolesc Psychopharmacol* 3:99-114, 1993.

Dinkmeyer D, McKay G: *Systematic training for effective parenting (STEP),* Circle Pines, Minn., 1975. American Guidance Services.

Dumas JE: Treating antisocial behavior in children: child and family approaches, *Clin Psychol Rev* 9:197-222, 1989.

Erickson MF, Sroufe LA, Egeland B: *The relationship between quality of attachment and behavior problems in pre-school in a high-risk sample.* In Bretherton I, Waters E, editors: *Growing points of attachment theory and research, Monographs of the society for research in child development* 50 Serial No. 209, 1989.

Fergusson DM, Horwood J, Lynskey MT: Prevalence and comorbidity of DSM-III-R diagnoses in a birth cohort of 15 year olds, *J Am Acad Child Adolesc Psychiatry* 32:1127-1134, 1993.

Green WH: *Principles of psychopharmacotherapy and specific drug treatments.* In Lewis M, editor: *Child and adolescent psychiatry: a comprehensive textbook,* Baltimore, 1991, Williams & Wilkins.

Gurman AS, Kniskern DP: *Handbook of family therapy,* vol 1, New York, 1981, Brunner/Mazel.

Kellam SG et al: The course and malleability of aggressive behavior from early first grade into middle school: results of a developmental epidemiologically-based preventive trial, *J Child Psychol Psychiatry* 35:259-281, 1994.

Kemph JP et al: Treatment of aggressive children with clonidine: results of an open pilot study, *J Am Acad Child Adolesc Psychiatry* 32:577-581, 1994.

Lochman JE, Lenhart LA: Anger coping intervention for aggressive children: conceptual models and outcome effects, *Clin Psychol Rev* 13:785-805, 1993.

McMahon RJ: Diagnosis, assessment, and treatment of externalizing problems in children: the role of longitudinal data, *J Consult Clin Psychol* 62:901-917, 1994.

Patterson GR: Orderly change in a stable world: the antisocial trait as a chimera, *J Consult Clin Psychol* 61:911-919, 1993.

Polyson J, Kimball W: *Social skills training with physically aggressive children.* In Finch AJ, Nelson WM, Ott ES, editors: *Cognitive-behavioral procedures with children and adolescents,* Boston, 1993, Allyn & Bacon.

Sanson A et al: Precursors of hyperactivity and aggression, *J Am Acad Child Adolesc Psychiatry* 32:1207-1216, 1993.

Satterfield J et al: Prediction of antisocial behavior in attention-deficit hyperactivity disorder boys from aggression/defiance scores, *J Am Acad Child Adolesc Psychiatry* 33:185-190, 1994.

Schroeder C, Goolsby E, Stangler S: Preventive services in a private pediatric practice, *J Clin Child Psychol* 4:32-33, 1975.

Thomas A, Chess S: *Temperament and development,* New York, 1977 Brunner/Mazel.

Verhulst FC, Koot HM: *The stability of externalizing behaviors in an epidemiological sample.* In Remschmidt H, Schmidt MH, editors: *Developmental psychopathology,* Lewiston, N.Y., 1992, Hogrefe & Huber Publishers.

Chapter 14

American Medical Association: *Rationale and recommendations: depression (severe or recurrent) and suicide.* In *AMA guidelines for adolescent preventative services,* Chicago, 1993, author.

American Psychiatric Association: *Diagnostic and statistical manual of mental disorders,* ed 4, Washington DC, 1994, American Psychiatric Press.

Becker RE: Depression in schizophrenia, *Hosp Commun Psychiatry* 39:1269-1275, 1988.

Berlin IN: Suicide among American Indian adolescents: an overview, *Suicide Life Threat Behav* 17:218-232, 1987.

Brent DA: Firearms and adolescent suicide: a community case control study, *Am J Dis Child* 147:1066-1071, 1993a.

Brent DA: Psychiatric risk factors for adolescent suicide: a case control study, *J Am Acad Child Adolesc Psychiatry* 32:521-529, 1993b.

Brent DA: Stressful life events, psychopathology and adolescent suicide: a case control study, *Suicide Life Threat Behav* 23:179-187, 1993c.

Brownstein M: Contacting the family after a suicide, *Can J Psychiatry* 37:208, April 1992.

deMan AF, Labreche-gauthier L, Leduc CP: Parent-child relationships and suicidal ideation in French-Canadian adolescents, *J Genet Psychol* 154:17-23, 1992.

Gould MS, Shaffer D: The impact of suicides in television movies: evidence of imitation, *N Engl J Med* 315:690-694, 1986.

Hendren RL: *Assessment and interviewing strategies for suicidal patients over the life cycle.* In Blumenthal SJ, Kupfer DJ, editors: *Suicide over the life cycle: risk factors, assessment, and treatment for suicidal patients,* Washington DC, 1990, American Psychiatric Press.

Hendren RL, Blumenthal SJ: Adolescent suicide: recognition and management in the forensic setting, *Forensic Rep* 2:47-63, 1989.

Hunington DD, Bender WN: Adolescents with learning disabilities at risk? Emotional well being, depression, suicide, *J Learn Disab* 26:159-166, 1993.

Kaplan H, Sadock B, Grebb JA: *Kaplan and Sadock's synopsis of psychiatry,* ed 7, Baltimore, Md., 1994, Williams and Wilkins.

Kashden J et al: Impulsivity in suicidal and non-suicidal adolescents, *J Abnorm Child Psychol* 21:339-353, 1993.

Lewinsohn P et al: Psychosocial characteristics of adolescents with a history of suicide attempt, *J Am Acad Child Adolesc Psychiatry* 32:60-68, 1993.

Million T: *Disorders of personality DSMIII:axis II,* New York, 1981, Wiley.

Motto JA, Heilborn DC, Hustes RP: Development of a clinical instrument to estimate suicide risk, *Am J Psychiatry* 142:680-686, 1988.

Pfeffer CR: *The suicidal child,* New York, 1986, Guilford Press.

Pfeffer CR: Risk factors associated with youth suicide: a clinical perspective, *Psychiatric Ann* 18:652-656, 1988.

Pfeffer CR: Suicidal behavior in children and adolescents: a clinical and research perspective, *Yale J Biol Med* 63:325-332, 1990.

Roose SP, Glassman AH, Walsh BT: Depression, delusions and suicide, *Am J Psychiatry* 140:1159-1162, 1983.

Shaffer D: Suicide in childhood and early adolescence, *J Child Psychol Psychiatry* 15:275-291, 1974.

Shafii M et al: Psychological autopsy of completed suicide in children and adolescents, *Am J Psychiatry* 142:1061-1064, 1985.

Stone MH: Paradoxes in the management of suicidality in borderline patients, *Am J Psychiatry* 140:1159-1162, 1983.

US Bureau of the Census: *Statistical abstract of the United States.* In *The national data book,* Washington, DC, 1993, author.

Chapter 15

Bailey GW: Children, Adolescents and Substance Abuse, *J Am Acad Child Adolesc Psychiatry* 31:1041-1045, 1992.

Chapter 16

American Academy of Child and Adolescent Psychiatry Committee on Rights and Legal Matters: *Guidelines for the clinical evaluation of child and adolescent sexual abuse,* Washington DC, 1988, author.

Black CA, Deblassie RR: Sexual abuse in the male children and adolescents: indicators, effects, and treatment, *Adolescence* 28:123-133, 1993.

Briere JN: *Child abuse trauma: theory and treatment of the lasting effects,* Newbury Park, Calif., 1992, Sage Publications.

Cohen E, MacKenzie MD, Yates MA: HEADSS, a psychosocial risk assessment instrument: implications for designing effective intervention programs for runaway youth, *J Adolesc Health* 12:539-544, 1991.

Crouch JL, Milner JS: Effects of child neglect on children, *Criminal Justice and Behavior* 20:49-65, 1993.

Daie N, Witztum E, Eleff M: Long-term effects of sibling incest, *J Clin Psychiatry* 50:428-431, 1989.

DeBellis MD et al: Hypothalamic-pituitary-adrenal axis dysregulation in sexually abused girls, *J Clin Endocrinol Metab* 78:249-255.

Dubowitz H, Black M, Harrington D: The diagnosis of child sexual abuse, *Am J Dis Child* 146:688-693, 1992.

Faller KC: Possible explanations for child sexual abuse allegations in divorce, *Am J Orthopsychiatry* 61:86-91, 1991.

Faller KC: Extrafamilial sexual abuse, *Child Adolesc Psychiatr Clin North Am* 3:713-727, 1994.

Finkelhor D: *Child sexual abuse: new theory and research,* New York, 1984, The Free Press.

Finkelhor D: The traumatic impact of child sexual abuse, *Am J Orthopsychiatry* 55:530-541, 1985.

Finkelhor D: Sexual abuse in a national survey of adult men and women: prevalence, characteristics, and risk factors, *Child Abuse Negl* 14:19-28, 1990.

Friedemann VM, Morgan MK: *Interviewing sexual abuse victims using anatomical dolls: the professional's guidebook,* Eugene, Ore., 1985, Migima Designs.

Gibbons M, Vincent EC: Childhood sexual abuse, *Am Fam Physician* 49:125-135, 1994.

Glod C: Long-term consequences of childhood physical and sexual abuse, *Arch Psychiatr Nurs* 7:163-173, 1993.

Green AH: Child sexual abuse: immediate and long-term effects and intervention, *J Am Acad Child Adolesc Psychiatry* 32:890-902, 1993.

Helfer RE: The neglect of our children, *Pediatr Clin North Am* 37:923-943, 1990.

Hegar RL, Zuravin SJ, Orme JG: Factors predicting severity of physical child abuse injury: a review of the literature, *J Interpersonal Violence* 9:170-183, 1994.

Hoekelman RA: A pediatrician's view: doom and gloom again—what we can do about it, *Pediatr Ann* 21:471-472, 1992.

Hibbard RA, Hartman G: Genitalia in human figure drawings: childrearing practices and child sexual abuse, *J Pediatr* 116:822-828, 1990.

Jennings KT: *Female child molesters: a review of the literature.* In Elliott M, editor: *Female sexual abuse of children,* New York, 1994, Guilford Press.

Juvenile Law Center: *Child abuse and the law,* ed 3, Philadelphia, 1987, author.

Kaplan SJ: *Physical abuse and neglect.* In Lewis M, editor: *Child and adolescent psychiatry: a comprehensive textbook,* Baltimore, 1991, Williams and Wilkins.

Lanning K: *Child molesters: a behavioral analysis.* In *Deviant and criminal sexuality,* Washington DC, 1991, National Center for the Analysis of Violent Crime; Federal Bureau of Investigation, U.S. Department of Justice.

Margolin L: Sexual abuse by grandparents, *Child Abuse Negl* 16:735-741, 1992.

Matthews JK: *Working with female sexual abusers.* In Elliott M: *Female sexual abuse of children,* New York, 1994, Guilford Press.

Newberger EH: Child physical abuse, *Prim Care* 20:317-327, 1993.

Risin LI, Koss MP: The sexual abuse of boys: prevalence and descriptive characteristics of childhood victimizations, *J Interpersonal Violence* 2:309-323, 1987.

Rosenberg DA, Krugman RD: Epidemiology and outcome of child abuse, *Ann Rev Med* 42:217-224, 1991.

Rowan EL, Rowan JB, Langelier P: Women who molest children, *Bull Am Acad Psychiatry Law* 18:79-83, 1990.

Smith H, Israel E: Sibling incest: a study of the dynamics of 25 cases, *Child Abuse Negl* 11:101-108, 1987.

Sobel MJ, Meyer LC: *Family and couple interactional patterns in cases of father/daughter incest.* In *Sexual abuse of children: selected readings,* Washington DC, 1980, National Center of Child Abuse and Neglect; Children's Bureau, U.S. Department of Health and Human Services Publication No. (OHDS) 78-30161.

Sorenson T, Snow B: How children tell: the process of disclosure in child sexual abuse, *Child Welfare* 52:3-15, 1991.

Srnec P: Children, violence, and intentional injuries, *Crit Care Nurs Clin North Am* 3(3)471-478, 1991.

Summit RC: The child sexual abuse accommodation syndrome, *Child Abuse Negl* 7:177-193, 1983.

Terr L: *Childhood trauma.* In Michels R, editor: *Psychiatry,* Philadelphia, 1992, J.B. Lippincott.

Tharinger D: Impact of child sexual abuse on developing sexuality, *Prof Psychol Res Pract* 21:331-337, 1990.

Walker CE, Bonner BL, Kaufman KL: *The physically and sexually abused child: evaluation and treatment,* New York, 1988, Pergamon Press.

Westen D: Physical and sexual abuse in adolescent girls with borderline personality disorder, *Am J Orthopsychiatry* 60:55-66, 1990.

Wolfe DA: *Child abuse: implications for child development and psychopathology,* Newbury Park, Calif., 1987, Sage Publications.

Wright S: Physical and emotional abuse and neglect of preschool children: a literature review, *Aust Occup Ther J* 41:55-63, 1994.

Zuravin AJ, DiBlasio FA: Child-neglecting adolescent mothers: how do they differ from their non-maltreating counterparts? *J Interpersonal Violence* 7:471-489, 1992.

Chapter 17

Aman MG: *Drugs and learning in mentally retarded persons.* In Burrows GD, Werry JS, editors: *Advances in human psychopharmacology,* vol 3, Greenwich, Conn., 1984, JAI Press.

Aman MG, Singh NN: Methylphenidate in severely retarded residents and the clinical significance of stereotypic behavior, *Appl Res Mental Retardation* 3:1-14, 1982.

Aman MG, Singh NN: *Aberrant behavior checklist and manual,* New York, 1986, Slosson Educational Publications.

Aman MG et al: Preliminary study of imipramine in profoundly retarded residents, *J Autism Dev Dis* 16:263-273, 1986.

American Psychiatric Association: *Diagnostic and statistical manual of mental disorders,* ed 4, Washington, DC, 1994, American Psychiatric Press.

Bregman J: Current developments in the understanding of mental retardation. II. Psychopathology, *J Am Acad Child Adolesc Psychiatry* 30:861-872, 1991.

Carr EG: The motivation of self-injurious behavior: a review of some hypotheses, *Psychol Bull* 84:800-816, 1977.

Chandler M, Gualtieri CT, Fahs JJ: *Other psychotropic drugs.* In Aman MG, Singh NN, editors: *Psychopharmacology of the developmental disabilities,* New York, 1988, Springer-Verlag.

Handen BL et al: Adverse side effects of Ritalin among mentally retarded children with ADHD, *J Am Acad Child Adolesc Psychiatry* 30:241-245, 1991.

Harris JC: *Neurobiological factors in self-injurious behavior.* In Luiselli JK, Matson JL, Singh NN, editors: *Self-injurious behavior: analysis, assessment, and treatment,* New York, 1992, Springer-Verlag.

Linscheid TR: *Aversive stimulation.* In Luiselli J, Matson JL, Singh NN, editors: *Self-injury: analysis, assessment, and treatment,* New York, 1992, Springer-Verlag.

Lovell RW, Reiss AL, Dual diagnoses: psychiatric disorders in developmental disabilities, *Pediatr Clin North Am* 40:579-592, 1993.

Matson JL: *The PIMRA manual,* Orland Park, Ill., 1988, International Diagnostic Systems.

Matson JL: A scale for evaluating emotional disorders in severely and profoundly retarded persons: development of the Diagnostic Assessment for the Severely Handicapped (DASH) scale, *Br J Psychiatry* 159:404-409, 1991.

Popper CW: *Disorders usually first evident in infancy, childhood, or adolescence.* In Talbott JA, Hales RE, Yudofsky SC, editors: *American Psychiatric Press textbook of psychiatry,* Washington, DC, 1988, American Psychiatric Press.

Pyles DAM, Bailey JS: *Behavioral diagnostic interventions,* In Luiselli JK, Matson JL, Singh NN, editors: *Self-injury: analysis, assessment, and treatment,* New York, 1992, Springer-Verlag.

Reiss S: *The Reiss screen for maladaptive behavior test manual,* Orland Park, Ill., 1988, International Diagnostic Systems.

Repp AC, Singh NN: *Perspectives on the use of nonaversive and aversive interventions for persons with developmental disabilities,* Sycamore, Ill., 1990, Sycamore Publishing.

Ricketts RW: Clinical effects of buspirone on intractable self-injury in adults with mental retardation, *J Am Acad Child Adolesc Psychiatry* 33:270-276, 1994.

Ricketts RW et al: Fluoxetine treatment of severe self-injury in young adults with mental retardation, *J Am Acad Child Adolesc Psychiatry* 32:865-869, 1993.

Ricketts RW et al: Opioid antagonists. II. Clinical effects in the treatment of self-injury in individuals with developmental disabilities, *J Dev Physical Disabil* 5:17-28, 1993.

Rutter M, Tizard J, Whitmore K: *Education, health, and behavior,* New York, 1970, Wiley.

Singh NN, Ellis CR, Singh YN: *Medication management.* In Cipani E, Spooner F, editors: *Curricular and instructional approaches for persons with severe handicaps,* Boston, 1994, Allyn & Bacon.

Singh NN, Guernsey TF, Ellis CR: Drug therapy for persons with developmental disabilities: legislation and litigation, *Clin Psychol Rev* 12:665-679, 1992.

Singh NN, Singh NN, Ellis CR: Psychopharmacology of self-injury. In Luiselli JK, Matson JL, Singh NN, editors: *Self-injury: assessment, analysis, and treatment,* New York, 1992, Springer-Verlag.

Singh NN, Winton ASW: *Behavioral pharmacology.* In Luiselli JK, editor: *Behavioral medicine and developmental disabilities,* New York, 1989, Springer-Verlag.

Singh NN et al: Assessment and diagnosis of mental illness in persons with mental retardation: methods and measures, *Behav Mod* 15:419-443, 1991.

Singh NN et al: *Collaboration of disciplines.* In Matson JL, editor: *Handbook of hyperactivity in children,* Boston, 1993, Allyn & Bacon.

Singh NN et al: Does diminished dopaminergic neurotransmission increase pica? *J Child Adolesc Psychopharmacol* 4:93-99, 1994.

Singh YN et al: Opioid antagonists. I. Pharmacology and rationale for use in treating self-injury, *J Dev Physical Disabil* 5:5-15, 1993.

Sprague RL et al: The dyskinesia identification system—coldwater (DIS-CO): a tardive dyskinesia rating scale for the developmentally disabled, *Psychopharmacol Bull* 20:328-338, 1984.

Van Houten R, Axelrod S: *Behavior analysis and treatment,* New York, 1984, Plenum.

Chapter 18

Friedman SB, Fisher M, Schonberg SK: *Comprehensive adolescent health care,* St Louis, 1992, Quality Medical Publishing.

Hofmann AD, Becker RD, Gabriel HP: *The hospitalized adolescent,* New York, 1976, Macmillan.

Kubler-Ross E: *On death and dying,* New York, 1970, Macmillan.

Levine MD et al: *Developmental-behavioral pediatrics,* Philadelphia, 1983, Saunders.

McCollum AT: *The chronically ill child: a guide for parents and professionals,* New Haven, 1975, Yale University Press.

Moos RH, Moos BS: *Family environment scale,* California, 1986, Consulting Psychologists Press.

Noshpitz J: *Understanding the school child's ethics.* In Silber T, editor: *Ethical issues in the treatment of children and adolescents,* New Jersey, 1983, Slack.

Schowalter J, Ferholt J, Mann N: *The adolescent patient's decision to die.* In Silber T, editor: *Ethical issues in the treatment of children and adolescents,* New Jersey, 1983, Slack.

Chapter 19

Adnopoz JA, Forsyth BWC, Nagler SF: Psychiatric aspects of HIV infection and AIDS on the family, *Child Adolescent Psychiatr Clin North Am* 3:543-555, 1994.

The Alan Guttmacher Institute: *Facts in brief: teenage reproductive health in the United States,* Washington DC, 1994, author.

Brookman RR: *Adolescent sexual behavior.* In Holmes et al, editors: *Sexually Transmitted Diseases,* ed 2, New York, 1990, McGraw-Hill.

Brookman RR: When your teen-age patient is pregnant, *Pediatr Management* 3:29-36, 1992.

Brooks-Gunn JR, Furstenberg F: Coming of age in the era of AIDS: puberty, sexuality, and contraception, *Milbank Q* 68(Suppl 1):59-84, 1990.

Bull C: Drawing the line, *Advocate* 655:27-28, 1994.

Cobliner WG: *Prevention of adolescent pregnancy: a developmental perspective.* In McAnary E, Stick L, editors: *Pregnancy and child bearing during adolescence,* New York, 1981, Alan R. Liss.

D'Angelo LJ et al: Human immunodeficiency virus infection in urban adolescents: can we predict who is at risk? *Pediatrics* 88:982-986, 1991.

Ehrhardt AA, Baker SW: *Fetal androgens, human central nervous system differentiation and sex behavior differences.* In Friedman RC et al, editors: In *Sex Differences in Behavior,* New York, 1974, John Wiley and Sons.

Erickson EH: *Identity and the life cycle.* In Klein GS, editor: *Psychological issues, monograph 1,* New York, 1959, International Universities Press.

Erickson EH: *Childhood and Society,* ed 2, New York, 1963, Williams & Wilkins.

Falco KL: *Psychotherapy with lesbian clients: theory into practice,* New York, 1991, Brunner/Mazel.

Ford ME, Linney JA: Comparative analysis of juvenile sexual offenders, violent nonsexual offenders, and status offenders, *J Interpersonal Violence* 10:56-70, 1995.

Freud S: *The standard edition of the complete psychological works of Sigmund Freud,* London, 1957, Hogarth Press.

Gagnon JH, Simon W: *Sexual conduct,* Chicago, 1973, Aldine Publishing.

Green R: *Sexual identity conflict in children and adults,* New York, 1974, Basic Books.

Greydanus DE, Dewdney D: Homosexuality in adolescence, *Semin Adolesc Med* 1:117-129, 1985.

Greyudanus DE et al: Sexual dysfunction in adolescents, *Semin Adolesc Med* 1:177-87, 1985.

Hamburg BA: *Chronic illness.* In Levine MD et al, editors: *Developmental Behavioral Pediatrics,* Philadelphia, 1983, WB Saunders.

Hazelwood RR et al: *Autoerotic fatalities,* Lexington, Mass., 1983, D.C. Heath.

Imperato-McGinley J et al: *The impact of androgens on the evolution of male gender identity.* In Kogan SJ, Hafez ESE, editors: *Pediatric andrology,* Boston, 1981, Martinus Nijhoff Publishers.

Isay R: *Being homosexual,* New York, 1989, Farrar, Straus & Giroux.

Johnson TC: Assessment of sexual behavior problems in preschool-aged and latency-aged children, *Child Adolesc Psychiatric Clin North Am* 2:431-449, 1993.

Kirkpatrick M, Morgan C: *Psychoanalytic psychotherapy of female homosexuality.* In Marmor J, editor: *Homosexual behavior a: modern appraisal,* New York, 1980, Basic Books.

Klinger RL, Cabaj RB: *Characteristics of gay and lesbian relationships.* In Odham J, Riba M, editors: *American Psychiatric Association annual review of psychiatry,* Washington DC, 1993, American Psychiatric Press.

Litt I, Vaughan V: *Adolescence.* In Behrman R, editor: *Nelson textbook of pediatrics,* Philadelphia, 1989, WB Saunders.

Lowry R, Holzman D, Truman B: Substance use and HIV related sexual behaviors among high school students: are they related? *Am J Public Health* 84:1116-1120, 1994.

Maier HW: *Three theories of child development,* New York, 1965, Harper and Row.

McWhirter DP: *Biological theories of sexual orientation.* In Odham J, Riba M, editors: *American Psychiatric Association annual review of psychiatry,* Washington DC, 1993, American Psychiatric Press.

Meyer-Bahlburg HFL: Psychobiologic research on homosexuality, *Child Adolesc Psychiatry Clin North Am* 2:489-500, 1993.

Mishel W: *A social learning view of sex differences and behavior.* In Maccoby E, editor: *The development of sex differences,* Stanford, 1966, Stanford University Press.

Money J, Pranzarone GF: Development of paraphilia in childhood and adolescence, *Child Adolesc Psychiatry Clin North Am* 2:463-475, 1993.

Murdock G: *Social structure,* New York, 1960, Macmillan.

Piaget J, Inhelder B: *The growth of logical thinking from childhood to adolescence,* New York, 1958, Basic Books.

Report of the secretary's task force on youth suicide, Rockville, Md., 1989, Alcohol, Drug Abuse, and Mental Health Administration, DHHS publication no. 89-1621.

Smith S, McClaugherty LO: Adolescent homosexuality: a primary care perspective, *Am Fam Physician* 48:33-36, 1993.

Stall R et al: Alcohol and drug use during sexual activity and compliance with safe sex guidelines for AIDS: the AIDS behavioral research project, *Health Educ Q,* 13:359-371, 1986.

Stein TS: *Overview of new developments in understanding homosexuality.* In Odham J, Riba M, editors: *American psychiatric association annual review of psychiatry,* Washington DC, 1993, American Psychiatric Press.

Tremble B, Schneider M, Appathurai C: *Growing up gay or lesbian in a multicultural context.* In Herdt G, editor: *Gay and lesbian youth,* New York: 1989, Harrington Park Press.

Troiden RR: The formation of homosexual identity, *J Homosex* 17:43-73, 1989.

Whiting B, Edwards CP: A cross cultural analysis of sex differences in behavior of children aged three through 11, *J Soc Psychol* 91:171-188, 1973.

Wilson PM: *Black culture and sexuality.* In Lister L, editor: *Human sexuality, ethnoculture and social work,* New York, 1986, Hawthorne Press.

Womack WM: Gay and lesbian youth, *AACAP News: The Newsletter of the American Academy of Child and Adolescent Psychiatry* 25:7, 1994.

Zucker KJ: *Gender identity disorders in children: clinical descriptions and natural history.* In Blanchard R, Steiner BW, editors: *Clinical management of gender identity disorders in children and adults,* Washington DC, 1990a, American Psychiatric Press.

Zucker KJ: *Treatment of gender identity disorders in children.* In Blanchard R, Steiner BW, editors: *Clinical management of gender identity disorders in children and adults,* Washington DC, 1990b, American Psychiatric Press.

Zucker KJ, Green R: Gender identity disorders, In Lewis M, editor: *Child and adolescent psychiatry: a comprehensive textbook,* Baltimore: Williams & Wilkins, 1991.

Zucker KJ, Green R: Psychological and familial aspects of gender identity disorder, *Child Adolesc Psychiatry Clin North Am* 2:513-542, 1993.

Chapter 20

American Psychiatric Association: *Diagnostic and statistical manual for mental disorders,* ed 4, Washington DC, 1994, American Psychiatric Press.

Ames LB: *Your three year old: friend or enemy,* New York, 1976, Dell.

Bowlby J: *Attachment and loss,* vol 1, *Attachment,* New York, 1969, Basic Books.

David RB: *Sleep disorders.* In David RB, editor: *Pediatric Neurology for the Clinician,* Norwalk, Conn., 1992. St Louis, 1992, Mosby.

Fitzpatrick KM, Boldizar JP: The prevalence and consequences of exposure to violence among African-American youth, *J Am Acad Child Adolesc Psychiatry* 32:424-430, 1993.

Fleisher DR: Diagnosis and treatment of disorders of defecation in children, *Pediatric Gastroenterology: Pediatric Annals* Nov. 1976.

Fraiberg SH: *The magic years,* New York, 1959, Scribners.

Gage RB: Consequences of children's exposure to spouse abuse, *Pediatr Nurs* 16:258-260, 1990.

Gardner RA: *Boys and girls book about divorce,* New York, 1970, J. Aronson.

Harlow HF: Love in infant monkeys, *Sci Am* 200:68-74, 1959.

Jaffe PG, Hurley DJ, Wolfe D: Children's observations of violence. I. Critical issues in child development and intervention planning (review), *Can J Psychiatry* 35:466-470, 1990.

Koocher GP, Gudas LJ: *Grief and loss in childhood.* In Walker CE, Roberts MC, editors: *Handbook of clinical child psychology,* ed 2, New York, 1992, Wiley & Sons.

Levine M et al: *Developmental and behavioral pediatrics,* Philadelphia, Pa., 1992, Saunders.

Richters JE, Martinex P: The NIMH community violence project. I. Children as victims of and witnesses to violence, *Psychiatry* 56: 7-21, 1993.

Steele B: *Parental abuse of infants and small children.* In Anthony E, Benedek T, editors: *Parenthood: its psychology and psychopathology,* Boston, 1970, Little, Brown, & Co.

Wallerstein J: *Second chances,* New York, 1990, Houghton Mifflin.

Index

A

α_2-Adrenergic agonists, 79
AAMD Adaptive Behavioral Scales, 29
ABC; see Aberrant Behavior Checklist
Aberrant Behavior Checklist, 29, 271
Abnormal Involuntary Movement Scale, 166-167
Abnormal sexual behaviors
  assessment of, 294
  types of, 296-297
ABS; *see* AAMD Adaptive Behavioral Scales
Abuse of children, 245-261; *see also* Specific types of abuse
  general notes on assessment of, 247
  interventions and treatments of, 260
  role of primary care physician in, 260
  sequelae of, 246-247
  symptoms of, 246
Achenbach's Child Behavior Checklist, 5, 194, 198-199
Achievement tests, 27-28
ACTeRS; *see* Attention Deficit Disorder Comprehensive Teacher Rating Scale
Addison's disease, anorexia nervosa and, 146
Adenosine, generalized anxiety disorder and, 100
ADHD; *see* Attention deficit/hyperactivity disorder
ADHDIT; *see* Attention deficit/hyperactivity disorder—inattentive type
ADI; *see* Autistic Diagnostic Interview
ADIS-C; *see* Anxiety Disorders Interview Schedule for Children
Adolescence, 9
ADOS; *see* Autism Diagnostic Observation Schedule
Aggression
  developmental disabilities and, 273-274
  diagnoses associated with, 217
  intractable, 221
  oppositional defiant disorder and, 215
  pervasive developmental disorder and, 217
  problematic, 215-217
    attention deficit/hyperactivity disorder and, 216-217, 220
    conduct disorder and, 215-216
Aggressive behavior, 211-223
  antipsychotics and, 221
  β-blockers and, 220-221
  depressive disorder and, 220
  GABA neurotransmission and, 221
  guidelines for referral for, 221-222
  haloperidol and, 221
  lithium and, 221
Aggressive behavior—cont'd
  pharmacotherapy for, 220-221
  problematic, 215-217
  propanolol and, 221
  psychosis and, 220
  treatment of, 217-221
  treatment stages of, 217
  working with the school and, 219
Agoraphobia, panic disorder and, 103, 104-105
Agraphia, 174; *see also* Disorder of written expression
  with alexia, 174 aphasic, 174
  apraxic, 174
  pure, 174
  spatial, 174
AIMS; *see* Abnormal Involuntary Movement Scale
Akathisia, developmental disabilities and, 271
Akineton; *see* Biperiden
Alcohol, substance abuse and, 238, 242
Alcoholics Anonymous, 242, 244
Alexia, agraphia with, 174
Alprozalam
  generalized anxiety disorder and, 100
  panic disorder and, 106
  separation anxiety disorder and, 112
  γ-aminobutyric acid dysfunction, generalized anxiety disorder and, 100
Amitriptyline, depression and, 131
Amphetamines, substance abuse and, 242, 244
Amyl nitrates, substance abuse and, 238
Anabolic steroids, substance abuse and, 238
Anger management for children, 220
Anorexia nervosa, 16, 145-147
  Addison's disease and, 146
  antipsychotic medications and, 147
  Crohn's disease and, 146
  depression and, 147
  DSM-IV diagnostic criteria for, 145
  Eriksonian goal in, 147
  fluoxetine and, 147
  parenteral alimentation and, 147
  paroxetine and, 147
  pica and, 145
  prognosis of, 147
  regional enteritis and, 146
  sepsis and, 147
  treatment of, 147
  Turner's syndrome and, 146
Antecedent treatment strategies, 269
Anticonvulsants, 92-93, 165

Antidepressant agents
- in bipolar disorders, 139
- bulimia nervosa and, 150-151
- depression and, 131
- depressive disorders and, 129-130
- developmental disabilities and, 271
- generalized anxiety disorder and, 100
- heterocyclic, 58

Antiepileptics, 271
Antimanics, 272
Antipsychotics, 165, 271
- in aggressive children, 221
- in bipolar disorders, 137-138
- in anorexia nervosa, 147

Anxiety disorders, 97-119
- developmental disabilities and, 271
- diagnostic instruments for, 25-26
- primary treatment of, 118
- substance abuse and, 242

Anxiety Disorders Interview Schedule for Children, 25-26
Anxiolytics, 271
APGAR score, 7
Aphasia, developmental, 172
Aphasic agraphia, 174
Apraxic agraphia, 174
Artane; *see* Trihexyphenidyl
Asperger's disorder, 14, 59-61, 197
- assessment of, 61
- comparison of autistic disorder with, 60-61
- diagnostic criteria for, 59, 61
- DSM-IV diagnostic criteria for, 60
- prevalence of, 59

Assessment, 3-5; *see also* Specific disorder
Ataxia, 62
At-risk infant, 189-210
- Achenbach's Child Behavior Checklist and, 194
- Clinical Adaptive Test/Clinical Linguistic Auditory Milestone Scale and, 194-196
- diagnostic classifications of, 194-197
- DSM-IV disorders diagnosable in, 197
- failure to thrive and, 197, 200
- feeding and eating disorders and, 197, 200
- Functional Emotional Assessment Scale for Infancy and Early Childhood, 194
- laboratory assessment for, 194
- physical examination of, 193-194
- prevention of, 203
- reactive attachment disorder and, 200-202
- screening tests for, 194-197
- social isolation and, 200
- treatment of, 202-203
- Woman Infant Child program and, 200

Attention Deficit Disorder Comprehensive Teacher Rating Scale, 27
Attention deficit/hyperactivity disorder, 4-5, 14, 69-81, 197
- α_2-adrenergic agonists and, 79
- brain imaging in, 43-44
- bupropion and, 79
- buspirone and, 79
- clonidine and, 79, 80
- clonidine skin patch and, 79, 80
- cognitive behavioral therapy and, 76
- combined type, 70
- conduct disorder and, 72-73
- Conners Rating Scales and, 75
- Conners Teacher Report Form and, 80
- depression and, 127
- desipramine and, 78-79
- developmental disabilities and, 271
- dextroamphetamine and, 77-78, 80
- diagnostic criteria for, 70-71
- diagnostic instruments for, 27-28 differential diagnosis and, 74
- disruptive behavior disorders and, 14
- drugs used to treat, 72-73
- DSM-IV diagnostic criteria for, 70
- educational interventions and, 76-77
- EEG and, 73, 80
- Feingold Diet and, 73
- fluoxetine and, 79
- guanfacine and, 79
- Hyperactivity Index and, 75
- imipramine and, 78-79, 80
- L-tryptophan and, 72
- learning disorders and, 181
- major depressive disorder and, 127-128
- methylphenidate and, 77-78, 80
- mimimal brain damage and, 72-73
- monoamine oxidase inhibitors and, 72
- MRI and, 72
- nontraditional treatment and, 80
- oppositional defiant disorder and, 74
- parent training and, 76
- pemoline and, 77-78, 80
- PET scans and, 72
- pharmacologic treatment and, 77-80
  - side effects, 77-80
- pharmacotherapy and, 80
- predominantly hyperactive-inattentive type, 70
- predominantly inattentive type, 70
- problematic aggression and, 216-217
- quantitative EEG and, 73, 80
- schizophrenia and, 155, 163
- serotoninergic agents and, 79
- substance abuse and, 237, 242
- treatment of, 76
- tricyclic antidepressants and, 78-79, 80
  - ECG, 78-79
- Wechsler Intelligence Scale for Children-Revised, 75

Attribution Questionnaire, 27
Attunement, autistic disorder and, 56
Atypical autism, 52
Autism
  atypical, 59
  high-functioning, 59
Autism Diagnostic Observation Schedule, 56
Autistic behavior, disorders associated with, 52
Autistic Diagnostic Interview, 55-56
Autistic disorder, 14, 50-59
  attunement and, 56
  brain imaging in, 42-43
  comparison of Asperger's disorder and, 60-61
  comparison of Rett's disorder and, 63
  diagnostic criteria for, 51-52
  differential diagnosis of, 56
  DSM-IV diagnostic criteria for, 50
  Duchenne's muscular dystrophy and, 52 fragile X syndrome, 52
  hydrocephalus and, 52
  infantile spasms and, 52
  intersubjectivity and, 56
  intrauterine rubella infections and, 52
  Möbius' syndrome and, 52
  neurofibromatosis and, 52
  neuropsychologic testing for, 56
  pemoline and, 77
  phenylketonuria and, 52
  postnatal herpes infection and, 52
  prevalence of, 52
  Public Law 94-142, Individuals with Disabilities Act B and, 76
  Rehabilitation Act of 1973, 76
  schizophrenia and, 51
  treatment of, 56-59
  tuberous sclerosis and, 52
Autistic Disturbances of Affective Contact, 49
Autoimmune mechanisms in schizophrenia, 159

B

BAS; *see* Behavioral activation system
Batelle Developmental Inventory, 194
Bayley Scales of Infant Development, 194
BDI; *see* Beck Depression Inventory
Beck Depression Inventory, 26, 127
Behavior management training for parents, 218-219
Behavior modification and developmental disabilities, 268
Behavior Rating Instrument for Autistic and Atypical Children, 25
Behavioral activation system, 89
Behavioral inhibition system, 89
Behavioral therapy and developmental disabilities, 268
Benadryl; *see* Diphenhydramine
Benzodiazepines
  generalized anxiety disorder and, 100, 118
  panic disorder and, 106
  posttraumatic stress disorder and, 118
  schizophrenia and, 165
  selective mutism and, 113, 118
  separation anxiety disorder and, 118
  social phobia and, 116, 118
  substance abuse and, 238
Benzotropine mesylate, 164, 271
Beta blockers
  aggressive behavior and, 220-221
  social phobia and, 116
Binge-eating disorder, DSM-IV diagnostic criteria for, 149
Bipolar affective disorders, brain imaging in, 45
Bipolar disorders, 132-140
  antipsychotic agents and, 137
  attention deficit/hyperactivity disorder and, 133, 137
  carbamazepine and, 137-140
  cerebral vascular accidents and, 137
  cocaine and, 137
  conduct disorder and, 133, 137
  corticosteroids and, 137
  cyclothymia in, 132-133, 139
  developmental disorders and, 264
  dextroamphetamine and, 137
  diagnostic criteria for, 133-136
  differential diagnosis of, 137
  DSM-IV diagnostic criteria for, 134-136
  dysphoric mania in, 133
  fluoxetine and, 137
  haloperidol and, 137
  head trauma and, 137
  hyperthyroidism and, 137
  hypomanic episodes, 132-133
  isoniazid and, 137
  lithium and, 137-140
  methylphenidate and, 137
  manic episode in, 132-133
  mixed episode in, 132
  multiple sclerosis and, 137
  seizure disorders and, 137
  suicide in, 228
  thalamic tumors and, 137
  thiothixene and, 137
  treatment of, 137-140
  valproate and, 138-140
Birth, 7
BIS; *see* Behavioral inhibiton system
Bonding, 8
Borderline personality disorder
  DSM-IV diagnostic criteria for, 257
  suicide in, 228

Brain imaging, 33-45
developmental factors in, 34
in attention deficit/hyperactivity disorder, 43-44
in autistic disorders, 42-43
in childhood schizophrenia, 44
in dyslexia, 43
in fragile X syndromes, 43
in mood disorders, 45
in Rett's disorder, 43
in Tourette's disorder, 44
BRIACC; *see* Behavior Rating Instrument for Autistic and Atypical Children
Bulimia nervosa, 148-151
antidepressant medication and, 150-151
bupropion and, 150
"chipmunk cheeks" in, 149
cognitive behavior therapy and, 150-151
desipramine and, 150-151
diabetic ketoacidosis and, 150
DSM-IV diagnostic criteria for, 148
Erikson stages and, 150
erosion of dental enamel in, 149
fluoxetine and, 150-151
insulin-dependent diabetes mellitus and, 150 ipecac use in, 149
Kleine-Levin syndrome and, 150
Kluver-Bucy syndrome and, 150
monoamine oxidase inhibitors and, 150
nonpurging type, 148
pica and, 145
Prader-Willi syndrome and, 150
purging type, 148
Russell's sign, 149, 150
treatment of, 150-151
Bupropion, 131
attention deficit/hyperactivity disorder and, 79
bulimia nervosa and, 150
Buspirone
attention deficit/hyperactivity disorder and, 79
developmental disabilities and, 272, 275
generalized anxiety disorder and, 100, 118
panic disorder and, 106
separation anxiety disorder and, 118
social phobia and, 116
Butane, substance abuse and, 238

C

Cannabis, substance abuse and, 238
Carbamazepine
autistic disorders and, 59
bipolar disorders and, 138
developmental disabilities and, 272
posttraumatic stress disorder and, 109, 118
CAEF; *see* Children's Anxiety Evaluation Form
Carburetor cleaner, substance abuse and, 238
CARS; *see* Childhood Autism Rating Scale
CAS; *see* Childhood Assessment Schedule
CAT/CLAMS; *see* Clinical Adaptive Test/Clinical Linguistic Milestone Scale
CAT Scale; *see* Children's Action Tendency Scale
Catapres TTS-1; *see* Clonidine
CBCL; *see* Child Behavior Checklist
CBT; *see* Cognitive Behavioral Therapy
CD; *see* Conduct disorder
CDI; *see* Children's Depression Inventory
CDRSR; *see* Children's Depression Rating Scale-Revised
CEDRI; *see* Clinical Eating Disorder Rating Instrument
Cerebral vascular accident, as cause of mania, 137
CHADD; *see* Children with Attention Deficit Disorder
CHEOPS; *see* Children's Hospital of Eastern Ontario Pain Scale
Child's World Questions, 253
Child abuse and physical neglect, 31
Child Assessment Schedule, 23
Child Behavior Checklist, 16, 24
Achenbach's, 194
Child Depression Inventory, 23
Child maltreatment, 247
Childhood Autism Rating Scale, 25, 55
Childhood disintegrative disorder, 14, 64-66, 197
differential diagnosis of, 66
disintegrative psychosis and, 64
DSM-IV diagnostic criteria for, 64
Heller syndrome and, 64
treatment of, 66
Childhood schizophrenia, brain imaging in, 44
Children with Attention Deficit Disorder, 69
Children's Action Tendency Scale, 28
Children's Anxiety Evaluation Form, 26
Children's Depression Inventory, 26, 127
Children's Depression Rating Scale-Revised, 26
Children's Hospital of Eastern Ontario Pain Scale, 30
Children's Protective Services, 93, 201
"Chipmunk cheeks," bulimia nervosa and, 149
Chlorpromazine, 165, 271
Chronic illness
childhood developmental considerations and, 278-279
dimensions of the patient and family and, 281
factors of nonadherence to medical regimen and, 279
illness specific variables and, 281-282
Kübler-Ross grief stages, 279-281
process of acceptance and, 279-281
role of consultant in, 284
use of resources in, 282-284
Chronic vocal or motor tic disorders, DSM-IV diagnostic criteria for, 310

Clinical Adaptive Test/Clinical Linguistic Milestone Scale, 194-196
scoring test, 195-196
Clinical Eating Disorder Rating Instrument, 29
Clinical judgment, 20-21
Clomipramine
autistic disorder and, 59
obsessive-compulsive disorder and, 103, 118
Clonazepam
developmental disorders and, 271
panic disorder and, 106
posttraumatic stress disorder and, 109
separation anxiety disorder and, 118
social phobia and, 116
Clonidine
attention deficit/hyperactivity disorder and, 79, 80
autistic disorder and, 58
conduct disorder and, 92
oppositional defiant disorder and, 92
posttraumatic stress disorder and, 109, 118
skin patch, 79, 80
Clozapine, 271
Cocaine
as cause of mania, 137
substance abuse and, 238
Codeine, substance abuse and, 238, 242
Cogentin; *see* Benztropine mesylate
Cognitive behavioral therapy
attention deficit/hyperactivity disorder and, 76
bulimia nervosa and, 150-151
conduct disorder and, 93
generalized anxiety disorder and, 118
oppositional defiant disorder and, 92
panic disorder and, 118
posttraumatic stress disorder and, 109, 118
selective mutism and, 118
separation anxiety disorder and, 118
social phobia and, 118
specific phobia and, 118
Communication disorders, 14
learning disorders and, 182
Computed tomography, 33, 35
Computer-analyzed EEGs in schizophrenia, 158
Conduct disorder, 72-73, 83-95
Achenbach Child Behavior Checklist and, 91
adolescent-onset type, 86, 88, 216
anticonvulsants and, 92-93
attention deficit/hyperactivity disorder and, 91
behavioral activation system and, 89
behavioral inhibition system and, 89
benzodiazepines and, 92-93
beta blockers and, 92-93
buspirone and, 92-93
calcium channel blockers and, 92-93
carbamazepine and, 92-93
Conduct disorder—cont'd
childhood-onset type, 86, 88-89, 216
Children's Protective Services, 93
chlorpromazine and, 93
clonidine and, 92-93
cognitive behavioral therapy and, 93
Conners Teacher Rating Scale and, 91
developmental disabilities and, 273-274
diagnostic criteria for, 86-90
differential diagnosis of, 90
dopamine β-hydroxylase, 89
DSM-IV diagnostic criteria for, 86, 216, 252
diphenylhydantoin and, 93
EEG and, 92
haloperidol and, 93
interventions for, 94-95
lithium and, 92-93
major depressive disorder and, 127-128
molindone and, 93
neuroleptics and, 92-93
physical abuse and, 251
problematic aggression and, 215-217
oppositional defiant disorder and, 83-87
separation anxiety disorder and, 111
schizophrenia and, 162
substance abuse and, 242
suicide in, 228, 230, 231
thioridazine and, 93
treatment of, 92-95
Conners Parent Questionnaire, 16
Conners Parent Rating Scale-Revised, 24, 27
Conners rating scales, 5, 75, 80
Conners Teacher Rating Scale-Revised, 24, 27
Conners Teacher Report Form, 80
Continuous Performance Test, 28
Coprophagia, 274
Corticosteroids, as cause of mania, 137 Crohn's disease, anorexia nervosa and, 146
CT; *see* Computed tomography
Cushing's syndrome in schizophrenia, 161
Cycle of violence, 249
Cyclothymia, 132
Cyclothymic disorder, DSM-IV diagnostic criteria for, 136

D

DA; *see* Dextroamphetamine
DBH; *see* Dopamine β-hydroxylase
DC:03; *see* Diagnostic Classification of Mental and Developmental Disorders of Infancy and Early Childhood
Death and dying, 312-313
Dementia, childhood disintegrative disorder and, 64,66

Dental enamel, erosion of, 149
Denver Developmental Screening Test, 8
Denver Developmental Screening Test II, 8, 194
Depersonalization, schizophrenia and, 157-158
Depression
  attention deficit/hyperactivity disorder and, 127
  amitriptyline and, 131
  antidepressant agents and, 131
  bupropion and, 131
  causes of, 129
  desipramine and, 131
  developmental disabilities and, 274
  diagnostic instruments for, 26
  doxepin and, 131
  fluoxetine and, 131
  fluvoxamine and, 131
  imipramine and, 131
  nefazadone and, 131
  nortriptyline and, 131
  paroxetine and, 131
  sertraline and, 131
  TCAs and, 130
  trazodone and, 131
  venlafaxine and, 131
Depressive disorder NOS, 122
Depressive disorders, 121-140
  diagnostic criteria for, 123-127
  differential diagnosis of, 127-128
  treatment of, 128-131
Desipramine
  attention disorder/hyperactivity disorder and, 78-79
  autistic disorder and, 59
  bulimia nervosa, 150-151
  depression and, 131
Developmental disabilities, 263-275
  Aberrant Behavior Checklist and, 271
  aggression and, 273-274
  akasthisia and, 271
  antecedent treatment strategies and, 269
  antidepressants and, 271
  antiepileptics and, 271
  antimanics and, 272
  antipsychotics and, 271 anxiety disorders and, 264
  anxiolytics and, 271
  attention deficit/hyperactivity disorder and, 272
  behavior modification and, 268
  behavioral therapy and, 268
  benzotropine and, 271
  biperiden and, 271
  bipolar disorders and, 264
  buspirone and, 264
  carbamazepine and, 272
  chlorpromazine and, 271
  clonazepam and, 271
  clozapine and, 271
Developmental disabilities—cont'd
  conduct disorders and, 273-274
  coprophagia and, 274
  depression and, 274
  dextroamphetamine and, 272
  differential reinforcement of alternate behavior and, 269
  differential reinforcement of incompatible behavior and, 269
  differential reinforcement of other behavior and, 269
  Dyskinesia Identification System-Coldwater and, 271
  ethopropazine and, 271
  felbamate and, 271
  fluoxetine and, 271, 275
  fluphenazine and, 271
  gabapentin and, 271
  geophagia and, 274
  haloperidol and, 271
  de Lange's syndrome and, 274-275
  Lesch-Nyhan syndrome and, 274-275
  lithium and, 273
  loxapine and, 271
  mesoridazine and, 271
  methylphenidate and, 272
  naloxone and, 273
  naltrexone and, 273
  negative reinforcement interventions and, 269
  obsessive-compulsive disorder and, 263, 274
  opioid antagonists and, 273
  pervasive developmental disorder and, 274-275
  phenytoin and, 272
  pica and, 274
  positive reinforcement interventions and, 269
  prevalence of, 264
  procyclidine and, 271
  psychopharmacotherapy and, 270-273
  psychotherapy and, 273
  punishment and, 269-270
  risperidone and, 271
  rumination disorder and, 274
  self-injury and, 274-275
  socioenvironmental therapy and, 273
  specific behavioral disorders and, 273-275
    stimulants and, 271-272
  tardive dyskinesia and, 271
  thioridazine and, 271
  thiothixene and, 271
  trifluoperazine and, 271
  trihexyphenidyl and, 271
  treatment of, 267-273
  valproic acid and, 272
Developmental history, 7-8

Developmental Screening Inventory Revised, 194
Dexedrine; *see* Dextroamphetamine
Dextroamphetamine, 77-78, 80, 137
Diabetic ketoacidosis and, 150
Diagnostic and Statistical Manual of Mental Disorders, Fourth Edition, 14-15, 19; *see also* Specific disorder
Diagnostic and Statistical Manual of Mental Disorders, Third Edition, 13, 23, 24
Diagnostic Assessment for the Severely Handicapped, 30, 267
Diagnostic Classification of Mental and Developmental disorders of Infancy and Early Childhood, 197
Diagnostic categories, 47-185
Diagnostic formulation, 12-13
Diagnostic instruments, 19-31; *see also* Specific instruments
  types of, 22-31
    disorder-specific, 25-31
    general, 22-25
Diagnostic Interview for Children and Adolescents-Revised, 23
Diagnostic Interview Schedule for Children-Revised, 23
Diagnostic interviews, 22
DICA-R; *see* Diagnostic Interview for Children and Adolescents-Revised
Differential reinforcement of alternate behavior, 268-269
Differential reinforcement of incompatible behavior, 268-269
Differential reinforcement of other behavior, 268-269
Diphenhydramine, 164
DISC-R; *see* Diagnostic Interview Schedule for Children-Revised
Disintegrative psychosis, childhood disintegrative disorder and, 64
Disorder of social competence, learning disorders and, 182
Disorder of written expression, 174-175
  DSM-IV diagnostic criteria for, 170
Disruptive behavior disorders, 93
  pharmacotherapy for, 92
Dissociative identity disorder, DSM-IV diagnostic criteria for, 258
Divorce, 313-314
Dopamine β-hydoxylase, conduct disorder and, 89
Doxepin, 131
DRA; *see* Differential reinforcement of alternate behavior
DRI; *see* Differential reinforcement of incompatible behavior
DRO; *see* Differential reinforcement of other behavior
DSM-III; *see Diagnostic and Statistical Manual of Mental Disorders, Third Edition*
DSM-III-R, 23-25
DSM-IV; *see Diagnostic and Statistical Manual of Mental Disorders, Fourth Edition*
Dyscalculia, 175-176; *see also* Mathematics disorder
  graphic, 175-176
  ideognostic, 175-176
  lexical, 175-176
  operational, 175-176
  practognostic, 175-176
  verbal, 175-176
Dysgraphia, 174
Dyskinesia Identification System-Coldwater, 271
Dyskinesias, 59
Dyslexia, 172-174
  brain imaging in, 43
Dysphoric mania, 133
Dysthymic disorder, 122-123
  DSM-IV diagnostic criteria for, 124, 250
    early onset, 124
    late onset, 124

E

Early Language Milestone Scale, 194
EAT; *see* Eating Attitudes Test
Eating Attitudes Test, 29
Eating Disorder Examination, 28-29
Eating Disorder Inventory-2, 29
Eating disorders, 15, 141-151
  diagnostic instruments for, 28-29
  eriksonian stages and, 142
ECA; *see* Epidemiological catchment area
ECBI; *see* Eyberg Child Behavior Inventory
Ecologic context of assessment, 21-22
EDE; *see* Eating Disorder Examination
EDI-2; *see* Eating Disorder Inventory-2
Elimination disorders, 14
Emotional abuse, 248-249
Encopresis, 15, 308-309
  DSM-IV diagnostic criteria for, 309
Enuresis, 8, 15, 307-308
  DSM-IV diagnostic criteria for, 307
Epidemiological catchment area, 106
Eriksonian stages
  anorexia nervosa and, 147
  bulimia nervosa and, 150
  eating disorders and, 142
Erikson's stages of sexuality, 289
Ether, substance abuse and, 238
Ethopropazine, 271
Exhibitionism, DSM-IV diagnostic criteria for, 299
Extrafamilial sexual abuse, 256
Eyberg Child Behavior Inventory, 28

F

Failure to thrive, 197, 200
Familial dysfunction, separation anxiety disorder and, 111
Family dysfunction, chronic, 230
Family Environmental Scale, 27
Family history, 9-10
FDA; *see* Food and Drug Administration
FEAS/IEC; *see* Functional Emotional Assessment Scale for Infancy and Early Childhood
Feeding and care disorders, 14
Feeding and eating disorders, DSM-IV diagnostic criteria for, 200, 248
Feeding disorder of infancy or early childhood, 142-143, 197
  DSM-IV diagnostic criteria for, 143
Feingold diet, 73
Felbamate, 271
FES; *see* Family Environmental Scale
Fetal Alcohol Syndrome, 7, 191
Fetishism, DSM-IV diagnostic criteria for, 299
Fluphenazine, 165
Fluoxetine
  anorexia nervosa and, 147
  attention deficit/hyperactivity disorder and, 79
  autistic disorder and, 59
  depression and, 131
  developmental disabilities and, 271, 275
  obsessive-compulsive disorder and, 103
  schizophrenia and, 165
  social phobia and, 116
Fluphenazine, 271
Fluvoxamine, 103,131
Food and Drug Administration, 77
Fragile X syndrome
  autistic disorder and, 52
  brain imaging in, 43
  learning disorders and, 181
Frankl Behavior Rating Scale, 30
Freud, Anna, 190
Freud's stages of sexuality, 289
Freon, substance abuse and, 238
Frotteurism, DSM-IV diagnostic criteria for, 299
Functional Emotional Assessment Scale for Infancy and Early Childhood, 194
Functional magnetic resonance imaging, 41-42

G

GAD; *see* Generalized Anxiety Disorder
GABA dysfunction, 100
GABA neurotransmission, 221
Gabapentin, 271
Gait apraxia, 62
Gasoline, substance abuse and, 238
Gateway drugs for substance abuse, 240
Gay sexual orientation, 288, 289, 293-295
Gender identity, core, 287-288
Gender identity disorder, 16
  DSM-IV diagnostic criteria for, 297-298
Gender role behavior, 287-288
Gender role identity, 287-288
Generalized anxiety disorder, 98-100
  adenosine and,100
  alprazolam and, 100
  antidepressants and, 100
  assessment of, using Revised Children's Manifest Anxiety Scale, 100
  benzodiazepines and, 100
  buspirone and, 100
  diagnostic criteria for, 99
  differential diagnosis of, 100
  DSM-IV diagnostic criteria for, 98
  GABA dysfunction and, 100
  noradrenaline and, 100
  overanxious disorder and, 99
  social phobia and, 115
  treatment of, 100, 118
Geopagia, developmental disabilities and, 274
Gesell Preschool Test, 194
GID; *see* Gender identity disorder
Glue, 238
Grief
  death and dying and, 312-313
  divorce and, 313-314
  separation and, 311-314
Grief reaction, acute, 312
Growth hormone, panic disorder and, 103
Guanfacine, 79

H

Hairballs; *see* Trichobezoars
Haldol; *see* Haloperidol
Hallucinations, 160
Hallucinogens, 238
Haloperidol, 58-59, 165
  developmental disabilities and, 271
Hashish, 238
HEADSS questions, 254
Head trauma, as cause of mania, 137
Heller syndrome, childhood disintegrative disorder and, 64
Heroin, 238, 242
HI; *see* Hyperactivity Index
High-functioning autism, 59
History, 9-10
HIV; *see* Human immunodeficiency virus
Homosexuality, 288, 289, 293-295

Human imunodeficiency virus, 160, 191, 207-208
Hyperactivity Index, 75
Hyperlexia, 55, 174
Hyperthyroidism, as cause of mania, 13
Hypomanic episode
in bipolar disorders, 132-133
DSM-IV diagnostic criteria for, 135

I

ICD; *see* International Classification of Diseases
Imaginary friends, 315-316
Imaginary Urine Drug Screen, 242
Imipramine
attention deficit/hyperactivity disorder and, 77-78, 80
depression and, 131
separation anxiety disorder and, 112
Impulse control for children, 220
Individuals with Disabilities Education Act, 172, 175, 183
Infancy, 7
Infant developmental screening tests, 194
Infant Monitoring Questionnaire, 194
Infant Psychiatry, 190
Infant psychiatry
crack baby and, 207
Fraiberg, Selma, and, 190
Freud, Anna, and 190
History of, 190
HIV and, 190-191, 207-208
Mahler, Margaret, and, 190
multiple births and, 208-209
neonatal intensive care unit and, 204-207
special concerns of, 204-209
Winnecott, D.W., and, 190
Inhalants, 238
Insulin-dependent diabetes mellitus, bulimia nervosa and, 150
Intelligence quotient, 5, 14
autism and, 57
Interactive Model of Child Abuse, 249-251
Intermittent explosive disorder, 216
DSM-IV diagnostic criteria for, 217
International Classification of Diseases, 22
Interview, 10-11
Interview for Aggression, 28
Interview Schedule for Children, 24
Intrafamilial sexual abuse, 255
IOWA-Conners Rating Scale, 27
ISC; *see* Interview Schedule for Children
Isoniazid, as cause of mania, 137
Issues of confidentiality, substance abuse and, 241

K

K-SADS; *see* Schedule for Affective Disorders and Schizophrenia for School-Age Children
K-SADS-E; *see* Schedule for Affective Disorders and Schizophrenia for School-Age Children
K-SADS-P; *see* Schedule for Affective Disorders and Schizophrenia for School-Age Children
K-TEA; *see* Kaufman test battery
Kanner, Leo, 49, 52, 169
Kaufman (K-TEA) test battery, 27-28
Kemadrin; *see* Procyclidine
Klein-Levin syndrome, bulimia nervosa and 150
Kluver-Bucy syndrome, bulimia nervosa and, 150
Kübler-Ross grief stages, 279-281

L

de Lange's syndrome, 274-275
Language disorder, receptive-expressive, 62
Learning disability, 172
Learning disorders, 14, 169-185; *see also* Specific disorder
attention deficit/hyperactivity disorder and, 181, 182
biophysical causes of, 176
cognitive processes and, 178-180
communicative disorders and, 182
conduct disorders and, 182
CT and, 177
disorders of social competence and, 182
EEGs and, 176-177
fragile X syndrome and, 181
MRI and, 177
QEEGs and, 177
obsessive-compulsive disorder and, 182
oppositional defiant disorder and, 182
Orton-Gillingham-based programs and, 184
pervasive developmental disorders and, 182
Prospective Study of Reading, 180
Retrospective Study of Learning Disabilities, 180
separation anxiety disorder and, 112
Tourette's syndrome and, 181
treatment of, 183-184
Turner's syndrome and, 181
Lesbian sexual orientation, 288, 289, 293-295
Lesch-Nyhan syndrome, 274-275
Leyton Obsessional Inventory-Child Version, obsessive-compulsive disorder and, 102
Librium, substance abuse and, 238
Lithium
aggressive behavior and, 221
autistic disorders and, 59
bipolar disorders and, 138
developmental disorders and, 273

Lithium—cont'd
posttraumatic stress disorder and, 109, 118
schizophrenia and, 165
Loxapine, 165, 271
Loxitane; *see* Loxapine, 165
LSD, substance abuse and, 238, 242

M

Magic, 316
Magnetic resonance imaging, 33, 34, 35-39
functional, 41-42
Magnetic resonance spectroscopy, 42
Mahler, Margaret, 190
Major depressive disorder, 45, 121-132
physical abuse, 251
suicide in, 228
Major depressive episode
DSM-IV diagnostic criteria for, 123, 251
mixed episode and, 135
social phobia and, 118
Mania, medical causes of, 137
Manic episode
in bipolar disorders, 132-133
DSM-IV diagnostic criteria for, 134
MAOIs; *see* Monoamine oxidase inhibitors
Masturbation, 295-296
Matching Familiar Figures Test, 28
Mathematics disorder, 174-175
DSM-IV diagnostic criteria for, 170
MBD; *see* Minimal brain damage; minimal brain dysfunction
MDD; *see* Major depressive disorder
Medical history, 7
Mellaril; *see* Thioridazine
Mental retardation, 14, 172, 197
aggression and, 217
diagnostic instruments for, 29-30
pica and, 145
schizophrenia and, 163
Mental status examination, 11-12
Mescaline, substance abuse and, 238
Mesoridazine, 271
Methamphetamine, substance abuse and, 238
Methandrosterolone, substance abuse and, 238
Methaqualone, substance abuse and, 238
Methylphenidate, 77-78, 80, 137, 237, 272
Miller Assessment for Preschoolers, 194
Minimal brain damage, 69, 72-73, 172
Minimal brain dysfunction, 43-44
Minnesota Child Development Inventory, 194
Mitral valve prolapse, panic disorder and, 105
Mixed episode
in bipolar disorders, 132
DSM-IV diagnostic criteria for, 135
Moban; *see* Molindone
Molindone, 165
Mood disorders, 121-140
antidepressant agents and, 139
antidepressant treatment of, 130
attention deficit/hyperactivity disorder and, 127-128
Beck Depression Inventory and, 127
brain imaging and, 45
Childhood Depression Inventory and, 127
conduct disorder and, 127-128
other anxiety disorders and, 15
Weinberg Screening Affective Scale and, 127
Monoamine oxidase inhibitors, 72, 118, 130, 150
Motor skills disorders, 14
MPH; *see* Methylphenidate
MRI; *see* Magnetic resonance imaging
MRS; *see* Magnetic resonance spectroscopy
Multidimensionally impaired syndrome, 163
Multiple sclerosis, as cause of mania, 137

N

NA; *see* Narcotics Anonymous
Navane; *see* Thiothixene
Naloxone, 273
Naltrexone
autistic disorders and, 59
developmental disabilities, 273
Nandrolone decanoate, substance abuse and, 238
Narcotics Anonymous, 242, 244
National Institute for Drug Abuse, 238
"Nattering," discipline and, 218
Nefazadone, 131
Negative reinforcement interventions and developmental disabilities, 269
Neglect, 247-248
Neonatal Behavioral Assessment Scale, 194, 197
Neonatal period, 7
Neurocognitive tests, 28
Neuroleptic-induced disorder, 111
Neuroleptic malignant syndrome, 163
Neuroleptics
autistic disorder and, 58-59
posttraumatic stress disorder and, 109
Neurotransmitter dysfunction, panic disorder and, 103
Neurological Examination of the Fullterm Newborn Infant, 197
Newborn Individualized Developmental Care and Assessment Program, 194, 197
NIDA; *see* National Institute for Drug Abuse
NIDCAP; *see* Newborn Individualized Developmental Care and Assessment Program
Nightmares, 314-315
Nitrous oxide, substance abuse and, 238
Noradrenalin, generalized anxiety disorder and, 100

Normal sexual behaviors, 292-293
Nortriptyline, 131

O

OAD; *see* Overanxious disorder
Observational Scale of Behavioral Distress, 30
Obsessive-compulsive disorder, 100-103
  clomipramine and, 103
  cognitive behavioral therapy and, 102
  developmental disabilities and, 263, 274
  diagnostic criteria for, 100
  differential diagnosis, 102
  DSM-IV diagnostic criteria for, 101
  fluoxetine and, 103
  Leyton Obsessional Inventory-Child Version and, 102
  paroxetine and, 103
  pervasive developmental disorders and, 102
  sertaline and, 103
  Tourette's disorder and, 102
  treatment of, 102-103
  with poor insight, 101
  Yale-Brown Obsessive Compulsive Scale and, 102
Opiate antagonist, autistic disorder and, 59
Opiates, substance abuse and, 238
Opioid antagonists and developmental disabilities, 273
OCD; *see* Obsessive-compulsive disorder
ODD; *see* Oppositional defiant disorder
Oppositional defiant disorder, 3, 83-95
  attention deficit/hyperactivity disorder and, 74
  cognitive behavioral therapy and, 92
  diagnostic criteria for, 84-87
  DSM-IV diagnostic criteria for, 84, 215
  problematic aggression and, 215, 217
  schizophrenia and, 162
Orap; *see* Pimozide
OSBD; *see* Observational Scale of Behavioral Distress
Overanxious disorder, generalized anxiety disorder and, 99
Oxycodone, substance and, 238

P

Pain disorder, diagnostic instruments for, 30
Paired Associate Learning Task, 28
Panic attacks; *see* Panic disorder
Panic disorder, 103-106, 118
  agoraphobia without history of, DSM-IV diagnostic criteria for, 105
  alprazolam and, 106
  benzodiazepines and, 106
  buspirone and, 106
  clonazepam and, 106
Panic disorder—cont'd
  diagnostic criteria, 103
  differential diagnosis and, 106
  growth hormone and, 103
  mitral valve prolapse and 105
  neurotransmitter dysfunction and, 103
  school phobia and, 106
  SSRIs and, 106
  thyroid-stimulating hormone and, 103
  thyrotropin-releasing hormone and, 103
  treatment of, 106
    primary, 118
  tricyclic antidepressants and, 106
  with agoraphobia, DSM-IV diagnostic criteria for, 104
  without agoraphobia, DSM-IV diagnostic criteria for, 104
Paraphilias, 298-299
Parenteral alimentation, anorexia nervosa and, 147
Parents, behavior management training for, 2180219
Paroxetine, 103, 131, 147
Parsidol; *see* Ethopropazine
PBCL; *see* Procedure Behavior Checklist
PBRS; *see* Procedure Behavior Rating Scale
PCP, substance abuse and, 238
PDD; *see* Pervasive developmental disorders
Peabody Individual Achievement Test-Revised, 27-28
Peabody Picture Vocabulary Test, 194
Pedophilia, DSM-IV diagnostic criteria for, 300
Pemoline, 77, 80
Perphenazine, 165
Pervasive developmental disorders, 14, 49-67, 197
  aggression and, 217
  developmental disabilities and, 274-275
  diagnostic instruments for, 25
  obsessive-compulsive disorder and, 102
  pica and, 145
  schizophrenia and, 155
Pervasive developmental disorder NOS, 49-50, 52
PET; *see* Positron emission tomograph
Peyote, substance abuse and, 238
Phenobarbital, 272
Physical abuse, 249-250
  conduct disorder and, 251
  cycle of violence and, 249
  dysthymic disorder, 250
  Interactive Model of Child Abuse, 249-251
  major depressive episode, 251
Pica, 143, 144-145
  anorexia nervosa and, 144
  bulimia nervosa and, 144
  developmental disabilities and, 274
  DSM-IV diagnostic criteria for, 144
  mental retardation and, 144
  pervasive developmental disorder and, 144

Pica—cont'd
  Toxocara canis and, 145
  trichobezoars and, 145
Pimozide, 165
Positive reinforcement interventions and developmental disabilities, 269
Positron emission tomography, 33, 40-42
  attention deficit/hyperactivity disorder and, 72
  schizophrenia and, 158, 160
Posttraumatic stress disorder, 16, 106-109, 118
  acute, 107
  benzodiazepine and, 118
  carbamazepine and, 109, 118
  chronic, 107
  clonazepam and, 109
  clonidine and, 109, 118
  cognitive behavioral therapy and, 109, 118
  diagnostic criteria of, 106
  differential diagnosis of, 108-109
  DSM-IV diagnostic criteria for, 107, 317
  fluoxetine and, 109
  genralized anxiety disorder and, 100
  lithium and, 109, 118
  monoamine oxidase inhibitors and, 118
  neuroleptics and, 109
  propranolol and, 118
  SSRIs and, 109, 118
  suicide in, 230
  trauma and, 316-318
  tricyclic antidepressants and, 109, 118
  treatment of, 109
    primary, 118
  with delayed onset, 107
PPQ; *see* Varni/Thompson Pediatric Pain Questionnaire
Practice Guideline for the Treatment of Patients with Bipolar Disorder, 137
Prader-Willi syndrome, bulimia nervosa and, 150
Pregnancy, 7
Preschool age, 8
Problematic aggression, 215-217
Problems of Behavior, 169
Procedure Behavior Check List, 30
Procedure Behavior Rating Scale, 30
Procyclidine, 271
Prolixin; *see* Fluphenazine
Prpanolol, aggressive behavior and, 220
Prout-Strohmer Assessment System, 30
Prout-Strohmer Personality Inventory, 30
PSAS; *see* Prout-Strohmer Assessment System
PSPI; *see* Prout-Strohmer Personality Inventory
Psychiatric diagnosis, 13-16; *see also* Specific disorder
Psychiatric examination, 5-6
Psychopathology Instrument for Mentally Retarded Adults, 30
Psychosis, brief reactive and schizophreniform, 58-59
Psychotic disorders, other, 15
PTSD; *see* Posttraumatic stress disorder
Puberty, 9
Public Law 94-142, Individuals with Disabilities Act, 76
Punishment and developmental disabilities, 269-270

R

Rating scales and behavior checklists, 24
RCMAS; *see* Revised Children's Manifest Anxiety Scale
Reactive attachment disorder, 14-15
  disinhibited type, 249
  DSM-IV diagnostic criteria for, 197, 201, 248
  inhibited type, 249
Reading disorder
  DSM-IV diagnostic criteria for, 170
  features, 173-174
Rehabilitation Act of 1973, section 504, 76
Reiss Screen for Maladaptive Behavior, 30
Retardation, severe psychomotor, 62
Rett's disorder, 14, 61-64
  brain imaging in, 43
  comparison of autistic disorder and, 63
  diagnostic criteria of, 61-62
  DSM-IV diagnostic criteria of, 62
Revised Behavior Problem Checklist, 24
Revised Children's Manifest Anxiety Scale, 26, 100
Rispersal; *see* Risperidone
Riperidone, 271
Ritalin; *see* Methylphenidate
Ritvo-Freeman Real Life Rating Scale, 25
Rosenblith Revision of the Graham Behavior Test for Neonates, 197
Rumination disorder, 143-144
  developmental disabilities and, 274
  DSM-IV diagnostic criteria for, 144
    anorexia nervosa and, 144
    bulimia nervosa and, 144
    mental retardation and, 144
    pervasive developmental disorder and, 144
Russell's sign, bulimia nervosa and, 149,150

S

SAD; *see* Separation anxiety disorder
Schedule for Affective Disorders and Schizophrenia for School-age children, 23-24, 25, 26, 27
  epidemiologic version, 23, 27, 159
  present-episode version, 23
Schizoaffective disorder, 153, 162
Schizophrenia, 153-168
  Abnormal Involuntary Movement Scale and, 164, 165-166

Schizophrenia—cont'd
anticonvulsants and, 165
antipsychotic medications and, 163
attention deficit/hyperactivity disorder, 155, 163
autoimmune mechanisms in, 159
benzopdiazepines and, 165
benztropine mesylate and, 164
childhood, 153
chlorpromazine and, 165
clozapine and, 163, 164
agranulocytosis and, 164
comparison of autistic disorder and, 160-161
computer analyzed EEGs and, 158, 160
conduct disorder and, 162
CT and, 158, 160
Cushing's syndrome and, 161
depersonalization and, 157-158
diagnostic criteria of, 153-158
diphenhydramine and, 164
DSM-IV diagnostic criteria for, 154
continuous, 154
episodic with interepisode residual symptoms, 154
episodic with no interepisode residual symptoms, 154
other or unspecified pattern, 154
single episode in full remission, 154
single episode in partial remission, 154
tardive dyskinesias and, 164
fluoxetine and, 165
fluphenazine and, 165
hallucinations and, 153, 160
haloperidol and, 164, 165
K-SADS-E and, 159
lithium and, 165
loxapine and, 165
medical conditions that may mimic, 161
mental retardation and, 162
molindone and, 165
MRI and, 158, 160
neuroleptic malignant syndrome and, 163, 164
oppositional defiant disorder and, 162
other psychotic disorders, 15
perphenazine and, 165
pervasive developmental disorders and, 155, 160-161
PET studies and, 158, 160
pimozide and, 165
psychomimetic agents and, 161-162
psychosis and, 153
risperidone and, 163, 164
schizotypal personality disorder and, 162
subtypes of, DSM-IV diagnostic criteria for, 156
suicide in, 228
thioridazine and, 165
Schizophrenia—cont'd
thiothixene and, 165
thyrotoxicosis and, 161
treatment of, 163
phases of, 164
trifluoperazine and, 165
trihexyphenidyl and, 164
Schizophrenic subtypes, DSM-IV diagnostic criteria for, 157
Schizophreniform disorder, 153, 162
School history, 9
School refusal, social phobia and, 115
Sedative hypnotics, substance abuse and, 238
Seizure disorder, as cause of mania, 137
Selective mutism, 15, 112-113
benzodiazepine and, 113, 118
clonazepam and, 113
cognitive behavior therapy and, 113
diagnostic criteria for, 112
differential diagnosis, 113
DSM-IV diagnostic criteria for, 112
fluoxetine and, 113
mental retardation and, 113
pervasive development disorder and, 113
phenelzine and, 113
schizophrenia and, 113
sertraline and, 113
SSRIs and, 113, 118
treatment of, 113
primary, 118
Self-help and advocacy groups, 244
Self-injury and developmental disabilities, 274-275
Self-Report Delinquency Scale, 28
Semistructured diagnostic interviews, 23-24
Separation and grief, 311-314
Separation anxiety disorder, 14, 15, 109-112, 118
alprozalam and, 112
benzodiazepine and, 112, 118
buspirone and, 118
clonazepam and, 112
cognitive behavioral therapy and, 112, 118
conduct disorder and, 111
diagnostic criteria for, 109
differential diagnosis for, 111
DSM-IV diagnostic criteria for, 110, 311
early onset, 110, 197
familial dysfunction and, 111
imipramine and, 111
learning disorders and, 111
neuroleptic-induced disorder and, 111
oppositional defiant disorder and, 111
pervasive developmental disorder and, 111
posttraumatic stress disorder and, 111
psychotic disorders and, 111
serotonin-selective reuptake inhibitors and, 112, 118

Separation anxiety disorder—cont'd
  substance abuse and, 111
  treatment of, 111
    primary, 118
Separation difficulties, 8
Sepsis, anorexia nervosa and, 147
Serentil; *see* Mesoridazine
Serotonin, generalized anxiety disorder and, 100
Serotonin-selective reuptake inhibitors, 101, 106, 109, 112, 118
Serotoninergic agents
  attention deficit/hyperactivity disorder and, 79
  obsessive-complusive disorders and, 102
Sertraline
  depression and, 131
  obsessive-compulsive disorders and, 102
  selective mutism and, 113
SESBI; *see* Sutter-Eyberg Student Behavior Inventory
Sexual abuse, 253-260
  extrafamilial, 256
  false allegations of, 259-260
  intrafamilial, 255
  role of the primary care physician in, 260
  sequelae of, 257-258
Sexual identity, 287
Sexual masochism, DSM-IV diagnostic criteria for, 301
Sexual orientation, 287
Sexual sadism, DSM-IV diagnostic criteria for, 301
Sexuality, 287-303
  cognitive theories of, 289-290
  coming out in gay and lesbian youth, 293
  development of, extrinsic factors in, 291-292
  development of, intrinsic-biologic factors in, 290-291
  Erikson's stages of, 289
  Freud's stages of, 289
  home and emotional climate continuum, 295
  normal development of, 290-293
  social learning theories of, 289
  Troiden's stages of, 290
Sexually aggressive behaviors, 296
Sexually transmitted diseases, 301
  pregnancy and, 301
Single-photon emission computed tomography, 33, 34, 39-40
Social competence, disorders of, 182
Social isolation, 200
Social phobia, 113-115, 118
  agoraphobia and, 115
  benzodiazepines and, 116, 118
  beta blockers and, 116
  buspirone and, 116
  clonazepam and, 116
  diagnostic criteria, 113
  differential diagnosis, 115
Social phobia—cont'd
  DSM-IV diagnostic criteria for, 114
  fluoxetine and, 116
  generalized, 114
  generalized anxiety disorder and, 115
  major depressive disorder and, 115
  neurotransmitters and, 116
  panic disorder with agoraphobia and, 115
  pharmacologic treatment and, 116, 118
  separation anxiety disorder and, 115
  sertaline and, 116
  school refusal and, 115
  social skills training and, 115
  specific phobias and, 115
  SSRIs and, 116, 118
  treatment of, 115
    primary, 118
  tricyclic antidepressants and, 116
  truancy and, 115
Social skills training, 115, 219-220
Socioenvironmental therapy for developmental disabilities, 273
SPBRS; *see* Strohmer-Prout Behavior Rating Scale
Specific phobia, 116-118
  CBT and, 118
  diagnostic criteria for, 116
  differential diagnosis for, 116-117
  DSM-IV diagnostic criteria for, 117
    animal type, 117
    blood-injection-injury type, 117
    natural environment type, 117
    other type, 117
    situational type, 117
  treatment of, 118
    primary, 118
SPECT; *see* Single-photon emission computed tomography
SSRIs; *see* Serotonin-selective reuptake inhibitors
SST; *see* Social skills training
STAIC; *see* State-Trait Anxiety Inventory for Children
Stanozolol, substance abuse and, 238
State-Trait Anxiety Inventory for Children, 23, 26
Stelazine; *see* Trifluoperazine
STEP; *see* Systematic Training for Effective Parenting
12-Step Programs, substance abuse and, 242, 243
Stimulants
  developmental disabilities, 271-272
  substance abuse and, 238
Stranger anxiety, 7
Stress, 305-320
  habits and, 309-311
Stressor scale, 307
Strohmer-Prout Behavior Rating Scale, 30
Structured diagnostic interviews, 23

Substance abuse, 237-244
alcohol and, 238, 242
Alcoholics Anonymous and, 242, 244
amphetamines and, 238
amyl nitrates and, 238
anabolic steroids and, 238
anxiety disorders and, 242
attention-deficit/hyperactivity disorder and, 237, 242
benzodiazepines and, 238
butane and, 238
cannabis and, 238
carburetor cleaner and, 238
cocaine and, 238, 242
codeine and, 238, 242
correction fluid and, 238
conduct disorder and, 242
DSM-IV diagnostic criteria for, 239
ether and, 238
freon and, 238
gasoline and, 238
gateway drugs for, 240
glue and, 238
hallucinogens and, 238
hashish and, 238
heroin and, 238, 242
Imaginary Urine Drug Screen and, 242
inhalants and, 238
issues of confidentiality, 241
librium and, 238
LSD and, 238, 242
marijuana and, 238, 242
mescaline and, 238
methalqualone, 238
methamphetamine and, 238
methylphenidate and, 237
methandrostenolone and, 238
nandrolone decanoate and, 238
Narcotics Anonymous and, 242, 244
National Institute of Drug Abuse and, 238
nitrous oxide and, 238
opiates and, 238
oxycodone and, 238
PCP and, 238
peyote and, 238
psilocybin and, 238
risk factors for, 240
sedative hypnotics and, 238
self-help and advocacy groups for, 244
stanozolol and, 238
12-Step programs and, 238
stimulants and, 238
suicide in, 238
tetrahydrocannabinol and, 243
tranquilizers and, 238
Substance abuse—cont'd
treatment methods for, 243
urine drug screening for, 241-243
Substance dependence, DSM-IV diagnostic criteria for, 239
Substance use disorders, 16
Suicidal child or adolescent, 225-235
Suicidal risk, 226-227
Suicide, 225-235
bipolar mood disorder and, 228
borderline personality and, 228
case analysis for, 234-235
common psychiatric diagnoses for, 227-228
conduct disorder and, 228
environmental stress and support of, 229-231
historical and genetic factors contributing to, 228
major depressive disorder and, 228
mental status and, 229
risk factors for, 227
schizophrenia and, 228
substance abuse in, 228
treatment plan and disposition of, 231-234
Sutter-Eyberg Student Behavior Inventory, 28

T

Tardive dyskinesia, 59
TCAs; *see* Tricyclic antidepressants
Teacher Report Form, 5
TEACCH; *see* Treatment and Education of Autistic and Related Communication Handicapped Children
Teenage pregnancy, 301-302
risk factors for, 302
Teenage sexual intimacy, risks associated with, 302-303
Thalamic tumors, as cause of mania, 137
THC; *see* Tetrahydrocannabinol
The Instructional Environmental Stage, 27
Thioridazine, 165
Thiothixene, 165
Thorazine; *see* Chlorpromazine
Thyroid-stimulating hormone, panic disorder and, 103
Thyrotoxicosis, schizophrenia and, 161
Thyrotropin-releasing hormone, panic disorder and, 103
Tic disorder NOS, DSM-IV diagnostic criteria for, 311
Tic disorders, 14
TIES; *see* The Instructional Environmental Stage
Toddlerhood, 8
Tourette's disorder
brain imaging in, 44
DSM-IV diagnostic criteria for, 310
learning disorders and, 181
obsessive-compulsive disorder and, 102
Tower of Hanoi Test, 56

Toxocara canis, pica and, 145
Tranquilizers, substance abuse and, 238
Transient tic disorder, DSM-IV diagnostic criteria for, 310
Transvestic fetishism, DSM-IV diagnostic criteria for, 300
Trauma
  community violence and, 318-319
  domestic violence and, 316-318
  witness to, 316-319
    posttraumatic stress disorder and, 316-318
Trazodone, 131
Treatment planning, 12-13
Treatment and Education of Autistic and Related Communication Handicapped Children, 58
TRF; *see* Teacher Report Form
Trichobezoars, pica and, 145
Tricyclic antidepressants
  attention deficit/hyperactivity disorders and, 78-79, 80
  depression and, 130
  generalized anxiety disorder and, 118
  panic disorder and, 106, 118
  posttraumatic stress disorder and, 109, 118
  social phobia and, 137
Trifluoperazine, 165
Trihexyphenidyl, 164
Trilafon; *see* Perphenazine
Troiden's stages of sexuality, 290
TRH; *see* Thyrotopin-releasing hormone
TSH; *see* Thyroid-stimulating hormone
Turner's syndrome, 147, 181

U

Urine drug screening for substance abuse, 241-243

V

VABS; *see* Vineland Adaptive Behavior Scales
Valproate, 138
Varni/Thompson Pediatric Pain Questionnaire, 30
Venlafaxine, 131
Vineland Adaptive Behavior Scales, 29, 194
Voyeurism, DSM-IV diagnostic criteria for, 300

W

WAIS; *see* Wechsler Adult Intelligence Scale
Walker-Rankin Rating Scale of Adaptive and Maladaptive Child Behavior in School, 27
WCST; *see* Wisconsin Card-Sorting Test
Weinberg Screening Affective Scale, 127
Wechsler Adult Intelligence Scale, 56
Wechsler Intelligence Scale for Children, 56
Wechsler Intelligence Scale for Children-Revised, 75
Wide Range Achievement Test-R, 27-28
WISC; *see* Wechsler Intelligence Scale for Children
Wisconsin Card-Sorting Test, 56
WISC-R; *see* Wechsler Intelligence Scale-Revised
Woodcock-Johnson Psychoeducational Battery, 27-28
WSAS; *see* Weinberg Screening Affective Scale

Y

Yale-Brown Obsessive Compulsive Scale, 102
YBOCS; *see* Yale-Brown Obsessive Compulsive Scale